Handbook
of
Difficult
Diagnosis

Handbook
of
Difficult
Diagnosis

Edited by

A. A. Louis, M.D.

Clinical Assistant Professor
Department of Neurology and
Neurological Sciences
Stanford University School of Medicine
Stanford, California

Associate Chief
Department of Neurology
Santa Clara Valley Medical Center
San Jose, California

CHURCHILL LIVINGSTONE
New York, Edinburgh, London, Melbourne

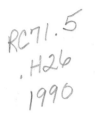

Library of Congress Cataloging-in-Publication Data

Handbook of difficult diagnosis / edited by A. A. Louis.
    p.   cm.
    Includes bibliographical references.
    ISBN 0-443-08677-X
    1. Diagnosis, Differential—Handbooks, manuals, etc. I. Louis,
A. A. (Anne A.)
    [DNLM: 1. Diagnosis, Differential—handbooks. WB 39 H2357]
    RC71.5.H26   1990
    616.07'5—dc20
    DNLM/DLC   89-71293
for Library of Congress   CIP

© **Churchill Livingstone Inc. 1990**

Distributed in the United Kingdom by Churchill Livingstone, Robert Stevenson House, 1–3 Baxter's Place, Leith Walk, Edinburgh EH1 3AF, and by associated companies, branches, and representatives throughout the world.

Accurate indications, adverse reactions, and dosage schedules for drugs are provided in this book, but it is possible that they may change. The reader is urged to review the package information data of the manufacturers of the medications mentioned.

The Publishers have made every effort to trace the copyright holders for borrowed material. If they have inadvertently overlooked any, they will be pleased to make the necessary arrangements at the first opportunity.

Acquisitions Editor: *Robert A. Hurley*
Copy Editor: *Bridgett Dickinson*
Production Designer: *Charlie Lebeda*
Production Supervisor: *Christina Hippeli*

Printed in the United States of America

First Published in 1990

To my family

Contributors

Joseph E. Andrews, M.D.
Formerly, Director of Kula Hospital, Maui, Hawaii

Philip H. Cogen, M.D., Ph.D.
Assistant Professor, Departments of Neurosurgery and Pediatrics, University of California, San Francisco, School of Medicine, San Francisco, California

Stanley C. Deresinski, M.D.
Clinical Associate Professor, Department of Medicine, Stanford University School of Medicine, Stanford, California; Associate Chief, Division of Infectious Diseases, Department of Medicine, Santa Clara Valley Medical Center, San Jose, California; Consultant in Infectious Disease, Sequoia Hospital, Redwood City, California

David A. Drachman, M.D.
Professor and Chairman, Department of Neurology, University of Massachusetts Medical School, Worcester, Massachusetts

Molly Fainstat, M.D.
Clinical Assistant Professor, Department of Medicine, Stanford University School of Medicine, Stanford, California; Associate Chief, Division of Rheumatology, Department of Medicine, Santa Clara Valley Medical Center, San Jose, California

Heidi E. Fleischmann, M.D.
Clinical Assistant Professor, Department of Dermatology, University of New Mexico School of Medicine, Albuquerque, New Mexico; formerly, Clinical Assistant Professor, Department of Dermatology, Stanford University School of Medicine, Stanford, California

Gabriel Garcia, M.D.
Assistant Professor and Chief of Clinical Gastroenterology, Division of Gastroenterology, Department of Medicine, Stanford University School of Medicine, Stanford, California

Gary M. Gray, M.D.
Professor, Division of Gastroenterology, Department of Medicine, Stanford University School of Medicine, Stanford, California

Christian Guilleminault, M.D.
Professor, Department of Psychiatry, Stanford University School of Medicine;
Associate Director, Sleep Disorders Clinic and Research Center, Stanford
University Medical Center, Stanford, California

Pramila R. Gupta, M.D.
Clinical Assistant Professor, Department of Neurology and Neurological
Sciences, Stanford University School of Medicine, Stanford, California

Anthony A. Haulk, M.D., FACP
Assistant Clinical Professor, Department of Family Practice, University of
California, Davis, School of Medicine, Davis, California

Jane E. Howard, M.D.
Dana Foundation Fellow, Department of Neurology and Neurological Sciences,
Stanford University School of Medicine, Stanford, California

Peter C. Johnson, M.D.
Chairman, Department of Neuropathology, Barrow Neurological Institute of St.
Joseph's Hospital and Medical Center, Phoenix, Arizona; formerly, Associate
Professor, Department of Pathology, University of Arizona College of Medicine,
Tucson, Arizona

Vicki Kalen, M.D.
Associate Professor, Department of Orthopaedics, University of Florida College
of Medicine, Gainesville, Florida

Brian R. Kaye, M.D.
Clinical Instructor, Department of Medicine, University of California, San
Francisco, School of Medicine, San Francisco, California; Attending Physician,
Rheumatology Clinic, Highland General Hospital, Oakland, California;
formerly, Fellow in Rheumatology, Santa Clara Valley Medical Center, San Jose,
California and Stanford University School of Medicine, Stanford, California

Thomas J. Kipps, M.D., Ph.D.
Associate Member, Molecular and Experimental Medicine, Research Institute of
Scripps Clinic; Staff Physician and Director of Clinical Flow Cytometry Lab,
Hematology/Oncology, Department of Medicine, Scripps Clinic and Research
Foundation, La Jolla, California

Mel Krajden M.D., FRCP(C)
Assistant Professor, Department of Microbiology, University of Toronto Faculty
of Medicine; Staff Microbiologist, Department of Microbiology, The Toronto
Hospital, Toronto, Ontario, Canada

John Laidlaw, FRCP(Edin)
Consultant Physician to Epilepsy Centre, Quarrier's Homes, Bridge of Weir,
Edinburgh, Scotland

R. Elaine Lambert, M.D.
Clinical Assistant Professor, Division of Immunology and Rheumatology,
Department of Medicine, Stanford University School of Medicine, Stanford,
California

Anne A. Louis, M.D.
Clinical Assistant Professor, Department of Neurology and Neurological Sciences, Stanford University School of Medicine, Stanford, California; Associate Chief, Department of Neurology, Santa Clara Valley Medical Center, San Jose, California

Jennifer McAfee, M.D.
Medical Director, Whatcom Diabetes Self-Management Center, Bellingham, Washington

David P. Nelson, M.D.
Medical Director, Heart and Lung Transplant Program, Arizona Heart Institute, Phoenix, Arizona

Sylvestre Quevedo, M.D.
Clinical Assistant Professor, Division of Nephrology, Department of Medicine, Stanford University School of Medicine, Stanford, California; Associate Chief, Division of Nephrology, Department of Medicine, Santa Clara Valley Medical Center, San Jose, California

Thomas A. Raffin, M.D.
Associate Professor and Assistant Chief of Medicine, Acting Chief, Division of Respiratory Medicine, Department of Medicine, Stanford University School of Medicine, Stanford, California

Luke M. Vaughan, M.D.
Head, Tumor Section, Division of Orthopaedic Surgery, Scripps Clinic and Research Foundation, La Jolla, California

Cody K. Wasner, M.D.
Clinical Assistant Professor, Division of Rheumatology, Department of Medicine, Oregon Health Sciences University School of Medicine, Portland, Oregon

Philip Wasserstein, M.D.
Clinical Assistant Professor, Department of Neurology and Neurological Sciences, Stanford University School of Medicine; Director, Neurology Outpatient Department, Department of Neurology and Neurological Sciences, Stanford University Medical Center, Stanford, California

Lorna Yamaguchi, M.D., FCCP
Director of Intensive Care, Departments of Anesthesia and Medicine, Santa Teresa Community Hospital, San Jose, California

Mark Yeager, M.D., Ph.D.
Assistant Member, Department of Molecular Biology, Research Institute of Scripps Clinic; Staff Cardiologist and Director of Cardiovascular Research, Division of Cardiovascular Diseases, Department of Medicine, Scripps Clinic and Research Foundation, La Jolla, California

Andrew R. Zolopa, M.D.
Post-Doctoral Fellow, Robert Wood Johnston Clinical Scholar's Program, Department of Medicine, Stanford University School of Medicine, Stanford, California

Preface

In *Handbook of Difficult Diagnosis* we have updated and annotated over 100 topics of differential diagnosis selected from 10 medical subspecialties in a format designed for quick access to referenced diagnostic possibilities and selected readings. The format and content are designed to supplement more general discussions of the selected topics and are to be used as an adjunct to traditional textbook approaches of differential diagnosis. With added clinical experience, common diagnoses are more easily recognized and problems of difficult diagnosis tend to appear less frequently. However, even with clinical experience, our evaluation of patients with a difficult diagnosis takes more time and often requires maximum use of diagnostic resources. Our purpose is to compile a useful handbook of referenced current information about selected signs, symptoms, and syndromes encountered in patients who may not clearly fit within a diagnostic category.

Each topic is introduced with a summary of common causes; less common causes are emphasized, particularly if disorders are considered treatable, life-threatening, or reflect recent information. For example, current concepts of HIV infection have significantly altered the order of diagnostic probabilities when evaluating a patient with lymphadenopathy, and the increasing prevalence of drug abuse has led to a number of new suspected nonatherosclerotic causes of stroke and myocardial infarction. We have mingled the diagnostic categories to provide the most meaningful agenda for each subspecialty area of consultation. For example, selected topics within Section II, Pulmonary, include diagnostic categories of symptoms (such as noncardiac causes of chest pain), mixed with diagnostic categories of signs (such as hemoptysis), and diagnostic categories of radiographic signs (such as the solitary pulmonary nodule). Because the medical literature is frequently consulted in problems of difficult diagnosis—and as clinical experience increases, the feeling of being current can decrease—we placed a major emphasis on referencing diagnostic possibilities with current literature. Each topic ends with annotated selected readings chosen for authority and clinical usefulness to serve as an update, review, or introduction to the current literature.

This quick-reference book for diagnostic possibilities reflects the needs and anxieties of the contributors. Most contributors are practicing subspecialists who also teach housestaff. As experienced clinicians, we do not always consciously rely, except for teaching purposes, on conventional frameworks of differential diagnosis. When confronted with problems of difficult diagnosis, we usually consult with medical journals, medical books, and each other. The selection and organization of *Handbook of Difficult Diagnosis* was strongly influenced by our subspecialty practice, housestaff, patient community, and these consultations. *Handbook of Difficult Diagnosis* is designed as a resource for consultations and as a stimulus for the physician to consider unusual diagnostic possibilities in the face of a difficult presentation.

A. A. Louis, M.D.

Acknowledgments

I am grateful to Joseph E. Andrews, my father, who introduced me to differential diagnosis; Colleen Crawford and Phyllis Shipway for earlier secretarial assistance; Edna Casem for untiring editorial assistance; JoAnn Ceranski for years of MEDLINE searches, proofing, and relentless editing, and who, together with Edna Casem, forged the final draft; and Eldora Polex and Barbara Wilson for years of library service. In addition, I wish to acknowledge colleagues, family, and friends who provided essential professional and personal support: Lois Andrews, Scott Casem, Molly Fainstat, Heidi E. Fleischmann, Gabriel Garcia, Terry Andrews Haljun, Anthony A. Haulk, Gary Hethcoat, Kathy Louis Hethcoat, Maie Herrick, Tracy Herrick, Judy Hogg, John R. Hotson, Vicki Kalen, Brian R. Kaye, Mel Krajden, R. Elaine Lambert, John G. Louis, Leah Louis, Sara Louis, Stan Louis, Jennifer McAfee, Kevin McGill, Thomas A. Raffin, Virginia W. Steel, Luke M. Vaughan, Sara Dean Villat, Cody K. Wasner, Lorna Yamaguchi, Mark Yeager. And special thanks to our Churchill Livingstone editors, Donna Balopole and Bridgett Dickinson, and, of course, Bob Hurley, who acquired this manuscript twice, rescued it once, and made it all come true.

Contents

IV ENDOCRINOLOGY   217

VII INFECTIOUS DISEASE   493

VIII DERMATOLOGY

I

CARDIOLOGY

1
Atherosclerotic Coronary Disease: Risk Factors

The Framingham Heart Study has identified certain risk factors that can be used to predict coronary artery disease. Such major risk factors include age, gender, total cholesterol level, high-density lipoprotein cholesterol level, systolic blood pressure, cigarette smoking, glucose intolerance, and left ventricular hypertrophy.[1,2] Other risk factors, although less common and somewhat controversial, have also been linked with coronary artery disease. Since many risk factors may be altered by treatment or life-style modification, their identification may result in prevention or blunting of the significant impact that the development of coronary artery disease creates in high-risk individuals.[3,4]

Major Risk Factors

Hypertension[5-8]
Smoking[9-12]
Elevated cholesterol[13-18]
Hyperlipoproteinemia[19-22]
Diabetes mellitus[23-27]
Increasing age[28]
Male sex[29,30]

Minor Risk Factors

Obesity[31,32]
Oral contraceptive use: particularly in women over 40 years of age[33,34]
Postmenopausal state[35]
Homocystinuria[36-38]
Emotional stress or Type A personality[39-41]
Family history[42-44]
Hypercalcemia[45]
Toxins: carbon disulfide,[46] aliphatic nitrates[47]
Myxedema[48]
Mediastinal radiation therapy[49]

Questionable Risk Factors

Soft water[50]
Hyperuricemia[51,52]
Vasectomy[53,54]
Hypocalcemia[55]
Ear lobe creases[56,57]
Corticosteroid use[58]
Coffee[59-61]
Alcohol[62-65]
Hemodialysis[66]
Sedentary life-style[67]
Thrombocytosis and increased blood viscosity[68]
Cold weather[69,70]

References

1. Wilson PW, Castelli WP, Kannel WB: Coronary risk prediction in adults (the Framingham Heart Study). Am J Cardiol 59:91G, 1987.
2. Raichlen JS, Healy B, Achuff SC, et al: Importance of risk factors in the angiographic progression of coronary artery disease. Am J Cardiol 57:66, 1986.
3. Gotto AM Jr: Interactions of the major risk factors for coronary heart disease. Am J Med 80(2A):48, 1986.
4. Superko HR, Wood PD, Haskell WL: Coronary heart disease and risk factor modification. Is there a threshold? Am J Med 78:826, 1985.
5. Schlant RC: Reversal of left ventricular hypertrophy by drug treatment of hypertension. Chest 88(S3):194S, 1985.
6. Connolly DC, Elveback LR, Oxman HA: Coronary heart disease in residents of Rochester, Minnesota, 1950–1975. III. Effect of hypertension and its treatment on survival of patients with coronary artery disease. Mayo Clin Proc 58:249, 1983.
7. Chobanian AV: The influence of hypertension and other hemodynamic factors in atherogenesis. Prog Cardiovasc Dis 26:177, 1983.
8. LeHeuzey JY, Guize L: Cardiac prognosis in hypertensive patients. Incidence of sudden death and ventricular arrhythmias. Am J Med 84:65, 1988.
9. Rosenberg L, Kaufman DW, Helmrich SP, et al: Myocardial infarction and cigarette smoking in women younger than 50 years of age. JAMA 253:2965, 1985.
10. Abbott RD, Yin Y, Reed DM, et al: Risk of stroke in male cigarette smokers. N Engl J Med 315:717, 1986.
11. Hallstrom AP, Cobb LA, Ray R: Smoking as a risk factor for recurrence of sudden cardiac arrest. N Engl J Med 314:271, 1986.
12. Weintraub WS, Klein LW, Seelaus PA, et al: Importance of total life consumption of cigarettes as a risk factor for coronary artery disease. Am J Cardiol 55:669, 1985.
13. Levy RI: Cholesterol and coronary artery disease. Am J Med 80(2A):18, 1986.
14. Stamler J, Wentworth D, Neaton JD: Prevalence and prognostic significance of hypercholesterolemia in men with hypertension. Am J Med 80(2A):33, 1986.

15. Martin MJ, Hulley SB, Browner WS, et al: Serum cholesterol, blood pressure, and mortality: implications from a cohort of 361,662 men. Lancet 2:933, 1986.
16. Roberts WC (ed): Reducing the blood cholesterol level reduces the risk of heart attack. Am J Cardiol 53:649, 1984.
17. Krauss RM, Lindgren FT, Williams PT, et al: Intermediate density lipoproteins and progression of coronary artery disease in hypercholesterolaemic men. Lancet 2:62, 1987.
18. Levy RI: Changing perspectives in the prevention of coronary artery disease. Am J Cardiol 57:17G, 1986.
19. Brunzell JD, Sniderman AD, Alberts JJ, et al: Apoproteins B and A-1 and coronary artery disease in humans. Arteriosclerosis 4:79, 1984.
20. Steinberg D: Lipoproteins and atherosclerosis. Arteriosclerosis 33:283, 1983.
21. Kreisberg RA: Lipids, lipoproteins, apolipoproteins, and atherosclerosis (editorial). Ann Intern Med 99:713, 1983.
22. Krauss RM: Relationship of intermediate and low-density lipoprotein subspecies to risk of coronary artery disease. Am Heart J 113:578, 1987.
23. Colwell JA, Winocour PD, Lopes-Virella M, et al: New concepts about the pathogenesis of atherosclerosis in diabetes mellitus. Am J Med 75(5B):67, 1983.
24. Ruderman NB, Haudenschild C: Diabetes as an atherogenic factor. Prog Cardiovasc Dis 26:373, 1984.
25. Kereiakes DJ, Naughton JL, Brundage B, et al: The heart in diabetes. West J Med 140:583, 1984.
26. Zavaroni I, Dall'Aglio E, Bonora E, et al: Evidence that multiple risk factors for coronary artery disease exist in persons with abnormal glucose tolerance. Am J Med 83:609, 1987.
27. Lemp GF, Vander-Zwaag R, Hughes JP, et al: Association between the severity of diabetes mellitus and coronary arterial atherosclerosis. Am J Cardiol 60:1015, 1987.
28. Aronow WS, Starling L, Etienne F, et al: Risk factors for coronary artery disease in persons older than 62 years in a long-term health care facility. Am J Cardiol 57:518, 1986.
29. Hazzard WR: Atherogenesis: why women live longer than men. Geriatrics 40(1):42, 1985.
30. Lerner DJ, Kannel WB: Patterns of coronary heart disease morbidity and mortality in the sexes: a 26-year follow-up of the Framingham population. Am Heart J 111:383, 1986.
31. Hubert HB, Feinleib M, McNamara PM, et al: Obesity as an independent risk factor for cardiovascular disease: a 26-year follow-up of participants in the Framingham Heart Study. Circulation 67:968, 1983.
32. Rhoads GG, Kagan A: The relation of coronary disease, stroke, and mortality to weight in youth and in middle age. Lancet 1:492, 1983.
33. Engel HJ, Engel E, Lichtlen PR: Coronary atherosclerosis and myocardial infarction in young women—role of oral contraceptives. Eur Heart J 4:1, 1983.
34. Hennekens CH, MacMahon B: Oral contraceptives and

myocardial infarction (editorial). N Engl J Med 296: 1166, 1977.

35. Stampfer MJ, Willett WC, Colditz GA, et al: A prospective study of postmenopausal estrogen therapy and coronary heart disease. N Engl J Med 313:1044, 1985.
36. Harker LA, Slichter SJ, Scott CR, et al: Homocystinemia: vascular injury and arterial thrombosis. N Engl J Med 291:537, 1974.
37. Wilcken DE, Reddy SG, Gupta VJ: Homocysteinemia, ischemic heart disease, and the carrier state for homocystinuria. Metabolism 32:363, 1983.
38. Murphy-Chutorian DR, Wexman MP, Grieco AJ, et al: Methionine intolerance: a possible risk factor for coronary artery disease. J Am Coll Cardiol 6:725, 1985.
39. Graboys TB: Stress and the aching heart (editorial). N Engl J Med 311:594, 1984.
40. Kannel WB, Eaker ED: Psychosocial and other features of coronary heart disease: insights from the Framingham Study. Am Heart J 112:1066, 1986.
41. Schneiderman N: Psychophysiologic factors in atherogenesis and coronary artery disease. Circulation 76 (Suppl):41, 1987.
42. Neufeld HN, Goldbourt U: Coronary heart disease: genetic aspects. Circulation 67:943, 1983.
43. Hamsten A, de Faire U: Risk factors for coronary artery disease in families of young men with myocardial infarction. Am J Cardiol 59:14, 1987.
44. Shea S, Ottman R, Gabrieli C, et al: Family history as an independent risk factor for coronary artery disease. J Am Coll Cardiol 4:793, 1984.
45. Roberts WC, Waller BF: Effect of chronic hypercalcemia on the heart. Am J Med 71:371, 1981.
46. Nurminen M, Mutanen P, Tolonen M, et al: Quantitated effects of carbon disulfide exposure, elevated blood pressure and aging on coronary mortality. Am J Epidemiol 115:107, 1982.
47. Morton WE: Occupational habituation to aliphatic nitrates and the withdrawal hazards of coronary disease and hypertension. J Occup Med 19:197, 1977.
48. Holvoet G, Gillebert TC, Piessens J, et al: Coronary artery surgery in patients with myxoedema. Acta Cardiol (Brux) 39:139, 1984.
49. Mittal B, Deutsch M, Thompson M, et al: Radiation-induced accelerated coronary arteriosclerosis. Am J Med 81:183, 1986.
50. Shaper AG, Packham RF, Pocock SJ: The British regional heart study: cardiovascular mortality and water quality. J Environ Pathol Toxicol 4:89, 1980.
51. Brand FN, McGee DL, Kannel WB, et al: Hyperuricemia as a risk factor of coronary heart disease: the Framingham study. Am J Epidemiol 121:11, 1985.
52. Fessel WJ: High uric acid as an indicator of cardiovascular disease. Am J Med 68:401, 1980.
53. Goldacre MJ, Holford TR, Vessey MP: Cardiovascular disease and vasectomy. N Engl J Med 308:805, 1983.
54. Walker AM, Jick H, Hunter JR, et al: Vasectomy and non-fatal myocardial infarction. Lancet 1:13, 1981.
55. Levine SN, Rheams CN: Hypocalcemic heart failure. Am J Med 78:1033, 1985.

56. Gutiu I, el Rifai C, Mallozi M: Relation between diagonal ear lobe crease and ischemic chronic heart disease and the factors of coronary risk. Med Interne 24:111, 1986.
57. Elliott WJ: Ear lobe crease and coronary artery disease. Am J Med 75:1024, 1983.
58. Nashel DJ: Is atherosclerosis a complication of long-term corticosteroid treatment? Am J Med 80:925, 1986.
59. LaCroix AZ, Mead LA, Liang KY, et al: Coffee consumption and the incidence of coronary heart disease. N Engl J Med 315:977, 1986.
60. Heyden S, Tyroler HA, Heiss G, et al: Coffee consumption and mortality. Arch Intern Med 138:1472, 1978.
61. Yano K, Rhoads GG, Kagan A: Coffee, alcohol, and risk of coronary heart disease among Japanese men living in Hawaii. N Engl J Med 297:405, 1977.
62. Klatsky AL, Armstrong MA, Friedman GD: Relations of alcoholic beverage use to subsequent coronary artery disease hospitalization. Am J Cardiol 58:710, 1986.
63. Criqui MH: The roles of alcohol in the epidemiology of cardiovascular diseases. Acta Med Scand 717 (Suppl):73, 1987.
64. Eichner ER: Alcohol, stroke, and coronary artery disease. Am Fam Physician 37(3):217, 1988.
65. Kelbaek H, Heslet L, Skagen K, et al: Hemodynamic effects of alcohol at rest and during upright exercise in coronary artery disease. Am J Cardiol 61:61, 1988.
66. Rostand SG, Gretes JC, Kirk KA, et al: Ischemic heart disease in patients with uremia undergoing maintenance hemodialysis. Kidney Int 16:600, 1979.
67. Crow RS, Rautaharju PM, Prineas RJ, et al: Risk factors, exercise fitness and electrocardiographic response to exercise in 12,866 men at high risk of symptomatic coronary heart disease. Am J Cardiol 57:1075, 1986.
68. Marcus AJ: Aspirin as an antithrombotic medication (editorial). N Engl J Med 309:1515, 1983.
69. Rogot E, Padgett SJ: Associations of coronary and stroke mortality with temperature and snowfall in selected areas of the United States, 1962–1966. Am J Epidemiol 103:565, 1976.
70. Hattenhauer M, Neill WA: The effect of cold air inhalation on angina pectoris and myocardial oxygen supply. Circulation 51:1053, 1975.

Selected Readings

Cheitlin MD: Finding the high-risk patient with coronary artery disease. JAMA 259:2271, 1988.
Author suggests an approach which limits the use of coronary angiography to patients with functional evidence of large areas of myocardium at risk from the next event. Clinical findings that would provide indications for coronary arteriography include (1) angina unacceptable to the patient despite medical management, (2) significant left main coronary artery or extensive two- or three-vessel disease suspected clinically in patients with stable or unstable angina, (3) extensive myocardial ischemia or potential extensive myocardial dysfunction as manifested on exercise testing, and (4) depressed left ventricular function (ejection fraction less than 45%).

Connolly DC, Elveback LR: Coronary heart disease in

residents of Rochester, Minnesota. VI. Hospital and post-hospital course of patients with transmural and subendocardial myocardial infarction. Mayo Clin Proc 60:375, 1985.
Study of 1,221 patients, 30 years of age or older, who had a myocardial infarction as the first manifestation of coronary heart disease.

Criqui MH: Epidemiology of atherosclerosis: an updated overview. Am J Cardiol 57:18C, 1986.
Review of the major risk factors of atherosclerosis and coronary artery disease.

Glueck CJ: Role of risk factor management in progression and regression of coronary and femoral artery atherosclerosis. Am J Cardiol 57:35G, 1986.
Results of studies that show the importance of reduction of lipids and lipoprotein cholesterol in treatment and prevention of coronary atherosclerosis.

Kromhout D, Bosschieter EB, de Lezenne Coulander C: The inverse relation between fish consumption and 20-year mortality from coronary heart disease. N Engl J Med 312:1205, 1985.
Study concluding that mortality from coronary heart disease was decreased by more than half in patients who ate at least 30 grams of fish per day.

Leon AS: Physical activity levels and coronary heart disease. Analysis of epidemiologic and supporting studies. Med Clin North Am 69:3, 1985.
Absolute proof of the contributing role of physical inactivity is not possible; however, epidemiologic studies strongly suggest that habitual physical exercise offers partial protection against primary or secondary events of coronary artery disease.

Moore RD, Pearson TA: Moderate alcohol consumption and coronary artery disease. Medicine 65:242, 1986.
Data for an inverse association between moderate alcohol consumption and coronary artery disease.

Phillipson BE, Rothrock DW, Connor WE, et al: Reduction of plasma lipids, lipoproteins, and apoproteins by dietary fish oils in patients with hypertriglyceridemia. N Engl J Med 312:1210, 1985.
This study concludes that fish oils and fish may be useful components of diets for the treatment of hypertriglyceridemia.

Sokil AB: Approach to the management of coronary artery disease in the elderly. Clin Geriatr Med 4:111, 1988.
A clinical review of current concepts of diagnosis and management of coronary artery disease in the elderly with an emphasis on atypical presentations of angina pectoris and myocardial infarction seen in this population. Problems with related drug therapy in the elderly are also discussed.

Sullivan JM, Vander-Zwaag R, Lemp GF, et al: Postmenopausal estrogen use and coronary atherosclerosis. Ann Intern Med 108:358, 1988.
A major study presents data suggesting that postmenopausal estrogen replacement is a significant independent protective factor and that postmenopausal estrogen treatment reduces the risk for angiographically significant coronary artery disease.

2

Coronary Artery Insufficiency and Myocardial Infarction: Nonatherosclerotic Causes

Patients with angina pectoris and/or myocardial infarction usually have atherosclerotic coronary disease. Except for congenital coronary anomalies in children, other causes of coronary artery disease leading to coronary artery insufficiency are rarely considered.[1] However, in patients with few or no obvious risk factors, such as in the younger patient, rarer conditions other than congenital anomalies can lead to clinically significant coronary artery insufficiency. The etiology of nonatherosclerotic coronary artery disease generally falls into categories that include nonatherosclerotic cardiac causes, embolic causes, inflammatory or infectious disease, and some hypercoagulable states.

Cardiac Causes of Coronary Artery Insufficiency

Coronary artery spasm[2]: Prinzmetal's angina, methylergonovine-induced,[3] spontaneous spasm during angina,[4] following coronary angioplasty,[5] diltiazem withdrawal,[6] catheter-induced spasm,[7] cocaine,[8–10] dextran,[11] nitrate withdrawal seen in workers in the nitrate industry who have symptoms on weekends presumed secondary to coronary spasm, chemotherapy,[12] pheochromocytoma.[13]
Anomalous coronary arteries [14–17]
Left coronary artery from anterior sinus of Valsalva
Coronary arteriovenous fistula[18]
Coronary artery aneurysms[19–21]
Coronary artery trauma[22]
Muscle bands over coronary arteries
Cardiac transplantation[23]

Juvenile intimal sclerosis
Hypertrophic cardiomyopathy[24]
Coronary artery dissection: e.g., due to aortic dissection or trauma

Coronary Artery Embolic Obstruction[26]

Endocarditis
Cardiac myxoma[25]
Paradoxical emboli: patent foramen ovale and an atrial septal defect[27]
Cardiac valve abnormalities: aortic stenosis,[28] aortic regurgitation,[29] mitral valve prolapse, prosthetic valves
Tumor emboli[30]
Right atrial thrombus
Myocardial contusion[31,32]
Coronary artery bypass surgery: air embolus, laceration, ligation
Coronary arteriography[33]

Inflammatory and Infectious Causes of Coronary Artery Insufficiency

Connective tissue diseases: rheumatoid arthritis, ankylosing spondylitis, systemic lupus erythematosus,[34–36] Wegener's granulomatosis, pseudoxanthoma elasticum, Ehlers-Danlos syndrome, Marfan syndrome[37]
Infectious causes: syphilis,[38] luetic arteritis, diphtheria, viral[39]
Polyarteritis nodosa
Coronary angiitis[40]
Rheumatic fever
Takayasu's disease[41]
Drug-induced arteritis: methysergide, birth control pills
Mucocutaneous lymph node syndrome[42]: Kawasaki disease[43–46]

Miscellaneous Causes of Coronary Artery Insufficiency

Systemic causes of hypoxia: prolonged hypotension, carbon monoxide poisoning[47]
Hematologic disorders[48]: anemia, sickle cell disease,[49,50] thrombocytic thrombotic purpura, myeloproliferative syndromes, disseminated intravascular thrombosis, hyperglobulinemia, hemophilia[51]
Postpartum coronary artery hyperplasia
Hypothyroidism
Inherited disorders[52]: mucopolysaccharidosis,[53] homocystinuria, Fabry's disease, neurofibromatosis,[54] Friedreich's ataxia, Hurler syndrome[55]

Amyloidosis[56,57]
Radiation therapy[58–60]
Carcinoid

References

1. Cheitlin MD, McAllister HA, de Castro CM: Myocardial infarction without atherosclerosis. JAMA 231:951, 1975.
2. Shepherd JT, Vanhoutte PM: Spasm of the coronary arteries: causes and consequences (the scientist's viewpoint). Mayo Clin Proc 60:33, 1985.
3. de la Morena G, Castello R, Barba J, et al: Methylergonovine-induced spasm of saphenous vein coronary bypass graft. Chest 87:545, 1985.
4. Yoshino F, Unoki T, Fukagawa K, et al: Left main coronary artery spasm: angiographic demonstration during spontaneous angina. Am J Cardiol 55:585, 1985.
5. Davis GS, Hollman J: Coronary artery spasm following percutaneous transluminal coronary angioplasty. Cleve Clin J Med 54:207, 1987.
6. Kozeny GA, Ragona BP, Bansal VK, et al: Myocardial infarction with normal results of coronary angiography following diltiazem withdrawal. Am J Med 80:1184, 1986.
7. Roberts DJ, Isner JM, Deckelbaum LI, et al: Acute myocardial infarction, normal coronary arteries, and catheter-induced spasm. Am J Cardiol 58:360, 1986.
8. Rod JL, Zucker RP: Acute myocardial infarction shortly after cocaine inhalation. Am J Cardiol 59:161, 1987.
9. Simpson RW, Edwards WD: Pathogenesis of cocaine-induced ischemic heart disease. Arch Pathol Lab Med 110:479, 1986.
10. Ascher EK, Stauffer JC, Gaasch WH: Coronary artery spasm, cardiac arrest, transient electrocardiographic Q waves and stunned myocardium in cocaine-associated acute myocardial infarction. Am J Cardiol 61:939, 1988.
11. Klugmann S, Salvi A, Valente M, et al: Coronary artery spasm after administration of dextran 40: implications concerning percutaneous transluminal coronary angioplasty. Am Heart J 111:1202, 1986.
12. Kleiman NS, Lehane DE, Geyer CE Jr, et al: Prinzmetal's angina during 5-fluorouracil chemotherapy. Am J Med 82:566, 1987.
13. Goldbaum TS, Henochowicz S, Mustafa M, et al: Pheochromocytoma presenting with Prinzmetal's angina. Am J Med 81:921, 1986.
14. Kimbiris D, Iskandrian AS, Segal BL, et al: Anomalous aortic origin of coronary arteries. Circulation 58:606, 1978.
15. Edelstein J, Juhasz RS: Myocardial infarction in the distribution of a patent anomalous left circumflex coronary artery. Cathet Cardiovasc Diagn 10:171, 1984.
16. Levin DC, Fellows KE, Abrams HL: Hemodynamically significant primary anomalies of the coronary arteries. Circulation 58:25, 1978.
17. Heifetz SA, Robinowitz M, Mueller KH, Virmani R:

Total anomalous origin of the coronary arteries from the pulmonary artery. Pediatr Cardiol 7:11, 1986.

18. Brooks CH, Bates PD: Coronary artery-left ventricular fistula with angina pectoris. Am Heart J 106:404, 1983.
19. Swaye PS, Fisher LD, Litwin P, et al: Aneurysmal coronary artery disease. Circulation 67:134, 1983.
20. Befeler B, Aranda MJ, Embi A, et al: Coronary artery aneurysms: study of the etiology, clinical course, and effect on left ventricular function and prognosis. Am J Med 62:597, 1977.
21. Zalman F, Andia AM, Wu KT, et al: Atherosclerotic coronary artery aneurysm progressing to coronary artery fistula: presentation as myocardial infarction with continuous murmur. Am Heart J 114:427, 1987.
22. Haas GE, Parr GV, Trout RG, Hargrove WC III: Traumatic coronary artery fistula. J Trauma 26:854, 1986.
23. Mason JW, Strefling A: Small vessel disease of the heart resulting in myocardial necrosis and death despite angiographically normal coronary arteries. Am J Cardiol 44:171, 1979.
24. Maron BJ, Epstein SE, Roberts WC: Hypertrophic cardiomyopathy and transmural myocardial infarction without significant atherosclerosis of the extramural coronary arteries. Am J Cardiol 43:1086, 1979.
25. de Morais C, Falzoni R, Alves VA: Myocardial infarct due to a unique atrial myxoma with epithelial-like cells and systemic metastases. Arch Pathol Lab Med 112:185, 1988.
26. Prizel KR, Hutchins GM, Bulkley BH: Coronary artery embolism and myocardial infarction. Ann Intern Med 88:155, 1978.
27. Edoga JK, Widmann WD, McLean ER: Paradoxical embolism to the superior mesenteric artery. Clin Cardiol 10:54, 1987.
28. Lombard JT, Selzer A: Valvular aortic stenosis. A clinical and hemodynamic profile of patients. Ann Intern Med 106:292, 1987.
29. Nitenberg A, Foult JM, Antony I, et al: Coronary flow and resistance reserve in patients with chronic aortic regurgitation, angina pectoris, and normal coronary arteries. J Am Coll Cardiol 11:478, 1988.
30. Ackermann DM, Hyma BA, Edwards WD: Malignant neoplastic emboli to the coronary arteries: report of two cases and review of the literature. Hum Pathol 18:955, 1987.
31. Lau OJ, Shabbo FP, Smyllie J: Acute left anterior descending coronary artery occlusion following blunt chest injury. Injury 16:55, 1984.
32. Anto MJ, Cokinos SG, Jonas E: Acute anterior wall myocardial infarction secondary to blunt chest trauma. Angiology 35:802, 1984.
33. Kennedy JW: Complications associated with cardiac catheterization and angiography. Cathet Cardiovasc Diagn 8:5, 1982.
34. Korbet SM, Schwartz MM, Lewis EJ: Immune complex deposition and coronary vasculitis in systemic lupus erythematosus. Am J Med 77:141, 1984.
35. Takatsu Y, Hattori R, Sakaguchi K, et al: Acute myo-

cardial infarction associated with systemic lupus erythematosus documented by coronary arteriograms. Chest
88:147, 1985.
36. Doherty NE, Siegel RJ: Cardiovascular manifestations
of systemic lupus erythematosus. Am Heart J 110:1257,
1985.
37. Bruno L, Tredici S, Mangiavacchi M, et al: Cardiac,
skeletal, and ocular abnormalities in patients with Marfan's syndrome and in their relatives. Br Heart J 51:220,
1984.
38. Holmes MD, Brant-Zawadzki MM, Simon RP: Clinical
features of meningovascular syphilis. Neurology 34:
553, 1984.
39. Spodick DH: Infection and infarction. Acute viral (and
other) infection in the onset, pathogenesis, and mimicry
of acute myocardial infarction. Am J Med 81:661, 1986.
40. Parrillo JE, Fauci AS: Necrotizing vasculitis, coronary
angiitis, and the cardiologist (editorial). Am Heart J
99:547, 1980.
41. Hall S, Barr W, Lie JT, et al: Takayasu arteritis.
Medicine 64:89, 1985.
42. Fukushige J, Nihill MR, McNamara DG: Spectrum of
cardiovascular lesions in mucocutaneous lymph node
syndrome: analysis of eight cases. Am J Cardiol 45:98,
1980.
43. Kato H, Ichinose E, Kawasaki T: Myocardial infarction
in Kawasaki disease: clinical analyses in 195 cases. J
Pediatr 108:923, 1986.
44. Onouchi Z, Shimazu S, Kiyosawa N, et al: Aneurysms
of the coronary arteries in Kawasaki disease. An angiographic study of 30 cases. Circulation 66:6, 1982.
45. Suzuki A, Kamiya T, Ono Y, et al: Myocardial ischemia
in Kawasaki disease: follow-up study by cardiac catheterization and coronary angiography. Pediatr Cardiol
9:1, 1988.
46. Nakano H, Saito A, Ueda K, Nojima K: Clinical characteristics of myocardial infarction following Kawasaki
disease: report of 11 cases. J Pediatr 108:198, 1986.
47. Ebisuno S, Yasuno M, Yamada Y, et al: Myocardial
infarction after acute carbon monoxide poisoning: case
report. Angiology 37:621, 1986.
48. Penner JA: Hypercoagulation and thrombosis. Med
Clin North Am 64:743, 1980.
49. Barrett O Jr, Saunders DE Jr, McFarland DE, Humphries JO: Myocardial infarction in sickle cell anemia.
Am J Hematol 16:139, 1984.
50. Martin CR, Cobb C, Tatter D, et al: Acute myocardial
infarction in sickle cell anemia. Arch Intern Med
143:830, 1983.
51. Small M, Jack AS, Lowe GDO, et al: Coronary artery
disease in severe haemophilia. Br Heart J 49:604, 1983.
52. Neufeld HN, Goldbourt U: Coronary heart disease:
genetic aspects. Circulation 67:943, 1983.
53. Fong LV, Menahem S, Wraith JE, Chow CW: Endocardial fibroelastosis in mucopolysaccharidosis type VI.
Clin Cardiol 10:362, 1987.
54. Halper J, Factor SM: Coronary lesions in neurofibromatosis associated with vasospasm and myocardial infarction. Am Heart J 108:420, 1984.

55. Brosius FC III, Roberts WC: Coronary artery disease in the Hurler syndrome. Am J Cardiol 47:649, 1981.
56. Roberts WC, Waller BF: Cardiac amyloidosis causing cardiac dysfunction: analysis of 54 necropsy patients. Am J Cardiol 52:137, 1983.
57. Smith RR, Hutchins GM: Ischemic heart disease secondary to amyloidosis of intramyocardial arteries. Am J Cardiol 44:413, 1979.
58. Gottdiener JS, Katin MJ, Borer JS, et al: Late cardiac effects of therapeutic mediastinal irradiation. N Engl J Med 308:569, 1983.
59. ODonnell L, ONeill T, Toner M, et al: Myocardial hypertrophy, fibrosis and infarction following exposure of the heart to radiation for Hodgkin's disease. Postgrad Med J 62:1055, 1986.
60. Dunsmore LD, LoPonte MA, Dunsmore RA: Radiation-induced coronary artery disease. J Am Coll Cardiol 8:239, 1986.

Selected Readings

Castello R, Alegria E, Merino A, et al: Syndrome of coronary artery spasm of normal coronary arteries. Clinical and angiographic features. Angiology 39:8, 1988.
Clinical and angiographic features of 77 patients with coronary artery spasm and angiographically normal coronary arteries were compared to 35 patients with coronary spasm and angiographically defined coronary artery disease. Angina at rest was a main clinical feature of spasm in patients with normal coronary arteries. Stress testing was found helpful in predicting which patients with spasm would have coronary lesions.

Feldman RL, Hill JA, Whittle JL, et al: Electrocardiographic changes with coronary artery spasm. Am Heart J 106:1288, 1983.
Diagnosis of transient ischemia secondary to coronary spasm should not be excluded based on the absence of ECG changes during rest angina.

Khan AH, Haywood LJ: Myocardial infarction in nine patients with radiologically patent coronary arteries. N Engl J Med 291:427, 1974.
Data suggest that coronary artery spasm or subsequently resolved platelet thrombi may be part of the pathogenesis.

Magnetic resonance imaging of the cardiovascular system. Present state of the art and future potential. Council on Scientific Affairs. Report of the Magnetic Resonance Imaging Panel. JAMA 259:253, 1988.
Informative discussion with interesting speculations about the future use of MRI of the cardiovascular system.

Morales AR, Romanelli R, Boucek RJ: The mural left anterior descending coronary artery, strenuous exercise, and sudden death. Circulation 62:230, 1980.
Clinical studies suggest that systolic constriction of the left anterior descending coronary artery may precipitate death in selected subjects.

Pasternak RC, Thibault GE, Savoia M, et al: Chest pain with angiographically insignificant coronary arterial obstruction. Am J Med 68:813, 1980.
Mortality and morbidity were low in this group of patients.

Przybojewski JZ, Becker PH: Angina pectoris and acute

myocardial infarction due to "slow-flow phenomenon" in nonatherosclerotic coronary arteries: a case report. Angiology 37:751, 1986.

Brief outline of the various aspects of the pathophysiology of angina pectoris in a patient, as well as the concept of the reduced vasodilator reserve.

Rosenblatt A, Selzer A: The nature and clinical features of myocardial infarction with normal coronary arteriogram. Circulation 55:578, 1977.

Study suggesting that thromboembolism with lysis or recanalization might be the most common cause of myocardial infarction in patients with a normal coronary arteriogram.

3
Angina-like Chest Pain: Cardiac and Noncardiac Causes

Acute chest pain in the adult population immediately raises the possibility of life-threatening myocardial ischemia secondary to atherosclerotic coronary artery disease. Although life-threatening acute chest pain syndromes often reflect vascular compromise, it is not always secondary to coronary artery disease. Other serious cardiac and noncardiac disorders, such as aortic stenosis, aortic dissection, or pulmonary embolus, can produce vascular compromise and angina-like chest pain.[1] Chronic chest pain is less likely to be caused by life-threatening disorders and more likely to be caused by something other than coronary artery disease.[2] In the older adult, gastroesophageal reflux-associated chest pain is a common cause of both acute and chronic noncardiac chest pain.[3] In the young person, musculoskeletal chest wall pain syndromes commonly cause angina-like syndromes. However, if chest pain in a young person does sound ischemic, rarer congenital cardiovascular abnormalities should be considered.[4]

Pain arising from any anatomic structure (skin, bones, lungs, esophagus, stomach, spleen, pancreas, gall bladder) in the vicinity of the heart can mimic angina pectoris. Some cardiologic diseases may also be associated with pain that mimics angina. A careful history with attention to type of pain, onset, radiation, associated features, factors exacerbating or relieving the pain, and duration can usually distinguish most of these causes.[5]

Musculoskeletal Pain Syndromes That Mimic Angina Pectoris

Musculoskeletal chest pain: chest wall syndrome most common cause,[6,7] particularly in adolescents[8]
Costochondritis:[9] Tietze's syndrome
Cervical radiculitis or osteoarthritis
Rib fractures[10]
Thoracic root pain
Thoracic outlet syndrome[11,12]
Sternocostoclavicular hyperostosis[13,14]
Herpes zoster (shingles)
Peripheral neuropathies
Trauma
Arthritis: involving articulations of ribs, sternum, and thoracic spine
Neoplasm: involving ribs, pleura, sternum[15]
Sternoclavicular joint infection[16]

Gastrointestinal Causes of Anginal Chest Pain

Esophageal spasm[17-19]: may be the etiology in 10 to 30% of patients presenting to the emergency room with chest pain[20]
Other esophageal disorders[21,22]: reflux esophagitis, achalasia, esophageal perforation or rupture,[23,24] Mallory-Weiss syndrome, Schatzki's ring, strictures, esophageal diverticulum, hiatus hernia
Peptic ulcer disease
Cholecystitis and cholelithiasis[25,26]
Pancreatitis[27]
Splenic flexure syndrome
Aortoesophageal fistula: mid-thoracic pain with severe gastrointestinal bleeding[28]

Psychiatric Causes of Anginal Chest Pain

Anxiety: panic disorder[29-32]
Depression
Hyperventilation: common etiology of noncardiac chest pain that can often be proven by having the patient elicit the pain during hyperventilation[33]

Cardiac neurosis[34,35]
Secondary gain

Pulmonary Causes of Anginal Chest Pain

Pleurodynia: pleuritic pain is exacerbated with inspiration[36]

Precordial catch or Texidor's Twinge[37]: sharp pain at the cardiac apex, possibly arising from the parietal pleura

Pleural effusion

Pulmonary hypertension: pain may be angina due to right ventricular ischemia

Pneumonia

Pulmonary embolism: usually presents with pleuritic chest pain[38]

Pneumothorax

Neoplasm: mediastinal, lung, pleura

Mediastinal emphysema

Pneumomediastinum[39]

Cardiovascular Causes of Anginal Chest Pain

Prinzmetal's angina: coronary artery spasm can occur with or without atherosclerotic lesions and can mimic or produce myocardial ischemia.[40]

Pericarditis: pericarditis after myocardial infarction may be mistaken for angina pectoris; pericardial pain is exacerbated by inspiration in contrast to angina pectoris, which does not vary with respiration. A friction rub may also be heard.[41,42]

Dressler's syndrome[43-45]

Postpericardiotomy syndrome[46]

Thoracic aortic aneurysm dissection

Premature beats[47]

Hypertrophic cardiomyopathy

Valvular heart disease: mitral valve prolapse,[48-50] aortic stenosis, aortic regurgitation, mitral stenosis, aortic stenosis. In the absence of associated coronary artery disease, the chest pain of mitral stenosis, aortic stenosis, and aortic regurgitation may indeed be due to myocardial ischemia due to the increased myocardial oxygen demand.

Central venous catheter malposition[51]

Myocarditis: acute viral myocarditis can cause myocardial damage and mimic acute myocardial infarction.[52]

Metastatic disease to the heart[53,54]

Chemotherapy: bleomycin infusions[55,56]

Congenital absence of pericardium: rare[57]

References

1. Rutledge JC, Amsterdam EA: Differential diagnosis and clinical approach to the patient with acute chest pain. Cardiol Clin 2:257, 1984.
2. Levine HJ: Difficult problems in the diagnosis of chest pain. Am Heart J 100:108, 1980.
3. Holtz A, Castell DO: Chest pain associated with esophageal disease. Postgrad Med 83(5):315, 1988.
4. Click RL, Spittell JA, Jr, Puga FJ: Chest pain in a young woman. Mayo Clin Proc 63:368, 1988.
5. Magarian GJ, Hickam DH: Noncardiac causes of angina-like chest pain. Prog Cardiovasc Dis 29:65, 1986.
6. Epstein SE, Gerber LH, Borer JS: Chest wall syndrome. A common cause of unexplained cardiac pain. JAMA 241:2793, 1979.
7. Fam AG, Smythe HA: Musculoskeletal chest wall pain. Can Med Assoc J 133:379, 1985.
8. Pantell RH, Goodman BW Jr: Adolescent chest pain: a prospective study. Pediatrics 71:881, 1983.
9. Wolf E, Stern S: Costosternal syndrome. Its frequency and importance in differential diagnosis of coronary heart disease. Arch Intern Med 136:189, 1976.
10. Kattan KR: What to look for in rib fractures and how. JAMA 243:262, 1980.
11. Woods WW: Thoracic outlet syndrome. West J Med 128:9, 1978.
12. Godfrey NF, Halter DG, Minna DA, et al: Thoracic outlet syndrome mimicking angina pectoris with elevated creatine phosphokinase values. Chest 83:461, 1983.
13. Kohler H, Uehlinger E, Kutzner J, et al: Sternocostoclavicular hyperostosis: painful swelling of the sternum, clavicles, and upper ribs. Ann Intern Med 87:192, 1977.
14. Chigira M, Maehara S, Nagase M, et al: Sternocostoclavicular hyperostosis. A report of nineteen cases, with special reference to etiology and treatment. J Bone Joint Surg (Am) 68:103, 1986.
15. LaBan MM, Newman JM: Occult sternal metastasis identified by laminography in patients with chest pain. Arch Phys Med Rehabil 65:203, 1984.
16. Seviour PW, Dieppe PA: Sternoclavicular joint infection as a cause of chest pain. Br Med J (Clin Res) 288:133, 1984.
17. Chobanian SJ, Benjamin SB, Curtis DJ, et al: Systematic esophageal evaluation of patients with noncardiac chest pain. Arch Intern Med 146:1505, 1986.
18. Davies HA, Jones DB, Rhodes J: "Esophageal angina" as the cause of chest pain. JAMA 248:2274, 1982.
19. Dart AM, Davies HA, Lowndes RH, et al: Oesophageal spasm and angina: diagnostic value of ergometrine (ergonovine) provocation. Eur Heart J 1:91, 1980.
20. Richter JE, Castell DO: Diffuse esophageal spasm: a reappraisal. Ann Intern Med 100:242, 1984.
21. Mellow MH: A gastroenterologist's view of chest pain. Curr Probl Cardiol 7(10):7, 1983.
22. Richter JE, Castell DO: Esophageal disease as a cause of noncardiac chest pain. Adv Intern Med 33:311, 1988.
23. Uehara DT, Dymowski JJ, Schwartz J, Turnbull TL:

Chest pain, shock, and pneumomediastinum in a previously healthy 56 year old man (clinical conference). Ann Emerg Med 16:359, 1987.

24. Jaworski A, Fischer R, Lippmann M: Boerhaave's syndrome. Computed tomographic findings and diagnostic considerations. Arch Intern Med 148:223, 1988.

25. Laing FC: Diagnostic evaluation of patient with suspected cholecystitis. Surg Clin North Am 64:3, 1984.

26. Fein AB, Rauch RF II, Bowie JD, et al: Value of sonographic screening for gallstones in patients with chest pain and normal coronary arteries. AJR 146:337, 1986.

27. Moossa AR: Diagnostic tests and procedures in acute pancreatitis. N Engl J Med 311:639, 1984.

28. Khawaja FI, Varindani MK: Aortoesophageal fistula. Review of clinical, radiographic, and endoscopic features. J Clin Gastroenterol 9:342, 1987.

29. Katon W: Panic disorder and somatization. Am J Med 77:101, 1984.

30. Beitman BD, Lamberti JW, Mukerji V, et al: Panic disorder in patients with angiographically normal coronary arteries. A pilot study. Psychosomatics 28:480, 1987.

31. Ballenger JC: Unrecognized prevalence of panic disorder in primary care, internal medicine, and cardiology. Am J Cardiol 60:39J, 1987.

32. Beitman BD, Basha I, Flaker G, et al: Atypical or nonanginal chest pain. Panic disorder or coronary artery disease? Arch Intern Med 147:1548, 1987.

33. Lum LC: Hyperventilation syndromes in medicine and psychiatry: a review. J R Soc Med 80:229, 1987.

34. Costa PT Jr: Influence of the normal personality dimension of neuroticism on chest pain symptoms and coronary artery disease. Am J Cardiol 60:20J, 1987.

35. Young LD, Barboriak JJ, Anderson AJ: Chest pain and behavior in suspected coronary artery disease. Cardiology 75:10, 1988.

36. Branch WT Jr, McNeil BJ: Analysis of the differential diagnosis and assessment of pleuritic chest pain in young adults. Am J Med 75:671, 1983.

37. Miller AJ, Texidor TA: "Precordial catch," a neglected syndrome of precordial pain. JAMA 159:1364, 1955.

38. Hull RD, Raskob GE, Carter CJ, et al: Pulmonary embolism in outpatients with pleuritic chest pain. Arch Intern Med 148:838, 1988.

39. Rose WD, Veach JS, Tehranzdeh J: Spontaneous pneumomediastinum as a cause of neck pain, dysphagia, and chest pain. Arch Intern Med 144:392, 1984.

40. Scardi S, Pivotti F, Pandullo C, et al: Exercise-induced intermittent angina and ST-segment elevation in Prinzmetal's angina. Eur Heart J 9:102, 1988.

41. Sternbach GL: Pericarditis. Ann Emerg Med 17:214, 1988.

42. Bellinger RL, Vacek JL: A review of pericarditis. 1. Causes, manifestations, and diagnostic techniques. Postgrad Med 82(2):95, 1987.

43. Kossowsky WA, Lyon AF, Spain DM: Reappraisal of the postmyocardial infarction Dressler's syndrome. Am Heart J 102:954, 1981.

44. Lichstein E, Arsura E, Hollander G, et al: Current incidence of postmyocardial infarction (Dressler's) syndrome. Am J Cardiol 50:1269, 1982.
45. Williams RK, Nagle RE, Thompson RA: Postcoronary pain and the postmyocardial infarction syndrome. Br Heart J 51:327, 1984.
46. Engle MA, Zabriskie JB, Senterfit LB, et al: Viral illness and the postpericardiotomy syndrome. Circulation 62:1151, 1980.
47. Madsen JK, Srensen JN, Kromann-Andersen B, et al: Ventricular premature beats on Holter monitoring in patients admitted with chest pain, in whom acute myocardial infarction is not confirmed. The prognostic value and relationship to scars or ischemia on thallium-201 scintigraphy. Clin Cardiol 10:305, 1987.
48. Spears PF, Koch KL, Day FP: Chest pain associated with mitral valve prolapse. Arch Intern Med 146:796, 1986.
49. Gottlieb SH: Mitral valve prolapse: from syndrome to disease. Am J Cardiol 60:53J, 1987.
50. Cheng TO: Mitral valve prolapse. Dis Mon 33:481, 1987.
51. Webb JG, Simmonds SD, Chan-Yan C: Central venous catheter malposition presenting as chest pain. Chest 89:309, 1986.
52. Miklozek CL, Crumpacker CS, Royal HD, et al: Myocarditis presenting as acute myocardial infarction. Am Heart J 115:768, 1988.
53. Cacciapuoti F, Arpino G, Davino M: Reliability of echocardiography in the detection of metastatic malignant pericardial masses. Int J Cardiol 18:109, 1988.
54. Leung CY, Cummings RG, Reimer KA, Lowe JE: Chondrosarcoma metastatic to the heart. Ann Thorac Surg 45:291, 1988.
55. White DA, Schwartzberg LS, Kris MG, Bosl GJ: Acute chest pain syndrome during bleomycin infusions. Cancer 59:1582, 1987.
56. Hancock EW: Chest pain during cancer chemotherapy. Hosp Pract 20(7):93,96, 1985.
57. Chapman JE Jr, Rubin JW, Gross CM, Janssen ME: Congenital absence of pericardium: an unusual cause of atypical angina. Ann Thorac Surg 45:91, 1988.

Selected Readings

Castell DO: Diagnosis of noncardiac chest pain in older patients. Geriatrics 40(10):61, 1985.

Author discusses the work-up of noncardiac chest pain in older patients with an emphasis on evaluating gastrointestinal causes of chest pain. The focus is on the clinical usefulness of the following modalities: barium swallow, gall bladder studies, intraesophageal acid infusion, and intraesophageal edrophonium chloride stimulation.

Constant J: The clinical diagnosis of nonanginal chest pain: the differentiation of angina from nonanginal chest pain by history. Clin Cardiol 6:11, 1983.

A nonanginal chest pain category of history taking is suggested to avoid diagnoses such as "atypical chest pain" and "atypical angina."

Eagle KA, Quertermous T, Kritzer GA, et al: Spectrum of conditions initially suggesting acute aortic dissection but with negative aortograms. Am J Cardiol 57:322, 1986.

Study defining the actual differential diagnosis of aortic dissection and the frequency of false-negative aortographic findings, as well as contrasting the clinical features of patients with and without dissection.

Goldman L: Acute chest pain: emergency room evaluation. Hosp Pract 21(7):94A, 1986.

Discussion of the concept of "stepdown" or intermediate care unit for some patients in which myocardial infarction is a possible but not likely diagnosis.

Goldman L, Cook EF, Brand DA, et al: A computer protocol to predict myocardial infarction in emergency department patients with chest pain. N Engl J Med 318:797, 1988.

A computer protocol was constructed to improve triage to the coronary care unit of patients presenting with chest pain. Data from 1,379 patients at two hospitals were used to construct a protocol to predict the presence of myocardial infarction. The protocol was prospectively tested in 4,770 patients at four hospitals and showed a significantly higher specificity in predicting the presence or absence of infarction than physicians deciding whether to admit patients to the coronary care unit. The authors conclude that, even though the computer based protocol was capable of producing accurate estimates of the probability of myocardial infarction, this information should not be used to override careful clinical judgment in individual cases.

Hedges JR, Kobernick MS: Detection of myocardial ischemia/infarction in the emergency department patient with chest discomfort. Emerg Med Clin North Am 6:317, 1988.

An update of current concepts and a review of the literature of decision-making when evaluating the patient with chest pain in the emergency room. Reliance on individual clinical impression is still the most significant guide to admission decisions. Usefulness of intermediate care units and outpatient follow-up and evaluation of myocardial ischemia or alternative diagnoses for noncardiac chest pain, particularly gastrointestinal and psychiatric causes, are discussed.

Iskandrian AS, Heo J, Hakki AH: Angina: DX of atypical presentations in the elderly. Geriatrics 41(10):51, 1986.

Authors suggest that pretest probability of coronary heart disease is helpful in interpreting exercise test results in the elderly. Marked ST-segment depression in multiple leads is a strong indication of extensive coronary disease, particularly when it occurs early during exercise and when it is associated with a blunted or hypotensive blood pressure response. In general, coronary artery disease occurs in 90% of patients with typical angina pectoris, in 50% of patients with atypical angina pectoris, and in only 10% of patients with non-anginal chest pain in this study.

Katon W, Hall ML, Russo J, et al: Chest pain: relationship of psychiatric illness to coronary arteriographic results. Am J Med 84:1, 1988.

Seventy-four patients with chest pain without a previous history of cardiovascular disease received psychiatric evaluations immediately after coronary arteriography. Patients with chest pain and negative coronary arteriograms were significantly younger and had a higher number of associated autonomic symptoms, such as tachycardia, dyspnea, dizziness, and paresthesias. Psychiatric diagnoses in decreasing frequency included panic disorders, major depression, and phobias.

Katz PO, Dalton CB, Richter JE, et al: Esophageal testing of patients with noncardiac chest pain or dysphagia. Results of three years' experience with 1161 patients. Ann Intern Med 106:593, 1987.

Data from 910 patients referred for clinical esophageal manometry for evaluation of noncardiac chest pain were reviewed. This study found the nutcracker esophagus a significant manometric marker for noncardiac chest pain. Manometric abnormalities were statistically more common in patients with dysphagia. Achalasia and nonspecific esophageal motility disorders were the most common abnormalities in patients with dysphagia.

Kaul S, Lilly DR, Gascho JA, et al: Prognostic utility of the exercise thallium-201 test in ambulatory patients with chest pain: comparison with cardiac catheterization. Circulation 77:745, 1988.

A study that attempted to determine the prognostic utility of the exercise thallium-201 stress test in ambulatory patients with chest pain who were also referred for cardiac catheterization. Data from a 4- to 8- year follow-up of 383 patients who underwent both exercise thallium-201 stress testing and cardiac catheterization for 1978 to 1981 were included. Authors conclude that a combination of both catheterization and exercise thallium-201 data provides superior information to either test used alone.

Madsen JK, Stubgaard M, Utne HE, et al: Prognosis and thallium-201 scintigraphy in patients admitted with chest pain without confirmed acute myocardial infarction. Br Heart J 59:184, 1988.

A study that included exercise and rest thallium scintingraphy and exercise electrocardiography on 158 patients less than 76 years of age admitted with chest pain and suspected acute myocardial infarction. Data suggest that thallium scintigraphy alone or in combination with exercise electrocardiography can identify groups of high- and low-risk patients in whom acute myocardial infarction is suspected.

Malliani A, Lombardi F: Consideration of the fundamental mechanisms eliciting cardiac pain (editorial). Am Heart J 103:575, 1982.

Concise commentary on gross anatomy of cardiac nociceptive pathways and peripheral mechanisms.

Oh JK, Miller FA, Shub C, et al: Evaluation of acute chest pain syndromes by two-dimensional echocardiography: its potential application in the selection of patients for acute reperfusion therapy. Mayo Clin Proc 62:59, 1987.

Authors found two-dimensional echocardiography particularly useful when electrocardiographic changes were absent and suggest that this technique may provide useful information in the initial noninvasive assessment of chest pain.

Owens GM: Chest pain. Prim Care 13:55, 1986.

A clinical review of multiple causes of chest pain from the perspective of the primary care physician. Emphasis is placed on differentiating the patient with acute chest pain who is an emergency from the majority of patients with chest pain who present in the physician's office.

Peters L, Maas L, Petty D, et al: Spontaneous noncardiac chest pain. Evaluation by 24-hour ambulatory esophageal motility and pH monitoring. Gastroenterology 94:878, 1988.

A study of 24 patients with chronic, daily, substernal chest pain in whom noncardiac causes were suspected. A 24-hour ambulatory esophageal motility and pH system were tested because patients in this group rarely experience spontaneous chest pain in the laboratory. Authors suggest that ambulatory esophageal motility and pH monitoring are useful in the evaluation of noncardiac chest pain. They found that the majority of chest pain episodes did not correlate with either motility or pH abnormalities, but that pH abnormalities correlated with chest pain episodes more commonly than esophageal motility abnormalities.

Sasaki H, Charuzi Y, Beeder C, et al: Utility of echocardiography for the early assessment of patients with nondiagnostic chest pain. Am Heart J 112:494, 1986.

This study suggests that in patients presenting with nondiagnostic chest pain, an early assessment of regional wall motion by two-dimensional echocardiography can differentiate patients with myocardial ischemia or early infarction from those with nonischemic pain when it is performed during an episode of chest pain.

Semble EL, Wise CM: Chest pain: a rheumatologist's perspective. South Med J 81:64, 1988.

Helpful clinical review from a rheumatologist's perspective that covers musculoskeletal disorders causing chest pain, including Tietze's syndrome, chest wall pain syndromes, fibrositis, inflammatory arthritic conditions, cervical osteoarthritis, and diseases of the thoracic spine.

Spears PF, Koch KL: Esophageal disorders in patients with chest pain and mitral valve prolapse. Am J Gastroenterol 81:951, 1986.

A study of 19 patients with mitral valve prolapse and chest pain with esophageal manometry in whom no significant coronary artery disease was found at cardiac catheterization. The authors found evidence of diffuse esophageal spasm in five patients, hypertensive lower esophageal sphincter-motility disorders in two patients, and hypotensive lower esophageal sphincters in five patients. Authors suggest esophageal disorders may provide an explanation for chest pain in certain patients with mitral valve prolapse.

Takaoka K, Yasue H, Horio Y: Possible role of coronary spasm in acute myocardial infarction precipitated by hyperventilation. Br Heart J 59:256, 1988.

A case report of a 65-year-old man with acute myocardial infarction precipitated by hyperventilation. His chronic phase coronary arteriogram showed almost normal coronary arteries; however, an acetylcholine injection into the left coronary artery induced circumflex artery spasm associated with chest pain and ST-segment elevation. Authors suggest that in the absence of endothelium, the response of smooth muscle to acetylcholine is constriction.

4
ECG Patterns: Disorders That Can Simulate Myocardial Ischemia and Infarction

Pseudoinfarct and pseudoischemic ECG changes are ECG patterns that can simulate myocardial ischemia and infarction. Such ECG patterns can occur in a wide variety of clinical situations. Some pseudoinfarct ECG changes reflect normal, physiologic, or positional variants. Other such ECG changes can offer electrophysiologic clues to underlying cardiac disease without coronary artery disease or noncardiac disease. Chest pain is a frequent clinical accompaniment of both myocardial ischemic-induced ECG changes and several serious disorders, such as pericarditis and pulmonary embolism, which can be associated with pseudoinfarct or pseudoischemic changes. If pseudoinfarct patterns are misdiagnosed, normal patterns, such as normal Q-wave variants, may result in a diagnosis of "electrocardiographogenic disease"; or serious underlying cardiovascular or pulmonary pathology, such as cardiomyopathies or acute pulmonary embolism, can be missed.[1]

Apical hypertrophy[2]
Aneurysm: the ST elevation of ventricular aneurysms may suggest myocardial injury. The history should reveal a previous myocardial infarction.
Athletic heart syndrome[3–5]
Metastatic disease[6]
Cardiomyopathies[7,8]: hypertrophic[9]
Cerebrovascular accident and subarachnoid hemorrhage[10–12]: can have dramatic T-wave changes
Chest deformity
Complex congenital heart disease
Drugs: digoxin is the best example of a drug that may cause ECG changes suggesting myocardial

ischemia; other examples include quinidine, procainamide, isuprel, and epinephrine.[13]

Electrolyte abnormalities[14-16]

Hyperventilation[17]: chest tightness due to anxiety may accompany hyperventilation syndrome.

"Juvenile" T-wave pattern

Left bundle branch block and left anterior hemiblock[18]: left bundle branch block mimics anteroseptal myocardial infarction; left anterior hemiblock mimics inferior myocardial infarction.[19]

Left tension pneumothorax[20]

Misplaced ECG leads[21]

Mitral valve prolapse[22,23]

Myocarditis

Neuromuscular disease: muscular dystrophies[24-27]

Normal variant

Pancreatitis[28]

Pericarditis[29,30]: although the ECG changes of pericarditis may suggest transmural ischemia, pain is usually pleuritic.[31]

Pneumothorax: ECG may be particularly misleading if taken in the supine position; it is helpful to perform ECG in erect position.[32,33]

"Poor" R-wave progression[34]: i.e., late R/S transition may mimic anteroseptal myocardial infarction.

Preexcitation syndromes[35]: may mimic anteroseptal or inferior myocardial infarction[36]

Pregnancy[37]: ECG changes are common, and chest pain may be due to pressure of the uterus against the diaphragm.[38]

Pulmonary diseases[39]: chronic obstructive pulmonary disease, pneumonia

Pulmonary embolism[40,41]: ECG usually shows nonspecific ST-T wave changes, and the chest pain is usually pleuritic.

Valvular heart disease [42,43]

Ventricular hypertrophy[44,45]: severe left ventricular hypertrophy may mimic anteroseptal myocardial infarction; right ventricular hypertrophy with severe right axis deviation may mimic diaphragmatic infarction.[46-50]

Miscellaneous stimuli: eating, drinking ice water, posture, fear, and pain

References

1. Goldberger AL: Normal and noninfarct Q waves. Cardiol Clin 5:357, 1987.
2. Vacek JL, Davis WR, Bellinger RL, McKiernan TL:

Apical hypertrophic cardiomyopathy in American patients. Am Heart J 108:1501, 1984.

3. Huston TP, Puffer JC, Rodney WM: The athletic heart syndrome. N Engl J Med 313:24, 1985.

4. Valle GA, Lemberg L: An acute cardiovascular event in an endurance-trained athlete. Heart Lung 17:216, 1988.

5. Abdulatif M, Fahkry M, Naguib M, et al: Multiple electrocardiographic anomalies during anaesthesia in an athlete. Can J Anaesth 34:284, 1987.

6. Conetta R, Gitler B: Electrocardiographic anterior wall pseudoinfarction pattern caused by a metastatic brain tumor. NY State J Med 87:125, 1987.

7. Gau GT, Goodwin JF, Oakley CM, et al: Q waves and coronary arteriography in cardiomyopathy. Br Heart J 34:1034, 1972.

8. McMartin DE, Flowers NC; Clinical-electrocardiographic correlations in diseases of the myocardium. Cardiovasc Clin 8(3):191, 1977.

9. Kumar S: Persistent ST-segment elevation in hypertrophic subaortic stenosis. Arch Intern Med 142:1957, 1982.

10. Gould L, Reddy CVR, Kollali M, et al: Electrocardiographic normalization after cerebral vascular accident. J Electrocardiol 14:191, 1981.

11. Samra SK, Kroll DA: Subarachnoid hemorrhage and intraoperative electrocardiographic changes simulating myocardial ischemia—anesthesiologist's dilemma. Anesth Analg 64:86, 1985.

12. Tobias SL, Bookatz BJ, Diamond TH: Myocardial damage and electrocardiographic changes in acute cerebrovascular hemorrhage: a report of three cases and review. Heart Lung 16:521, 1987.

13. Sundqvist K, Atterhog JH, Jogestrand T: Effect of digoxin on the electrocardiogram at rest and during exercise in healthy subjects. Am J Cardiol 57:661, 1986.

14. VanderArk CR, Ballantyne F III, Reynolds EW Jr: Electrolytes and the electrocardiogram. Cardiovasc Clin 5(3):268, 1973.

15. Khardori R, Cohen B, Taylor D, et al: Electrocardiographic finding simulating acute myocardial infarction in a compound metabolic aberration. Am J Med 78:529, 1985.

16. Surawicz B, Mangiardi ML: Electrocardiogram in endocrine and metabolic disorders. Cardiovasc Clin 8(3):243, 1977.

17. Shteingardt IUN, Melnik TG, Porovskii IAV: Pseudoischemic changes in the ECG caused by hyperventilation. Kardiologiia 23(10):54, 1983.

18. Hultgren HN, Craige E, Fujii J, et al: Left bundle branch block and mechanical events of the cardiac cycle. Am J Cardiol 52:755, 1983.

19. Flowers NC; Left bundle branch block: a continuously evolving concept. J Am Coll Cardiol 9:684, 1987.

20. Werne CS, Sands MJ: Left tension pneumothorax masquerading as anterior myocardial infarction. Ann Emerg Med 14:164, 1985.

21. Hill NE, Goodman JS: Importance of accurate placement of precordial leads in the 12-lead electrocardiogram. Heart Lung 16:561, 1987.

22. Jeresaty RM: Mitral valve prolapse. JAMA 254:793, 1985.
23. Joyner CR, Cornman CR: The mitral valve prolapse syndrome: clinical features and management. Cardiovasc Clin 16:233, 1986.
24. Perloff JK, Roberts WC, de Leon AC Jr, et al: The distinctive electrocardiogram of Duchenne's progressive muscular dystrophy. Am J Med 42:179, 1967.
25. Olofsson BO, Forsberg H, Andersson S, et al: Electrocardiographic findings in myotonic dystrophy. Br Heart J 59:47, 1988.
26. Wintzen AR, Schipperheyn JJ: Cardiac abnormalities in myotonic dystrophy. Electrocardiographic and echocardiographic findings in 65 patients and 34 of their unaffected relatives. Relation with age and sex and relevance for gene detection. J Neurol Sci 80:259, 1987.
27. Yamamoto S, Matsushima H, Suzuki A, et al: A comparative study of thallium-201 single-photon emission computed tomography and electrocardiography in Duchenne and other types of muscular dystrophy. Am J Cardiol 61:836, 1988.
28. Bdker B, Kelbaek H, Jensen SM, Godtfredsen J: Electrocardiographic changes in patients with upper abdominal pain admitted to a surgical ward. Am J Cardiol 60:1188, 1987.
29. Wanner WR, Schaal SF, Bashore TM, et al: Repolarization variant vs acute pericarditis. Chest 83:180, 1983.
30. Burma GM, Emerman CL: Pericarditis mimicking acute myocardial infarction. Am J Emerg Med 4:262, 1986.
31. Tilley WS, Harston WE: Inadvertent administration of streptokinae to patients with pericarditis. Am J Med 81:541, 1986.
32. Keller N, Szaff M, Sykulski R: Electrocardiographic changes in spontaneous left pneumothorax. Acta Med Scand 221:499, 1987.
33. Kounis NG, Mallioris CN, Karavias D, et al: Unusual electrocardiographic changes in intrathoracic conditions. Acta Cardiol (Brux) 42:179, 1987.
34. DePace NL, Colby J, Hakki AH, et al: Poor R wave progression in the precordial leads: clinical implications for the diagnosis of myocardial infarction. J Am Coll Cardiol 2:1073, 1983.
35. Chung KY, Walsh TJ, Massie E: Wolff-Parkinson-White syndrome. Am Heart J 69:116, 1965.
36. Rinne C, Klein GJ, Sharma AD, Yee R: Clinical usefulness of the 12-lead electrocardiogram in the Wolff-Parkinson-White syndrome. Cardiol Clin 5:499, 1987.
37. Sullivan JM, Ramanathan KB: Management of medical problems in pregnancy—severe cardiac disease. N Engl J Med 313:304, 1985.
38. Mulders LG, Boers GH, Prickartz-Wijdeveld MM, Hein PR: A study of maternal ECG characteristics before and during intravenous tocolysis with beta-sympathicomimetics. Effects of i.v. tocolysis on maternal ECG characteristics. Acta Obstet Gynecol Scand 66:417, 1987.
39. Ferrer MI: Clinical and electrocardiographic correlations in pulmonary heart disease (cor pulmonale). Cardiovasc Clin 8(3);215, 1977.
40. Stein PD, Dalen JE, McIntyre KM, et al: The electro-

cardiogram in acute pulmonary embolism. Prog Cardiovasc Dis 17:247, 1975.

41. Denton TA, Litvack F, Siegel RJ: Pseudoinfarction in patients with massive pulmonary embolism. West J Med 145:98, 1986.
42. Siegel RJ, Roberts WC: Electrocardiographic observations in severe aortic valve stenosis: correlative necropsy study to clinical, hemodynamic, and ECG variables demonstrating relation to 12-lead QRS amplitude to peak systolic transaortic pressure gradient. Am Heart J 103:210, 1982.
43. Rios JC, Leet C: Electrocardiographic assessment of valvular heart disease. Cardiovasc Clin 8(3):161, 1977.
44. Murphy ML, Thenabadu PN, DeSoyza N, et al: Reevaluation of electrocardiographic criteria for left, right and combined cardiac ventricular hypertrophy. Am J Cardiol 53:1140, 1984.
45. McKenna WJ, Borggrefe M, England D, et al: The natural history of left ventricular hypertrophy in hypertrophic cardiomyopathy: an electrocardiographic study. Circulation 66:1233, 1982.
46. Kimura M, Matsushita S, Nakahara K, et al: Evaluation of electrocardiographic criteria for left ventricular hypertrophy based on anatomical comparison. J Electrocardiol 20:369, 1987.
47. Hutchins SW, Murphy ML, Dinh H: Recent progress in the electrocardiographic diagnosis of ventricular hypertrophy. Cardiol Clin 5:455, 1987.
48. Lehtonen J, Sutinen S, Ikaheimo M, Paakko P: Electrocardiographic criteria for the diagnosis of right ventricular hypertrophy verified at autopsy. Chest 93:839, 1988.
49. Scognamiglio R, Fasoli G, Bruni A, Dalla-Volta S: Observations on the capability of the electrocardiogram to detect left ventricular function in chronic severe aortic regurgitation. Eur Heart J 9:54, 1988.
50. Chia BL, Choo M: Pseudo-infarction ECG pattern due to extreme right ventricular hypertrophy. J Electrocardiol 19:189, 1986.

Selected Readings

Hancock EW: ECG casebook. Acute chest pain and abnormal R-wave progression. Hosp Pract 18(12):75, 1983.
"Poor R wave progression" is an electrocardiographic diagnosis that is a frequent source of misunderstanding or overinterpretation.

Kopitsky RG, Geltman EM: Lack of myocardial necrosis despite clinical and electrocardiographic criteria of acute transmural infarction. Am J Med 83:589, 1987.
The evolution of "pathologic" Q waves with ST segment elevation is diagnostic of transmural myocardial infarction. This study describes a patient with severe myocardial ischemia and electrocardiographic evidence that suggested acute transmural myocardial infarction in a patient in whom significant myocardial necrosis was adequately excluded.

Krikler DM: Historical aspects of electrocardiography. Cardiol Clin 5:349, 1987.

Historical perspective covering the development of the human electrocardiogram from 1901, when it first became clinically relevant.

Levy D, Bailey JJ, Garrison RJ, et al: Electrocardiographic changes with advancing age. A cross-sectional study of the association of age with QRS axis, duration, and voltage. J Electrocardiol 20(Suppl):44, 1987.

A study that examined ECG changes that occur in the elderly using a healthy reference population derived from subjects followed prospectively in the Framingham Heart Study found significant sex differences. Mean values and correlations with age for the PR duration, QRS duration and axis, S wave voltage, V1 and R wave voltage and V5 are presented. Findings in elderly men included QRS narrowing, left QRS axis shift, and loss of S V1 and R V5 amplitude. Findings in elderly women were limited to a leftward QRS axis shift.

Miller DH, Kligfield P, Schreiber TL, Borer JS: Relationship of prior myocardial infarction to false-positive electrocardiographic diagnosis of acute injury in patients with chest pain. Arch Intern Med 147:257, 1987.

This study compared the predictive value of ST segment elevation with ST segment depression in the diagnosis of evolving myocardial infarction in 100 consecutive patients admitted with a minimum of 30 minutes of chest pain to a coronary unit of New York Hospital. Eight-four percent (26/31) of patients with ST segment elevation evolved myocardial infarction; 48% (13/27) of patients with ST segment depression evolved myocardial infarctions. Authors conclude that patients with chest pain and ST segment elevation have about twice the likelihood of developing a myocardial infarction than patients with ST segment depression.

Nesto RW, Kowalchuk GJ: The ischemic cascade: temporal sequence of hemodynamic, electrocardiographic, and symptomatic expressions of ischemia. Am J Cardiol 59:23C, 1987.

Current concepts of the pathophysiology of myocardial ischemia correlated with clinical symptoms of angina pectoris and electrocardiographic changes.

5

Congestive Heart Failure: Major Etiologic Categories

Congestive heart failure is a common syndrome of depressed myocardial function resulting in decreased cardiac output.[1] Since signs and symptoms of congestive heart failure are often nonspecific and underlying causes include a wide variety of abnormalities, accurate etiologic diagnosis is often difficult.[2] The usual form of heart failure is a heart muscle that has reduced contractility, causing a reduced cardiac output and perfusion of blood that is inadequate to meet metabolic needs of peripheral tissues.[3] Two major etiologic categories of congestive heart failure are (1) primary cardiac disorders that decrease the heart's ability to meet the metabolic needs of the body, and (2) disorders, which are usually systemic, that increase the workload of the heart. The major factors that govern myocardial workload and also determine left ventricular performance and myocardial oxygen consumption are (1) decreased intrinsic heart muscle contractility, (2) increased preload or left atrial filling pressure, (3) increased afterload such as occurs with decreased systemic blood pressure and increased systemic vascular resistance, and (4) increased heart rate such as occurs in compensatory response to increased sympathetic tone and circulating catecholamines.[3]

Factors Associated With Heart's Inability to Meet Metabolic Needs

Myocardial infarction[4]: mitral regurgitation due to papillary muscle dysfunction,[5] ventricular aneurysm,[6,7] ventricular rupture

Arrhythmias[8,9]: bradyarrhythmias, tachyarrhythmias or asystole[10,11]

Pericarditis: particularly with tamponade

Myocarditis: multiple etiologies, recently a frequent autopsy finding in AIDS patients[12,13]

Cardiomyopathy: hypertensive, idiopathic, ischemic, restrictive, hypertrophic, familial[14–21]

Valvular disease: e.g., aortic stenosis,[22,23] mitral valve prolapse[24,25]

Endocarditis[26]: particularly in association with valve dysfunction and myocardial abscesses.

Myocardial contusion: as occurs with chest trauma

Hypothyroidism

Cardiac transplant rejection

Carcinoid syndrome[27,28]: tricuspid stenosis and/or regurgitation[29]

Cardiac tumors: primary and metastatic[30–33]

Toxins: e.g., alcohol, cobalt, snake and insect venoms,[34] halogenated hydrocarbons,[35] carbon monoxide[36]

Drugs: drugs that decrease myocardial contractility,

e.g., disopyramide,[37] doxorubicin,[38–40] beta-block-ers,[41] chloroquine,[42] verapamil,[43] cyclophos-phamide[44]

Congenital heart malformations: tetralogy of Fallot, aortic coarctation, ventral septal defect, Ebstein's malformation[45]

Factors Associated With an Increased Work Load on the Heart

Noncompliance with drug therapy

Excessive salt intake: dietary and also drugs with salt retaining properties, e.g., indomethacine and ste-roids

Fluid overload: transfusions

Accelerated hypertension

Endocarditis: as a consequence of systemic infection, i.e., sepsis

Aortic dissection[46–52]: causing acute aortic insuffi-ciency

Fistulae: aortopulmonary fistula,[53] Osler-Weber-Rendu disease or hemorrhagic hereditary telangi-ectasia[54]

High output states: anemia,[55] pregnancy,[56] arterio-venous fistula, hemodialysis, beriberi,[57] Paget's dis-ease, hyperthyroidism,[58,59] multiple myeloma[60]

Pulmonary hypertension[61,62] leading to cor pulmon-ale: pulmonary embolism, pancreatitis,[63] acute res-piratory distress syndrome, chronic obstructive pul-monary disease

References

1. Moe GW, Armstrong PW: Congestive heart failure. Can Med Assoc J 138:689, 1988.
2. Franciosa JA: Eidemiologic patterns, clinical evaluation, and long-term prognosis in chronic congestive heart failure. Am J Med 80:14, 1986.
3. Parmley WW: Pathophysiology of congestive heart fail-ure. Am J Cardiol 56:7A, 1985.
4. Weisman HF, Healy B: Myocardial infarct expansion, infarct extension, and reinfarction: pathophysiologic concepts. Prog Cardiovasc Dis 30:73, 1987.
5. Nunley DL, Starr JA: Papillary muscle rupture compli-cating acute myocardial infarction. Am J Surg 145:574, 1983.
6. Louagie Y, Alouini T, Lesperance J, Pelletier LC: Left ventricular aneurysm with predominating congestive heart failure. A comparative study of medical and surgical treatment. J Thorac Cardiovasc Surg 94:571, 1987.
7. Cohen DE, Vogel RA: Left ventricular aneurysm as a coronary risk factor independent of overall left ventric-ular function. Am Heart J 111:23, 1986.

8. Meinertz T, Hofmann T, Kasper W, et al: Significance of ventricular arrhythmias in idiopathic dilated cardiomyopathy. Am J Cardiol 53:902, 1984.
9. Gallagher JJ: Tachycardia and cardiomyopathy: the chicken-egg dilemma revisited. J Am Coll Cardiol 6:1172, 1985.
10. Deedwania PC: Significance of arrhythmias in congestive heart failure. Postgrad Med 83(4):223, 228, 1988.
11. Parmley WW: Factors causing arrhythmias in chronic congestive heart failure. Am Heart J 114:1267, 1987.
12. Lash AD, Wittman AL, Quismorio FP Jr: Myocarditis in mixed connective tissue disease: clinical and pathologic study of three cases and review of the literature. Semin Arthritis Rheum 15:288, 1986.
13. Anderson DW, Virmani R, Reilly JM, et al; Prevalent myocarditis at necropsy in the acquired immunodeficiency syndrome. J Am Coll Cardiol 11:792, 1988.
14. Johnson RA, Palacios I: Dilated cardiomyopathies of the adult. (Two parts.) N Engl J Med 307:1051, 307:1119, 1982.
15. Pantely GA, Bristow JD: Ischemic cardiomyopathy. Prog Cardiovasc Dis 27:95, 1984.
16. Fein FS, Sonnenblick EH: Diabetic cardiomyopathy. Prog Cardiovasc Dis 27:255, 1985.
17. Regan TJ: Alcoholic cardiomyopathy. Prog Cardiovasc Dis 27:141, 1984.
18. Cohen IS, Anderson DW, Virmani R, et al: Congestive cardiomyopathy in association with the acquired immunodeficiency syndrome. N Engl J Med 315:628, 1986.
19. Berko BA, Swift M: X-linked dilated cardiomyopathy. N Engl J Med 316:1186, 1987.
20. James TN, Cobbs BW, Coghlan HC, et al: Coronary disease, cardioneuropathy, and conduction system abnormalities in the cardiomyopathy of Friedreich's ataxia. Br Heart J 57:446, 1987.
21. Shah PM, Abelmann WH, Gersh BJ: Cardiomyopathies in the elderly. J Am Coll Cardiol 10(2 Suppl A):77A, 1987.
22. Cheitlin MD, Gertz EW, Brundage BH, et al: Rate of progression of severity of valvular aortic stenosis in the adult. Am Heart J 98:689, 1979.
23. Dineen E, Brent BN: Aortic valve stenosis: comparison of patients with those without chronic congestive heart failure. Am J Cardiol 57:419, 1986.
24. Grenadier E, Alpan G, Keidar S, et al: The prevalence of ruptured chordae tendineae in the mitral valve prolapse syndrome. Am Heart J 105:603, 1983.
25. Naggar CZ, Pearson WN, Seljan MP: Frequency of complications of mitral valve prolapse in subjects aged 60 years and older. Am J Cardiol 58:1209, 1986.
26. Weinstein L: Life-threatening complications of infective endocarditis and their management. Arch Intern Med 146:953, 1986.
27. Tornebrandt K, Eskilsson J, Nobin A: Heart involvement in metastatic carcinoid disease. Clin Cardiol 9:13, 1986.
28. Ross EM, Roberts WC: The carcinoid syndrome: comparison of 21 necropsy subjects with carcinoid heart disease to 15 necropsy subjects without carcinoid heart disease. Am J Med 79:339, 1985.

29. Blick DR, Zoghbi WA, Lawrie GM, Verani MS: Carcinoid heart disease presenting as right-to-left shunt and congestive heart failure: successful surgical treatment. Am Heart J 115:201, 1988.
30. Kutalek SP, Panidis IP, Kotler MN, et al: Metastatic tumors of the heart detected by two-dimensional echocardiography. Am Heart J 109:343, 1985.
31. DAngelo GJ, Kish GF, Sardesai PG, Tan WS: Cardiac tumors in 19 years of private practice. Am Surg 53:105, 1987.
32. Cairns P, Butany J, Fulop J, et al: Cardiac presentation of non-Hodgkin's lymphoma. Arch Pathol Lab Med 111:80, 1987.
33. Constantino A, West TE, Gupta M, Loghmanee F: Primary cardiac lymphoma in a patient with acquired immune deficiency syndrome. Cancer 60:2801, 1987.
34. Rowe SF, Greer KE, Hodge RH Jr: Electrocardiographic changes associated with multiple yellow jacket stings. South Med J 72:483, 1979.
35. Garriott J, Petty CS: Death from inhalant abuse: toxicological and pathological evaluation of 34 cases. Clin Toxicol 16:305, 1980.
36. Turino GM: Effect of carbon monoxide on the cardiorespiratory system. Circulation 63:253A, 1981.
37. Podrid PJ, Schoeneberger A, Lown B: Congestive heart failure caused by oral disopyramide. N Engl J Med 302:614, 1980.
38. Gottdiener JS, Mathisen DJ, Borer JS, et al: Doxorubicin cardiotoxicity: assessment of late left ventricular dysfunction by radionuclide cineangiography. Ann Intern Med 94:430, 1981.
39. Torti FM, Bristow MR, Howes AE, et al: Reduced cardiotoxicity of doxorubicin delivered on a weekly schedule. Ann Intern Med 99:745, 1983.
40. Buzdar AU, Marcus C, SmithTL, Blumenschein GR: Early and delayed clinical cardiotoxicity of doxorubicin. Cancer 55:2761, 1985.
41. Goldstein S: Propranolol therapy in patients with acute myocardial infarction: the beta-blocker heart attack trial. Circulation 67(Suppl I):53, 1983.
42. Ratliff NB, Estes ML, Myles JL, et al: Diagnosis of chloroquine cardiomyopathy by endomyocardial biopsy. N Engl J Med 316:191, 1987.
43. Packer M, Meller J, Medina N, et al: Hemodynamic consequences of combined beta-adrenergic and slow calcium channel blockade in man. Circulation 65:660, 1982.
44. Goldberg MA, Antin JH, Guinan EC, Rappeport JM: Cyclophosphamide cardiotoxicity: an analysis of dosing as a risk factor. Blood 68:1114, 1986.
45. Areias JC, Valente I: Congenital heart malformations associated with dilated cardiomyopathy. Int J Cardiol 17:83, 1987.
46. Griffith GL, Todd EP: Acute aortic dissection. South Med J 78:1487, 1985.
47. Haverich A, Miller DC, Scott WC, et al: Acute and chronic aortic dissections—determinants of long-term outcome for operative survivors. Circulation 72:II22, 1985.

48. Dalen JE, Howe JP III: Dissection of the aorta. Current diagnostic and therapeutic approaches. JAMA 242: 1530, 1979.
49. Hitter E, Ranquin R, Mortelmans L, Parizel G: Diagnosis of aortic dissection. Comparison of investigatory methods—case report. Angiology 38:859, 1987.
50. Ruberti U, Odero A, Arpesani A, et al: Acute aortic dissection. Personal experience, J Cardiovasc Surg (Torino) 29:70, 1988.
51. Lyons J, Gershlick A, Norell M, et al: Intravenous digital subtraction angiography in the diagnosis and management of acute aortic dissection. Eur Heart J 8:186, 1987.
52. Gustavsson CG, Gustafson A, Albrechtsson U, et al: Diagnosis and management of acute aortic dissection, clinical and radiological follow-up. Acta Med Scand 223:247, 1988.
53. Butman SM, Kumar KL, Froelicher V: Acquired atherosclerotic aortopulmonary fistula presenting as new-onset congestive heart failure. Am J Med 80:530, 1986.
54. Montejo-Baranda M, Perez M, DeAndres J, et al: High out-put congestive heart failure as first manifestation of Osler-Weber-Rendu disease. Angiology 35:568, 1984.
55. Varat MA, Adolph RJ, Fowler NO: Cardiovascular effects of anemia. Am Heart J 83:415, 1972.
56. Homans DC: Peripartum cardiomyopathy. N Engl J Med 312:1432, 1985.
57. Pereira VG, Masuda Z, Katz A, et al: Shoshin beriberi: report of two successfully treated patients with hemodynamic documentation. Am J Cardiol 53:1467, 1984.
58. Symons C: Thyroid heart disease (editorial). Br Heart J 41:257, 1979.
59. Feldman T, Borow KM, Sarne DH, et al: Myocardial mechanics in hyperthyroidism: importance of left ventricular loading conditions, heart rate and contractile state. J Am Coll Cardiol 7:967, 1986.
60. Rimon D, Lurie M, Storch S, et al: Cardiomyopathy and multiple myeloma. Complications of scleredema adultorum. Arch Intern Med 148:551, 1988.
61. Tatum VD, Light RW: Approach to the diagnosis of secondary pulmonary hypertension: the chest roentgenograma as a diagnostic tool. Heart Lung 15:352, 1986.
62. Janicki JS, Weber KT, Likoff MJ, Fishman AP: The pressure-flow response of the pulmonary circulation in patients with heart failure and pulmonary vascular disease. Circulation 72;1270, 1985.
63. Miyashiro A, Grosberg SJ, Wapnick S: Reversible pulmonary hypertension and cardiac failure with chronic recurrent pancreatitis. Chest 71:669, 1977.

Selected Readings

Bigger JT Jr: Why patients with congestive heart failure die: arrhythmias and sudden cardiac death. Circulation 75:IV28, 1987.

A high incidence of sudden cardiac death in patients with congestive heart failure is attributed to ventricular arrhythmias. This review focuses on the prevalence, prognostic implications, precipitating factors and current concepts of therapy for arrhythmias in congestive heart failure. Abnormalities that promote ventricular arrhythmias, including electrical, mechanical, humoral and electrolyte abnormalities, are discussed.

Cohn JN, Levine TB, Olivari MT, et al: Plasma norepinephrine as a guide to prognosis in patients with chronic congestive heart failure. N Engl J Med 311:819, 1984.
A study suggesting that the plasma norepinephrine concentration measured from a resting venous blood sample provides a guide to prognosis in patients with chronic congestive heart failure.

Dunnigan A, Staley NA, Smith SA, et al: Cardiac and skeletal muscle abnormalities in cardiomyopathy: comparison of patients with ventricular tachycardia or congestive heart failure. J Am Coll Cardiol 10:608, 1987.
Cardiac muscle and skeletal muscle biopsies from 22 patients with cardiomyopathy were compared. Data demonstrated abnormalities of both cardiac and skeletal muscle that were similar in patients with initial symptoms secondary to ventricular tachycardia or congestive heart failure. The authors suggest that these patients with cardiomyopathy may have a generalized myopathy.

Eriksson H, Svardsudd K, Caidahl K, et al: Early heart failure in the population. The study of men born in 1913. Acta Med Scand 223:197, 1988.
A multivariate analysis of characteristics possibly associated with congestive heart failure was performed among 644 men, all 67 years of age and randomly selected from the general population. Factors believed to correlate significantly with congestive heart failure in this population included smoking habits, hypertension, body weight, and serum insulin.

Factor SM, Sonnenblick EH: The pathogenesis of clinical and experimental congestive cardiomyopathies: recent concepts. Prog Cardiovasc Dis 27:395, 1985.
Concise review.

Forrester JS, Diamond G, Chatterjee K, et al: Medical therapy of acute myocardial infarction by application of hemodynamic subsets. Two parts. N Engl J Med 295:1356; 295:1404, 1976.
Classic discussion of hemodynamic monitoring. Well referenced.

Francis GS: Neurohumoral mechanisms involved in congestive heart failure. Am J Cardiol 55:15A, 1985.
Review of the roles of the sympathetic nervous system and the renin-angiotensin-aldosterone system.

Gross JS, Neufeld RR, Libow LS, et al: Autopsy study of the elderly institutionalized patient. Review of 234 autopsies. Arch Intern Med 148:173, 1988.
A study of clinical and autopsy records of 234 elderly patients who died during a 14-year period in a chronic care institution found that the most common causes of death in decreasing frequency were bronchopneumonia, congestive heart failure, metastatic carcinoma, pulmonary embolism, myocardial infarction, cerebrovascular accident, unknown cause, and a miscellaneous group. Highest diagnostic error rate was in the underdiagnosis of pulmonary embolism.

Lutz JE: A XII century description of congestive heart failure. Am J Cardiol 61:494, 1988.
Historical perspective.

Mancini DM, LeJemtel TH, Factor S, et al: Central and peripheral components of cardiac failure. Am J Med 80(2B):2, 1986.

Discussion of myocardial and congestive failure as processes resulting in chronic heart failure.

Marantz PR, Tobin JN, Wassertheil-Smoller S, et al: The relationship between left ventricular systolic function and congestive heart failure diagnosed by clinical criteria. Circulation 77:607, 1988.

Current concepts and clinical definitions of congestive heart failure with an emphasis on the relationship between left ventricular systolic function and congestive heart failure. Useful discussion.

McKee PA, Castelli WP, McNamara PM, et al: The natural history of congestive heart failure: the Framingham Study. N Engl J Med 285:1441, 1971.

A study of the natural history of congestive heart failure in a large population who were initially free of the disease.

Parrillo JE, Aretz HT, Palacios I, et al: The results of transvenous endomyocardial biopsy can frequently be used to diagnose myocardial diseases in patients with idiopathic heart failure. Endomyocardial biopsies in 100 consecutive patients revealed a substantial incidence of myocarditis. Circulation 69:93, 1984.

Authors review the results of transvenous endomyocardial biopsy in 74 patients with congestive heart failure of unknown etiology and in 26 patients with constrictive or restrictive cardiovascular characteristics. Useful pathologic diagnoses in patients with congestive heart failure included myocarditis, vasculitis, doxorubicin cardiomyopathy, and congestive cardiomyopathy. Useful pathologic diagnoses in patients with restrictive cardiomyopathy included radiation-induced cardiomyopathy, endomyocardial fibrosis, amyloidosis, or no myocardial disease.

Ruggie N: Congestive heart failure. Med Clin North Am 70:829, 1986.

A useful clinical review.

Schmaltz AA, Apitz J, Hort W: Dilated cardiomyopathy in childhood: problems of diagnosis and long-term follow-up. Eur Heart J 8:100, 1987.

Clinical profile and course of children aged 2 to 17 years with dilated cardiomyopathy, which excluded those with endocardial fibroelastosis and myocarditis by endomyocardial biopsy, found that the main complications were rhythm disturbances and thrombus formation. No definite predictors of survival were identified.

Srebro J, Karliner JS: Congestive heart failure. Curr Probl Cardiol 11:301, 1986.

Another useful clinical review.

Stone PH, Raabe DS, Jaffe AS, et al: Prognostic significance of location and type of myocardial infarction: independent adverse outcome associated with anterior location. J Am Coll Cardiol 11:453, 1988.

A study to determine the prognostic significance of location of myocardial infarction compared prognosis in anterior infarction with inferior infarction. Authors found that patients with anterior infarction demonstrated a lower left ventricular ejection fraction and a higher incidence of subsequent congestive heart failure than patients with inferior wall infarctions.

6
Cardiomegaly: A Differential Diagnosis

Cardiomegaly, or an enlarged heart, is a common radiographic finding during the initial evaluation of acute or chronic heart failure; occasionally cardiomegaly is an incidental finding, such as can occur with asymptomatic hypertrophic cardiomyopathy, or at autopsy, particularly after sudden death. The major etiologies of cardiomegaly overlap with the etiologies of heart failure, particularly when associated with cardiomyopathy. Major categories include intrinsic disorders of the myocardium, volume overload states, pressure overload states, and rare etiologies, such as pericardial disorders, aneurysms, and neoplasia. Pericardial cysts, pericardial fat pads, and mediastinal masses can mimic cardiomegaly.[1,2]

Intrinsic Disorders of the Myocardium

Congestive (dilated) cardiomyopathy[3-9]: multiple etiologies, such as infections, connective tissue diseases, nutritional deficiencies, disorders of metabolism, endocrinopathies, peritoneal dialysis,[10] toxins, hypersensitivity, postpartum,[11] genetic,[12] burns,[13] and neuromuscular diseases.[14] Also see Chapter 5: Congestive Heart Failure.

Ischemic cardiomyopathy: as a consequence of multiple myocardial infarctions

Restrictive cardiomyopathy: amyloidosis,[15,16] glycogen storage disease, scleredema adultorum,[17,18] sarcoidosis,[19] hemochromatosis[20]

Idiopathic[21,22]

Volume Overload States

Aortic valve regurgitation

Mitral valve regurgitation[23]

Tricuspid valve regurgitation: most often due to dilation of the right ventricle and tricuspid annulus as a consequence of right ventricular failure[24]

Congenital heart disease[25,26]: ventricular septal defect,[27] patent ductus arteriosus,[28] atrial septal defect

37

Athletic heart: reflects hemodynamic loading in endurance athletes[29]

Pressure Overload States

Hypertensive cardiomyopathy[30]

Aortic stenosis: left ventricular pressure overload[31]

Mitral stenosis[32]: right ventricular pressure overload is due to secondary pulmonary hypertension.

Tricuspid stenosis: right atrial enlargement leads to prominence of the right heart border on chest radiograph.

Pulmonic stenosis: significant cardiac enlargement is uncommon except in end-stage pulmonic stenosis in which the right ventricle and atrium are markedly dilated.

Hypertrophic cardiomyopathies[33]: common cause of sudden death in young athletes[34]

Coarctation

Acromegaly: presumably due to associated hypertension but many patients also have myocardial fibrosis, myocarditis, and small vessel atherosclerosis

Chronic renal failure[35]

Pericardial Disorders

Pericardial effusion[36,37]

Pericardial cysts[38]: usually congenital and occur at the cardiophrenic angle

Pericardial tumors[39]: primary, metastatic; also see Neoplastic Disorders, below

Pericardial fat from exogenous steroids

Hypothyroidism[40]

Constrictive pericarditis: equalization and elevation of intracardiac diastolic pressures. About two-thirds of patients have cardiomegaly.[41] Also see Chapter 8: Acute Pericarditis.

Aneurysmal Disorders

Ventricular aneurysms[42]: often postmyocardial infarction

Atrial aneurysms: rare congenital lesion

Mycotic aneurysms

Coronary artery aneurysms[43,44]

Neoplastic Disorders

Primary neoplastic disorders[45,46]

Myxomas[47,48]: heart failure and embolization are the most frequent presentations.

Sarcomas[49]

Lymphoma: primary cardiac lymphomas are very rare; however, they may be expected to increase in the acquired immune deficiency syndrome (AIDS) population.[50,51]

Rare cardiac neoplasms: lipomas, angiomas, fibromas, hamartomas, teratomas, rhabdomyomas,[52] pheochromocytomas,[53,54] histiocytomas,[55] mesotheliomas[56]

Secondary metastatic tumors[57–59]

Metastatic tumors: 16 times more common than primary cardiac tumors; lung,[60] breast, lymphoma,[61] and malignant melanoma[62] are the most common metastatic carcinomas

References

1. Maze SS, Robinson F, Stevens JE, Mervis B: A huge mediastinal abscess masquerading as cardiomegaly: the value of non-invasive investigations. Thorax 38:155, 1983.
2. Paling MR, Williamson BR: Epipericardial fat pad: CT findings. Radiology 165:335, 1987.
3. Johnson RA, Palacios I: Dilated cardiomyopathies of the adult. (Two parts.) N Engl J Med 307:1051; 307:1119, 1982.
4. Dec GW Jr, Palacios IF, Fallon JT, et al: Active myocarditis in the spectrum of acute dilated cardiomyopathies. N Engl J Med 312:885, 1985.
5. Fallon JT: Myocarditis and dilated cardiomyopathy: different stages of the same disease? Cardiovasc Clin 18:155, 1988.
6. Griffin ML, Hernandez A, Martin TC, et al: Dilated cardiomyopathy in infants and children. J Am Coll Cardiol 11:139, 1988.
7. Kopecky SL, Gersh BJ: Dilated cardiomyopathy and myocarditis: natural history, etiology, clinical manifestations, and management. Curr Probl Cardiol 12:569, 1987.
8. Ghali JK, Shanes JG: A review of dilated cardiomyopathy. Compr Ther 13:46, 1987.
9. Kawai C, Matsumori A, Fujiwara H: Myocarditis and dilated cardiomyopathy. Annu Rev Med 38:221, 1987.
10. Feldman AM, Fivush B, Zahka KG, et al: Congestive cardiomyopathy in patients on continuous ambulatory peritoneal dialysis. Am J Kidney Dis 11:76, 1988.
11. Adler AK, Davis MR: Peripartum cardiomyopathy: two case reports and a review. Obstet Gynecol Surv 41:675, 1986.
12. Vincenzo-Fragola P, Autore C, Picelli A, et al: Familial idiopathic dilated cardiomyopathy. Am Heart J 115:912, 1988.
13. Mukherjee GD, Basu PG, Roy S, Seal M: Cardiomegaly following extensive burns. Ann Plast Surg 19:378, 1987.
14. Hoshio A, Kotake H, Saitoh M, et al: Cardiac involve-

ment in a patient with limb-girdle muscular dystrophy. Heart Lung 16:439, 1987.

15. Eriksson P, Backman C, Eriksson A, et al: Differentiation of cardiac amyloidosis and hypertrophic cardiomyopathy. A comparison of familial amyloidosis and polyneuropathy and hypertrophic cardiomyopathy by electrocardiography and echocardiography. Acta Med Scand 221:39, 1987.

16. Benson MD, Wallace MR, Tejada E, et al: Hereditary amyloidosis: description of a new American kindred with late onset cardiomyopathy. Appalachian amyloid. Arthritis Rheum 30:195, 1987.

17. Olson LJ, Reeder GS, Noller KL, et al: Cardiac involvement in glycogen storage disease III: morphologic and biochemical characterization with endomyocardial biopsy. Am J Cardiol 53:980, 1984.

18. Rimon D, Lurie M, Storch S, et al: Cardiomyopathy and multiple myeloma. Complications of scleredema adultorum. Arch Intern Med 148:551, 1988.

19. Lemery R, McGoon MD, Edwards WD: Cardiac sarcoidosis: a potentially treatable form of myocarditis. Mayo Clin Proc 60:549, 1985.

20. Olson LJ, Baldus WP, Tajik AJ: Echocardiographic features of idiopathic hemochromatosis. Am J Cardiol 60:885, 1987.

21. Gillum RF: Idiopathic cardiomyopathy in the United States, 1970–82. Am Heart J 111:752, 1986.

22. Gravanis MB, Ansari AA: Idiopathic cardiomyopathies. A review of pathologic studies and mechanisms of pathogenesis. Arch Pathol Lab Med 111:915, 1987.

23. Bergeron GA: Minimally symptomatic patients with ruptured chordae tendineae due to myxomatous degeneration of the mitral valve. Am J Med 81:333, 1986.

24. Waller BF: Etiology of pure tricuspid regurgitation. Cardiovasc Clin 17:53, 1987.

25. Copel JA, Pilu G, Kleinman CS: Congenital heart disease and extracardiac anomalies: associations and indications for fetal echocardiography. Am J Obstet Gynecol 154:1121, 1986.

26. Kirk AJ, Pollock JC: Concomitant cor triatriatum and coronary sinus total anomalous pulmonary venous connection. Ann Thorac Surg 44:203, 1987.

27. Ellis JH IV, Moodie DS, Sterba R, Gill CC: Ventricular septal defect in the adult: natural and unnatural history. Am Heart J 114:115, 1987.

28. Page GG: Patent ductus arteriosus in the premature neonate. Heart Lung 14:156, 1985.

29. Hauser AM, Dressendorfer RH, Vos M, et al: Symmetric cardiac enlargement in highly trained endurance athletes: a two-dimensional echocardiographic study. Am Heart J 109:1038, 1985.

30. Topol EJ, Traill TA, Fortuin NJ: Hypertensive hypertrophic cardiomyopathy of the elderly. N Engl J Med 312:277, 1985.

31. Pelech AN, Dyck JD, Trusler GA, et al: Critical aortic stenosis. Survival and management. J Thorac Cardiovasc Surg 94:510, 1987.

32. Sullivan ID, Robinson PJ, de Leval M, et al: Membranous supravalvular mitral stenosis: a treatable form of congenital heart disease. J Am Coll Cardiol 8:159, 1986.

33. Leon MB, Cohen LS: Hypertrophic cardiomyopathy. DM 28:7, 1981.
34. Maron BJ, Epstein SE, Roberts WC: Causes of sudden death in competitive athletes. J Am Coll Cardiol 7:204, 1986.
35. Alexander J, Mehlman DJ, Talano JV: Cardiomegaly with chronic renal failure. Arch Intern Med 144:101, 1984.
36. McKenna RJ Jr, Ali MK, Ewer MS, et al: Pleural and pericardial effusions in cancer patients. Curr Probl Cancer 9:1, 1985.
37. Suzuki S, Tajimi T, Takeshita A, et al: Isolated right heart purulent pericarditis forming a large mediastinal mass. Chest 93:667, 1988.
38. Patel BK, Markivee CR, George EA: Pericardial cyst simulating intracardiac mass. AJR 141:292, 1983.
39. Millman A, Meller J, Motro M, et al: Pericardial tumor or fibrosis mimicking pericardial effusion by echocardiography. Ann Intern Med 86:434, 1977.
40. Shenoy MM, Goldman JM: Hypothyroid cardiomyopathy: echocardiographic documentation of reversibility. Am J Med Sci 294:1, 1987.
41. Puvaneswary M, Singham KT, Singh J: Constrictive pericarditis: clinical, hemodynamic and radiological correlation. Australas Radiol 26:53, 1982.
42. Hochman JS, Platia EB, Healy Bulkley B: Endocardial abnormalities in left ventricular aneurysms. Ann Intern Med 100:29, 1984.
43. Baker PB, Keyhani-Rofagha S, Graham RL, et al: Dissecting hematoma (aneurysm) of coronary arteries. Am J Med 80:317, 1986.
44. Adkins GF, Steele RH: Left coronary artery dissection: an unusual presentation. Br Heart J 55:411, 1986.
45. Bear PA, Moodie DS: Malignant primary cardiac tumors. The Cleveland Clinic experience, 1956 to 1986. Chest 92:860, 1987.
46. Reece IJ, Cooley DA, Frazier OH, et al: Cardiac tumors. Clinical spectrum and prognosis of lesions other than classical benign myxoma in 20 patients. J Thorac Cardiovasc Surg 88:439, 1984.
47. Semb BKH: Surgical considerations in the treatment of cardiac myxoma. J Thorac Cardiovasc Surg 87:251, 1984.
48. Smith C: Tumors of the heart. Arch Pathol Lab Med 110:371, 1986.
49. Janigan DT, Husain A, Robinson NA: Cardiac angiosarcomas. Cancer 57:852, 1986.
50. Constantino A, West TE, Gupta M, Loghmanee F: Primary cardiac lymphoma in a patient with acquired immune deficiency syndrome. Cancer 60:2801, 1987.
51. Cairns P, Butany J, Fulop J, et al: Cardiac presentation of non-Hodgkin's lymphoma. Arch Pathol Lab Med 111:80, 1987.
52. Fischer DR, Beerman LB, Park SC, et al: Diagnosis of intracardiac rhabdomyoma by two-dimensional echocardiography. Am J Cardiol 53:978, 1984.
53. Saad MF, Frazier OH, Hickey RC, et al: Intrapericardial pheochromocytoma. Am J Med 75:371, 1983.
54. Scott I, Parkes R, Cameron DP: Phaeochromocytoma and cardiomyopathy. Med J Aust 148:94, 1988.

55. Terashima K, Aoyama K, Nihei K, et al: Malignant fibrous histiocytoma of the heart. Cancer 52:1919, 1983.
56. Takeda K, Ohba H, Hyodo H, et al: Pericardial mesothelioma: hyaluronic acid in pericardial fluid. Am Heart J 110:486, 1985.
57. Lagrange JL, Despins P, Spielman M, et al: Cardiac metastases. Cancer 58:2333, 1986.
58. Skhvatsabaja LV: Secondary malignant lesions of the heart and pericardium in neoplastic disease. Oncology 43:103, 1986.
59. Johnson M, Soulen RL: Echocardiography of cardiac metastases. AJR 141:677, 1983.
60. Quraishi MA, Costanzi JJ, Hokanson J: The natural history of lung cancer with pericardial metastases. Cancer 51:740, 1983.
61. Chou ST, Arkles LB, Gill GD, et al: Primary lymphoma of the heart. Cancer 52:744, 1983.
62. Hanley PC, Shub C, Seward JB, et al: Intracavitary cardiac melanoma diagnosed by endomyocardial left ventricular biopsy. Chest 84:195, 1983.

Selected Readings

Amsterdam EA, Laslett L, Holly R: Exercise and sudden death. Cardiol Clin 5:337, 1987.

A study to define mechanisms of exercise-associated sudden death found that cardiovascular disease is present in most patients who die during exercise. In patients less than 35 years old, hypertrophic cardiomyopathy and congenital coronary anomalies are the most common conditions. In patients older than 35 years old, coronary artery disease or recognizable coronary risk factors are most common.

Kitzman DW, Scholz DG, Hagen PT, et al: Age-related changes in normal human hearts during the first 10 decades of life. Part II (Maturity): a quantitative anatomic study of 765 specimens from subjects 20 to 99 years old. Mayo Clin Proc 63:137, 1988.

Heart weights, ventricular wall thicknesses, and valve circumferences were measured in normal hearts of 765 autopsy specimens in persons aged 20 to 99 years. Body weight was the best predictor of heart weight. Ventricular septal thickness increased significantly between the third and tenth decade, with the mean ratio of septal-to-left ventricular free wall thicknesses exceeding 1.20, an important consideration in the evaluation of hypertrophic cardiomyopathy in elderly patients. Aortic valve circumference surpassed pulmonary valve circumference in the fourth decade and neared the size of the mitral valve by the tenth decade of life.

Kragel AH, Roberts WC: Sudden death and cardiomegaly unassociated with coronary, valvular, congenital or specific myocardial disease. Am J Cardiol 61:659, 1988.

Autopsy studies of eight patients who died suddenly disclosed cardiomegaly without a specific cause of death. In six of the eight patients, the most likely cause for cardiomegaly was systemic hypertension. None of these six patients had evidence of coronary artery narrowing or valvular, myocardial, congenital or pericardial heart disease. Authors present this report as the first reported series of patients with sudden death and systemic hypertension in the absence of significant narrowing of one or more epicardial coronary arteries.

Schoenfeld MH, Supple EW, Dec GW Jr, et al: Restrictive

cardiomyopathy versus constrictive pericarditis: role of endomyocardial biopsy in avoiding unnecessary thoracotomy.
Circulation 75:1012, 1987.

*The role of right ventricular endomyocardial biopsy was examined
in patients with evidence of constrictive/restrictive physiology in 54
patients. Specific sources of restrictive cardiomyopathy, such as amyloidosis and myocarditis, were identified in 14 (77%) patients avoiding a diagnostic thoracotomy, which would have been necessary to
rule out pericardial constriction in patients without specific pathologic findings.*

Shah PM, Abelmann WH, Gersh BJ: Cardiomyopathies
in the elderly. J Am Coll Cardiol, 10(Suppl A):77A, 1987.

*This review focuses on characteristic features of cardiomyopathy
in the elderly. A syndrome of clinical heart failure with reduced
diastolic compliance and preserved systolic function found more commonly in the elderly is discussed. Dilated and restrictive cardiomyopathies were not commonly found in the elderly.*

Wigle ED, Sasson Z, Henderson MA, et al: Hypertrophic
cardiomyopathy. The importance of site and the extent of
hypertrophy. A review. Prog Cardiovasc Dis 28:1, 1985.

*Clinical and pathophysiologic review of hypertrophic cardiomy-
opathy.*

7
Cardiac Arrhythmias: Cardiac and Noncardiac Causes

Arrhythmias are most commonly seen in the setting
of acute myocardial infarction[1] and congestive heart
failure.[2] However, it is not uncommon for an individual to have a life-threatening arrhythmia without
recognizable clinical heart disease.[3] Clinical arrhythmias are either bradyarrhythmias or tachyarrhythmias. Tachyarrhythmias may be supraventricular or
ventricular.[4] Cardiac arrhythmias result from abnormalities of impulse initiation, conduction, or a combination of these abnormalities.[5] Since any process
that leads to myocardial cellular hypoxia and/or dis-

ruption of normal tissue anatomy and biochemistry can cause cardiac arrhythmias, the possible causes of arrhythmias are myriad. Major etiologic categories include cardiac abnormalities, drugs, and electrolyte abnormalities.

Cardiac Abnormalities That Cause Arrhythmias

Myocardial infarction[6,7]: Both atrial and ventricular arrhythmias are common following an acute myocardial infarction.[8,9]

Congestive heart failure: sudden death often attributed to ventricular arrhythmias[10-13]

Atherosclerotic coronary artery disease[14-17]

Cardiomyopathy[18-20]: e.g., hypertrophic, dilated

Restrictive and infiltrative myocardial disease: amyloidosis[21]

Infectious endocarditis

Myocarditis

Pericarditis[22]

Cardiac aneurysm: ventricular[23] or atrial

Primary conduction system disorders: prolonged Q-T syndromes,[24-28] sinus node dysfunction,[29] preexcitation syndromes,[30] and other inherited conduction system disorders[31]

Variant angina pectoris[32]

Valvular disease: aortic stenosis,[33] mitral stenosis, mitral regurgitation,[34] mitral valve prolapse,[35-37] tricuspid prolapse[38]

Postcardiac surgery[39]

Cardiac trauma[40,41]

Neoplasms: cardiac metastases more common than primary tumors[42,43]

Congenital heart disease: e.g., septal defects, tetralogy of Fallot[44-47]

Iatrogenic: e.g., pacemaker-induced[48,49]

Common Drugs Associated With Arrhythmias

Cardioactive drugs[50]: digoxin,[51-53] procainamide,[54] quinidine,[55] verapamil,[56] and others; virtually all antiarrhythmic drugs can induce or worsen arrhythmias[57-59]

Psychotropic drugs: lithium, antidepressants,[60-62] phenothiazines, Ecstasy (3,4-methylenedioxy-methamphetamine)[63]

Caffeine[64]

Nicotine[65,66]

Alcohol[67-70]

Chemotherapeutic agents: doxorubicin[71,72]

Anticonvulsants: carbamazepine,[73] dilantin

Aminophylline[74–77]

Anesthetics[78,79]: ketamine,[80] nitrous oxide[81]

Sulphonylurea drugs[82]

Diuretics: thiazide diuretics deplete potassium and magnesium, which can result in cardiac arrhythmias.[83]

Sympathomimetics: e.g., see list under Drugs that Can Cause Hypertension in Chapter 94, Hypertension: Renovascular and Other Secondary Causes in Section IX, Renal and Electrolyte Consultations.

Other Precipitating Factors of Arrhythmias

Electrolyte abnormalities[84,85]: hyperkalemia,[86] hypokalemia, hypocalcemia, hypomagnesemia,[87] and hypermagnesemia

pH abnormalities: acidosis or alkalosis

Hypoxemia

Hypercarbia

Hypotension: particularly a sudden acute drop of blood pressure

Infection

Pulmonary disease: pneumonia, chronic obstructive disease,[88] asthma[89]

Pulmonary embolism

Gastrointestinal disease: pancreatitis, gall bladder disease

Anemia

Weight loss[90,91]: arrhythmias that have been associated with low quality protein diet supplements can be prevented with use of high-quality protein, vigorous mineral supplementation, and potassium supplementation.

Malnutrition: a common occurrence in hospitalized patients; nutritional supplementation may have significant cardiac implications[92]

Hemodialysis[93–95]

Pregnancy[96]

Athletic heart syndrome[97,98]

Endocrine dysfunction[99]: thyrotoxicosis,[100] pheochromocytoma, myxedema

Neurogenic causes: subarachnoid hemorrhage,[101] stroke,[102] dysautonomic syndromes, carotid sinus hypersensitivity, seizures[103]

Spinal cord injury: acute cervical spinal cord injury is associated with acute autonomic imbalance and arrhythmias.[104]

Sleep apnea[105]

Arrhythmias occurring in normal individuals[106]

Marfan syndrome[107]
Electrocution[108]
Acute elevation of blood pressure[109]
Stress[110,111]

References

1. Lazzara R, Scherlag BJ: Generation of arrhythmias in myocardial ischemia and infarction. Am J Cardiol 61:20A, 1988.
2. Francis GS: Development of arrhythmias in the patient with congestive heart failure: pathophysiology, prevalence and prognosis. Am J Cardiol 57:3B, 1986.
3. Hosenpud JD, McAnulty JH, Niles NR: Unexpected myocardial disease in patients with life threatening arrhythmias. Br Heart J 56:55, 1986.
4. Schmidt PJ, Ezri MD, Denes P: Cardiac arrhythmias—update 1987. Dis Mon 33:365, 1987.
5. Rosen MR: Mechanisms for arrhythmias. Am J Cardiol 61:2A, 1988.
6. Bigger JT Jr: Relation between left ventricular dysfunction and ventricular arrhythmias after myocardial infarction. Am J Cardiol 57:8B, 1986.
7. Bolli R, Fisher DJ, Entman ML: Factors that determine the occurrence of arrhythmias during acute myocardial ischemia. Am Heart J 111:261, 1986.
8. Salerno JA, Klersy C, Vigano M, et al: Ventricular tachycardia in post-myocardial infarction patients. Preoperative and intraoperative mapping. Eur Heart J, 7(Suppl A):157, 1986.
9. Gottlieb SH, Ouyang P, Gottlieb SO: Death after acute myocardial infarction: interrelation between left ventricular dysfunction, arrhythmias, and ischemia. Am J Cardiol 61:7B, 1988.
10. Deedwania PC: Significance of arrhythmias in congestive heart failure. Postgrad Med 83(4):223, 1988.
11. Bigger JT Jr: Why patients with congestive heart failure die: arrhythmias and sudden cardiac death. Circulation 75:IV28, 1987.
12. Pitt B: Evaluation of the patient with congestive heart failure and ventricular arrhythmias. Am J Cardiol 57:19B, 1986.
13. Parmley WW, Chatterjee K: Congestive heart failure and arrhythmias: an overview. Am J Cardiol 57:34B, 1986.
14. Blevins RD, Kerin NZ, Frumin H, et al: Arrhythmia control and other factors related to sudden death in coronary disease patients at intermediate risk. Am Heart J 111:638, 1986.
15. Lazzara R, Scherlag BJ: Electrophysiologic basis for arrhythmias in ischemic heart disease. Am J Cardiol 53:1B, 1984.
16. Carboni GP, Lahiri A, Cashman PM, Raftery EB: Mechanisms of arrhythmias accompanying ST-segment depression on ambulatory monitoring in stable angina pectoris. Am J Cardiol 60:1246, 1987.
17. Blevins RD, Kerin NZ, Frumin H, et al: Arrhythmia control and other factors related to sudden death in

coronary disease patients at intermediate risk. Am Heart J 111:638, 1986.

18. McKenna WJ, Krikler DM, Goodwin JF: Arrhythmias in dilated and hypertrophic cardiomyopathy. Med Clin North Am 68:983, 1984.
19. Holmes J, Kubo SH, Cody RJ, et al: Arrhythmias in ischemic and nonischemic dilated cardiomyopathy: prediction of mortality by ambulatory electrocardiography. Am J Cardiol 55:146, 1985.
20. Neri R, Mestroni L, Salvi A, Camerini F: Arrhythmias in dilated cardiomyopathy. Postgrad Med J 62:593, 1986.
21. Smith TJ, Kyle RA, Lie JT: Clinical significance of histopathologic patterns of cardiac amyloidosis. Mayo Clin Proc 59:547, 1984.
22. Spodick DH: Frequency of arrhythmias in acute pericarditis determined by Holter monitoring. Am J Cardiol 53:842, 1984.
23. Hochman JS, Platia EB, Healy Bulkley B: Endocardial abnormalities in left ventricular aneurysms. Ann Intern Med 100:29, 1984.
24. Schwartz PJ: The idiopathic long Q-T syndrome (editorial). Ann Intern Med 99:561, 1983.
25. Schwartz PJ: Idiopathic long QT syndrome: progress and questions. Am Heart J 109:399, 1985.
26. Moss AJ, Schwartz PJ, Crampton RS, et al: The long QT syndrome: a prospective international study. Circulation 71:17, 1985.
27. Surawicz B: The QT interval and cardiac arrhythmias. Annu Rev Med 38:81, 1987.
28. Kossmann CE: The long Q-T interval and syndromes. Adv Intern Med 32:87, 1987.
29. Alpert MA, Flaker GC: Arrhythmias associated with sinus node dysfunction. JAMA 250:2160, 1983.
30. Prystowsky EN, Miles WM, Heger JJ, et al: Preexcitation syndromes. Med Clin North Am 68:831, 1984.
31. Guntheroth WG, Motulsky AG: Inherited primary disorders of cardiac rhythm and conduction. Prog Med Genet 5:381, 1983.
32. Kerin NZ, Rubenfire M, Willens HJ, et al: The mechanism of dysrhythmias in variant angina pectoris: occlusive versus reperfusion. Am Heart J 106:1332, 1983.
33. Kostis JB, Tupper B, Moreyra AE, et al: Aortic valve replacement in patients with aortic stenosis. Effect on cardiac arrhythmias. Chest 85:211, 1984.
34. Kligfield P, Hochreiter C, Kramer H, et al: Complex arrhythmias in mitral regurgitation with and without mitral valve prolapse: contrast to arrhythmias in mitral valve prolapse without mitral regurgitation. Am J Cardiol 55:1545, 1985.
35. Pratt CM, Young JB, Wierman AM, et al: Complex ventricular arrhythmias associated with the mitral valve prolapse syndrome. Am J Med 80:626, 1986.
36. Ware JA, Magro SA, Luck JC, et al: Conduction system abnormalities in symptomatic mitral valve prolapse: an electrophysiologic analysis of 60 patients. Am J Cardiol 53:1075, 1984.
37. Kligfield P, Levy D, Devereux RB, Savage DD: Ar-

rhythmias and sudden death in mitral valve prolapse. Am Heart H 113:1298, 1987.

38. Raichlen JS, Brest AN: Tricuspid valve prolapse. Cardiovasc Clin 17:97, 1987.

39. Waldo AL, Henthorn RW, Epstein AE, et al: Diagnosis and treatment of arrhythmias during and following open heart surgery. Med Clin North Am 68:1153, 1984.

40. Cheitlin MD, Abbott JA: The internist's role in the recognition and management of cardiovascular trauma. Med Clin North Am 63:201, 1979.

41. Beresky R, Klingler R, Peake J: Myocardial contusion: when does it have clinical significance? J Trauma 28:64, 1988.

42. Burday MJ, Lombardi AC: Cardiac tumors. Am Fam Physician 37(2):301, 1988.

43. Leung CY, Cummings RG, Reimer KA, Lowe JE: Chondrosarcoma metastatic to the heart. Ann Thorac Surg 45:291, 1988.

44. Daliento L, Corrado D, Buja G, et al: Rhythm and conduction disturbances in isolated, congenitally corrected transposition of the great arteries. Am J Cardiol 58:314, 1986.

45. Deanfield J, McKenna W, Rowland E: Local abnormalities of right ventricular depolarization after repair of tetralogy of Fallot: a basis for ventricular arrhythmia. Am J Cardiol 55:522, 1985.

46. Musewe NN, Smallhorn JF, Moes CA, et al: Echocardiographic evaluation of obstructive mechanism of tetralogy of Fallot with restrictive ventricular septal defect. Am J Cardiol 61:664, 1988.

47. Flanagan MF, Foran RB, Van Praagh R, et al: Tetralogy of Fallot with obstruction of the ventricular septal defect: spectrum of echocardiographic findings. J Am Coll Cardiol 11:386, 1988.

48. Phibbs B, Mariott HJ: Complications of permanent transvenous pacing. N Engl J Med 312:1428, 1985.

49. Kowey PR, Friehling TD, Kline RA, Engel TR: Pacing-induced angina pectoris and induction of ventricular arrhythmias in coronary artery disease. Am J Cardiol 58:90, 1986.

50. Taliercio CP, Olney BA, Lie JT: Myocarditis related to drug hypersensitivity. Mayo Clin Proc 60:463, 1985.

51. Smith TW, Antman EM, Friedman PL, et al: Digitalis glycosides: mechanisms and manifestations of toxicity. Prog Cardiovasc Dis 27:21, 1984.

52. Minson RB, McRitchie RJ: Digoxin in the 1980s. Med J Aust 147:403, 410, 1987.

53. Fisch C, Knoebel SB: Digitalis cardiotoxicity. J Am Coll Cardiol 5(Suppl A):91A, 1985.

54. Strasberg B, Sclarovsky S, Erdberg A, et al: Procainamide-induced polymorphous ventricular tachycardia. Am J Cardiol 47:1309, 1981.

55. Koenig W, Schinz AM: Spontaneous ventricular flutter and fibrillation during quinidine medication. Am Heart J 105:863, 1983.

56. Schwartz JB, Jeang M, Raizner AE, et al: Accelerated junctional rhythms during oral verapamil therapy. Am Heart J 107:440, 1984.

57. Smith WM, Gallagher JJ: "Les torsades de pointes": an unusual ventricular arrhythmia. Ann Intern Med 93:578, 1980.
58. Torres V, Flowers D, Somberg JC: The arrhythmogenicity of antiarrhythmic agents. Am Heart J 109: 1090, 1985.
59. Woosley RL, Roden DM: Pharmacologic causes of arrhythmogenic actions of antiarrhythmic drugs. Am J Cardiol 59:19E, 1987.
60. Boehnert MT, Lovejoy FJ Jr: Value of the QRS duration versus the serum drug level in predicting seizures and ventricular arrhythmias after an acute overdose of tricyclic antidepressants. N Engl J Med 313:474, 1985.
61. Herrmann HC, Kaplan LM, Bierer BE: Q-T prolongation and torsades de pointes ventricular tachycardia produced by the tetracyclic antidepressant agent maprotiline. Am J Cardiol 51:904, 1983.
62. Pellinen TJ, Farkkila M, Heikkila J, Luomanmaki K: Electrocardiographic and clinical features of tricyclic antidepressant intoxication. A survey of 88 cases and outlines of therapy. Ann Clin Res 19:12, 1987.
63. Dowling GP, McDonough ET III, Bost RO: "Eve" and "Ecstasy." A report of five deaths associated with the use of MDEA and MDMA. JAMA 257:1615, 1987.
64. Sutherland DJ, McPherson DD, Renton KW, et al: The effect of caffeine on cardiac rate, rhythm, and ventricular repolarization. Chest 87:319, 1985.
65. Davis MJE, Hockings BEF, El Dessouky MAM, et al: Cigarette smoking and ventricular arrhythmia in coronary heart disease. Am J Cardiol 54:282, 1984.
66. Benowitz NL, Jones RT, Jacob P III: Additive cardiovascular effects of nicotine and ethanol. Clin Pharmacol Ther 40:420, 1986.
67. Engel TR, Luck JC: Effect of whiskey on atrial vulnerability and "holiday heart." J Am Coll Cardiol 1:816, 1983.
68. Gribaldo RS, Pomini GS, Sale F, et al: Arrhythmias and left ventricular function in chronic alcoholics with alcoholic cirrhosis. Am J Cardiol 56:825, 1985.
69. McCall D: Alcohol and the cardiovascular system. Curr Probl Cardiol 12:1, 1987.
70. Criqui MH: The roles of alcohol in the epidemiology of cardiovascular diseases. Acta Med Scand 717 (Suppl):73, 1987.
71. Friess GG, Boyd JF, Geer MR, Garcia JC: Effects of first-dose doxorubicin on cardiac rhythm as evaluated by continuous 24-hour monitoring. Cancer 56:2762, 1985.
72. Raina A, Ferrante F, Bisol A, et al: Cardiotoxicity during chemotherapy for advanced gastroenteric tumors. Tumori 73:359, 1987.
73. Boesen F, Andersen EB, Jensen EK, et al: Cardiac conduction disturbances during carbamazepine therapy. Acta Neurol Scand 68:49, 1983.
74. Dutt AK, de Soyza ND, Au WY, et al: The effect of aminophylline on cardiac rhythm in advanced chronic obstructive pulmonary disease: correlation with serum theophylline levels. Eur J Respir Dis 64:264, 1983.

75. Patel AK, Skatrud JB, Thomsen JH: Cardiac arrhythmia due to oral aminophylline in patients with chronic obstructive pulmonary disease. Chest 80:661, 1981.
76. Bigi R, Camerone G, Corradetti C, et al: Effect of combined use of intravenous salbutamol and aminophylline on cardiac rhythm in chronic obstructive lung disease. Respiration 51:119, 1987.
77. Eiriksson CE Jr, Writer SL, Vestal RE: Theophylline-induced alterations in cardiac electrophysiology in patients with chronic obstructive pulmonary disease. Am Rev Respir Dis 135:322, 1987.
78. Greenan J: Cardiac dysrhythmias and heart rate changes at induction of anaesthesia: a comparison of two intravenous anticholinergics. Acta Anaesthesiol Scand 28:182, 1984.
79. Atlee JL III: Anaesthesia and cardiac electrophysiology. Eur J Anaesthesiol 2:215, 1985.
80. Faithfull NS, Poelman C, Dhasmana KM, Erdmann W: Ketamine-induced dysrhythmia and its antagonism: a case report. Eur J Anaesthesiol 4:287, 1987.
81. Roizen MF, Plummer GO, Lichtor JL: Nitrous oxide and dysrhythmias. Anesthesiology 66:427, 1987.
82. Huupponen R: Adverse cardiovascular effects of sulphonylurea drugs. Clinical significance. Med Toxicol 2:190, 1987.
83. Caralis PV, Perez-Stable E: Electrolyte abnormalities and ventricular arrhythmias. Drugs 31(Suppl 4):85, 1986.
84. Nordrehaug JE: Malignant arrhythmia in relation to serum potassium in acute myocardial infarction. Am J Cardiol 56:20D, 1985.
85. Packer M, Gottlieb SS, Kessler PD: Hormone-electrolyte interactions in the pathogenesis of lethal cardiac arrhythmias in patients with congestive heart failure. Am J Med 80(4A):23, 1986.
86. Vellodi A, Bini RM: Malignant ventricular arrhythmias caused by hyperkalaemia complicating the Kasabach-Merritt syndrome. J R Soc Med 81:167, 1988.
87. Berkelhammer C, Bear RA: A clinical approach to common electrolyte problems: 4. Hypomagnesemia. Can Med Assoc J 132:360, 1985.
88. Conradson TB, Eklundh G, Olofsson B, et al: Cardiac arrhythmias in patients with mild-to-moderate obstructive lung disease. Chest 88:537, 1985.
89. Emerman CL, Crafford WA, Vrobel TR: Ventricular arrhythmias during treatment for acute asthma. Ann Emerg Med 15:699, 1986.
90. Van Itallie TB, Yang MU: Cardiac dysfunction in obese dieters: a potentially lethal complication of rapid, massive weight loss. Am J Clin Nutr 39:695, 1984.
91. Amatruda JM, Biddle TL, Patton ML, et al: Vigorous supplementation of a hypocaloric diet prevents cardiac arrhythmias and mineral depletion. Am J Med 74:1016, 1983.
92. Webb JG, Kiess MC, Chan-Yan CC: Malnutrition and the heart. Can Med Assoc J 135:753, 1986.
93. Weber H, Schwarzer C, Stummvoll HK, et al: Chronic hemodialysis: high risk patients for arrhythmias? Nephron 37:180, 1984.

94. Forsstrom J, Forsstrom J, Heinonen E, et al: Effects of haemodialysis on heart rate variability in chronic renal failure. Scand J Clin Lab Invest 46:665, 1986.
95. Wizemann V, Kramer W, Funke T, Schutterle G: Dialysis-induced cardiac arrhythmias: fact or fiction? Importance of preexisting cardiac disease in the induction of arrhythmias during renal replacement therapy. Nephron 39:356, 1985.
96. Rotmensch HH, Rotmensch S, Elkayam U: Management of cardiac arrhythmias during pregnancy. Current concepts. Drugs 33:623, 1987.
97. Coelho A, Palileo E, Ashley W, et al: Tachyarrhythmias in young athletes. J Am Coll Cardiol 7:237, 1986.
98. Caru B, Mauri L, Andreuzzi B, et al: Arrhythmias in sport. Eur Heart J 8(Suppl D):47, 1987.
99. Surawicz B, Mangiardi ML: Electrocardiogram in endocrine and metabolic disorders. Cardiovasc Clin 8:243, 1977.
100. Forfar JC, Miller HC, Toft AD: Occult thyrotoxicosis: a correctable cause of "idiopathic" atrial fibrillation. Am J Cardiol 44:9, 1979.
101. Andreoli A, di Pasquale G, Pinelli G, et al: Subarachnoid hemorrhage: frequency and severity of cardiac arrhythmias. A survey of 70 cases studied in the acute phase. Stroke 18:558, 1987.
102. Taylor IC, Stout RW: Are cardiac arrhythmias important in stroke? Age Ageing 12:217, 1983.
103. Gilchrist JM: Arrhythmogenic seizures: diagnosis by simultaneous EEG/ECG recording. Neurology 35:1503, 1985.
104. Lehmann KG, Lane JG, Piepmeier JM, Batsford WP: Cardiovascular abnormalities accompanying acute spinal cord injury in humans: incidence, time course, and severity. J Am Coll Cardiol 10:46, 1987.
105. Guilleminault C, Connolly ST, Winkle RA: Cardiac arrhythmia and conduction disturbance during sleep in 400 patients with sleep apnea syndrome. Am J Cardiol 52:490, 1983.
106. Barrett PA, Peter CT, Swan HJ, et al: The frequency and prognostic significance of electrocardiographic abnormalities in clinically normal individuals. Prog Cardiovasc Dis 23:299, 1981.
107. Chen S, Fagan LF, Nouri S, et al: Ventricular dysrhythmias in children with Marfan's syndrome. Am J Dis Child 139:273, 1985.
108. Housinger TA, Green L, Shahangian S, et al: A prospective study of myocardial damage in electrical injuries. J Trauma 25:122, 1985.
109. Sideris DA, Kontoyannis DA, Michalis L, et al: Acute changes in blood pressure as a cause of cardiac arrhythmias. Eur Heart J 8:45, 1987.
110. Dimsdale JE, Ruberman W, Carleton RA, et al: Sudden cardiac death. Stress and cardiac arrhythmias. Circulation 76:I198, 1987.
111. Cinciripini PM: Cognitive stress and cardiovascular reactivity. II. Relationship to atherosclerosis, arrhythmias, and cognitive control. Am Heart J 112:1051, 1986.

Selected Readings

Akhtar M, Tchou PJ, Jazayeri M: Mechanisms of clinical tachycardias. Am J Cardiol 61:9A, 1988.
Current concepts of the pathophysiology of cardiac arrhythmias. Normal and abnormal mechanisms are reviewed.

Commerford PJ, Lloyd EA: Arrhythmias in patients with drug toxicity, electrolyte, and endocrine disturbances. Med Clin North Am 68:1051, 1984.
A well-referenced review of common drug-, electrolyte-, and endocrine-related disturbances. The common rhythm disturbances related to electrolyte imbalance are due predominantly to potassium abnormalities.

Coumel P, Leclercq HF, Leenhardt A: Arrhythmias as predictors of sudden death. Am Heart J 114:929, 1987.
An important review of methods of evaluating arrhythmias and identifying arrhythmias that indicate risk for sudden death. Authors stress the role of intervention in provoking lethal events, particularly the arrhythmogenic effect of powerful antiarrhythmic drugs. Ischemia in coronary patients was found to provoke cardiac arrest or an electromechanical dissociation more often than a ventricular tachycardia or fibrillation.

Hammill SC, Sugrue DD, Gersh BJ, et al: Clinical intracardiac electrophysiologic testing: technique, diagnostic indications, and therapeutic uses. Mayo Clin Proc 61:478, 1986.
A review discussing methods of electrophysiologic testing and their clinical applications.

Hinkle LE Jr, Thaler HT, Merke DP, et al: The risk factors for arrhythmic death in a sample of men followed for 20 years. Am J Epidemiol 127:500, 1988.
Risk factors for arrhythmic death were determined in a group of 301 men, aged 54 to 62 years, who were followed prospectively from 1963 to 1984. Sixty-five of 148 deaths were manifested by abrupt fatal ventricular arrhythmias. Multivariate analysis of factors at initial examination found the following significantly related to arrhythmic death: abnormal patterns of QRS conduction, level of blood pressure, number of cigarettes currently smoked, chronic myocardial ischemia, chronic airway disease, and failure to exercise.

Holmes J, Kubo SH, Cody RJ, et al: Arrhythmias in ischemic and nonischemic dilated cardiomyopathy: prediction of mortality by ambulatory electrocardiography. Am J Cardiol 55:146, 1985.
Study suggesting that complex ventricular arrhythmias represent an independent mortality risk factor in patients with severe dilated cardiomyopathy.

Horowitz LN, Kay HR, Kutalek SP, et al: Risks and complications of clinical cardiac electrophysiologic studies: a prospective analysis of 1,000 consecutive patients. J Am Coll Cardiol 9:1261, 1987.
Complications of clinical cardiac electrophysiologic studies were prospectively evaluated in 1,000 consecutive patients studied in 1 laboratory. Complications included one death, arterial injury, thrombophlebitis, systemic arterial embolism, pulmonary embolus, cardiac perforation, catheter-induced permanent complete atrioventricular (AV) block, atrial fibrillation, and severe proarrhythmic events. Authors conclude that, despite complications, risks are small and acceptable.

Kennedy HL, Whitlock JA, Sprague MK, et al: Long-term follow-up of asymptomatic healthy subjects with frequent and complex ventricular ectopy. N Engl J Med 312:193, 1985.
Study concluding that asymptomatic healthy subjects with frequent and complex ventricular ectopy have the same prognosis as that of the healthy U.S. population.

Lampert S, Lown B, Graboys TB, et al: Determinants of survival in patients with malignant ventricular arrhythmia associated with coronary artery disease. Am J Cardiol 67:791, 1988.
Long-term survival data in patients with coronary artery disease and a history of malignant ventricular arrhythmia derived from a 9-year follow-up of a group of 161 patients.

Levy D, Anderson KM, Savage DD, et al: Risk of ventricular arrhythmias in left ventricular hypertrophy: the Framingham Heart Study. Am J Cardiol 60:560, 1987.
The association of ventricular arrhythmias with left ventricular hypertrophy was examined in 6,218 participants in the Framingham Heart Study. ECG and echocardiographic criteria for left ventricular hypertrophy were compared. After adjustment for age, sex, systolic blood pressure, valvular heart disease, angina pectoris, and acute myocardial infarction, the association of echocardiographic, but not ECG left ventricular hypertrophy with ventricular arrhythmia, remained significant.

Marinchek RA, Friehling TD, Kowey PR: Diagnosis and treatment of cardiac rhythm disorders in the elderly. Clin Geriatr Med 4:83, 1988.
A review of arrhythmias in the elderly with a focus on practical issues such as diagnostic devices, treatment modalities, and decision-making, including a helpful review of normal variations in the elderly.

Morganroth J: Ambulatory Holter electrocardiography: choice of technologies and clinical uses. Ann Intern Med 102:73, 1985.
Review of the origin of the Holter monitor, its clinical role, and the importance of proper analysis technique.

Morganroth J: Noninvasive testing for ventricular arrhythmias. Postgrad Med 83(4):241, 1988.
A review of noninvasive testing techniques for classification and evaluation for ventricular arrhythmias. Indications for continuous Holter monitoring, exercise testing, and quantitative Holter monitoring are discussed.

Pannizzo F, Mercando AD, Fisher JD, Furman S: Automatic methods for detection of tachyarrhythmias by antitachycardia devices. J Am Coll Cardiol 11:308, 1988.
A review of current techniques and those under investigation for the detection of tachyarrhythmias.

Parmley WW, Chatterjee K: Congestive heart failure and arrhythmias: an overview. Am J Cardiol 57:34B, 1986.
Arrhythmias are common in patients with congestive heart failure, particularly in patients with ischemic heart disease. The degree of left ventricular dysfunction and complexity of present arrhythmias are significantly related to survival.

Samuels MA: Neurogenic heart disease: a unifying hypothesis. Am J Cardiol 60:15J, 1987.
Interesting discussion of electrocardiographic and cardiac abnormalities that occur with neurologic disease. It was previously

thought that neurologic disease caused electrophysiologic alterations without real heart disease. Current evidence of cardiac enzyme release and autopsy findings of myofibrillar degeneration suggest a strong neurogenic influence over cardiac function. Authors propose a unifying hypothesis bringing together clinical, physiologic, biochemical, and pathologic findings in neurogenic heart disease.

Slater W, Lampert S, Podrid PJ, Lown B: Clinical predictors of arrhythmia worsening by antiarrhythmic drugs. Am J Cardiol 61:349, 1988.

A retrospective clinical study of patients treated with antiarrhythmic agents. The study attempted to identify useful parameters that would predict aggravation of arrhythmia. Authors compared hemodynamic, pharmacologic, and electrophysiologic parameters and concluded that only the presenting arrhythmia and a left ventricular ejection fraction less that 35% identified patients at risk for drug-induced aggravation of arrhythmia.

Surawicz B: Noninvasive assessment of ventricular arrhythmias in clinical practice: prognostic implications. Can J Cardiol 2:285, 1986.

Useful review of indications for studying arrhythmias with an emphasis on prognostic implications of arrhythmias. Limitations of clinical decision-making and certain classifications of ventricular arrhythmias are discussed.

Syverud S: Cardiac pacing. Emerg Med Clin North Am 6:197, 1988.

Updated review of current pacemaker technology. Transcutaneous pacemakers now allow rapid institution of cardiac pacing in the emergency department or the prehospital setting.

Zipes DP (ed): Symposium on cardiac arrhythmias I. Med Clin North Am 68:793, 1984.

Monograph on cardiac arrhythmias.

8

Acute Pericarditis: Common and Less Common Causes

Acute inflammatory pericarditis is most often idiopathic or occurs in the setting of acute myocardial infarction. Pleuritic chest pain, dyspnea, pericardial friction rub, and ST-segment elevation on the ECG are common presenting symptoms and signs. There are a number of less common causes of pericarditis, which include infection, neoplasia, rheumatologic disorders, immune disorders, drugs, toxins, and iatrogenic complications. The clinical course varies with the underlying cause of pericarditis, ranging from a subclinical entity to potential life-threatening cardiac tamponade. Although any cause of pericarditis can lead to cardiac tamponade, malignant pericardial effusions probably are the most common cause of cardiac tamponade.[1,2]

Idiopathic: idiopathic benign pericarditis is the most common form of acute pericarditis.

Acute myocardial infarction: pericarditis occurs more frequently following anterior wall myocardial infarction.[3]

Late complication of myocardial infarction: rare[4]

Post-myocardial infarction pericarditis[5] (Dressler syndrome): fever, chest pain, pericarditis, pleurisy, pneumonitis with a tendency for symptoms to recur[6]

Postsurgical: cardiotomy or thoracotomy[7-9]

Radiation[10,11]: commonly seen after higher dose radiation therapy for Hodgkin's disease[12-14]

Uremia[15]

Chest trauma[16]

Dissecting aortic aneurysm: leaking into pericardial sac

Infectious

    Endocarditis[17]

    Bacterial[18]: staphylococcus,[19,20] *Haemophilus influenzae*,[21-23] meningococcus,[24,25] gonococcus, streptococcus, pneumococcus,[26] peptococcus,[27] legionella[28]

    Viral: infectious mononucleosis,[29] Coxsackie,[30] mumps, cytomegalovirus

    Rheumatic fever

    Parasitic: amebiasis,[31] toxoplasmosis, cryptococcus, histoplasmosis, echinococcus, dracunculosis

    Fungal: candida[32,33]

    Tuberculosis[34-36]: may occur with increased frequency in acquired immune deficiency syndrome[37,38]

Neoplastic[39-42]: see Chapter 6, p. 38.

    Primary pericardial neoplasm: rare

    Secondary pericardial neoplasm: most commonly from lung and breast carcinoma, lymphoma, leukemia[43]

Drugs and toxins: anticoagulants, daunorubicin, minoxidil,[44] dantrolene,[45] ibuprofen,[46] cytarabine,[47] silicone,[48] penicillin, phenytoin, hydralazine, procainamide, isoniazid, methysergide, cyclosporine[49]

Connective tissue disorders: rheumatoid arthritis,[50–53] systemic lupus erythematosus,[54,55] Still's disease,[56,57] mixed connective tissue disease,[58,59] periarteritis nodosa, giant cell arteritis, scleroderma[60]

Chronic renal disease and hemodialysis.

Inflammatory bowel disease[61]: ulcerative colitis[62–64]

Sarcoidosis[65,66]

Hypothyroidism: may be associated with cholesterol pericarditis[67]

Pancreatitis[68,69]

Familial Mediterranean fever

Pregnancy[70]

Postinstrumentation[71,72]

References

1. Sternbach GL: Pericarditis. Ann Emerg Med 17:214, 1988.
2. Krikorian JG, Hancock EW: Pericardiocentesis. Am J Med 65:808, 1978.
3. Galve E, Garcia-Del Castillo H, Evangalista A, et al: Pericardial effusion in the course of myocardial infarction: incidence, natural history, and clinical relevance. Circulation 73:294, 1986.
4. Ramsdale DR, Epstein EJ, Coulshed N: Constrictive pericarditis after myocardial infarction. Br Heart J 56:476, 1986.
5. Lichstein E: The changing spectrum of post-myocardial infarction pericarditis. Int J Cardiol 4:234, 1983.
6. Northcote RJ, Hutchison SJ, McGuinness JB: Evidence for the continued existence of the postmyocardial infarction (Dressler's) syndrome. Am J Cardiol 53:1201, 1984.
7. Kleiman NS, Verani MS, George S, et al: Right-to-left intracardiac shunt and constrictive pericarditis following coronary artery bypass surgery. Am Heart J 114:431, 1987.
8. Miedzinski LJ, Keren G: Serious infectious complications of open-heart surgery. Can J Surg 30:103, 1987.
9. Fyke FE III, Tancredi RG, Shub C, et al: Detection of intrapericardial hematoma after open heart surgery: the role of echocardiography and computed tomography. J Am Coll Cardiol 5:1496, 1985.
10. Gutierrez CA, Just-Viera JO: Clinical spectrum of radiation induced pericarditis. Am Surg 47:113, 1983.
11. Martin RG, Ruckdeschel JC, Chang P, et al: Radiation-related pericarditis. Am J Cardiol 35:216, 1975.
12. Applefeld MM, Cole JF, Pollock SH, et al: The late appearance of chronic pericardial disease in patients treated by radiotherapy for Hodgkin's disease. Ann Intern Med 94:338, 1981.

13. Lederman GS, Sheldon TA, Chaffey JT, et al: Cardiac disease after mediastinal irradiation for seminoma. Cancer 60:772, 1987.
14. Pohjola-Sintonen S, Totterman KJ, Salmo M, Siltanen P: Late cardiac effects of mediastinal radiotherapy in patients with Hodgkin's disease. Cancer 60:31, 1987.
15. Daugirdas JT, Leehey DJ, Popli S, et al: Subxiphoid pericardiostomy for hemodialysis-associated pericardial effusion. Arch Intern Med 146:1113, 1986.
16. Kron IL, Cox PM Jr: Cardiac injury after chest trauma. Crit Care Med 11:524, 1983.
17. Weinstein L: Life-threatening complications of infective endocarditis and their management. Arch Intern Med 146:953, 1986.
18. Johnson MA, Hirji MK, Hennig RC, et al: Pericardial abscess: diagnosis using two-dimensional echocardiography and CT. Radiology 159:419, 1986.
19. Suzuki S, Tajimi T, Takeshita A, et al: Isolated right heart purulent pericarditis forming a large mediastinal mass. Chest 93:667, 1988.
20. Sinzobahamvya N, Ikeogu MO: Purulent pericarditis. Arch Dis Child 62:696, 1987.
21. Buckingham TA, Wilner G, Sugar SJ: *Haemophilus influenzae* pericarditis in adults. Arch Intern Med 143:1809, 1983.
22. Schwartz KV, Guercio CA, Katz A: *Haemophilus influenzae* pericarditis. Conn Med 51:423, 1987.
23. Weingarten S, Weinberg H, Frang M, Meyer RD: *Haemophilus influenzae* pericarditis in two adults. West J Med 145:690, 1986.
24. van Dorp WT, van Rees C, van der Meer JW, Thompson J: Meningococcal pericarditis in the absence of meningitis. Infection 15:109, 1987.
25. Hardy DJ, Bartholomew WR, Amsterdam D: Pathophysiology of primary meningococcal pericarditis associated with *Neisseria meningitidis* group C. A case report and review of the literature. Diagn Microbiol Infect Dis 4:259, 1986.
26. Starling RC, Yu VL, Shillington D, et al: Pneumococcal pericarditis. Diagnostic usefulness of counterimmunoelectrophoresis and computed tomographic scanning. Arch Intern Med 146:1174, 1986.
27. Phelps R, Jacobs RA: Purulent pericarditis and mediastinitis due to *Peptococcus magnus*. JAMA 254:947, 1985.
28. Svendsen JH, Jnsson V, Niebuhr U: Combined pericarditis and pneumonia caused by Legionella infection. Br Heart J 58:663, 1987.
29. Mozes B, Pines A. Holtzman E, et al: Pericardial effusion as the sole manifestation of infectious mononucleosis. J Infect 11:149, 1985.
30. Hashimoto R, Ogata M, Koga Y, Toshima H: Clinical manifestations of acute Coxsackie-B viral myocarditis and pericarditis with a special reference to serum enzyme patterns and long-term prognosis. Kurume Med J 34:19, 1987.
31. Baid CS, Varma AR, Lakhotia M: A case of subacute effusive constrictive pericarditis with a probable amoebic aetiology. Br Heart J 58:296, 1987.
32. Kaufman LD, Seifert FC, Eilbott DJ, et al: Candida

pericarditis and tamponade in a patient with systemic lupus erythematosus. Arch Intern Med 148:715, 1988.

33. Kraus WE, Valenstein PN, Corey GR: Purulent pericarditis caused by *Candida*: report of three cases and identification of high-risk populations as an aid to early diagnosis. Rev Infect Dis 10:34, 1988.

34. Strang JIG: Tuberculous pericarditis in Transkei. Clin Cardiol 7:667, 1984.

35. Harris LF: Tuberculous pericarditis, a unique experience. Ala Med 57:16, 1987.

36. Sagrista-Sauleda J, Permanyer-Miralda G, Soler-Soler J: Tuberculous pericarditis: ten year experience with a prospective protocol for diagnosis and treatment. J Am Coll Cardiol 11:724, 1988.

37. D'Cruz IA, Sengupta EE, Abrahams C, et al: Cardiac involvement, including tuberculous pericardial effusion, complicating acquired immune deficiency syndrome. Am Heart J 112:1100, 1986.

38. Dalli E, Quesada A, Juan G, et al: Tuberculous pericarditis as the first manifestation of acquired immunodeficiency syndrome. Am Heart J 114:905, 1987.

39. Posner MR, Cohen GI, Skarin AT: Pericardial disease in patients with cancer. Am J Med 71:407, 1981.

40. Kralstein J, Frishman W: Malignant pericardial diseases: diagnosis and treatment. Am Heart J 113:785, 1987.

41. Donato DM, Sevin BU, Averette HE: Neoplastic pericarditis and gynecologic malignancies—a review of the literature. Obstet Gynecol Surv 41:473, 1986.

42. Vesterinen E, Kivinen S, Nieminen U: Cervical carcinoma complicated by malignant pericarditis. Acta Obstet Gynecol Scand 66:569, 1987.

43. Nowicka J, Haus O, Dzik T, et al: Pericarditis in the course of acute leukemia. Folia Haematol (Leipz) 114:220, 1987.

44. Evans CW, Tucker SC: Pericarditis: a complication of minoxidil therapy. South Med J 76:815, 1983.

45. Miller DH, Haas LF: Pneumonitis, pleural effusion, and pericarditis following treatment with dantrolene. J Neurol Neurosurg Psychiatry 47:553, 1984.

46. Boden WE, Sadaniantz A: Ventricular septal rupture during ibuprofen therapy for pericarditis after acute myocardial infarction. Am J Cardiol 55:1631, 1985.

47. Vaickus L, Letendre L: Pericarditis induced by high-dose cytarabine therapy. Arch Intern Med 144:1868, 1984.

48. Ratliff NB, McMahon JT, Shirey EK, et al: Silicone pericarditis. Cleve Clin Q 51:185, 1984.

49. Goldman MH, Barnhart G, Mohanakumar T, et al: Cyclosporine in cardiac transplantation. Surg Clin North Am 65:637, 1985.

50. Thould AK: Constrictive pericarditis in rheumatoid arthritis. Ann Rheum Dis 45:89, 1986.

51. Jurik AG, Graudal H: Pericarditis in rheumatoid arthritis. A clinical and radiological study. Rheumatol Int 6:37, 1986.

52. Persellin ST, Ramirez G, Moatamed F: Immunopathology of rheumatic pericarditis. Arthritis Rheum 25:1054, 1982.

53. Franssen MJ, Boerbooms AM, van de Putte LB: Polychondritis and rheumatoid arthritis. Case report and review of the literature. Clin Rheumatol 6:453, 1987.
54. Doherty NE, Siegel RJ: Cardiovascular manifestations of systemic lupus erythematosus. Am Heart J 110:1257, 1985.
55. Ansari A, Larson PH, Bates HD: Cardiovascular manifestations of systemic lupus erythematosus: current perspective. Prog Cardiovasc Dis 27:421, 1985.
56. Jamieson TW: Adult Still's disease complicated by cardiac tamponade. JAMA 249:2065, 1983.
57. Wouters JM, van de Putte LB: Adult-onset Still's disease: clinical and laboratory features, treatment and progress of 45 cases. Q J Med 61:1055, 1986.
58. Alpert MA, Goldberg SH, Singsen BH, et al: Cardiovascular manifestations of mixed connective tissue disease in adults. Circulation 68:1182, 1983.
59. Nunoda S, Mifune J, Ono S, et al: An adult case of mixed connective tissue disease associated with perimyocarditis and massive pericardial effusion. Jpn Heart J 27:129, 1986.
60. Follansbee WP: The cardiovascular manifestations of systemic sclerosis (scleroderma). Curr Probl Cardiol 11:241, 1986.
61. Patwardhan RV, Heilpern J, Brewster AC, et al: Pleuropericarditis: an extraintestinal complication of inflammatory bowel disease. Arch Intern Med 143:94, 1983.
62. Gould L, Patel C, Betzu R, et al: Pericarditis and ulcerative colitis. Am Heart J 111:802, 1986.
63. Pang JA: Acute pericarditis. An unusual presentation of an exacerbation of ulcerative colitis. Med J Aust 143:356, 1985.
64. Farley JD, Thomson AB, Dasgupta M: Pericarditis and ulcerative colitis. J Clin Gastroenterol 8:567, 1986.
65. Rubenstein I, Baum GL, Hiss Y: Cardiac tamponade as the presenting symptom of sarcoidosis. Am Heart J 109:1387, 1985.
66. Liss HP: Pleuropericarditis in sarcoidosis. South Med J 79:258, 1986.
67. Kelly JK, Butt JC: Fatal myxedema pericarditis in a Christian Scientist. Am J Clin Pathol 86:113, 1986.
68. Louie S, McGahan JP, Frey C, et al: Pancreatic pleuropericardial effusions. Arch Intern Med 145:1231, 1985.
69. Jones B, Haponik EF, Katz R: Fibrinous pericarditis: an uncommon complication of acute pancreatitis. South Med J 80:377, 1987.
70. Sachs BP, Lorell BH, Mehrez M, Damien N: Constrictive pericarditis and pregnancy. Am J Obstet Gynecol 154:156, 1986.
71. Knauer CM, Fogel MR: Pericarditis: complication of esophageal sclerotherapy. A report of three cases. Gastroenterology 93:287, 1987.
72. Almassi GH, Chapman PD, Troup PJ, et al: Constrictive pericarditis associated with patch electrodes of the automatic implantable cardioverter-defibrillator. Chest 92:369, 1987.

Selected Readings

Bellinger RL, Vacek JL: A review of pericarditis. 1. Causes, manifestations, and diagnostic techniques. 2. Specific pericardial disorders. Postgrad Med 82(2):95; 82(2):105, 1987.
Clinical review of pericardial disease that discusses multiple etiologies, diagnosis, and treatment.

Callahan JA, Seward JB, Tajik AJ: Cardiac tamponade: pericardiocentesis directed by two-dimensional echocardiography. Mayo Clin Proc 60:344, 1985.
Echocardiography provides a unique means of diagnosing and managing pericardial effusions.

Callahan JA, Seward JB, Nishimura RA, et al: Two-dimensional echocardiographically guided pericardiocentesis: experience in 117 patients. Am J Cardiol 55:476, 1985.
Two-dimensional echocardiographic imaging of the heart and pericardial fluid can help perform a safe and effective pericardiocentesis.

Fowler NO, Harbin AD III: Recurrent acute pericarditis: follow-up study of 31 patients. J Am Coll Cardiol 7:300, 1986.
Data from 31 patients with recurrent pericarditis observed for 2 to 19 years is presented. Etiologies of pericarditis that became recurrent in decreasing frequency include idiopathic pericarditis, postoperative or post-traumatic pericarditis, postinfarction pericarditis, and anticoagulant pericarditis. Three patients developed cardiac tamponade in the initial attack, but none developed cardiac tamponade during recurrences. Recurrent chest pain was a major disabling feature.

Jerjes-Sanchez C, Ibarra-Perez C, Ramirez-Rivera A, et al: Dressler-like syndrome after pulmonary embolism and infarction. Chest 92:115, 1987.
Clinical and echocardiographic data in 46 patients after acute myocardial effusion were evaluated. M-mode echocardiograms were performed 24 hours, 72 hours, and 5 days after acute myocardial infarction. Early acute pericarditis was found in 19 (41%) of the patients. Pericardial effusion was detected in 29 (63%) of patients. Authors conclude that pericardial effusion is observed frequently after acute myocardial infarction and that echocardiographic studies are helpful in the diagnosis.

Karjalainen J, Heikkila J: "Acute pericarditis": myocardial enzyme release as evidence for myocarditis. Am Heart J 111:546, 1986.
A clinical study of the relationship between serial ECG ST-T wave changes considered typical of acute pericarditis and serum cardiac enzyme levels in 18 young men with symptoms of acute infectious disease. Authors conclude that the serial ECG changes of ST-segment elevation with subsequent T wave inversions associated with acute infection are caused by acute myocardial injury and myocarditis reflected by myocardial enzyme release.

Little AG, Ferguson MK: Pericardioscopy as adjunct to pericardial window. Chest 89:53, 1986.
Authors indicate that pericardioscopy is a safe intervention in patients with central tumors and pericardial effusion in whom subxiphoid pericardial window is not clearly diagnostic at the time of surgery.

Permanyer-Miralda G, Sagrista-Sauleda J, Soler-Soler J:

Primary acute pericardial disease: a prospective series of 231 consecutive patients. Am J Cardiol 56:623, 1985.

This study concludes that the evaluation of primary acute pericardial disease must be systemically individualized for a maximal diagnostic yield.

Pierard LA, Albert A, Henrard L, et al: Incidence and significance of pericardial effusion in acute myocardial infarction as determined by two-dimensional echocardiography. J Am Coll Cardiol 8:517, 1986.

Pericardial effusion was frequently seen by two-dimensional echocardiography after acute myocardial infarction, and this finding was associated with a higher incidence of complications and cardiac death.

Sagrista-Sauleda J, Permanyer-Miralda G, Candell-Riera J, et al: Transient cardiac constriction: an unrecognized pattern of evolution in effusive acute idiopathic pericarditis. Am J Cardiol 59:961, 1987.

Features of cardiac constriction in 16 of 177 patients with effusive acute idiopathic pericarditis are described. Results of cardiac catheterization and clinical follow-up suggest that some patients may go through a transient phase of cardiac constriction at the end of the effusive period of acute idiopathic pericarditis. Better understanding of these clinical features may avoid unnecessary pericardiectomies.

Schoenfeld MH, Supple EW, Dec GW Jr, et al: Restrictive cardiomyopathy versus constrictive pericarditis: role of endomyocardial biopsy in avoiding unnecessary thoracotomy. Circulation 75:1012, 1987.

The differentiation of restrictive cardiomyopathy from constrictive pericarditis remains difficult. The role of right ventricular endomyocardial biopsy in defining the underlying process was examined in 54 patients with evidence of constrictive/restrictive physiology. Endomyocardial biopsy was found useful in identifying a large subset of patients with specific forms of restrictive cardiomyopathy in whom thoracotomy was avoided.

Sechtem U, Tscholakoff D, Higgins CB: MRI of the abnormal pericardium. AJR 147:245, 1986.

A retrospective study evaluated the use of MRI in the diagnosis of pericardial disease in 63 patients with pericardial abnormalities of clinically suspected pericardial disease. MRI estimates of pericardial effusion correlated well with echocardiographic estimations. MRI demonstrated fibrinous adhesions in uremic pericarditis, was helpful in the diagnosis of constrictive pericarditis versus restrictive cardiomyopathy, correctly detected hemopericardium, and was useful in documenting the presence of pericardial cysts. Authors conclude that the MRI will provide important additional information when diagnosis cannot be made by other noninvasive imaging techniques.

Somolinos M, Violan S, Sanz R, Marrero P: Early pericarditis after acute myocardial infarction: a clinical echocardiographic study. Crit Care Med 15;648, 1987.

Clinical and echocardiographic data were evaluated in 46 patients after acute myocardial infarction (AMI). Authors observed that pericardial effusion is a frequent finding following AMI and that an echocardiographic study can help in the diagnosis of early acute pericarditis following AMI.

9
Bloody Pericardial Effusions: Major Causes

Acute myocardial infarction and acute aortic dissection are the most common causes of acute hemopericardium leading to cardiac tamponade.[1] When the accumulation of blood in the pericardium is subacute or gradual, an underlying neoplastic or infectious process, such as tuberculosis, is a common cause. Since a significant amount of blood can accumulate within the pericardium, aspiration of bloody fluid during pericardiocentesis can sometimes appear as though the ventricular cavity has been penetrated, particularly when pericardial effusions with significantly high hematocrits are aspirated.[2]

Neoplasms[3]
    Metastatic carcinoma[4]: melanoma, lymphoma, leukemia, breast carcinoma, and lung carcinoma; the bloody effusion is often nonclotting
    Primary cardiac neoplasms: mesothelioma, sarcoma
Aortic dissection[5]
Postcardiac surgery[6]
Myocardial rupture: due to trauma or infarction
Tuberculosis[7]
Pseudoaneurysms[1]: aortic and cardiac
Myocardial infarction[8] without rupture
Rheumatoid arthritis[9]
Systemic lupus erythematosus
Chest trauma: may cause bloody and/or chylous effusion if the thoracic duct is ruptured
Anticoagulant therapy[10,11]

References

1. Olson LJ, Edwards WD, Olney BA, et al: Hemorrhagic cardiac tamponade: A clinicopathologic correlation. Mayo Clin Proc 59:785, 1984.
2. Krikorian JG, Hancock EW: Pericardiocentesis. Am J Med 65:808, 1978.
3. Theologides A: Neoplastic cardiac tamponade. Semin Oncol 5:181, 1978.

4. Posner MR, Cohen GI, Skarin AT: Pericardial disease in patients with cancer. Am J Med 71:407, 1981.
5. Saner HE, Gobel FL, Nicoloff DM, Edwards JE: Aortic dissection presenting as pericarditis. Chest 91:71, 1987.
6. Wickstrom PH, Monson BK, Helseth HK: Delayed postoperative bloody pericardial effusion. Minn Med 68:19, 1985.
7. Strang JIG: Tuberculous pericarditis in Transkei. Clin Cardiol 7:667, 1984.
8. Low RI, Arthur A, Kelly PB, et al: Clotted hemopericardium postmyocardial infarction presenting as effusive constrictive pericarditis. Am Heart J 109:905, 1985.
9. John JT Jr, Hough A, Sergent JS: Pericardial disease in rheumatoid arthritis. Am J Med 66:385, 1979.
10. Karim AH, Salomon J: Constrictive pericarditis after myocardial infarction. Sequela of anticoagulant-induced hemopericardium. Am J Med 79:389, 1985.
11. Scheetz A: Constrictive pericarditis after myocardial infarction: sequela of anticoagulant-induced hemopericardium (letter). Am J Med 81:948, 1986.

Selected Readings

D'Cruz IA, Kensey K, Campbell C, et al: Two-dimensional echocardiography in cardiac tamponade occurring after cardiac surgery. J Am Coll Cardiol 5:1250, 1985.
Two-dimensional echocardiograms of 11 patients who required surgical relief of cardiac tamponade complicating cardiac surgery are reviewed.

Pierard LA, Albert A, Henrard L, et al: Incidence and significance of pericardial effusion in acute myocardial infarction as determined by two-dimensional echocardiography. J Am Coll Cardiol 8:517, 1986.
Study concluding that pericardial effusion was frequently seen by two-dimensional echocardiography after acute myocardial infarction, and this presence is associated with increased occurrence of complications and cardiac death.

Viquerat CE, Hansen RM, Botvinick EH, et al: Undrained bloody pericardial effusion in the early postoperative period after coronary bypass surgery: a prospective blood pool study. Am Heart J 110:335, 1985.
This study reports the generally benign occurrence of blood postoperative mediastinal effusions, the frequent accumulation of substantial amounts of undrained sanguineous fluid, and the lack of connection between the presence and/or amount of pericardial blood and the postperiocardiotomy syndrome.

10
Cervical Sounds: Conditions That Can Mimic Carotid Bruits

Atheromatous lesions in the carotid arteries are an important cause of embolic cerebrovascular infarction. Although these lesions often cause carotid bruits, some of the most severe carotid stenoses may produce no audible bruit. Most carotid bruits are due to turbulence caused by atherosclerotic disease. The most common clinically significant cervical bruit is heard near the angle of the jaw and arises from lesions within or near the carotid bifurcation.[1] Many commonly auscultated noises in the neck mimic atherosclerotic carotid disease.

Venous Hums

Venous hums are continuous sounds due to nonpulsatile venous blood flow usually heard along the borders of the sternocleidomastoid muscle and clavicles. Venous hums are softer during the Valsalva maneuver and louder during expiration.

Children and young adults
High cardiac output: anemia, pregnancy, thyrotoxicosis, arteriovenous fistula, fever, Paget's disease, hemodialysis,[2] beriberi, exercise

Transmitted Cardiac Murmurs[3]

Aortic stenosis: the murmur of aortic stenosis may mask a faint sound caused by carotid artery disease.
Aortic regurgitation
Mitral regurgitation: e.g., due to ruptured chordae tendineae
Atherosclerosis of innominate, subclavian, and vertebral arteries
Patent ductus arteriosus
Tricuspid insufficiency[4]

Nonatheromatous
Disease Causing
Carotid Bruits

Carotid artery loops and kinks
Fibromuscular dysplasia[5,6]
Carotid artery-cavernous sinus fistula[7]
Arteriovenous malformations
Extrinsic compression of cervical carotid artery[8]
Carotid arteritis[9]: syphilis, tuberculosis
Vasculitis
Carotid tumors
Carotid aneurysms[10]
Carotid artery trauma[11]
Carotid surgery: i.e., postcarotid endarterectomy[12]
Thyroid disease: thyroid bruit mistaken for carotid
   bruit
Glomus jugular tumor[13]

References

1. Fields WS: The asymptomatic carotid bruit—operate or not? Stroke 9:269, 1978.
2. Wheeler SD: Long-term hemodialysis and supraclavicular bruits. JAMA 247:1026, 1982.
3. Hurst JW, Hopkins LC, Smith RB III: Noises in the neck (editorial). N Engl J Med 302:862, 1980.
4. Amidi M, Irwin JM, Salerni R, et al: Venous systolic thrill and murmur in the neck: a consequence of severe tricuspid insufficiency. J Am Coll Cardiol 7:942, 1986.
5. Wesen CA, Elliott BM: Fibromuscular dysplasia of the carotid arteries. Am J Surg 151:448, 1986.
6. Smith DC, Smith LL, Hasso AN: Fibromuscular dysplasia of the internal carotid artery treated by operative transluminal balloon angioplasty. Radiology 155:645, 1985.
7. Harris AE, McMenamin PG: Carotid artery—cavernous sinus fistula. Arch Otolaryngol 110:618, 1984.
8. Etheredge SN, Effeney DJ, Ehrenfeld WK: Symptomatic extrinsic compression of the cervical carotid artery. Arch Neurol 41:672, 1984.
9. Howard GF III, Ho SU, Kim KK, et al: Bilateral carotid artery occlusion resulting from giant cell arteritis. Ann Neurol 15:204, 1984.
10. Mas JL, Goeau C, Bousser MG, et al: Spontaneous dissecting aneurysms of the internal carotid and vertebral arteries—two case reports. Stroke 16:125, 1985.
11. Brown MF, Graham JM, Feliciano DV, et al: Carotid artery injuries. Am J Surg 144:748, 1982.
12. Hines GL, Harvey V: The post endarterectomy carotid bruit. Evaluation by Duplex scan. Am Surg 51:570, 1985.
13. Kinney SE, Sebek BA: Rare tumors of the skull base and temporal bone. Am J Otol (Suppl):135, 1985.

Selected Readings

Barry R, Nel CJ: Comparison of duplex Doppler scanning with contrast angiography in carotid artery disease. S Afr Med J 72:851, 1987.

A retrospective study to determine the long-term prognosis of patients with asymptomatic, hemodynamically significant internal carotid lesions compared 640 neurologically asymptomatic patients who demonstrated pressure-significant lesions as measured by ocular pneumoplethysmography with 348 patients with carotid bruits without pressure-significant lesions, i.e., with normal ocular pneumoplethysmography. Annual stroke rate and annual event rate (stroke and transient ischemic attack) were significantly higher in those patients with pressure-significant carotid occlusive lesions than those without pressure significant carotid occlusive lesions.

Bogousslavsky J, Despland PA, Regli F: Asymptomatic tight stenosis of the internal carotid artery: long-term prognosis. Neurology 36:861, 1986.
Study suggesting that the low risk of unheralded ipsilateral infarct questions the usefulness of prophylactic endarterectomy.

Cote R, Barnett HJM, Taylor DW: Internal carotid occlusion: A prospective study. Stroke 14:898, 1983.
A prospective study of 47 patients with internal carotid occlusion who presented without any or only mild neurologic deficit.

Darazs B, Hesdorffer CS, Butterworth AM, Ziady F: The possible etiology of the vibratory systolic murmur. Clin Cardiol 10:341, 1987.
Authors evaluated the relationship between the presence of left ventricular bands and systolic murmurs. A prospective analysis of patients with a classic vibratory systolic murmur (Still's murmur), such as is commonly found in children and young adults, was performed. Echocardiographic studies found two types of ventricular bands, one of which was believed related to Still's murmur. Such possible murmur-related ventricular bands were noted to cross the left ventricular outflow tract, possibly causing turbulence and a murmur.

Donaldson MC, Sabine C, Showah AT, Bucknam CA: Recent experience with the asymptomatic cervical bruit. Arch Surg 122:893, 1987.
Another view on the prognosis of the asymptomatic cervical bruit. A retrospective review of 418 patients referred to a noninvasive vascular laboratory with a follow-up of 23.7 months obtained for 370 patients. Risk of neurologic morbidity was highest in patients with advanced carotid stenosis. Authors suggest that low morbidity performance of carotid endarterectomy in selected surgical candidates with advanced carotid stenosis is reasonable.

Ford CS, Howard VJ, Howard G, et al: The sex difference in manifestations of carotid bifurcation disease. Stroke 17:877, 1986.
Study suggesting that women are probably predisposed to develop carotid bruit, even without carotid stenosis.

Ford CS, Frye JL, Toole JF, et al: Asymptomatic carotid bruit and stenosis. A prospective follow-up study. Arch Neurol 43:219, 1986.
Authors found that myocardial infarctions occurred more often and were more commonly the cause of death than cerebral infarctions in patients with asymptomatic carotid bruit and stenosis.

Gutierrez IZ, Makula PA, Gage AA: The asymptomatic carotid bruit. Am Surg 51:388, 1985.
Authors conclude that patients with an asymptomatic hemodynamically significant carotid bruit have a high risk of developing a stroke and suggest surgical treatment.

Lo LY, Ford CS, McKinney WM, et al: Asymptomatic bruit, carotid and vertebrobasilar transient ischemic attacks—a clinical and ultrasonic correlation. Stroke 17:65, 1986.

In this patient population, ipsilateral plaque ulceration occurred in half of those with symptomatic carotid bruits, but in only 10% of those with asymptomatic carotid bruits.

Perler BA, Carr J, Williams GM: Oculoplethysmography and supraorbital Doppler evaluation of carotid disease. A reappraisal. Am Surg 51:107, 1985.

Discussion of the variety of noninvasive tests presently available for the evaluation of patients with suspected extracranial cerebrovascular disease.

Ropper AH, Wechsler LR, Wilson LS: Carotid bruit and the risk of stroke in elective surgery. N Engl J Med 307:1388, 1982.

Results of prospective study of 735 patients who underwent elective surgery demonstrates a low incidence of stroke in patients with and without bruits.

Rothstein J, Hilger PA, Boies LR Jr: Venous hum as a cause of reversible factitious sensorineural hearing loss. Ann Otol Rhinol Laryngol 94:267, 1985.

Authors speculate that hearing loss in a patient with venous hum was factitious and represented a masking effect from the venous hum.

Sutton KC, Dai WS, Kuller LH: Asymptomatic carotid artery bruits in a population of elderly adults with isolated systolic hypertension. Stroke 16:781, 1985.

Study supporting the hypothesis that asymptomatic cervical bruits are an indication of systemic vascular disease.

Theodotou B, Mahaley MS Jr: Complications following carotid endarterectomy for all indications: report of 192 operations. Surg Neurol 24:484, 1985.

Study pointing out the need to separate patients who have undergone endarterectomy into presenting groups before comparing with other studies having similar postoperative observations.

11
Aortoarterial Emboli: Cardiac and Noncardiac Sources

In most cases of cerebral or systemic embolism, the heart is the source.[1] The cause of cardiac embolization can sometimes be found with echocardiography.[2] However, if the patient with an embolic event has no previous history of cardiac disease and has a normal cardiac physical examination, chest radiograph, and ECG, it is unlikely that the heart is the source of embolization.[3]

Cardiogenic Emboli

Acute myocardial infarction[4,5]

Atrial fibrillation: nonrheumatic atrial fibrillation is the most frequent substrate for brain embolism.[6-11]

Rheumatic mitral valve disease[12]

Mural thrombi[13-16]: ventricular aneurysm,[17,18] cardiomyopathy[19-21]

Cardiac surgery: prosthetic valves,[22-26] cardiac sutures, intraoperative embolism, air embolism, postoperative idiopathic hypertrophic subaortic stenosis (IHSS) myomectomy, transvenous pacing[27]

Atherosclerotic disease with and without myocardial infarction[28]

Aortic valve disease[29-31]

Infectious endocarditis[32-37]

Marantic endocarditis[38,39]: nonbacterial thrombotic endocarditis

Paradoxical emboli[40-42]

Mitral valve prolapse[43-46]

Cardiac tumors: myxoma,[47-50] rhabdomyomas, metastatic

Mitral annulus calcification[51]

Cardiac catheterization[52]

Cardiopulmonary bypass[53]

**Noncardiogenic
Emboli**

Aneurysms, ulcerated atheromatous plaques, and suture lines are major sources of noncardiogenic emboli.

Carotid artery disease: see also Chapter 10, Cervical Sounds: Conditions Which Can Mimic Carotid Bruits.
Cardiac procedures: angiography, catheterization[54]
Mural thrombi within aortic aneurysms
Noncardiac tumor emboli[55-57]
Aortoarteritis[58]
Fibromuscular dysplasia[59]
Cervical trauma and manipulation
Vertebral artery injury,[60] anomaly[61]
Fat emboli: associated with trauma[62]
Neoplastic emboli[63]
Air embolism: related to central venous catheterization[64-67]
Systemic lupus erythematosus[68]

References

1. Rem JA, Hachinski VC, Boughner DR, et al: Value of cardiac monitoring and echocardiography in TIA and stroke patients. Stroke 16:940, 1985.
2. Lovett JL, Sandok BA, Giuliani ER, et al: Two-dimensional echocardiography in patients with focal cerebral ischemia. Ann Intern Med 95:1, 1981.
3. Greenland P, Knopman DS, Mikell FL, et al: Echocardiography in diagnostic assessment of stroke. Ann Intern Med 95:51, 1981.
4. Weinreich DJ, Burke JF, Pauletto FJ: Left ventricular mural thrombi complicating acute myocardial infarction. Long-term follow-up with serial echocardiography. Ann Intern Med 100:789, 1984.
5. Puletti M, Cusmano E, Testa MG, et al: Incidence of systemic thromboembolic lesions in acute myocardial infarction. Clin Cardiol 9:331, 1986.
6. Sherman DG, Goldman L, Whiting RB, et al: Thromboembolism in patients with atrial fibrillation. Arch Neurol 41:708, 1984.
7. Kannel WB, Abbott RD, Savage DD, et al: Epidemiologic features of chronic atrial fibrillation: the Framingham study. N Engl J Med 306:1018, 1982.
8. Petersen P, Godtfredsen J: Embolic complications in paroxysmal atrial fibrillation. Stroke 17:622, 1986.
9. Kelley RE, Berger JR, Alter M, et al: Cerebral ischemia and atrial fibrillation: prospective study. Neurology 34:1285, 1984.
10. Sherman DG: Atrial fibrillation and stroke: the view from neurology. Adv Exp Med Biol 214:283, 1987.
11. Cardiogenic brain embolism. Cerebral Embolism Task Force. Arch Neurol 43:71, 1986.
12. Easton JD, Sherman DG: Management of cerebral embolism of cardiac origin. Stroke 11:433, 1980.

13. Meltzer RS, Visser CA, Fuster V: Intracardiac thrombi and systemic embolization. Ann Intern Med 104:689, 1986.
14. Arvan S: Mural thrombi in coronary artery disease. Recent advances in pathogenesis, diagnosis, and approaches to treatment. Arch Intern Med 144:113, 1984.
15. Reeder GS, Tajik AJ, Seward JB: Left ventricular mural thrombus: two-dimensional echocardiography diagnosis. Mayo Clin Proc 56:82, 1981.
16. Stratton JR, Resnick AD: Increased embolic risk in patients with left ventricular thrombi. Circulation 75:1004, 1987.
17. Reeder GS, Lengyel M, Tajik AJ, et al: Mural thrombus in left ventricular aneurysm: incidence, role of angiography, and relation between anticoagulation and embolization. Mayo Clin Proc 56:77, 1981.
18. Nixon JV: Left ventricular mural thrombus. Arch Intern Med 143:1567, 1983.
19. Fuster V, Gersh BJ, Giuliani ER, et al: The natural history of idiopathic dilated cardiomyopathy. Am J Cardiol 47:525, 1981.
20. Taliercio CP, Seward JB, Driscoll DJ, et al: Idiopathic dilated cardiomyopathy in the young: clinical profile and natural history. J Am Coll Cardiol 6:1126, 1985.
21. Narvaez R, Strauss C, Kotler MN, et al: Embolization of a large left ventricular thrombus during two-dimensional and color flow Doppler examination in idiopathic dilated cardiomyopathy. Am J Cardiol 60:402, 1987.
22. Gersh BJ, Schaff HV, Vatterott PJ, et al: Results of triple valve replacement in 91 patients: perioperative mortality and long-term follow-up. Circulation 72:130, 1985.
23. Zussa C, Ottino G, di Summa M, et al: Porcine cardiac bioprostheses: evaluation of long-term results in 990 patients. Ann Thorac Surg 39:243, 1985.
24. Garcia-Del Castillo H, Larrousse-Perez E, Murtra-Ferre M, et al: Strut fracture and disk embolization of a Bjork-Shiley mitral valve prosthesis. Am J Cardiol 55:597, 1985.
25. Adams PC, Cohen M, Chesebro JH, Fuster V: Thrombosis and embolism from cardiac chambers and infected valves. J Am Coll Cardiol 8(Suppl B):76B, 1986.
26. Edmunds LH Jr: Thrombotic and bleeding complications of prosthetic heart valves. Ann Thorac Surg 44:430, 1987.
27. Phibbs B, Marriott HJ: Complications of permanent transvenous pacing. N Engl J Med 312:1428, 1985.
28. Thompson PL, Robinson JS: Stroke after acute myocardial infarction: relation to infarct size. Br Med J 2:457, 1978.
29. Brockmeier LB, Adolph RJ, Gustin BW, et al: Calcium emboli to the retinal artery in calcific aortic stenosis. Am Heart J 101:32, 1981.
30. Pleet AB, Massey EW, Vengrow ME: TIA, stroke, and the bicuspid aortic valve. Neurology 31:1540, 1981.
31. Czer LS, Matloff JM, Chaux A, et al: The St. Jude valve: analysis of thromboembolism, warfarin-related hemorrhage, and survival. Am Heart J 114:389, 1987.
32. Pruitt AA, Rubin RH, Karchmer AW, et al: Neurologic

complications of bacterial endocarditis. Medicine 57: 329, 1978.
33. Alsip SG, Blackstone EH, Kirklin JW, et al: Indications for cardiac surgery in patients with active infective endocarditis. Am J Med 78(6B):138, 1985.
34. Lerner PI: Neurologic complications of infective endocarditis. Med Clin North Am 69:385, 1985.
35. Dean RH, Waterhouse G, Meacham PW, et al: Mycotic embolism and embolomycotic aneurysms. Neglected lessons of the past. Ann Surg 204:300, 1986.
36. Young EJ, Klima M, Goldberg J, et al: Culture-negative endocarditis with purpura and arterial emboli. South Med J 79:493, 1986.
37. Weinstein L: Life-threatening complications of infective endocarditis and their management. Arch Intern Med 146:953, 1986.
38. Kooiker JC, MacLean JM, Sumi SM: Cerebral embolism, marantic endocarditis, and cancer. Arch Neurol 33:260, 1976.
39. Weisberg LA: Nonseptic cardiogenic cerebral embolic stroke: clinical-CT correlations. Neurology 35:896, 1985.
40. Loscalzo J: Paradoxical embolism: clinical presentation, diagnostic strategies, and therapeutic options. Am Heart J 112:141, 1986.
41. Jones HR, Caplan LR, Come PC, et al: Paradoxical cerebral emboli: an occult cause of stroke (abstract). Ann Neurol 10:105, 1981.
42. Langdon TJ, Bandyk DF, Olinger GN, et al: Multiple paradoxical emboli. J Vasc Surg 4:284, 1986.
43. Schnee MA, Bucal AA: Fatal embolism in mitral valve prolapase. Chest 83:285, 1983.
44. Sandok BA, Giuliani ER: Cerebral ischemic events in patients with mitral valve prolapse. Stroke 13:448, 1982.
45. Jackson AC, Boughner DR, Barnett HJM: Mitral valve prolapse and cerebral ischemic events in young patients. Neurology 34:784, 1984.
46. Egeblad H, Soelberg-Srensen P: Prevalence of mitral valve prolapse in younger patients with cerebral ischaemic attacks. A blinded controlled study. Acta Med Scand 216:385, 1984.
47. Sandok BA, von Estorff I, Guiliani ER: CNS embolism due to atrial myxoma. Clinical features and diagnosis. Arch Neurol 37:485, 1980.
48. Macaulay VM, Crawford PJ, McKeran R: Atrial myxoma presenting with cerebral haemorrhage. Postgrad Med J 61:331, 1985.
49. Branch CL Jr, Laster DW, Kelly DL Jr: Left atrial myxoma with cerebral emboli. Neurosurgery 16:675, 1985.
50. Talley JD, Wenger NK: Atrial myxoma: overview, recognition, and management. Compr Ther 13:12, 1987.
51. Jespersen CM, Egeblad H: Mitral annulus calcification and embolism. Acta Med Scand 222:37, 1987.
52. B-Lundqvist C, Olsson SB, Varnauskas E: Transseptal left heart catheterization, a review of 278 studies. Clin Cardiol 9:21, 1986.
53. Padayachee TS, Parsons S, Theobold R, et al: The detection of microemboli in the middle cerebral artery

during cardiopulmonary bypass: a transcranial Doppler ultrasound investigation using membrane and bubble oxygenators. Ann Thorac Surg 44:298, 1987.

54. Dawson DM, Fischer EG: Neurologic complications of cardiac catheterization. Neurology 27:496, 1977.
55. Kearsley JH, Tattersall MHN: Cerebral embolism in cancer patients. Q J Med 51:279, 1982.
56. Bloch RS, Jacobs LA, Lewis LS, Bernys CF: Malignant tumor embolism: a rare presentation of malignant disease. J Cardiovasc Surg (Torino) 27:630, 1986.
57. Lefkovitz NW, Roessmann U, Kori SH: Major cerebral infarction from tumor embolus. Stroke 17:555, 1986.
58. Wickremasinghe HR, Peiris JB, Thenabadu PN, et al: Transient emboligenic aortoarteritis. Arch Neurol 35:416, 1978.
59. So EL, Toole JF, Moody DM, et al: Cerebral embolism from septal fibromuscular dysplasia of the common carotid artery. Ann Neurol 6:75, 1979.
60. Katirji MB, Reinmuth OM, Latchaw RE: Stroke due to vertebral artery injury. Arch Neurol 42:242, 1985.
61. Berry AD III, Kepes JJ, Wetzel MD: Segmental duplication of the basilar artery with thrombosis. Stroke 19:256, 1988.
62. Schwartz DA, Finkelstein SD, Lumb GD: Fat embolism to the cardiac conduction system associated with sudden death. Hum Pathol 19:116, 1988.
63. Ackermann DM, Hyma BA, Edwards WD: Malignant neoplastic emboli to the coronary arteries: report of two cases and review of the literature. Hum Pathol 18:955, 1987.
64. Seidelin PH, Stolarek IH, Thompson AM: Central venous catheterization and fatal air embolism. Br J Hosp Med 38:438, 1987.
65. Roe BB: Air embolism prevention. Ann Thorac Surg 44:212, 1987.
66. Griffiths DM, Gough MH: Gas in the hepatic portal veins. Br J Surg 73:172, 1986.
67. Robicsek F, Duncan GD: Retrograde air embolization in coronary operations. J Thorac Cardiovasc Surg 94:110, 1987.
68. Gorelick PB, Rusinowitz MS, Tiku M, et al: Embolic stroke complicating systemic lupus erythematosus. Arch Neurol 42:813, 1985.

Selected Readings

Anderson DC: Brain cardioembolism. Issues in diagnosis and management. Postgrad Med 82(3):48, 1987.

Clinical review of current concepts in diagnosis and treatment of cardioembolism. Authors suggest that echocardiography is of limited diagnostic usefulness and should be limited to young patients and older patients with clinical heart disease.

Biller J, Johnson MR, Adams HP Jr, et al: Echocardiographic evaluation of young adults with nonhemorrhagic cerebral infarction. Stroke 17:608, 1986.

Etiologies diagnosed by echocardiography in nine cases of young adult nonhemorrhagic cerebral infarction in decreasing frequency included paradoxical embolism, right atrial myxoma, rheumatic mi-

tral valve vegetation, myxomatous mitral valve, and left atrial en-largement associated with decreased left ventricular function.

Bogousslavsky J, Hachinski VC, Boughner DR, et al: Cardiac and arterial lesions in carotid transient ischemic attacks. Arch Neurol 43:223, 1986.
Results of a study recommending the search for a potential cardiac source of emboli in patients with carotid transient ischemic attacks and known heart disease.

Bogousslavsky J, Hachinski VC, Boughner DR, et al: Clinical predictors and arterial lesions in carotid transient ischemic attacks. Arch Neurol 43:229, 1986.
Study concluding that important information regarding etiology can be drawn from the clinical characteristics of transient ischemic attacks.

Erbel R, Rohmann S, Drexler M, et al: Improved diagnostic value of echocardiography in patients with infective endocarditis by transoesophageal approach. A prospective study. Eur Heart J 9:43, 1988.
A prospective study of the clinical value of transoesophageal two-dimensional echocardiography (TOE) was compared with transthoracic two-dimensional echocardiography (TTE) in patients with suspected infective endocarditis. Ninety-six patients were studied with TOE and TTE. TOE was found superior to TTE in detecting vegetations in suspected infective endocarditis, particularly during earlier stages when the vegetations were small.

Fisher DF Jr, Clagett GP, Brigham RA, et al: Dilemmas in dealing with the blue toe syndrome: aortic versus peripheral source. Am J Surg 148:836, 1984.
Study of peripheral lesion exploration in patients with blue toe syndrome.

Gagliardi R, Benvenuti L, Frosini F, et al: Frequency of echocardiographic abnormalities in patients with ischemia of the carotid territory—a preliminary report. Stroke 16:118, 1985.
Mitral valve prolapse was not seen in this series in patients with a probable carotid source on angiography.

Graus F, Rogers LR, Posner JB: Cerebrovascular complications in patients with cancer. Medicine 64:16, 1985.
A well-referenced monograph that discusses the incidence and causes of cerebrovascular disease in a large cancer population.

Kessler C, Henningsen H, Reuther R, et al: Identification of intracardiac thrombi in stroke patients with indium-111 platelet scintigraphy. Stroke 18:63, 1987.
A study reviewing the usefulness of platelet scintigraphy (PSC) with indium-111-labeled platelets as an adequate method for the detection of intracardiac thrombi in patients with heart disease. PSC of the heart and neck vessels was performed in 27 stroke patients with suspected cardiac embolism who were then compared to 10 control patients with atherosclerotic lesions of the carotid arteries without evidence of heart disease. Thirteen pathologic conditions were identified by PSC in the 27 stroke patients. Two-dimensional echocardiography revealed pathologic findings in 8 of 13 patients with positive heart PSC findings.

Kornberg E: Lumbar artery aneurysm with acute aortic occlusion resulting from chiropractic manipulation: a case report. Surgery 103:122, 1988.
Case report describing an acute aortic occlusion after chiropractic

manipulation in a 44-year-old man with chronic back pain. A lumbar artery aneurysm was associated with a distal aortic occlusion.

Lutas EM, Roberts RB, Devereux RB, et al: Relation between the presence of echocardiographic vegetations and the complication rate in infective endocarditis. Am Heart J 112:107, 1986.

This study concludes that valve cusp or chordal rupture and/or premature mitral valve closure are associated with congestive heart failure and the need for surgery.

Takamoto T, Kim D, Urie PM, et al: Comparative recognition of left ventricular thrombi by echocardiography and cineangiography. Br Heart J 53:36, 1985.

The study suggests that cross-sectional echocardiography is more reliable than cineangiography in recognizing thrombi.

Todnem K, Vik-Mo H: Cerebral ischemic attacks as a complication of heart disease: the value of echocardiography. Acta Neurol Scand 74:323, 1986.

The usefulness of echocardiography in detecting heart disease and possible emboli was studied in 194 patients with transitory cerebral ischemic attacks or stroke. Ninety-five of these patients had heart disease, and 63 had positive echocardiographic findings. Thirty-five patients had heart disease as a probable source for systemic embolism. In 25 patients, clinically undetected cardiac disorders were found; unsuspected aortic and mitral valve disease were the most frequent findings.

Weisberg LA: Nonseptic cardiogenic cerebral embolic stroke: clinical-CT correlations. Neurology 35:896, 1985.

Thirty-five patients with nonseptic cardiogenic cerebral emboli were studied. CT correlations were made with the clinical course. CT showed evidence of cerebral infarct in all cases and evidence of hemorrhagic infarct in nine cases.

PULMONARY

12
Cough: Common and Uncommon Causes

A cough is a reflex mechanism that attempts to cleanse the tracheobronchial system and is a common manifestation of acute and chronic pulmonary disease. Acute self-limiting coughs are usually secondary to viral upper respiratory tract infections; chronic and persistent coughs are usually secondary to chronic bronchitis or postnasal drip. Such historical facts as duration of cough, characterization of cough, smoking history, environmental or occupational exposures, allergies, asthma, and recent upper respiratory tract infections can usually establish the diagnosis.

The cough reflex is usually associated with common pulmonary disorders that irritate the pharynx, larynx, trachea, bronchi and sinuses. Other less likely pulmonary and nonpulmonary disorders can also initiate a cough by irritating the tracheobronchial tree or can cause a cough by irritating certain regions of the pleura, stomach, pericardium, diaphragm, or tympanic membrane involved in the cough reflex pathway. Therefore, if the cause of cough is not obvious, particularly when the cough persists beyond several weeks, or with a new or changing cough in a cigarette smoker, consider neoplastic, infectious, and mechanical sources of cough along the cough reflex pathway.[1-4]

Viral infections: usually cause an acute, reversible cough
Chronic bronchitis
Bronchial asthma[5]
Postnasal drip[6]
Tobacco smoking: commonly associated with acute bronchitis and chronic obstructive pulmonary disease
Nasal polyps: usually associated with postnasal drip
Sinusitis[7]
Pulmonary infection: acute or chronic along the

tracheobronchial tree or other less common pathways of the cough reflex[8,9]

Neoplastic disorders: particularly endobronchial bronchogenic carcinoma

Psychogenic habit cough[10]

Occupational exposures: occupational dust, gases, fumes[11,12]

Drug abuse: marijuana smoking, cocaine[13,14]

Esophageal reflux

Left ventricular failure

Broncholithiasis: stones from calcified peribronchial lymph nodes that erode into the tracheobronchial tree, most commonly associated with infections such as tuberculosis and histoplasmosis[15]

Elongated uvula

Tonsillitis

Enlarged tonsils

Lingual tonsillitis: lingual tonsils may be visible only with the use of laryngeal mirror[16]

External auditory canal disorders: impacted cerumen, inflammation, foreign body

Pleural inflammation

Pulmonary infarction

Postexercise cough[17,18]

Esophageal cyst[19]

Angiotensin-converting enzyme inhibitors: captopril and enalapril[20-22]

Miscellaneous causes of pulmonary fibrosis: idiopathic pulmonary fibrosis, sarcoidosis, pneumoconiosis[23]

References

1. Irwin RS, Rosen MJ, Braman SS: Cough. A comprehensive review. Arch Intern Med 137:1186, 1977.
2. Widdicombe J: The neural reflexes in the airways. Eur J Respir Dis 144 (Suppl):1, 1986.
3. Widdicombe JG: Mechanism of cough and its regulation. Eur J Respir Dis 61 (Suppl 110):11, 1980.
4. Brashear RE: Cough: diagnostic considerations with normal chest roentgenograms. J Fam Pract 15:979, 1982.
5. Strachan DP, Anderson HR, Bland JM, Peckham C: Asthma as a link between chest illness in childhood and chronic cough and phlegm in young adults. Br Med J 296:890, 1988.
6. Irwin RS, Pratter MR, Holland PS, et al: Postnasal drip causes cough and is associated with reversible upper airway obstruction. Chest 85:346, 1984.
7. Sacha RF, Tremblay NF, Jacobs RL: Chronic cough, sinusitis, and hyperreactive airways in children: an often overlooked association. Ann Allergy 54:195, 1985.

8. Aluoch JA, Swai OB, Edwards EA, et al: Study of case-finding for pulmonary tuberculosis in outpatients complaining of a chronic cough at a district hospital in Kenya. Am Rev Respir Dis 129:915, 1984.
9. Baugh R, Gilmore BB Jr: Infectious croup: a critical review. Otolaryngol Head Neck Surg 95:40, 1986.
10. Gay M, Blager F, Bartsch K, et al: Psychhogenic habit cough: review and case reports. J Clin Psychiatry 48:483, 1987.
11. Korn RJ, Dockery DW, Speizer FE, et al: Occupational exposures and chronic respiratory symptoms. A population-based study. Am Rev Respir Dis 136:298, 1987.
12. Chapman RS, Calafiore DC, Hasselblad V: Prevalence of persistent cough and phlegm in young adults in relation to long-term ambient sulfur oxide exposure. Am Rev Respir Dis 132:261, 1985.
13. Tashkin DP, Coulson AH, Clark VA, et al: Respiratory symptoms and lung function in habitual heavy smokers of marijuana alone, smokers of marijuana and tobacco, smokers of tobacco alone, and nonsmokers. Am Rev Respir Dis 135:209, 1987.
14. Kissner DG, Lawrence WD, Selis JE, Flint A: Crack lung: pulmonary disease caused by cocaine abuse. Am Rev Respir Dis 136:1250, 1987.
15. Haines JD Jr: Coughing up a stone. What to do about broncholithiasis. Postgrad Med 83(3):83, 1988.
16. Puar RK, Puar HS: Lingual tonsillitis. South Med J 79:1126, 1986.
17. Banner AS, Green J, O'Connor M: Relation of respiratory water loss to coughing after exercise. N Engl J Med 311:883, 1984.
18. Banner AS, Chausow A, Green J: The tussive effect of hyperpnea with cold air. Am Rev Respir Dis 131:362, 1985.
19. Bowton DL, Katz PO: Esophageal cyst as a cause of chronic cough. Chest 86:150, 1984.
20. Bucknall CE, Neilly JB, Carter R, et al: Bronchial hyperreactivity in patients who cough after receiving angiotensin converting enzyme inhibitors. Br Med J 296:86, 1988.
21. Stoller JK, Elghazawi A, Mehta AC, Vidt DG: Captopril-induced cough. Chest 93:659, 1988.
22. Coulter DM, Edwards IR: Cough associated with captopril and enalapril. Br Med J 294:1521, 1987.
23. Braman SS, Corrao WM: Chronic cough. Diagnosis and treatment. Prim Care 12:217, 1985.

Selected Readings

Banner AS: Relationship between cough due to hypotonic aerosol and the ventilatory response to CO_2 in normal subjects. Am Rev Respir Dis 137:647, 1988.
This study tested the hypothesis that susceptibility of the tussive effect of hypotonic aerosol is related to the ventilatory response of CO_2. Findings suggest that the susceptibility to the tussive effect of hypotonic aerosol and CO_2 ventilatory responses are determined by a common neural mechanism.

Braman SS, Corraeo WM: Cough: differential diagnosis and treatment. Clin Chest Med 8:177, 1987.

Recommended clinical review of current concepts of pathophysiology and state of the art evaluation of cough.

Brashear RE: Cough: diagnostic considerations with normal chest roentgenograms. J Fam Pract 15:979, 1982.
Outpatient evaluation of cough. Well referenced.

Britten N, Davies JM, Colley JR: Early respiratory experience and subsequent cough and peak expiratory flow rate in 36-year-old men and women. Br Med J 294:1317, 1987.
This study found additional evidence for a causal relationship between childhood respiratory disease and adult respiratory disease. Measurements of peak expiratory flow rate and histories of respiratory symptoms were elicited in 3,261 cohort members. Lower peak expiratory flow and higher respiratory morbidity were independently associated with indices of poor social circumstances, cigarette smoking, poor home environment at age 2 years, and lower respiratory tract illness before age 10.

Cohen RM, Grant W, Lieberman P, et al: The use of methacholine inhalation, methacholine skin testing, distilled water inhalation challenge, and eosinophil counts in the evaluation of patients presenting with cough and/or nonwheezing dyspnea. Ann Allergy 56:308, 1986.
A study that suggests that total eosinophil counts (TEC) may predict which patients with cough or dyspnea will respond successfully to bronchodilator therapy.

Irwin RS, Curley FJ, Pratter MR: The effects of drugs on cough. Eur J Respir Dis 153 (suppl):173, 1987.
Helpful review of antitussive therapy that emphasizes differences in pathophysiology of pathologic and nonspecific cough mechanisms with implications for appropriate cough management.

Leith DE: The development of cough. Am Rev Respir Dis 131:S39, 1985.
Pathophysiology of cough in newborns.

McCool FD, Leith DE: Pathophysiology of cough. Clin Chest Med 8:189, 1987.
Current concepts of the pathophysiology of cough.

Poe RH, Israel RH, Utell MJ, et al: Chronic cough: bronchoscopy or pulmonary function testing? Am Rev Respir Dis 126:160, 1982.
A study suggesting pulmonary function testing has a higher yield than bronchoscopy in the evaluation of chronic cough.

Power JT, Stewart IC, Connaughton JJ, et al: Nocturnal cough in patients with chronic bronchitis and emphysema. Am Rev Respir Dis 130:999, 1984.
This study concludes that spontaneous cough during sleep in patients with chronic bronchitis and emphysema is usually suppressed and rarely awakens patients.

Puolijoki H, Lahdensuo A: Chronic cough as a risk indicator of broncho-pulmonary disease. Eur J Respir Dis 71:77, 1987.
This study evaluated 182 patients who were seen in a chest clinic with an unexplained cough. Twenty-nine patients (16%) developed asthma during a mean follow-up of 4.4 years. Chronic bronchitis was diagnosed in 18 patients (10%). Circadian changes in peak expiratory flow and total blood eosinophil counts were the best variables for predicting the risk of developing asthma in a patient with unexplained cough.

Sparrow D, O'Connor G, Colton T, et al: The relationship

of nonspecific bronchial responsiveness to the occurrence of respiratory symptoms and decreased levels of pulmonary function. The Normative Aging Study. Am Rev Respir Dis 135:1255, 1987.

Nonspecific bronchial responsiveness was evaluated by an abbreviated methacholine challenge test in 458 males. Cigarette smoking was significantly associated with a positive response to the methacholine challenge test. Statistical analyses of data suggest that increased level of nonspecific responsiveness is significantly associated with wheeze and cough symptoms and decreased levels of pulmonary function in men.

Stulbarg M: Evaluating and treating intractable cough— medical staff conference, University of California, San Francisco. West J Med 143:223, 1985.

Well-referenced discussion of the physiology, complications, differential diagnosis, and diagnostic approach to cough.

13

Dyspnea: Common and Less Common Causes

Dyspnea is an uncomfortable awareness of the act of breathing leading to a sensation described as breathlessness.[1] Multiple physiologic and psychological factors contribute to the sensation of acute and chronic dyspnea. Acute dyspnea is usually easily diagnosed with a history, physical examination and chest radiograph. Chronic dyspnea, one of the most common respiratory complaints of patients, can be more difficult to diagnose and can require pulmonary function testing, measurements of respiratory muscle strength, and cardiopulmonary exercise testing.[2]

Underlying causes of acute and chronic dyspnea reflect a wide range of disorders, from benign hyperventilation or anxiety syndromes to serious cardiovascular and pulmonary diseases, particularly those associated with disordered lung mechanics. Two major forms of disordered lung mechanics that result in pulmonary dyspnea are obstructive lung diseases and pulmonary edema causing increased lung stiffness. Dyspnea associated with chronic obstructive lung disease is usually easily distinguished from cardiac dyspnea. However, since stiff lungs underlie both cardiac dyspnea and restrictive lung disease, it is sometimes difficult to distinguish these two causes, particularly in patients with both pulmonary and cardiac disorders. Dyspnea related to intrinsic pulmonary vascular disease is less common and particularly difficult to diagnose.[1] Some other less common and poorly understood disorders associated with dyspnea are listed.

Psychogenic Causes

Hyperventilation syndrome[3,4]
Anxiety[5,6]

Obstructive Pulmonary Disease

Dyspnea is caused by increased airway resistance.
Bronchial asthma[7-11]
Chronic obstructive pulmonary disease (COPD): chronic bronchitis, emphysema, small airway disease[11,12]
Large airway obstruction: foreign body, neoplasm, external compression of the tracheobronchial airway, goiter[13-15]
Bronchiolitis

Restrictive Pulmonary Disease

Dyspnea is caused by increased lung stiffness.
Cardiogenic pulmonary edema: a major cause of cardiac dyspnea through lung stiffness
Noncardiogenic pulmonary edema: capillary leak, sepsis, aspiration, neurogenic, adult respiratory distress syndrome
Diffuse infiltrative diseases: infectious, occupational, neoplastic, immunologic, interstitial pneumonitis
Pleural diseases
Asbestos: causes a pleuroparenchymal disease[16]
Pneumothorax
Neoplasm: carcinoma of the lung[13]
Neuromuscular: Landry-Guillain-Barré syndrome, diaphragmatic disease, myasthenia gravis, muscular dystrophy, multiple sclerosis, spinal cord injury[17,18]

Pulmonary Vascular Disease

Pulmonary emboli
Pulmonary hypertension: primary and secondary causes[19,20]
Pulmonary venous and arterial disorders: systemic

lupus erythematosus and other collagen vascular disorders, sarcoidosis, other causes of diffuse pulmonary infiltrations and fibrosis[21-23]

Pulmonary vascular anomalies[24,25]

Miscellaneous and Less Common Associations

Skeletal deformities

Shock

Metabolic acidosis: may cause hyperventilation without the sensation of dyspnea

Anemia: severe anemia

Hypermetabolic states: exercise, fever, hyperthyroidism, pregnancy

Terminally ill cancer patients[26]

Drug-induced: bronchopulmonary pleural disease and other miscellaneous mechanisms[27-29]

Abnormal central nervous system regulation of respiration[30]

DaCosta's syndrome or neurocirculatory asthenia: symptoms of dyspnea with and without effort, fatigue; initially described in men in wartime, now commonly identified in civilians, and often encountered as a familial disorder[31]

Chest trauma[32]

Cardiac myxomas[33]

Obesity

References

1. Raffin TA, Theodore J: Separating cardiac from pulmonary dyspnea. JAMA 238:2066, 1977.
2. Mahler DA: Dyspnea: diagnosis and management. Clin Chest Med 8:215, 1987.
3. Gorman JM, Fyer MR, Goetz R, et al: Ventilatory physiology of patients with panic disorder. Arch Gen Psychiatry 45:31, 1988.
4. Robinson DP, Greene JW, Walker LS: Functional somatic complaints in adolescents: relationship to negative life events, self-concept, and family characteristics. J Pediatr 113:588, 1988.
5. Becklake MR: Organic or functional impairment. Overall perspective. Am Rev Respir Dis 129 (Suppl):S96, 1984.
6. Sivraprasad R, Payne CB Jr: Nonpulmonary causes of dyspnea. Radiol Clin North Am 22:463, 1984.
7. Burdon JGW, Juniper EF, Killian KJ, et al: The perception of breathlessness in asthma. Am Rev Respir Dis 126:825, 1982.
8. Yamamoto H, Inaba S, Nishimura M, et al: Relationship between the ability to detect added resistance at rest and breathlessness during bronchoconstriction in asthmatics. Respiration 52:42, 1987.
9. Baumann UA, Haerdi E, Keller R: Relations between

clinical signs and lung function in bronchial asthma: how is acute bronchial obstruction reflected in dyspnea and wheezing? Respiration 50:294, 1986.

10. Enarson DA, Vedal S, Schulzer M, et al: Asthma, asthmalike symptoms, chronic bronchitis, and the degree of bronchial hyperresponsiveness in epidemiologic surveys. Am Rev Respir Dis 136:613, 1987.

11. Govindaraj M: What is the cause of dyspnea in asthma and emphysema? Ann Allergy 59:63, 1987.

12. Gift AG, Plaut SM, Jacox A: Psychologic and physiologic factors related to dyspnea in subjects with chronic obstructive pulmonary disease. Heart Lung 15:595, 1986.

13. Mahler DA, Snyder PE, Virgulto JA, Loke J: Positional dyspnea and oxygen desaturation related to carcinoma of the lung. Up with the good lung. Chest 83:826, 1983.

14. Kramer DS, Brown GP, Schuller DE: Proximal airway obstruction presenting as dyspnea. A case of chondrosarcoma of the larynx. Postgrad Med 73(5):133, 1983.

15. Melliere D, Saada F, Etienne G, et al: Goiter with severe respiratory compromise: evaluation and treatment. Surgery 103:367, 1988.

16. Agostoni P, Smith DD, Schoene RR, et al: Evaluation of breathlessness in asbestos workers. Results of exercise testing. Am Rev Respir Dis 135:812, 1987.

17. Scharf S, Bye P, Pardy R, Macklem PT: Dyspnea, fatigue, and second wind. Am Rev Respir Dis 129 (Suppl):S88, 1984.

18. Olgiati R, Jacquet J, Di Prampero PE: Energy cost of walking and exertional dyspnea in multiple sclerosis. Am Rev Respir Dis 134:1005, 1986.

19. Koerner SK: Pulmonary hypertension: etiology and clinical evaluation. J Thorac Imaging 3:25, 1988.

20. Rich S, Dantzker DR, Ayres SM, et al: Primary pulmonary hypertension. A national prospective study. Ann Intern Med 107:216, 1987.

21. Jacobelli S, Moreno R, Massardo L, et al: Inspiratory muscle dysfunction and unexplained dyspnea in systemic lupus erythematosus. Arthritis Rheum 28:781, 1985.

22. Yousem SA, Hochholzer L: Pulmonary hyalinizing granuloma. Am J Clin Pathol 87:1, 1987.

23. Desigan G, Wang M, Wofford B, et al: Occult gastric cancer manifested by progressive shortness of breath in a young adult. South Med J 79:1173, 1986.

24. Davies SF, McQuaid KR, Iber C, et al: Extreme dyspnea from unilateral pulmonary venous obstruction. Demonstration of a vagal mechanism and relief by right vagotomy. Am Rev Respir Dis 136:184, 1987.

25. Stiller RJ, Soberman S, Turetsky A, et al: Agenesis of the pulmonary artery: an unusual cause of dyspnea in pregnancy. Am J Obstet Gynecol 158:172, 1988.

26. Reuben DB, Mor V: Dyspnea in terminally ill cancer patients. Chest 89:234, 1986.

27. Rosenow EC III: Drug-induced bronchopulmonary pleural disease. J Allergy Clin Immunol 80:780, 1987.

28. Brook G, Pain A: Major adverse reactions to a short course of daily rifampicin. Scand J Infect Dis 19:271, 1987.

29. O'Neill PA, Stark RD, Morton PB: Do prostaglandins have a role in breathlessness? Am Rev Respir Dis 132:22, 1985.
30. Przedborski S, Brunko E, Hubert M, et al: The effect of acute hemiplegia on intercostal muscle activity. Neurology 38:1882, 1988.
31. Paul O: DaCosta's syndrome or neurocirculatory asthenia. Br Heart J 58:306, 1987.
32. Landercasper J, Cogbill TH, Lindesmith LA: Long-term disability after flail chest injury. J Trauma 24:410, 1984.
33. DAngelo GJ, Kish GF, Sardesai PG, Tan WS: Cardiac tumors in 19 years of private practice. Am Surg 53:105, 1987.

Selected Readings

Becklake MR: Dyspnea. Organic or functional impairment. Am Rev Respir Dis 129:S96, 1984.
The difficult evaluation of functional versus organic dyspnea.

Burki NK: Dyspnea. Lung 165:269, 1987.
Well-referenced clinical review of current pathophysiology, current methods of testing, and therapeutic modalities available for management of dyspnea.

Cherniack NS, Altose MD: Mechanisms of dyspnea. Clin Chest Med 8:207, 1987.
A review of the various mechanisms of dyspnea, including a discussion integrating current concepts and methods of psychophysical testing of respiratory sensations that help to evaluate dyspnea.

Cockcroft A, Guz A: Breathlessness. Postgrad Med J 63:637, 1987.
A clinical review outlining current concepts of outpatient evaluation of dyspnea. Indications for using various respiratory function tests are reviewed.

DeMaria LC Jr, Cohen HJ: Characteristics of lung cancer in elderly patients. J Gerontol 42:540, 1987.
To define better the natural history of lung cancer in the elderly, a number of characteristics were retrospectively studied from three cohorts: ages 40 to 50, ages 51 to 69, and ages 70 and over. Compared with younger patients, the elderly were more likely to present with dyspnea, but less likely to complain of chest pain.

Eriksson H, Caidahl K, Larsson B, et al: Cardiac and pulmonary causes of dyspnea—validations of a scoring test for clinical–epidemiological use: the Study of Men Born in 1913. Eur Heart J 8:1007, 1987.
Within a population study of the natural history and epidemiology of congestive heart failure, a scoring test to differentiate heart disease from airway obstruction disorders was designed that the authors suggest may be useful for the often difficult distinction between cardiac and pulmonary disease in dyspneic patients.

Killian KJ: The objective measurement of breathlessness. Chest 88 (Suppl):S84, 1985.
A review of current direct and psychophysical methods used to measure breathlessness. Methods of psychophysical scaling are emphasized.

Mahler DA, Wells CK: Evaluation of clinical methods for rating dyspnea. Chest 93:580, 1988.

Review of available clinical methods such as self-ratings and questionnaires for rating dyspnea. Authors conclude that clinical ratings of dyspnea correlate significantly with physiologic parameters of lung function, and such clinical ratings may provide complementary quantitative information to measurements of lung function.

O'Neill PA, Stark RD, Morton PB: Do prostaglandins have a role in breathlessness? Am Rev Respir Dis 132:22, 1985.

Study of the effects of indomethacin on breathlessness during exercise suggests a possible role for prostanoids in the mechanisms that give rise to breathlessness.

Robinson RW, White DP, Zwillich CW: Relationship of respiratory drives to dyspnea and exercise performance in chronic obstructive pulmonary disease. Am Rev Respir Dis 136:1084, 1987.

Variabilities of dyspnea and exercise tolerance in subgroups of patients with COPD are evaluated with a particular focus on attempting to separate classic "blue bloaters" with attenuated respiratory drive who have been described as less dyspneic than the classic "pink puffers." The results of this study do not support the concept that depressed respiratory drives are associated with less dyspnea.

Scharf S, Bye P, Pardy R, et al: Dyspnea, fatigue, and second wind. Am Rev Respir Dis 129:S88, 1984.

A clinical investigation of the second wind phenomenon.

Siefkin AD: Dyspnea in the elderly: cardiac or pulmonary? Geriatrics 40(5):63, 1985.

Clinical review of current concepts and techniques helpful in evaluating dyspnea in the elderly. Dyspnea is a challenge in geriatrics because of the high incidence of pulmonary and cardiac disease, as well as factors associated with aging that commonly influence the feeling of breathlessness.

Sivraprasad R, Payne CB Jr: Nonpulmonary causes of dyspnea. Radiol Clin North Am 22:463, 1984.

A review of nonpulmonary causes of dyspnea including heart failure, anemia, and neuromuscular diseases.

Supplement: Exercise testing in the dyspneic patient. Am Rev Respir Dis 129 (Suppl):part 2, 1984.

An update and review of exercise testing to evaluate dyspnea.

Wasserman K, Casaburi R: Dyspnea: physiological and pathophysiological mechanisms. Annu Rev Med 39:503, 1988.

Well-referenced review of current concepts of physiology and pathophysiology of dyspnea. New developments in monitoring ventilation during exercise and the range of mechanisms that determine exercise ventilation and their testing are included in this excellent review.

Zema MJ, Masters AP, Margouleff D: Dyspnea: the heart or the lungs? Differentiation at bedside by use of the Valsalva maneuver. Chest 85:59, 1984.

A clinical demonstration of the Valsalva maneuver to identify left ventricular dysfunction in dyspneic patients.

14
Acute and Chronic Chest Pain: Noncardiac Causes

Since acute chest pain may be the initial manifestation of underlying cardiac disease, the initial evaluation is directed toward ruling out cardiac disease, particularly myocardial ischemia secondary to coronary artery disease.[1,2] Acute chest pain in the younger adult can be an early manifestation of an acute pulmonary embolism or, uncommonly, underlying viral or idiopathic pleuritic syndromes.[3] When chest pain becomes chronic, if angiographic studies of coronary arteries and other indicators of underlying cardiac disease fail to show objective evidence of heart disease, there are many possible causes of noncardiac chest pain.

Characterizing chest pain into pain that varies with respiration (pleuritic chest pain) and chest pain that does not vary with respiration may help narrow the wide spectrum of possibilities. In patients with non-pleuritic chronic chest pain, a variety of musculo-skeletal syndromes are commonly diagnosed, such as chest wall syndrome and costosternal syndrome.[4] Other major categories of noncardiac chest pain include esophageal disorders, as well as infectious, inflammatory, and neoplastic disorders involving pleura and various parts of the chest wall. An added diagnostic consideration includes a group of patients with certain cardiac disorders, such as mitral valve prolapse, in whom chest pain may seem inappropriate to objective findings.[5]

Musculoskeletal Syndromes	Costochondritis: Tietze's syndrome[6]
	Costosternal syndrome[7]
	Cervical osteoarthritis
	Focal arthritis conditions: particularly conditions that involve articulations of ribs, sternum, and thoracic spine
	Chest wall trauma
	Fibrositis

Psychogenic chest wall pain: anxiety, panic disorder[8-10]

Pseudoxanthoma elasticum[11]

Chest wall joint infections[12]

Sternocostoclavicular hyperostosis[13]

Esophageal Disorders

Esophageal angina can mimic pain of myocardial ischemia and is an important cause of many patients presenting with chest pain in the emergency room.[14]

Reflux esophagitis: demonstration of chest pain associated with an intraesophageal acid perfusion test is helpful diagnostically.[15,16]

Esophageal motor disorders: excessive esophageal contractions or esophageal spasms is a proposed mechanism.[15]

Boerhaave's syndrome: spontaneous esophageal rupture, vomiting, chest pain, and cardiovascular collapse.[17-19]

Pleural Syndromes

Pleuritic infarction secondary to pulmonary embolism[20]

Viral syndromes causing pleuritis

Idiopathic pleurisy

Other infectious causes of pleuritis: *Cryptococcus*, coccidioidomycosis, tuberculosis[21]

Neoplastic causes of pleuritis

Asbestosis

Pneumonia: Legionnaire's disease can mimic pulmonary embolism and pleurisy.[22,23]

Drug-induced pleuritis: methotrexate, 5-fluorouracil, mercury[24-26]

Pleural mesothelioma[27,28]

Familial Mediterranean fever[29]

Whipple's disease: pleuritic chest pain, chronic cough; pleural adhesions can be manifestations of this rare multisystem disease[30]

Vasculitis[31]

Cardiac Disorders

Cardiac disorders sometimes are associated with chest pain that seems disproportionate to objective evidence.

Pericarditis: may occur with chest pain and dyspnea

with ECG changes, that occasionally require the differentiation from myocardial infarction[32]
Mitral valve prolapse[33-35]
Hypertrophic cardiomyopathy
Aortic valve disease
Atypical angina syndrome[36]

Miscellaneous

Pneumothorax[37]
Pulmonary embolism: particularly in young adults[20]
Postherpetic radiculitis: shingles
Collagen vascular disease: systemic lupus erythematosus[38]
Pulmonary hypertension: primary and secondary
Mesenchymal hamartomatous nodules and cysts of the lung[39]
Pneumomediastinum[40]
Pulmonary cryptococcus: frequent pulmonary infection in patients with acquired immune deficiency syndrome (AIDS)[41]
Systemic infection: Q fever, coccidioidomycosis[42,43]
Aneurysm of subclavian artery[44]
Neoplasms

References

1. Ockene IS, Shay MJ, Alpert JS, et al: Unexplained chest pain in patients with normal coronary arteriograms. A followup study of functional status. N Engl J Med 303:1249, 1980.
2. Owens GM: Chest pain. Prim Care 13:55, 1986.
3. Branch WT Jr, McNeil BJ: Analysis of the differential diagnosis and assessment of pleuritic chest pain in young adults. Am J Med 75:671, 1983.
4. Fam AG, Smythe HA: Musculoskeletal chest wall pain. Can Med Assoc J 133:379, 1985.
5. Epstein SE, Gerber LH, Borer JS: Chest wall syndrome. A common cause of unexplained cardiac pain. JAMA 241:2793, 1979.
6. Levey GS, Calabro JJ: Tietze's syndrome: report of two cases and review of the literature. Arthritis Rheum 5:261, 1962.
7. Wolf E, Stern S: Costosternal syndrome: its frequency and importance in differential diagnosis of coronary heart disease. Arch Intern Med 136:189, 1976.
8. Dager SR, Saal AK, Comess KA, Dunner DL: Mitral valve prolapse and the anxiety disorders. Hosp Community Psychiatry 39:517, 1988.
9. Ballenger JC: Unrecognized prevalence of panic disorder in primary care, internal medicine, and cardiology. Am J Cardiol 60:39J, 1987.
10. Beitman BD, Basha I, Flaker G, et al: Atypical or nonanginal chest pain. Panic disorder or coronary artery disease? Arch Intern Med 147:1548, 1987.

11. Sane DC, Vidaillet HJ Jr, Burton CS III: Pitfalls of chest pain. Pseudoxanthoma elasticum. Chest 91:134, 1987.
12. Seviour PW, Dieppe PA: Sternoclavicular joint infection as a cause of chest pain. Br Med J 288:133, 1984.
13. Hallas J, Olesen KP: Sterno-costo-clavicular hyperostosis. A case report with a review of the literature. Acta Radiol 29:577, 1988.
14. Davies HA, Jones DB, Rhodes J: "Esophageal angina" as the cause of chest pain. JAMA 248:2274, 1982.
15. Castell DO: Diagnosis of noncardiac chest pain in older patients. Geriatrics 40(10):61, 1985.
16. Janssens J, Vantrappen G, Ghillebert G: 24-Hour recording of esophageal pressure and pH in patients with noncardiac chest pain. Gastroenterology 90:1978, 1986.
17. Singh GS, Slovis CM: "Occult" Boerhaave's syndrome. J Emerg Med 6:13, 1988.
18. Uehara DT, Dymowski JJ, Schwartz J, Turnbull TL: Chest pain, shock, and pneumomediastinum in a previously healthy 56-year-old man (clinical conference). Ann Emerg Med 16:359, 1987.
19. Bladergroen MR, Lowe JE, Postlethwait RW: Diagnosis and recommended management of esophageal perforation and rupture. Ann Thorac Surg 42:235, 1986.
20. Hull RD, Raskob GE, Carter CJ, et al: Pulmonary embolism in outpatients with pleuritic chest pain. Arch Intern Med 148:838, 1988.
21. Lee CH, Wang WJ, Lan RS, et al: Corticosteroids in the treatment of tuberculous pleurisy. A double-blind, placebo-controlled, randomized study. Chest 94:1256, 1988.
22. Woodhead MA, MacFarlane JT: Legionnaire's disease: a review of 79 community acquired cases in Nottingham. Thorax 41:635, 1986.
23. Fang GD, Yu VL, Vickers RM: Infections caused by the Pittsburgh pneumonia agent. Semin Respir Infect 2:262, 1987.
24. Urban C, Nirenberg A, Caparros B, et al: Chemical pleuritis as the cause of acute chest pain following high-dose methotrexate treatment. Cancer 51:34, 1983.
25. Clavel M, Simeone P, Grivet B: Cardiac toxicity of 5-fluorouracil. Review of the literature, 5 new cases. Presse Med 17:1675, 1988.
26. Giombetti RJ, Rosen DH, Kuczmierczyk AR, Marsh DO: Repeated suicide attempts by the intravenous injection of elemental mercury. Int J Psychiatry Med 18:153, 1988.
27. Antman KH, Corson JM: Benign and malignant pleural mesothelioma. Clin Chest Med 6:127, 1985.
28. Pisani RJ, Colby TV, Williams DE: Malignant mesothelioma of the pleura. Mayo Clin Proc 63:1234, 1988.
29. el Kassimi FA: Acute pleuritic chest pain with pleural effusion and plate atelectasis. Familial Mediterranean fever (periodic disease). Chest 91:265, 1987.
30. Symmons DP, Shepherd AN, Boardman PL, Bacon PA: Pulmonary manifestations of Whipple's disease. Q J Med 56:497, 1985.
31. Falk DK: Pulmonary disease in idiopathic urticarial vasculitis. J Am Acad Dermatol 11:346, 1984.

32. Sternbach GL: Pericarditis. Ann Emerg Med 17:214, 1988.
33. Schatz IJ: Understanding mitral valve prolapse (MVP). Herz 13:235, 1988.
34. Boudoulas H, Wooley CF: Mitral valve prolapse syndrome: neuro-endocrinological aspects. Herz 13:249, 1988.
35. Cheng TO: Mitral valve prolapse. DM 33:481, 1987.
36. Maseri A: The changing face of angina pectoris: practical implications. Lancet 1:746, 1983.
37. Chambers CE, Leaman DM: Management of acute chest pain syndrome. Crit Care Clin 5:415, 1989.
38. Brasington RD, Furst DE: Pulmonary disease in systemic lupus erythematosus. Clin Exp Rheumatol 3:269, 1985.
39. Mark EJ: Mesenchymal cystic hamartoma of the lung. N Engl J Med 315:1255, 1986.
40. Yellin A, Gapany-Gapanavicius M, Lieberman Y: Spontaneous pneumomediastinum: is it a rare cause of chest pain? Thorax 38:383, 1983.
41. Wasser L, Talavera W: Pulmonary cryptococcosis in AIDS. Chest 92:692, 1987.
42. Sawyer LA, Fishbein DB, McDade JE: Q fever: current concepts. Rev Infect Dis 9:935, 1987.
43. Tom PF, Long TJ, Fitzpatrick SB: Coccidioidomycosis in adolescents presenting as chest pain. J Adolesc Health Care 8:365, 1987.
44. Jauch KW, Riel KA, Lauterjung L, Berger H: Aneurysm of the arteria lusoria. Case report and review of the literature. Chirurg 59:418, 1988.

Selected Readings

Beitman BD, Mukerji V, Flaker G, Basha IM: Panic disorder, cardiology patients, and atypical chest pain. Psychiatr Clin North Am 11:387, 1988.
Current concepts of panic disorders and atypical chest pain in cardiology patients with angiographically normal coronary arteries. Authors suggest that many chest pain patients who appear in cardiology clinics who do not have heart disease may benefit from a psychiatric evaluation.

Constant J: The clinical diagnosis of nonanginal chest pain: the differentiation of angina from nonanginal chest pain by history. Clin Cardiol 6:11, 1983.
A nonanginal chest pain category of history taking is suggested to avoid diagnosis such as "atypical chest pain" and "atypical angina."

Goyal RK, Crist JR: Chest pain of esophageal etiology. Hosp Pract 23(9A):15, 1988.
Helpful clinical review of esophageal disorders known to cause chest pain. Authors discuss the difficult patient population with coexistent cardiac and esophageal disease.

Magarian GJ, Hickam DH: Noncardiac causes of angina-like chest pain. Prog Cardiovasc Dis 29:65, 1986.
Comprehensive, well-referenced major clinical review.

Nelson JB, Castell DO: Esophageal motility disorders. DM 34:297, 1988.
Comprehensive, well-referenced clinical monograph.

Peters L, Maas L, Petty D, et al: Spontaneous noncardiac chest pain. Evaluation by 24-hour ambulatory esophageal motility and pH monitoring. Gastroenterology 94:878, 1988.

Twenty-four patients with chronic, daily, substernal chest pain were studied with a prototype 24-hour ambulatory esophageal motility and pH system. Spontaneous chest pain was correlated with a pH less than 4 and abnormal motility changes. Although the majority of chest pain episodes did not have an association with motility or pH change, 59%, or 13 of 22 patients, had at least one chest pain episode that correlated with abnormal findings. Abnormal pH findings correlated with chest pain more frequently than abnormal esophageal motility.

Richter JE, Bradley LA, Castell DO: Esophageal chest pain: current controversies in pathogenesis, diagnosis, and therapy. Ann Intern Med 110:66, 1989.

State of the art review of current concepts and importance of esophageal abnormalities as a potential cause of recurrent noncardiac chest pain.

Richter JE, Castell DO: Esophageal disease as a cause of noncardiac chest pain. Adv Intern Med 33:311, 1988.

Comprehensive, well-referenced review with an emphasis on diagnostic modalities, including traditional barium swallow, esophageal motility studies, edrophonium and acid perfusion provocative testing, and 24-hour continuous patient monitoring and endoscopy.

Semble EL, Wise CM: Chest pain: a rheumatologist's perspective. South Med J 81:64, 1988.

Chest pain is frequently evaluated by rheumatologists once cardiac and esophageal causes of chest pain are ruled out. Musculoskeletal disorders that can result in chest pain are reviewed, including Tietze's syndrome, chest wall pain syndromes, fibrositis, inflammatory arthritis conditions, cervical osteoarthritis, and thoracic spine disease.

15
Wheezing: Common and Less Common Causes

Wheezing is a high-pitched, continuous lung sound that usually reflects a reduction in caliber of medium or large bronchial airways. Although asthma is the most common cause of wheezing, a wide spectrum of disorders from benign to life-threatening can cause airway obstruction. Major mechanisms of extrinsic and intrinsic airway obstruction include disorders that cause smooth muscle constriction, increased secretions, airway edema, mass lesions, foreign body obstruction, and vascular congestion. It is helpful to characterize wheezing as local or diffuse, episodic or chronic, inspiratory or expiratory, or associated with forced or passive respiration to identify the underlying cause.[1] For example, asthma and bronchitis usually cause wheezing that occurs before maximal expiration. When more common disorders are ruled out, less common causes can be benign or life-threatening. In young patients, causes of wheezing can range from benign, factitious wheezing to a life-threatening disorder, such as a pulmonary embolus. It is unusual for asthma to begin late in life; therefore, in elderly patients, other causes, such as chronic obstructive pulmonary disease, congestive heart failure, pulmonary aspiration, bronchogenic carcinoma, and pulmonary embolism, should be considered.[2]

Most Common Causes

Asthma[3,4]

Upper respiratory infections: common trigger of wheezing in asthma patients[4]

Exercise-induced asthma: many nonasthmatic, allergic rhinitis patients wheeze with exercise.[5,6]

Chronic obstructive pulmonary disease (COPD)

Drug-induced asthma: aspirin sensitivity usually occurs in adults with asthma and rhinosinusitis; it may occur with only rhinosinusitis.[7-9]

Pulmonary infections: viral, bacterial, aspiration[10,11]

Pulmonary edema: cardiac and noncardiac

Laryngeal or tracheal obstruction: croup, tracheostenosis, polyp, adenoma, neoplasm, adenopathy, foreign body obstruction, goiter[12-14]

Endobronchial obstruction: neoplasm, foreign body, adenopathy, aortic aneurysm, aortic arch anomaly[15,16]

Less Common Causes

Sinusitis: may underlie some cases of chronic asthma[17]

Pulmonary embolus[18]

Hypersensitivity lung disorders: thermophilic actinomyces, aspergillosis, tropical pulmonary eosinophilia[19,20]

Organic dust hypersensitivity: byssinosis, wood, bark or grain dust exposure, volcanic ash[21]

Chemical and drug-induced: toluene diisocyanate, platinum salts, nickel salts, soldering flux, polyvinyl chloride fumes, freebase smoking, aluminum ("potroom asthma"), beclomethasone aerosol, marijuana smoking, hazardous wastes, azodicarbonamide foaming agent, sulfur dioxide[22-31]

Occupational exposures: miners, farmers, industrial workers[32-34]

Parasitic invasion of the lung (larval stage): toxocariasis[35]

Factitious wheezing[36]

Psychogenic wheezing[37,38]

Vocal cord dysfunction: bilateral abductor paresis and laryngeal dyskinesias can masquerade as asthma.[39-42]

Emotional laryngeal wheezing[43]

Pneumothorax

Adult respiratory distress syndrome (ARDS)

Vasculitis: pulmonary polyarteritis nodosa[44]

Bronchial carcinoid[45]

Cystic fibrosis[46]

References

1. Hollingsworth HM: Wheezing and stridor. Clin Chest Med 8:231, 1987.
2. Braman SS, Davis SM: Wheezing in the elderly. Asthma and other causes. Clin Geriatr Med 2:269, 1986.
3. Shim CS, Williams MH Jr: Relationship of wheezing to the severity of obstruction in asthma. Arch Intern Med 143:890, 1983.
4. Busse WW: The precipitation of asthma by upper respiratory infections. Chest 87:44S, 1985.
5. Anderson SD: Current concepts of exercise-induced asthma. Allergy 38:289, 1983.
6. Suliaman F, Townley RG: The risk of allergy in asthma. Prim Care 14:475, 1987.
7. Lumry WR, Curd JG, Stevenson DD: Aspirin-sensitive asthma and rhinosinusitis: current concepts and recent advances. Ear Nose Throat J 63(2):66, 1984.
8. Virchow C, Szczeklik A, Bianco S, et al: Intolerance to tartrazine in aspirin-induced asthma: results of a multicenter study. Respiration 53:20, 1988.
9. Szczeklik A: Aspirin-induced asthma as a viral disease. Clin Allergy 18:15, 1988.
10. Postlethwaite R: Parvovirus infection in a family with wheeze in an adult. J R Coll Gen Pract 36:220, 1986.
11. Schroeckenstein DC, Busse WW: Viral "bronchitis" in childhood: relationship to asthma and obstructive lung disease. Semin Respir Infect 3:40, 1988.
12. Parrish RW, Banks J, Fennerty AG: Tracheal obstruction presenting as asthma. Postgrad Med J 59:775, 1983.
13. Lakin RC, Metzger WJ, Haughey BH: Upper airway

obstruction presenting as exercise-induced asthma. Chest 86:499, 1984.

14. Lloyd-Thomas AR, Bush GH: All that wheezes is not asthma. Anaesthesia 41:181, 1986.
15. Buckwalter J, Sasaki C, Kopf G, et al: Aortic wheeze: intermittent tracheal obstruction caused by a rare aortic arch anomaly. Ann Otol Rhinol Laryngol 92:383, 1983.
16. Lebow R, Mehta J, Dossett BE Jr, Archie D: One year of wheezing, cough after pneumonia. Hosp Pract 21(2):22, 1986.
17. Slavin RG: Relationship of nasal disease and sinusitis to bronchial asthma. Ann Allergy 49:76, 1982.
18. Sharma GVRK, Sasahara AA, McIntyre KM: Pulmonary embolism: the great imitator. DM 22:4, 1976.
19. Jones DA, Pillai DK, Rathbone BJ, et al: Persisting "asthma" in tropical pulmonary eosinophilia. Thorax 38:692, 1983.
20. Jederlinic PJ, Sicilian L, Gaensler EA: Chronic eosinophilic pneumonia. A report of 19 cases and a review of the literature. Medicine 67:154, 1988.
21. Buist AS, Vollmer WM, Johnson LR, et al: A four-year prospective study of the respiratory effects of volcanic ash from Mt. St. Helens. Am Rev Respir Dis 133:526, 1986.
22. Moller DR, McKay RT, Bernstein IL, Brooks SM: Persistent airways disease caused by toluene diisocyanate. Am Rev Respir Dis 134:175, 1986.
23. Chan-Yeung M: Occupational assessment of asthma. Chest 82:24S, 1982.
24. Rebhun J: Association of asthma and freebase smoking. Ann Allergy 60:339, 1988.
25. Wergeland E, Lund E, Waage JE: Respiratory dysfunction after potroom asthma. Am J Ind Med 11:627, 1987.
26. Shim C, Williams MH Jr: Cough and wheezing from beclomethasone aerosol. Chest 91:207, 1987.
27. Shim CS, Williams MH Jr: Cough and wheezing from beclomethasone dipropionate aerosol are absent after triamcinolone acetonide. Ann Intern Med 106:700, 1987.
28. Tashkin DP, Coulson AH, Clark VA, et al: Respiratory symptoms and lung function in habitual heavy smokers of marijuana alone, smokers of marijuana and tobacco, smokers of tobacco alone, and nonsmokers. Am Rev Respir Dis 135:209, 1987.
29. Ozonoff D, Colten ME, Cupples A, et al: Health problems reported by residents of a neighborhood contaminated by a hazardous waste facility. Am J Ind Med 11:581, 1987.
30. Whitehead LW, Robins TG, Fine LJ, Hansen DJ: Respiratory symptoms associated with the use of azodicarbonamide foaming agent in a plastics injection molding facility. Am J Ind Med 11:83, 1987.
31. Balmes JR, Fine JM, Sheppard D: Symptomatic bronchoconstriction after short-term inhalation of sulfur dioxide. Am Rev Respir Dis 136:1117, 1987.
32. Korn RJ, Dockery DW, Speizer EE, et al: Occupational exposures and chronic respiratory symptoms. A population-based study. Am Rev Respir Dis 136:298, 1987.

33. Dosman JA, Graham BL, Hall D, et al: Respiratory symptoms and pulmonary function in farmers. J Occup Med 29:38, 1987.
34. Costabel U: The alveolitis of hypersensitivity pneumonitis. Eur Respir J 1:5, 1988.
35. Taylor MR, Keane CT, O'Connor P, et al: The expanded spectrum of toxocaral disease. Lancet 1:692, 1988.
36. Downing ET, Braman SS, Fox MJ, Corrao WM: Factitious asthma. Physiological approach to diagnosis. JAMA 248:2878, 1982.
37. Brashear RE: Psychosomatic stridor and wheezing. Indiana Med 80:444, 1987.
38. Barnes SD, Grob CS, Lachman BS, et al: Psychogenic upper airway obstruction presenting as refractory wheezing. J Pediatr 109:1067, 1986.
39. Kivity S, Bibi H, Schwarz Y, et al: Variable vocal cord dysfunction presenting as wheezing and exercise-induced asthma. J Asthma 23:241, 1986.
40. Randolph C, Lapey A, Shannon DC: Bilateral abductor paresis masquerading as asthma. J Allergy Clin Immunol 81:1122, 1988.
41. Ramirez J, Leon I, Rivera LM: Episodic laryngeal dyskinesia. Clinical and psychiatric characterization. Chest 90:716, 1986.
42. Christopher KL, Wood RP II, Eckert RC, et al: Vocal-cord dysfunction presenting as asthma. N Engl J Med 308:1566, 1983.
43. Rodenstein DO, Francis C, Stanescu DC: Emotional laryngeal wheezing: a new syndrome. Am Rev Respir Dis 127:354, 1983.
44. Phanuphak P, Kohler PF: Onset of polyarteritis nodosa during allergic hyposensitization treatment. Am J Med 68:479, 1980.
45. Wynn SR, O'Connell EJ, Frigas E, et al: Exercise-induced "asthma" as a presentation of bronchial carcinoid. Ann Allergy 57:139, 1986.
46. Penketh AR, Wise A, Mearns MB, et al: Cystic fibrosis in adolescents and adults. Thorax 42:526, 1987.

Selected Readings

Banerjee DK, Lee GS, Malik SK, Daly S: Underdiagnosis of asthma in the elderly. Br J Dis Chest 81:23, 1987.
One hundred ninety-nine elderly men and women were assessed for pulmonary function and mental ability. One hundred twenty-one patients had a PEFR less than 70% of that predicted for age and height. Eighty-two patients had 15% or more improvement in their PEFR after being treated with 200 µg salbutamol. Only 6% of patients were previously receiving respiratory-related medication. Authors suggest that potentially reversible airway obstruction often may be overlooked or misdiagnosed in the elderly.

Bascom R, Fisher JF, Thomas RJ, et al: Eosinophilia, respiratory symptoms, and pulmonary infiltrates in rubber workers. Chest 93:154, 1988.
Case reports of respiratory illnesses associated with eosinophilia occurring in a group of workers exposed to fumes from a synthetic rubber-based curing operation. Cases illustrate the diversity of res-

piratory illnesses that may result from common workplace exposures and reinforce the importance of considering occupational exposures in diagnostic considerations, particularly when patients have peripheral eosinophilia.

Baughman RP, Loudon RG: Quantitation of wheezing in acute asthma. Chest 86:718, 1984.

Pulmonary sounds were studied in 20 patients with acute asthmatic attacks as they were being treated with bronchodilators. Analysis of sounds showed that improvement in forced expiratory volume in 1 second was usually associated with the proportion of the respiratory cycle occupied by wheezing (Tw/Ttot), and the sound frequency of the highest pitched wheeze reduced.

Baumann UA, Haerdi E, Keller R: Relations between clinical signs and lung function in bronchial asthma: how is acute bronchial obstruction reflected in dyspnea and wheezing? Respiration 50:294, 1986.

The degree of clinical manifestations and bronchial obstruction in acute asthma was correlated with lung function tests and clinical symptoms in 33 patients during acute attacks of bronchospasm induced by specific and nonspecific inhalation challenge tests and compared with results of similar challenge tests in 12 healthy subjects. About 60% of patients did not reveal wheezing or dyspnea in spite of marked bronchial obstruction. Authors conclude that the degree of bronchospasm can be underestimated if it is related only to subjective complaints and physical signs of expiratory wheezing. Serial lung function tests in certain conditions are suggested to avoid misdiagnosis.

Charbonneau G, Sudraud M, Racineux JL, et al: Forced expirations in normal subjects. Is the shape of the flow rate curve related to existence of a wheeze? Chest 92:825, 1987.

Shapes of flow rate curves from normal subjects during forced expiration were evaluated for a possible alteration of shape associated with the presence of wheezing. The presence of wheezes was correlated with two main shapes: a short onset until a sharp peak, followed by a fast exponential decay, and a triangular shape with a late-appearing wheeze.

Dodge R, Cline MG, Burrows B: Comparisons of asthma, emphysema, and chronic bronchitis diagnoses in a general population sample. Am Rev Respir Dis 133:981, 1986.

An analysis of cases of obstructive lung disease diagnosed during the first 8 years of a community study included 351 subjects who received a new diagnosis of asthma, emphysema, or chronic bronchitis from community physicians. Asthma developed more often in young subjects, emphysema in older subjects, and chronic bronchitis occurred in all groups. Authors suggest a physician bias for labeling male patients emphysematous and female patients asthmatic or bronchitic.

Enarson DA, Vedal S, Schulzer M, et al: Asthma, asthmalike symptoms, chronic bronchitis, and the degree of bronchial hyperresponsiveness in epidemiologic surveys. Am Rev Respir Dis 136:613, 1987.

The usefulness of bronchial hyperresponsiveness in identifying asthmatics was studied through questionnaires. Bronchial hyperresponsiveness was more closely associated with asthma than any other asthma-like symptoms explored by this questionnaire.

Gavriely N, Kelly KB, Grotberg JB, Loring SH: Forced

expiratory wheezes are a manifestation of airway flow limitation. J Appl Physiol 62:2398, 1987.

A clinical research study in normal subjects that describes a mechanical sequence of events involving forced expiratory wheezes and flow limitations with clinical applications, particularly for respiratory wheezes.

Gershel JC, Goldman HS, Stein REK, et al: The usefulness of chest radiographs in first asthma attacks. N Engl J Med 309:336, 1983.

Most first-time wheezers will not have findings on chest radiograph.

Kaplan BA, Mascie-Taylor CG: Asthma and wheezy bronchitis in a British national sample. J Asthma 24:289, 1987.

The relationship between biosocial factors and childhood asthma and wheezy bronchitis was examined in a British national sample. Asthma and wheezy bronchitis correlated with parental occupation, household amenities, and noncrowding in the home.

Kauffmann F, Neukirch F, Korobaeff M, et al: Eosinophils, smoking, and lung function. An epidemiologic survey among 912 working men. Am Rev Respir Dis 134:1172, 1986.

The relationship of eosinophilia in smokers with baseline lung function measurements was studied in a working population of 912 men. Absolute numbers of eosinophils were related significantly to a history of asthma and eczema in childhood as well as current tobacco consumption. Percentage of eosinophils, on the other hand, was related only to the occurrence of asthma and eczema.

Kraman SS: Lung sounds for the clinician. Arch Intern Med 146:1411, 1986.

New techniques for examining lung sounds are explored. An outline of recent work relating to vesicular lung sounds, crackles, and wheezes of interest both to researchers and to clinicians.

Pasterkamp H, Wiebicke W, Fenton R: Subjective assessment vs computer analysis of wheezing in asthma. Chest 91:376, 1987.

A clinical study comparing computer analysis with subjective assessments of wheezing severity made by four groups of health professionals, including pediatric residents, nurses, pediatricians, and physiotherapists. In contrast to a wide variability of interobserver and intraobserver assessment, the computer analysis provided an objective and reproducible characterization of wheezing in asthma.

Snider GL: Distinguishing among asthma, chronic bronchitis, and emphysema. Chest 87:35S, 1985.

A discussion of clinical factors differentiating asthma, chronic bronchitis, and emphysema.

Sparrow D, O'Connor G, Colton T, et al: The relationship of nonspecific bronchial responsiveness to the occurrence of respiratory symptoms and decreased levels of pulmonary function. The Normative Aging Study. Am Rev Respir Dis 135:1255, 1987.

Nonspecific bronchial responsiveness was assessed by an abbreviated methacholine challenge test in 458 male participants of the Normative Aging Study. Cigarette smoking was significantly associated with a positive methacholine response. Findings suggest that an increased level of nonspecific responsiveness is significantly associated with wheeze and cough symptoms and decreased levels of pulmonary function.

Strachan DP, Anderson HR, Bland JM, Peckham C:

Asthma as a link between chest illness in childhood and chronic cough and phlegm in young adults. Br Med J [Clin Res] 296:890, 1988.

This study evaluated the relationship between chest illnesses in childhood to age 7 and the prevalence of cough and phlegm in the winter reported at age 23 in a cohort of 10,557 British children born in 1 week in 1958. Pneumonia and asthma or wheezy bronchitis to age 7 were associated with a significant excess in the prevalence of chronic cough and phlegm at age 23, even after controlling for current smoking.

Wasserman SI: Basic mechanisms in asthma. Ann Allergy 60:477, 1988.

Current concepts of pathophysiology of asthma.

16
Pleural Effusions: Common and Uncommon Causes

A pleural effusion is an accumulation of fluid in the pleural cavity that occurs when a variety of systemic or local diseases disrupt the usual flow of liquid and solutes between parietal and visceral pleura.[1] Effusions may be either exudative or transudative. Exudative effusions are inflammatory fluid; transudative effusions are the result of an oncotic or hydrostatic imbalance. Exudative pleural effusions usually are diagnosed by additional pleural fluid studies, such as cytology, culture, and biopsy. Transudative pleural effusions are most commonly pulmonary manifestations of underlying disorders, such as congestive heart failure or hepatic or renal insufficiency. Exudative effusions are characterized by one or more of the following: (1) pleural-to-serum protein ratio over 0.5, (2) pleural-to-serum LDH ratio greater than 0.6, and (3) pleural LDH level greater than two-thirds upper limit of normal.[2] Infection is the most common cause of exudative pleural effusions.

Transudative Pleural Effusions

Congestive heart failure: most common cause of transudative effusions;[3] characteristic radiographic signs are enlarged cardiac silhouette and isolated right-sided or bilateral effusions[4,5]

Cirrhosis: effusions are usually unilateral and commonly right-sided.[6-8]

Renal failure: nephrotic syndrome, uremia[9]

Myxedema: hypothyroidism can be missed because patients often have other disorders, such as congestive heart failure, to explain the bilateral serous effusions seen in hypothyroidism.[10]

Pericardial disease: often left-sided effusions[11]

Hypoproteinemia

Meigs' syndrome: ascites and hydrothorax associated with ovarian or other pelvic tumor

Peritoneal dialysis

Postpartum pleural effusions: pleural effusion occurs frequently in the first 24 hours after delivery, usually without other signs of cardiopulmonary disorder.[12,13]

Subclavian venous catheterization: ipsilateral effusions probably relate to communication; contralateral effusions may occur from mediastinal leakage.[14]

Exudative Pleural Effusions

Bacterial pneumonia: common cause

Viral pneumonia

Parapneumonia (effusions accompanied by pneumonia): consider possible empyema associated with parapneumonic effusions.[15,16]

Tuberculosis: often predates clinical parenchymal findings; initial tuberculin skin tests and pleural biopsies can be negative initially[17-19]

Mycoplasma pneumonia[20]

Pulmonary embolism: although classically described as bloody exudates, characteristics of effusions with pulmonary embolism vary widely.[21]

Bronchogenic carcinoma: effusion often bloody[22]

Metastatic carcinoma: breast and lung are common

Lymphoma: Hodgkin's lymphoma, non-Hodgkin's lymphoma[23]

Other malignancy-related causes: pleural effusions are common in cancer patients, secondary to the neoplasm or related to other underlying disorders such as congestive heart failure, pulmonary infarction, or infection.[24,25]

Drug related: nitrofurantoin, methysergide, amiodarone[26,27]

Trauma: chylous effusions, subarachnoid-pleural effusions[28,29]

Post upper abdominal surgery: usually resolves within a few days of surgery

Radiation therapy

Mesothelioma: characteristic symptoms include chest pain, dyspnea, and large unilateral pleural effusions[30–32]

Asbestos pleural effusion: important to rule out bronchogenic carcinoma and mesothelioma[33–36]

Postpericardiotomy syndrome: clinical symptoms include fever and signs of pericarditis.[37]

Fungal infections: actinomycosis, histoplasmosis, and coccidioidomycosis[38]

Sarcoidosis: rare and usually associated with extensive parenchymal involvement[39,40]

Rheumatoid arthritis: cytologic characteristics parallel histology of rheumatoid nodules[41]

Systemic lupus erythematosus: drug-induced minoxidil, sulfasalazine[42–45]

Other collagen vascular diseases: scleroderma, Wegener's granulomatosis[46]

Acute pancreatitis: rarely, chest symptoms may dominate the clinical picture[47–49]

Chronic pancreatitis: large pleural effusions can develop with pancreatic pseudocysts that tract into the pleural space in chronic pancreatitis.[47,50]

Esophageal rupture: right-sided pleural effusions common with midesophageal rupture; left-sided pleural effusions common with distal esophageal rupture[51]

Familial Mediterranean fever (periodic paralysis)[52]

Miscellaneous surgical complications: reexpansion pulmonary edema following pneumothorax treatment[53,54]

Miscellaneous neoplasms: hairy cell leukemia, epithelioid hemangioendothelioma, Kaposi's sarcoma[55–57]

Pleural amyloidosis[58]

Waldenström's macroglobulinemia[59]

References

1. Rosa UW: Pleural effusion. How to avoid a diagnostic stalemate. Postgrad Med 75(5):253, 1984.
2. Light RW, MacGregor I, Luchsinger PC, et al: Pleural effusions: the diagnostic separation of transudates and exudates. Ann Intern Med 77:507, 1972.
3. Chetty KG: Transudative pleural effusions. Clin Chest Med 6:49, 1985.
4. Weiss JM, Spodick DH: Laterality of pleural effusions

in chronic congestive heart failure. Am J Cardiol 53:951, 1984.

5. Wiener-Kronish JP, Matthay MA, Callen PW, et al: Relationship of pleural effusions to pulmonary hemo-dynamics in patients with congestive heart failure. Am Rev Respir Dis 132:1253, 1985.

6. Vargas-Tank L, Escobar C, Fernandez G, et al: Massive pleural effusions in cirrhotic patients with ascites. Scand J Gastroenterol 19:294, 1984.

7. Verreault J, Lepage S, Bisson G, Plante A: Ascites and right pleural effusion: demonstration of a peritoneo-pleural communication. J Nucl Med 27:1706, 1986.

8. Eisenberg B, Velchik MG, Alavi A: Pleuroperitoneal communication in a patient with right pleural effusion and ascites diagnosed by technetium-99m sulfur colloid imaging. Clin Nucl Med 13:99, 1988.

9. Maher JF: Uremic pleuritis. Am J Kidney Dis 10:19, 1987.

10. Brown SD, Brashear RE, Schnute RB: Pleural effusion in a young woman with myxedema. Arch Intern Med 143:1458, 1983.

11. Weiss JM, Spodick DH: Association of left pleural effusion with pericardial disease. N Engl J Med 308:696, 1983.

12. Hughson WG, Friedman PJ, Feigin DS, et al: Postpar-tum pleural effusion: a common radiologic finding. Ann Intern Med 97:856, 1982.

13. Stark P, Pollack MS: Pleural effusions in the postpartum period. Radiologe 26:471, 1986.

14. Ciment LM, Rotbart A, Galbut RN: Contralateral ef-fusions secondary to subclavian venous catheters. Chest 83:926, 1983.

15. Varkey B: Pleural effusions caused by infection. Post-grad Med 80(5):213, 1986.

16. Light RW: Parapneumonic effusions and empyema. Clin Chest Med 6:55, 1985.

17. Woodring JH, Vandiviere HM, Fried AM, et al: Update: the radiographic features of pulmonary tuberculosis. AJR 146:497, 1986.

18. Rossi GA, Balbi B, Manca F: Tuberculous pleural effusions. Evidence for selective presence of PPD-spe-cific T-lymphocytes at site of inflammation in the early phase of the infection. Am Rev Respir Dis 136:575, 1987.

19. Bergroth V, Konttinen YT, Nordstrom D, et al: Lym-phocyte subpopulations, activation phenotypes, and spontaneous proliferation in tuberculous pleural effu-sions. Chest 91:338, 1987.

20. Nagayama Y, Sakurai N, Tamai K, et al: Isolation of *Mycoplasma pneumoniae* from pleural fluid and/or cere-brospinal fluid: report of four cases. Scand J Infect Dis 19:521, 1987.

21. Brown SE, Light RW: Pleural effusion associated with pulmonary embolization. Clin Chest Med 6:77, 1985.

22. Albain KS, Hoffman PC, Little AG, et al: Pleural involvement in stage IIIMO non-small-cell broncho-genic carcinoma. A need to differentiate subtypes. Am J Clin Oncol 9:255, 1986.

23. Das DK, Gupta SK, Ayyagari S, et al: Pleural effusions

in non-Hodgkin's lymphoma. A cytomorphologic, cytochemical, and immunologic study. Acta Cytol 31:119, 1987.

24. Prakash UB: Malignant pleural effusions. Postgrad Med 80(5):201, 1986.
25. Salcedo JR: Urinothorax: report of 4 cases and review of the literature. J Urol 135:805, 1986.
26. Gonzalez-Rothi RJ, Hannan SE, Hood CI, Franzini DA: Amiodarone pulmonary toxicity presenting as bilateral exudative pleural effusions. Chest 92:179, 1987.
27. Manolis AS, Tordjman T, Mack KD, Estes NA III: Atypical pulmonary and neurologic complications of amiodarone in the same patient. Report of a case and review of the literature. Arch Intern Med 147:1805, 1987.
28. Singhi P, Nayak US, Ghai S, et al: Rapidly filling pleural effusion due to a subarachnoid-pleural fistula. Clin Pediatr 26:416, 1987.
29. Brook MP, Dupree DW: Bilateral traumatic chylothorax. Ann Emerg Med 17:69, 1988.
30. Hillerdal G: Malignant mesothelioma 1982: review of 4710 published cases. Br J Dis Chest 77:321, 1983.
31. Antman KH, Corson JM: Benign and malignant pleural mesothelioma. Clin Chest Med 6:127, 1985.
32. Herbert A: Pathogenesis of pleurisy, pleural fibrosis, and mesothelial proliferation. Thorax 41:176, 1986.
33. Casey KR, Rom WN, Moatamed F: Asbestos-related diseases. Clin Chest Med 2:179, 1981.
34. Martensson G, Hagberg S, Pettersson K, Thiringer G: Asbestos pleural effusion: a clinical entity. Thorax 42:646, 1987.
35. Chandler KW: Asbestos-related pleuropulmonary disorders. Compr Ther 12:45, 1986.
36. Antman KH: Asbestos-related malignancy. CRC Crit Rev Oncol Hematol 6:287, 1986.
37. McClendon CE, Leff RD, Clark EB: Postpericardiotomy syndrome. Drug Intell Clin Pharm 20:20, 1986.
38. Swinburne AJ, Fedullo AJ, Wahl GW, Farnand B: Histoplasmoma, pleural fibrosis, and slowly enlarging pleural effusion in an asymptomatic patient. Am Rev Respir Dis 135:502, 1987.
39. Sharma OP, Ratto D: Pulmonary sarcoidosis: radiographic features. Clin Dermatol 4:96, 1986.
40. Watts R Jr, Thompson JR, Jasuja ML: Sarcoidosiss presenting with massive pleural effusion. IMJ 163:57, 1983.
41. Montes S, Guarda LA: Cytology of pleural effusions in rheumatoid arthritis. Diagn Cytopathol 4:71, 1988.
42. Segal AM, Calabrese LH, Ahmad M, et al: The pulmonary manifestations of systemic lupus erythematosus. Semin Arthritis Rheum 14:202, 1985.
43. Tunkel AR, Shuman M, Popkin M, et al: Minoxidil-induced systemic lupus erythematosus. Arch Intern Med 147:599, 1987.
44. Clementz GL, Dolin BJ: Sulfasalazine-induced lupus erythematosus. Am J Med 84:535, 1988.
45. Good JT Jr, King TE, Antony VB, et al: Lupus pleuritis. Clinical features and pleural fluid characteristics with special reference to pleural fluid antinuclear antibodies. Chest 84:714, 1983.

46. Hunninghake GW, Fauci AS: Pulmonary involvement in the collagen vascular diseases. Am Rev Respir Dis 119:471, 1979.
47. Light RW: Exudative pleural effusions secondary to gastrointestinal diseases. Clin Chest Med 6:103, 1985.
48. Basran GS, Ramasubramanian R, Verma R: Intrathoracic complications of acute pancreatitis. Br J Dis Chest 81:326, 1987.
49. Renner IG, Savage WT III, Pantoja JL, Renner VJ: Death due to acute pancreatitis. A retrospective analysis of 405 autopsy cases. Dig Dis Sci 30:1005, 1985.
50. Dewan NA, Kinney WW, O'Donohue WJ Jr: Chronic massive pancreatic pleural effusion. Chest 85:497, 1984.
51. Han SY, McElvein RB, Aldrete JS, Tishler JM: Perforation of the esophagus: correlation of site and cause with plain film findings. AJR 145:537, 1985.
52. el Kassimi FA: Acute pleuritic chest pain with pleural effusion and plate atelectasis. Familial Mediterranean fever (periodic disease). Chest 91:265, 1987.
53. Kim YK, Mohsenifar Z, Koerner SK: Lymphocytic pleural effusion in postpericardiotomy syndrome. Am Heart J 115:1077, 1988.
54. Mahfood S, Hix WR, Aaron BL, et al: Reexpansion pulmonary edema. Ann Thorac Surg 45:340, 1988.
55. Bevelaqua FA, Valensi Q, Hulnick D: Epithelioid hemangioendothelioma. A rare tumor with variable prognosis presenting as a pleural effusion. Chest 93:665, 1988.
56. Cooper C, Watts EJ, Smith AG: Salmonella septicemia and pleural effusion as presenting features of hairy cell leukemia. Br J Clin Pract 41:670, 1987.
57. Sivit CJ, Schwartz AM, Rockoff SD: Kaposi's sarcoma of the lung in AIDS: radiologic–pathologic analysis. AJR 148:25, 1987.
58. Knapp MJ, Roggli VL, Kim J, et al: Pleural amyloidosis. Arch Pathol Lab Med 112:57, 1988.
59. Monteagudo M, Lima J, Garcia-Bragado F, Alvarez J: Chylous pleural effusion as the initial manifestation of Waldenström's macroglobulinemia. Eur J Respir Dis 70:326, 1987.

Selected Readings

Bell RC, Andrews CP: Pleural effusions: meeting the diagnostic challenge. Geriatrics 40(4):101, 1985.
A clinical approach to evaluation of pleural effusions in the elderly. Major etiologies of complicated pleural effusions include infection, malignancies, and rheumatologic disorders.

Croonen AM, van der Valk P, Herman CJ, Lindeman J: Cytology, immunopathology, and flow cytometry in the diagnosis of pleural and peritoneal effusions. Lab Invest 58:725, 1988.
One hundred six pleural and peritoneal effusions were studied to investigate the usefulness of immunocytochemistry and flow cytometry to routine cytologic diagnosis. Marker profiles were formulated for the three most frequently occurring diagnoses: reactive mesothelial proliferation, adenocarcinoma, and malignant mesothelioma. Car-

cinoembryonic antigen was the most useful marker to differentiate between adenocarcinoma and malignant mesothelioma.

Cunha BA: Pneumonias acquired from others. 2. Radiographic findings, treatment. Postgrad Med 82(2):149, 1987.

Interesting review of a variety of radiographic patterns commonly seen with certain pneumonias. Infectious and noninfectious causes of infiltrates, miliary patterns, and pleural effusions are reviewed.

Feinsilver SH, Barrows AA, Braman SS: Fiberoptic bronchoscopy and pleural effusion of unknown origin. Chest 90:516, 1986.

Seventy patients who underwent fiberoptic bronchoscopy (FOB) for pleural effusions of unknown origin were reviewed. From this study, authors conclude that although pleural effusion of unknown origin is frequently caused by bronchogenic carcinoma, FOB in the absence of other indications for this procedure should not be considered a routine test.

Fontan-Bueso J, Verea-Hernando H, Garcia-Buela JP, et al: Diagnostic value of simultaneous determination of pleural adenosine deaminase and pleural lysozyme/serum lysozyme ratio in pleural effusions. Chest 93:303, 1988.

To determine the usefulness of adenosine deaminase (ADAp) and lysozyme/serum lysozyme (Lp/Ls) ratios in pleural effusions, simultaneous levels of ADAp and Lp/Ls were determined in 61 tuberculous, 41 malignant, 14 transudates, 5 uncomplicated parapneumonic, 6 empyematous, and 10 miscellaneous causes. By fixing the ADAp values at 33 U and Lp/Ls ratio at 1.2, authors felt they could differentiate tuberculous pleural effusion cases from nontuberculous effusions.

Hausheer FH, Yarbro JW: Diagnosis and treatment of malignant pleural effusion. Cancer Metastasis Rev 6:23, 1987.

A review of complications and special problems associated with pleural effusions in patients with known malignancy. Current diagnostic and therapeutic modalities are discussed.

Houston MC: Pleural fluid pH: diagnostic, therapeutic, and prognostic value. Am J Surg 154:333, 1987.

Forty-three CT examinations of patients referred for evaluation of pleural effusion were reviewed. Focal pleural masses or thick irregular pleura were consistently associated with malignancies. Authors suggest that it is useful to simultaneously image pleura, lungs, and mediastinum by CT for diagnosis, prognosis, staging, and determining optimal therapeutic approaches.

Hsu C: Cytologic detection of malignancy in pleural effusion: a review of 5,255 samples from 3,811 patients. Diagn Cytopathol 3:8, 1987.

A retrospective analysis of 5,255 pleural effusion specimens from 3,811 patients was performed to determine the accuracy of cytopathologic correlations with pleural biopsy, cytologic detection rate of malignancy, and distribution frequency of malignant effusions according to age groups. Cytopathologic correlations were considered 96.5% accurate. Carcinoma of the lung was the most common cause of malignant effusion. Adenocarcinoma of the lung was the most frequent type of malignancy found in pleural effusions. Lymphoreticular malignancies were the most common cause of malignancies in young adults.

Jay SJ: Diagnostic procedures for pleural disease. Clin Chest Med 6:33, 1985.

A systematic approach to the diagnosis of pleural effusions and selective use of tests.

Jay SJ: Pleural effusions. 1. Preliminary evaluation— recognition of the transudate. 2. Definitive evaluation of the exudate. Postgrad Med 80(5):164, 1986.

A two-part article that describes how to document the presence and location of pleural effusion, perform thoracentesis, and differentiate transudates from exudates.

Johnson EJ, Scott CS, Parapia LA, Stark AN: Diagnostic differentiation between reactive and malignant lymphoid cells in serous effusions. Eur J Cancer Clin Oncol 23:245, 1987.

A study of lymphoid cell components in a total of 34 pleural and ascitic aspirates were evaluated immunologically. The study suggests that reactive lymphocytes predominate in effusions from nonhematopoietic malignancies and benign conditions. Authors make a case of using immunologic lymphocyte typing as an adjunct to conventional diagnostic methods, particularly in those patients in whom invasive procedures are undesirable.

Johnston WW: The malignant pleural effusion. A review of cytopathologic diagnoses of 584 specimens from 472 consecutive patients. Cancer 56:905, 1985.

A 14-year experience of cytopathologic diagnoses of malignant pleural effusions was reviewed. Lung was the most common primary tumor type and organ site in both sexes. Malignancies found in males in decreasing frequency were lung, lymphoma/leukemia, gastrointestinal tract, genitourinary tract, and melanoma. Malignancies found in females in decreasing frequency were breast, genital tract (usually ovarian), lung, lymphoma/leukemia, and gastrointestinal tract.

Kochenour NK, Branch DW, Rote NS, Scott JR: A new postpartum syndrome associated with antiphospholipid antibodies. Obstet Gynecol 69:460, 1987.

Three women with antiphospholipid antibodies and a postpartum syndrome of pleuropulmonary disease, fever, and cardiac manifestations are described. Although each patient had either lupus anticoagulant or anticardiolipin antibodies or both, they did not have antinuclear antibodies or fulfill criteria for diagnosis of systemic lupus erythematosus. Authors suggest that patients with antiphospholipid antibodies are at risk for an autoimmune postpartum syndrome.

Maffessanti M, Tommasi M, Pellegrini P: Computed tomography of free pleural effusions. Eur J Radiol 7:87, 1987.

A major review of the usefulness, limitations, and indications for evaluating pleural fluid pH. Authors consider the major value of pleural fluid pH is to determine the need for chest tube drainage in parapneumonic effusions and to evaluate the response to sclerosing agents in patients with malignant pleural effusions.

Nordkild P, Kromann-Anderson H, Struve-Christensen E: Yellow nail syndrome—the triad of yellow nails, lymphedema, and pleural effusions. A review of the literature and a case report. Acta Med Scand 219:221, 1986.

A rare syndrome that presents as a triad of yellow nails, lymphedema, and pleural effusions is described. A review of the literature includes a summary of features found in 97 patients with this syndrome.

Ribera E, Ocana I, Martinez-Vazquez JM, et al: High level

of interferon gamma in tuberculous pleural effusion. Chest 93:308, 1988.

Authors studied interferon (IFN) gamma levels in pleural fluid and serum in 80 patients with pleural effusions; 30 patients with tuberculous pleurisy had high IFN gamma pleural fluid levels; whereas, patients with malignant, nonspecific, parapneumonic, and transudative effusions had low levels of IFN.

Rosa UW: Pleural effusion. How to avoid a diagnostic stalemate. Postgrad Med 75(5):253, 1984.

A systematic, selective approach to the myriad of options available to evaluate pleural fluid.

Rossi GA, Balbi B, Manca F: Tuberculous pleural effusions. Evidence for selective presence of PPD-specific T-lymphocytes at site of inflammation in the early phase of the infection. Am Rev Respir Dis 136:575, 1987.

Patients with tuberculous pleural effusions may be anergic to tuberculin purified-protein derivative (PPD). Authors present data to suggest that early skin anergy in tuberculous pleurisy may be associated with sequestration of PPD-reactive T-lymphocytes in the pleural spaces.

Ruskin JA, Gurney JW, Thorsen MK, Goodman LR: Detection of pleural effusions on supine chest radiographs. AJR 148:681, 1987.

A prospective study of anteroposterior supine radiographs in 34 patients was performed to determine the ability to detect pleural effusions on supine radiographs. Blunting of the costophrenic angle was the most frequent but least specific criterion for detecting pleural effusions on supine radiographs. Loss of hemidiaphragm and increased density of the hemithorax were considered helpful signs. Authors stress that a normal supine radiograph does not exclude a pleural effusion.

Sahn SA: Immunologic diseases of the pleura. Clin Chest Med 6:83, 1985.

A review of the heterogenous immunologic causes of pleural effusions including connective tissue diseases, postcardiac injury syndrome, sarcoidosis, malignancy, and drug reactions. Except for pleural effusions in patients with rheumatoid pleurisy and lupus pleuritis, the pleural fluid findings are usually nonspecific.

Tamura S, Nishigaki T, Moriwaki Y, et al: Tumor markers in pleural effusion diagnosis. Cancer 61:298, 1988.

Pleural fluid from 54 patients with lung cancer, 20 with malignancies other than lung cancer, 18 with tuberculous pleurisy, and 22 other benign diseases (other than tuberculosis) were evaluated for levels of carcinoembryonic antigen (CEA), ferritin, beta$_2$-microglobulin (BMG), acid-soluble glycoprotein (ASP), tisssue polypeptide antigen (TPA), adenosine deaminase (ADA), and immunosuppressive acidic protein (IAP). CEA levels were significantly higher in malignant effusions. No significant differences, however, were found in pleural fluid levels of ferritin, ASP, TPA, or IAP in malignant and benign conditions.

Wiener-Kronish JP, Goldstein R, Matthay RA, et al: Lack of association of pleural effusion with chronic pulmonary arterial and right atrial hypertension. Chest 92:967, 1987.

A retrospective study of nine patients and a prospective study of 18 patients with long-term right atrial or pulmonary arterial hypertension was undertaken to evaluate the influence of right atrial hypertension on the formation of transudative pleural effusions. Authors present data suggesting that chronic elevation of right atrial pressure or pulmonary arterial pressure or both is not enough cause to explain a pleural effusion.

Wiener-Kronish JP, Matthay MA: Pleural effusions associated with hydrostatic and increased permeability pulmonary edema. Chest 93:852, 1988.

State of the art review of current concepts of the pathophysiology of the transudative pleural effusion. Several clinical studies are reviewed, and authors include many useful clinical observations.

17
Infectious Pulmonary Infiltrates: Common and Uncommon Causes of Pneumonia in the Adult

Pneumonia is the most common cause of infectious disease death in the United States.[1,2] The most common infectious causes of pneumonia are pneumococcal pneumonia, *Mycoplasma pneumoniae*, and viral infections, respectively. Although there are endless reported causes of pneumonia, a few infectious causes stand out in frequency within given settings. (See Section VII, Chapters 74–76.)

Acute "Typical" Pneumonia in the Community: Common Causes

"Typical" pneumonia presents with the sudden onset of fever, chills, pleuritic chest pain, and purulent sputum and is often preceded by influenza.

Streptococcus pneumoniae: S. pneumoniae accounts for about 70% of bacterial pneumonia in the United States.[3–6]
Staphylococcus aureus[7,8]
Haemophilus influenzae[9,10]
Klebsiella pneumoniae
Anaerobic bacteria: less common[11]
Legionnaire's disease[12,13]

Pneumonia in the Elderly: Common Causes

Diagnosis of pneumonia in the elderly is often difficult because signs and symptoms are not as obvious. Common community-acquired pathogens in the elderly include *S. pneumoniae, Legionella pneumophila* and enteric gram-negative bacilli. Common hospital and institutional acquired pathogens in the elderly include *K. pneumoniae*, other enteric gram-negative bacilli, *L. pneumophila* and *S. pneumoniae*.[14,15,16]

S. pneumoniae: most common organism cultured in the elderly[17]

S. aureus: most common after influenza

K. pneumoniae: *K. pneumoniae* and *S. aureus* cause pneumonia more frequently in nursing homes than in the community.[17]

H. influenzae, type b[18,19]

L. pneumophila: Legionnaire's disease; infection acquired by inhalation of *Legionella* species-contaminated environmental aerosols, presenting usually as a bronchopneumonia that mimics other nosocomial pneumonias[20–22]

Influenza A virus: most common cause of viral pneumonia in the elderly; particularly dangerous to elderly patients with concomitant pulmonary, cardiovascular, or other debilitating disorders[23–25]

Tuberculosis: abnormal mentation, a common symptom in elderly men with tuberculosis; classic symptoms such as night sweats and weight loss more common in younger men[26–28]

Gram-negative bacilli[29,30]

Acute Atypical Pneumonia in the Community

Consider atypical pneumonia when the prodrome of headache, sore throat, dry cough, and malaise is subacute (3 to 4 days) and when there is marked dissociation between a relatively mild clinical picture and impressive radiographic findings.

M. pneumoniae: most common causes of atypical pneumonia in young adults; common clinical associations include chronic bronchitis, bullous myringitis, lower lobe infiltrates on radiograph[31–36]

Viral pneumonia (numerous viruses can cause pneumonia, but only a few are common)[37]: Influenza A, B,[38] adenovirus,[39] varicella-zoster,[40] primary measles, respiratory syncytial virus,[41,42] cytomegalovirus,[43–45] parainfluenza viruses[46]

L. pneumophila: Legionnaire's disease occurs most

commonly in smokers over 50 years of age. Common clinical associations include abdominal pain, mental confusion, and lobar consolidation on chest radiograph.[47-54]

Francisella tularensis: tularemic pneumonia occurs with exposure to rabbits or ticks; bloody, pleural effusions and hilar adenopathy are common clinical manifestations.[55-57]

Coxiella burnetii: Q fever pneumonia is caused by rickettsia, transmitted by dustborne infected aerosols of cows, sheep, or goats. Common clinical manifestations include myalgias, severe headache, and interstitial pulmonary infiltrates on radiograph.[58-60]

Chlamydia psittaci: psittacosis or ornithosis pneumonia occurs when infected bird material, such as turkey guana, is inhaled. Pleuritic chest pain and chest radiograph findings of lobar consolidation are common clinical associations.[61-66]

Polymicrobial bacteremic pneumonia: a rare, severe outcome of pyogenic organisms such as *S. aureus* and *S. pneumoniae* complicating community-acquired pneumonia[67]

Mixed aerobic bacteria: poor response to specific antibacterial therapy should suggest possible rare mixed potential pathogens[68]

Aspiration Pneumonia

Aspiration pneumonia is characterized by pneumonitis in a dependent segment of lung with necrosis or sometimes abscess formation. Most pathogens are anaerobic; leading species include *Bacteroides, Fusobacterium, Peptococcus*, and *Peptostreptococcus*. Aerobic bacteria often include *S. aureus*, gram-negative bacilli, particularly *Klebsiella* species and *Pseudomonas aeruginosa*.[69] Low pH gastric fluid, large volumes of aspirate, and certain more virulent pathogens worsen the prognosis.[70-72]

S. pneumoniae
Gram-positive cocci anaerobes: *Peptococcus, Peptostreptococcus*
S. aureus
Gram-negative bacilli: mainly *Klebsiella* and *P. aeruginosa*[73]
Gram-negative rod anaerobes: *B. fragilis*, fusobacterium
Enteric gram-negative aerobes

References

1. Centers for Disease Control: Table V. Years of potential life lost, deaths, and death rates, by cause of death and estimated number of physician contacts, by principal diagnosis, United States. MMWR 34:439, 1985.
2. Roth RM, Gleckman RA: Pneumonia in the elderly: a nursing home perspective. Am Fam Physician 31:131, 1985.
3. Perlino CA: Laboratory diagnosis of pneumonia due to *Streptococcus pneumoniae*. J Infect Dis 150:139, 1984.
4. Roberts RB: *Streptococcus pneumoniae*. p. 1589. In Mandell GL, Douglas RG Jr, Bennett JE (eds): Principles and Practices of Infectious Diseases. John Wiley & Sons, New York, 1979.
5. George AL Jr, Savage AM: Fatal group B streptococcal empyema in an adult. South Med J 80:1436, 1987.
6. Bibler MR, Rouan GW: Cryptogenic group A streptococcal bacteremia: experience at an urban general hospital and review of the literature. Rev Infect Dis 8:941, 1986.
7. Goodwin RA, Opal SM: Polymicrobial bacteremic pneumonia: report of three cases caused by *Staphylococcus aureus* and *Streptococcus pneumoniae*. Am Rev Respir Dis 136:1005, 1987.
8. Watanakunakorn C: Bacteremic *Staphylococcus aureus* pneumonia. Scand J Infect Dis 19:623, 1987.
9. Parker RH: *Haemophilus influenzae* respiratory infection in adults. 1. Recognition and incidence. Postgrad Med 73(3):179, 1983.
10. Broughton SJ, Warren RE: A review of *Haemophilus influenzae* infections in Cambridge 1975–1981. J Infect 9:30, 1984.
11. Swartz MA, Marino PL: Anaerobic bacterial pneumonia in an otherwise healthy young adult. Postgrad Med 77(1):87, 1985.
12. Holmberg H: Etiology of community-acquired pneumonia in hospital treated patients. Scand J Infect Dis 19:491, 1987.
13. Benson RF, Thacker WL, Wilkinson HW, et al: *Legionella pneumophila* serogroup 14 isolated from patients with fatal pneumonia. J Clin Microbiol 26:382, 1988.
14. Busby J, Caranasos GJ: Immune function, autoimmunity, and selective immunoprophylaxis in the aged. Med Clin North Am 69:465, 1985.
15. Krumpe PE, Knudson RJ, Parsons G, Reiser K: The aging respiratory system. Clin Geriatr Med 1:143, 1985.
16. Niederman MS, Fein AM: Pneumonia in the elderly. Clin Geriatr Med 2:241, 1986.
17. Garb JL, Brown RB, Garb JR, et al: Differences in etiology of pneumonias in nursing home and community patients. JAMA 240:2169, 1978.
18. Musher DM, Kubitschek KR, Crennan J, et al: Pneumonia and acute febrile tracheobronchitis due to *Haemophilus influenzae*. Ann Intern Med 99:444, 1983.
19. Woodhead MA, MacFarlane JT: *Haemophilus influenzae*

pneumonia in previously fit adults. Eur J Respir Dis 70:218, 1987.
20. Cotton EM, Strampfer MJ, Cunha BA: Legionella and mycoplasma pneumonia—a community hospital experience with atypical pneumonias. Clin Chest Med 8:441, 1987.
21. Kirby BD, Harris AA: Nosocomial Legionnaire's disease. Semin Respir Infect 2:255, 1987.
22. Schurmann D, Ruf B, Fehrenbach FJ, et al: Fatal Legionnaires' pneumonia: frequency of legionellosis in autopsied patients with pneumonia from 1969 to 1985. J Pathol 155:35, 1988.
23. Louria DB, Blumenfeld HL, Ellis JT, et al: Studies on influenza in the pandemic of 1957–1958. II. Pulmonary complications of influenza. J Clin Invest 38:213, 1959.
24. Cate TR: Clinical manifestations and consequences of influenza. Am J Med 82:15, 1987.
25. Ruben FL, Cate TR: Influenza pneumonia. Semin Respir Infect 2:122, 1987.
26. Alvarez S, Shell C, Berk SL: Pulmonary tuberculosis in elderly men. Am J Med 82:602, 1987.
27. Stead WW, To T: The significance of the tuberculin skin test in elderly persons. Ann Intern Med 107:837, 1987.
28. Morris CD, Nell H: Epidemic of pulmonary tuberculosis in geriatric homes. S Afr Med J 74:117, 1988.
29. Levison ME, Kaye D: Pneumonia caused by gram-negative bacilli: an overview. Rev Infect Dis 7 (Suppl 4):S656, 1985.
30. Morrison AJ Jr, Wenzel RP: Epidemiology of infections due to *Pseudomonas aeruginosa*. Rev Infect Dis 6 (Suppl 3):S627, 1984.
31. Dean NL: Mycoplasmal pneumonias in the community hospital. Clin Chest Med 2:121, 1981.
32. Luby JP: Pneumonias in adults due to mycoplasma, chlamydiae, and viruses. Am J Med Sci 294:45, 1987.
33. Moskal MJ: Mycoplasmal infections. Pulmonary and extrapulmonary manifestations. Postgrad Med 82(3):104, 1987.
34. Leigh MW, Clyde WA Jr: Chlamydia and mycoplasmal pneumonias. Semin Respir Infect 2:152, 1987.
35. Wheeler RR, Peacock JE Jr, Alford PT, McLean RL: Atypical community-acquired pneumonia: concurrent infection with *Chlamydia psittaci* and *Mycobacterium tuberculosis*. South Med J 80:402, 1987.
36. Garo B, Garre M, Quiot JJ, et al: *Mycoplasma pneumoniae* infections. A multicenter retrospective study of 182 cases. Presse Med 17:1475, 1988.
37. Glezen WP: Viral pneumonia as a cause and result of hospitalization. J Infect Dis 147:765, 1983.
38. Ruben FL, Cate TR: Influenza pneumonia. Semin Respir Infect 2:122, 1987.
39. Zahradnik JM: Adenovirus pneumonia. Semin Respir Infect 2:104, 1987.
40. Schlossberg D, Littman M: Varicella pneumonia. Arch Intern Med 148:1630, 1988.
41. Vikerfors T, Grandien M, Olcen P: Respiratory syncytial virus infections in adults. Am Rev Respir Dis 136:561, 1987.

42. Levenson RM, Kantor OS: Fatal pneumonia in an adult due to respiratory syncytial virus. Arch Intern Med 147:791, 1987.
43. Idell S, Johnson M, Beauregard L, et al: Pneumonia associated with rising cytomegalovirus antibody titres in a healthy adult. Thorax 38:957, 1983.
44. Weiss RL, Colby TV, Spruance SL, et al: Simultaneous cytomegalovirus and herpes simplex virus pneumonia. Arch Pathol Lab Med 111:242, 1987.
45. Pomeroy C, Englund JA: Cytomegalovirus: epidemiology and infection control. Am J Infect Control 15:107, 1987.
46. Henderson FW: Pulmonary infections with respiratory syncytial virus and the parainfluenza viruses. Semin Respir Infect 2:112, 1987.
47. Edelstein PH, Meyer RD: Legionnaire's disease. A review. Chest 85:114, 1984.
48. Leophonte P, Larios-Ramos L, Rouquet RM: Community-acquired pneumonia. Rev Prat 39:1570, 1989.
49. Fang GD, Yu VL, Vickers RM: Infections caused by the Pittsburgh pneumonia agent. Semin Respir Infect 2:262, 1987.
50. Muder RR, Yu VL, Woo AH: Mode of transmission of *Legionella pneumophila*. A critical review. Arch Intern Med 146:1607, 1986.
51. Korvick JA, Yu VL, Fang GD: Legionella species as hospital-acquired respiratory pathogens. Semin Respir Infect 2:34, 1987.
52. Doebbeling BN, Wenzel RP: The epidemiology of *Legionella pneumophila* infections. Semin Respir Infect 2:206, 1987.
53. Strampfer MJ, Cunha BA: Clinical and laboratory aspects of Legionnaire's disease. Semin Respir Infect 2:228, 1987.
54. Muder RR, Yu VL, Parry MF: The radiologic manifestations of Legionella pneumonia. Semin Respir Infect 2:242, 1987.
55. Penn RL, Kinasewitz GT: Factors associated with a poor outcome in tularemia. Arch Intern Med 147:265, 1987.
56. Evans ME: *Francisella tularensis*. Infect Control 6:381, 1985.
57. Evans ME, Gregory DW, Schaffner W, McGee ZA: Tularemia: a 30-year experience with 88 cases. Medicine 64:251, 1985.
58. Kosatsky T: Household outbreak of Q-fever pneumonia related to a parturient cat. Lancet 2:1447, 1984.
59. Langley JM, Marrie TJ, Covert A, et al: Poker players' pneumonia. An urban outbreak of Q fever following exposure to a parturient cat. N Engl J Med 319:354, 1988.
60. Sawyer LA, Fishbein DS, McDade JE: Q fever: current concepts. Rev Infect Dis 9:935, 1987.
61. Saikku P, Wang SP, Kleemola M, et al: An epidemic of mild pneumonia due to an unusual strain of *Chlamydia psittaci*. J Infect Dis 151:832, 1985.
62. Larson E, Nachamkin I: Chlamydial infections. Am J Infect Control 13:259, 1985.
63. Grayston JT, Kuo CC, Wang SP, Altman J: A new *Chlamydia psittaci* strain, TWAR, isolated in acute respiratory tract infections. N Engl J Med 315:161, 1986.

64. Lisby SM, Nahata MC: Recognition and treatment of chlamydial infections. Clin Pharm 6:25, 1987.
65. Wheeler RR, Peacock JE Jr, Alford PT, McLean RL: Atypical community-acquired pneumonia: concurrent infection with *Chlamydia psittaci* and *Mycobacterium tuberculosis*. South Med J 80:402, 1987.
66. Wainwright AP, Beaumont AC, Kox WJ: Psittacosis: diagnosis and management of severe pneumonia and multi organ failure. Intensive Care Med 13:419, 1987.
67. Goodwin RA, Opal SM: Polymicrobial bacteremic pneumonia: report of three cases caused by *Staphylococcus aureus* and *Streptococcus pneumoniae*. Am Rev Respir Dis 136:1005, 1987.
68. Brown RB, Sands M, Ryczak M: Community-acquired pneumonia caused by mixed aerobic bacteria. Chest 90:810, 1986.
69. Lode H: Microbiological and clinical aspects of aspiration pneumonia. J Antimicrob Chemother 21 (Suppl):83, 1988.
70. Chokshi SK, Asper RF, Khandheria BK: Aspiration pneumonia: a review. Am Fam Physician 33(3):195, 1986.
71. Kinni ME, Stout MM: Aspiration pneumonitis: predisposing conditions and prevention. J Oral Maxillofac Surg 44:378, 1986.
72. Bartlett JG: Anaerobic bacterial infections of the lung. Chest 91:901, 1987.
73. Padmanabhan K, Rajgopalan K, Yeo K, Dhar SR: Intracavitary mass in a patient with *Klebsiella pneumoniae*. Chest 93:187, 1988.

Selected Readings

Ajello GW, Bolan GA, Hayes PS, et al: Commercial latex agglutination tests for detection of *Haemophilus influenzae* type b and *Streptococcus pneumoniae* antigens in patients with bacteremic pneumonia. J Clin Microbiol 25:1388, 1987.

Usefulness of commercial latex agglutination kits for detection of H. influenzae *type b and* S. pneumoniae *antigens in serum and urine were studied. Results suggest that these kits are useful in diagnosing* H. influenzae *type b pneumonia, however, they are limited in their ability to diagnose* S. pneumoniae *pneumonia.*

Bartlett JG: Diagnosis of bacterial infections of the lung. Clin Chest Med 8:119, 1987.

Review of indications, controversies, limitations, and strengths of various diagnostic modalities. Modalities reviewed include sputum Gram stain and culture, transtracheal aspiration, transthoracic needle aspiration, and bronchoscopy.

Bartlett JG: Anaerobic bacterial infections of the lung. Chest 91:901, 1987.

State of the art clinical review.

British Thoracic Society and the Public Health Laboratory Service: Community-acquired pneumonia in adults in British hospitals in 1982–1983: a survey of etiology, mortality, prognostic factors and outcome. Q J Med 62:195, 1987.

Four hundred fifty-three adults with community-acquired pneumonia were evaluated. Microbiologic diagnoses were established in 67%; pathogens identified in decreasing frequency included S.

pneumoniae, M. pneumoniae, and influenza A virus. *Authors suggest their data support the view that most patients in the microbiologically-negative group (33%) had S.* pneumoniae *infection. Most useful diagnostic tests were blood cultures, sputum cultures, sputum pneumococcal antigen assays, and tests for serum mycoplasma specific IgM. Morbidity and mortality risk factors are analyzed.*

Campinos L, Duval G, Couturier M, et al: The value of early fibreoptic bronchoscopy after aspiration of gastric contents. Br J Anaesth 55:1103, 1983.
Authors make a case for usefulness of early fiberoptic bronchoscopic examination of gastric contents in suspected cases of gastric fluid aspiration.

Celis R, Torres A, Gatell JM, et al: Nosocomial pneumonia. A multivariate analysis of risk and prognosis. Chest 93:318, 1988.
One hundred twenty consecutive episodes of nosocomial pneumonia in 118 nonneutropenic adults admitted to a teaching hospital were investigated to determine prognostic risk factors. High risk organisms identified included Pseudomonas aeruginosa, Enterobacteriaceae *and other gram-negative bacilli,* Streptococcus faecalis, S. aureus, Candida *species,* Aspergillus *species, and episodes of polymicrobial pneumonia. Factors significantly contributing to a poor prognosis included tracheal intubation, depressed consciousness, underlying chronic lung disease, prior thoracic or upper abdominal surgery, large aspirations, and age older than 70 years.*

Cunha BA: Pneumonia acquired from others. 2. Radiographic findings, treatment. Postgrad Med 82(2):149, 1987.
Useful clinical discussion of radiographic features and differential diagnostic possibilities of pulmonary infection. Patterns discussed include miliary patterns, cavitary lesions, bilateral hilar adenopathy, pleural effusions, and pulmonary nodules. Infectious as well as noninfectious causes are discussed.

Faling LJ: New advances in diagnosing nosocomial pneumonia in intubated patients. Part I. Advances in preventing nosocomial pneumonia. Part II. Am Rev Respir Dis 137:253, 1988.
Two-part, state-of-the-art review of advances in diagnosing and preventing nosocomial pneumonia.

Fedullo AJ, Swinburne AJ: Relationship of patient age to clinical features and outcome for in-hospital treatment of pneumonia. J Gerontol 40:29, 1985.
Clinical observations that do not support some time-honored descriptions of pneumonia in the elderly.

Gleckman R, DeVita J, Hibert D, et al: Sputum gram stain assessment in community-acquired bacteremic pneumonia. J Clin Microbiol 26:846, 1988.
A prospective study was performed over a 4.5-year period to determine the ability of a sputum Gram stain to predict the cause of community-acquired bacterial pneumonia. Data from this study suggest that the morphology of pathogens identified on stained sputum can result in selecting appropriate monotherapy approximately 94% of the time within the study's defined criteria.

Gross JS, Neufeld RR, Libow LS, et al: Autopsy study of the elderly institutionalized patient. Review of 234 autopsies. Arch Intern Med 148:173, 1988.
Clinical and autopsy records of 234 patients who died during

14.5-year period at a chronic care institution were analyzed for accuracy of clinical determination of death. The most common causes of death in decreasing order of frequency were bronchopneumonia, congestive heart failure, metastatic carcinoma, pulmonary embolism, myocardial infarction, cerebrovascular accident, and a category of unknown and miscellaneous. The highest diagnostic error rate was the underdiagnosis of pulmonary embolism. Pneumonia was correctly diagnosed antemortem in 73% of patients.

Gross PA: Epidemiology of hospital-acquired pneumonia. Semin Respir Infect 2:2, 1987.

Nosocomial pneumonia is associated with a high mortality. This study suggests that major risk factors are increasing age, thoracoabdominal surgery, chronic lung disease, length of hospital stay, immunosuppressive therapy, and continuous ventilatory support.

Hager H, Verghese A, Alvarez S, Berk SL: *Branhamella catarrhalis* respiratory infections. Rev Infect Dis 9:1140, 1987.

B. catarrhalis, a normal commensal of the oropharynx, has been increasingly identified as an important etiology of bronchitis and bacterial pneumonia. The microbiologic, immunologic and clinical features of B. catarrhalis *infection are reviewed.*

Hershey CO, Panaro V: Round pneumonia in adults. Arch Intern Med 148:1155, 1988.

An interesting review of three adult patients with rounded densities on chest radiographs in whom the final diagnosis was a presumed lower respiratory tract infection. Usually described in children, "round pneumonias" have not often been characterized in adult patients.

Holmberg H: Etiology of community-acquired pneumonia in hospital treated patients. Scand J Infect Dis 19:491, 1987.

A 1-year prospective study of adult patients with community-acquired, radiologically verified, hospital treated pneumonia was performed at an infectious diseases department in Orebro, Sweden. Median age of 147 patients studied was 71 years. A pneumococcal etiology was established in 46.9% of patients. Less common, but not infrequent infections included H. influenzae A virus, M. pneumoniae, Legionnaire's disease, and B. catarrhalis.

Kerttula Y, Leinonen M, Koskela M, Makela PH: The etiology of pneumonia. Application of bacterial serology and basic laboratory methods. J Infect 14:21, 1987.

Newer bacterial and established viral serologic methods, as well as blood cultures, were studied in the diagnosis of 162 patients with community-acquired pneumonia. Specific etiology was obtained in 79 (49.4%) patients. Pneumococcus was the most common etiologic pathogen; others included H. influenzae, B. catarrhalis, Neisseria meningitidis, Chlamydia species, and Mycoplasma. In 58% of patients with viral pneumonia, there was evidence of mixed infection with bacteria.

Levin S: The atypical pneumonia syndrome. JAMA 251:945, 1984.

Current concepts with an historical perspective. Well referenced.

Levy M, Dromer F, Brion N, et al: Community-acquired pneumonia. Importance of initial noninvasive bacteriologic and radiographic investigations. Chest 93:43, 1988.

A 1-year epidemiologic survey of acute community-acquired pneumonia was prospectively investigated in 116 adult nonimmunocompromised patients to evaluate the importance of initial noninvasive investigations, such as blood cultures, quantitative sputum cultures, and chest radiographs. Quantitative sputum culture or blood culture resulted in a bacteriologic diagnosis in 44% of patients. Alveolar densities were associated with a bacterial infection in 90% of cases of known etiology. Authors suggest a pragmatic strategy of initial management of community-acquired pneumonia.

Luby JP: Pneumonia in adults due to mycoplasma, chlamydia, and viruses. Am J Med Sci 294:45, 1987.

Adult pneumonia due to mycoplasma, chlamydiae, and viruses are common. Recent trends are discussed, such as the emergence of a C. psittaci *strain (TWAR), which is passed from human to human. Current trends and problems in using antiviral agents are also discussed.*

MacFarlane JT, Miller AC, Roderick Smith WH, et al: Comparative radiographic features of community-acquired Legionnaires' disease, pneumococcal pneumonia, mycoplasma pneumonia, and psittacosis. Thorax 39:28, 1984.

Radiographic features of selected pulmonary infections.

Martin SJ, Hoganson DA, Thomas ET: Detection of *Streptococcus pneumoniae* and *Haemophilus influenzae* type b antigens in acute nonbacteremic pneumonia. J Clin Microbiol 25:248, 1987.

Commercially available latex agglutination and coagglutination reagents were evaluated for their ability to detect bacterial antigens in sera of 165 patients to determine their usefulness in the rapid diagnosis of pneumonia. No evidence of cross-reactivity or false-positive reactions was observed. Authors suggest that since a negative agglutination test may occur during nonbacteremic infections, these reagents should be used only in conjunction with standard bacteriologic tests.

McGarry T, Giosa R, Rohman M, Huang CT: Pneumatocele formation in adult pneumonia. Chest 92:717, 1987.

Three cases of adult patients with pneumatocele formation are reviewed. Although pneumatoceles are usually asymptomatic, they may enlarge and compress adjacent lung and mediastinum. Etiology, consequences, and treatment are discussed.

Murphy TF, Apicella MA: Nontypable *Haemophilus influenzae*: a review of clinical aspects, surface antigens, and the human immune response to infection. Rev Infect Dis 9:1, 1987.

Nontypable H. influenzae *is an established pathogen in both adults and children. Recent work has identified distinctions between nontypable and type b strains of* H. influenzae. *These organisms affect different patient populations and cause different infections with distinct surface antigen and genetic differences. The most common clinical manifestation of nontypable* H. influenzae *in adults is lower respiratory tract infection, particularly in the elderly with chronic bronchitis.*

Niederman MS: Strategies for the prevention of pneumonia. Clin Chest Med 8:543, 1987.

State-of-the-art methods of prophylaxis, including pneumococcal vaccines and topical antibiotics administered in the upper and lower airway, and other newer infection control methods are discussed.

Palmer DL: Microbiology of pneumonia in the patient at risk. Am J Med 76(5A):53, 1984.

Problems of diagnosis of pulmonary infection in the elderly.

Stratton CW: Bacterial pneumonias—an overview with

emphasis on pathogenesis, diagnosis, and treatment. Heart Lung 15:226, 1986.
Well-referenced state-of-the-art summary.

Tobin MJ: Diagnosis of pneumonia: techniques and problems. Clin Chest Med 8:513, 1987.
Clinical review of diagnostic strategies in patients suspected of having pneumonia. Problems and controversies regarding diagnostic modalities in patients with hospital-acquired pneumonia are particularly well reviewed.

Warner DO, Warner MA, Divertie MB: Open lung biopsy in patients with diffuse pulmonary infiltrates and acute respiratory failure. Am Rev Respir Dis 137:90, 1988.
The usefulness of open lung biopsy in patients with diffuse pulmonary infiltrates and acute respiratory failure was examined within the context of an 11-year experience with 80 patients. Open lung biopsy provided a specific diagnosis in 53 patients (66%). Fifteen patients (19%) suffered complications possibly related to open lung biopsy.

Winterbauer RH, Dreis DF: New diagnostic approaches to the hospitalized patient with pneumonia. Semin Respir Infect 2:57,1987.
A review of recent advances in invasive techniques such as fiberoptic bronchoscopy coupled with quantitative bacterial cultures and immunofluorescence demonstration of antibody-coated bacteria.

Wollschlager CM, Khan FA, Khan A: Utility of radiography and clinical features in the diagnosis of community-acquired pneumonia. Clin Chest Med 8:393, 1987.
A clinical review of the approach to the differential diagnosis of community-acquired pneumonia. Authors include a discussion of the altered differential diagnosis in patients with diabetes and alcoholism.

Woodhead MA, Macfarlane JT: Comparative clinical and laboratory features of legionella with pneumococcal and mycoplasma pneumonias. Br J Dis Chest 81:133, 1987.
Eighty-three cases of community-acquired pneumococcal pneumonia, 79 cases of legionella pneumonia and 62 cases of mycoplasma pneumonia were compared to identify clinical and laboratory features. Although no unique features were identified, some general trends included the following: (1) patients with mycoplasma tended to be younger and were more likely to have had prior antibiotics before referral; (2) in both pneumococcal and legionella pneumonia, multisystem features were common, including confusion, high fever, hyponatremia, and abnormal liver functions. High leukocyte counts were particularly common with pneumococcal pneumonia.

Woodhead MA, Macfarlane JT, McCracken JS, et al: Prospective study of the etiology and outcome of pneumonia in the community. Lancet 1:671, 1987.
A prospective 1-year study of community pneumonia in Nottingham evaluated 236 of 251 episodes of pneumonia. Acute radiographic changes were present in 93 (39%). Identified pathogens in 129 (55%) most frequently included S. pneumoniae, H. influenzae and influenza viruses. Uncommon pathogens included Mycoplasma *and* L. pneumophilia.

18

Noninfectious Pulmonary Infiltrates: Common and Uncommon Causes

Chest radiographic findings in the acutely ill patient with fever, productive sputum, and diagnostic laboratory findings are typically patterns of perihilar or interstitial pulmonary infiltrates. Even these typical radiographic patterns, with or without concomitant clinical findings, can be atypical presentations of noninfectious disorders. When chest radiographic patterns consist of peripheral infiltrates and unusual infections, such as actinomycosis or nocardiosis, are ruled out, noninfectious causes are a significant possibility.

Virtually every pattern of infiltrate—peripheral, perihilar, bilateral hilar, as well as nodules and effusions—have possible infectious and noninfectious causes.[1] Noninfectious pulmonary infiltrates of unknown etiology usually require biopsy and careful pathologic evaluation for diagnosis. Common infectious causes of pulmonary infiltrates are listed in Section II, Chapter 16: Pleural Effusions. Infectious and noninfectious causes of pulmonary infiltrates in patients with HIV infection and other immune compromise disorders are listed in Section VII, Chapters 75 and 76.

Common Noninfectious Causes

Neoplastic: neoplasia can simulate pneumonia, and pneumonia can simulate tumors.[2]
Primary and metastatic bronchogenic carcinoma
Lymphoma[3]
Diffuse carcinomatosis
Bronchiolar alveolar carcinoma[4]
Mycosis fungoides[5]
Radiation pneumonitis[6-10]
Trauma: lung contusion, hemorrhage
Pulmonary edema: cardiac, neurogenic, hypersensitivity

Atelectasis
Aspiration: chemical and lipoid pneumonitis[11]
Pulmonary embolism: pulmonary infarction[12]

**Less Common
Noninfectious Causes**

Drugs and toxins[13-15]
Drugs causing interstitial pneumonitis and fibrosis: cyclophosphamide, busulfan, BCNU (carmustine), melphalan, bleomycin, dantrolene, oxygen therapy, hydrocarbon aerosol[16-18]
Drugs causing pulmonary hypersensitivity and eosinophilia: nitrofurantoin, penicillin, methotrexate, sulfonamides, isoniazid, gold, streptomycin, procainamide, butane, humidifier aerosols and air conditioners, Fansidar, beryllium oxide[19-27]
Drugs causing pulmonary edema and pulmonary infiltrates: heroin, methadone, propoxyphene, thiazides, amiodarone[28]
Crack lung: pulmonary infiltrates and bronchospasm following cocaine inhalation[29]
Silicone pneumonitis: following subcutaneous injections of silicone[30]
Granulomas: sarcoidosis, Wegener's granulomatosis, eosinophil granuloma[31]
Allergic phenomena: bronchopulmonary aspergillosis, alveolitis, and chronic eosinophilic pneumonia[32-37]
Interstitial pneumonias: usual interstitial (UIP), desquamative interstitial (DIP), and lymphocytic interstitial pneumonia (LIP)[38-40]
Pneumoconioses: berylliosis, asbestosis, silicosis, Caplan's syndrome[41,42]
Rheumatoid nodules
Fat embolism[43]
Löffler's syndrome
Collagen vascular diseases: systemic lupus erythematosus, scleroderma, Sjögren's syndrome[44-46]
Other hypersensitivity pneumonitis[47]
Nonspecific and idiopathic pulmonary fibrosis[48]
Chronic bronchiolitis: bronchiolitis obliterans and organizing pneumonia[49,50]
Uremic pneumonitis[51-53]
Pulmonary alveolar proteinosis (PAP), alveolar phospholipoproteinosis[54,55]
Lipoma[56,57]
Vascular anomalies: Thoracic hemangiomatosis, pseudoaneurysm[58,59]

References

1. Cunha BA: Pneumonias acquired from others. 2. Radiographic findings, treatment. Postgrad Med 82(2):149, 1987.
2. Weingarten NM, Fred HL: Pneumonia simulating tumor of the lung. Am Fam Physician 26(6):117, 1982.
3. Schuurman HJ, Gooszen HC, Tan IW, et al: Low-grade lymphoma of immature T-cell phenotype in a case of lymphocytic interstitial pneumonia and Sjögren's syndrome. Histopathology 11:1193, 1987.
4. Axiotis CA, Jennings TA: Observations on bronchioloalveolar carcinomas with special emphasis on localized lesions. A clinicopathological, ultrastructural, and immunohistochemical study of 11 cases. Am J Surg Pathol 12:918, 1988.
5. Rubin DL, Blank N: Rapid pulmonary dissemination in mycosis fungoides simulating pneumonia. A case report and review of the literature. Cancer 56:649, 1985.
6. Gross NJ: Pulmonary effects of radiation therapy. Ann Intern Med 86:81, 1977.
7. Gibson PG, Bryant DH, Morgan GW, et al: Radiation-induced lung injury: a hypersensitivity pneumonitis? Ann Intern Med 109:288, 1988.
8. Frija J, Ferme C, Baud L, et al: Radiation-induced lung injuries: a survey by computed tomography and pulmonary function tests in 18 cases of Hodgkin's disease. Eur J Radiol 8:18, 1988.
9. Ikezoe J, Takashima S, Morimoto S, et al: CT appearance of acute radiation-induced injury in the lung. AJR 150:765, 1988.
10. Koga K, Kusumoto S, Watanabe K, et al: Age factor relevant to the development of radiation pneumonitis in radiotherapy of lung cancer. Int J Radiat Oncol Biol Phys 14:367, 1988.
11. Casademont J, Xaubet A, Lopez-Guillermo J, et al: Radiographic bilateral cavitary lesions in lipoid pneumonia. Eur Respir J 1:93, 1988.
12. Dunnick NR, Newman GE, Perlmutt LM, Braun SD: Pulmonary embolism. Curr Probl Diagn Radiol 17:197, 1988.
13. Batist G, Andrews JL Jr: Pulmonary toxicity of antineoplastic drugs. JAMA 246:1449, 1981.
14. Cooper JA Jr, White DA, Matthay RA: Drug-induced pulmonary disease. Part I. Cytotoxic drugs. Am Rev Respir Dis 133:321, 1986.
15. White DA, Orenstein M, Godwin TA, et al: Chemotherapy-associated pulmonary toxic reactions during treatment for breast cancer. Arch Intern Med 144:953, 1984.
16. Van Barneveld PW, Sleijfer DT, van der Mark TW, et al: Natural course of bleomycin-induced pneumonitis. A follow-up study. Am Rev Respir Dis 135:48, 1987.
17. Miller DH, Haas LF: Pneumonitis, pleural effusion, and pericarditis following treatment with dantrolene. J Neurol Neurosurg Psychiatry 47:553, 1984.
18. Perrone H, Passero MA: Hydrocarbon aerosol pneumonitis in an adult. Arch Intern Med 143:1607, 1983.

19. Searles G, McKendry RJ: Methotrexate pneumonitis in rheumatoid arthritis: potential risk factors. Four case reports and a review of the literature. J Rheumatol 14:1164, 1987.

20. Akoun GM, Gauthier-Rahman S, Mayaud CM, et al: Leukocyte migration inhibition in methotrexate-induced pneumonitis. Evidence for an immunologic cell-mediated mechanism. Chest 91:96, 1987.

21. Evans RB, Ettensohn DB, Fawaz-Estrup F, et al: Gold lung: recent developments in pathogenesis, diagnosis, and therapy. Semin Arthritis Rheum 16:196, 1987.

22. Lertratanakul Y, Budiman-Mak E, Dietz AA, et al: Gold pneumonitis. A case report with electron microscopy and electron probe analysis. Clin Exp Rheumatol 4:371, 1986.

23. Goldberg SK, Lipschutz JB, Ricketts RM, et al: Procainamide-induced lupus lung disease characterized by neutrophil alveolitis. Am J Med 76:146, 1984.

24. Cartwright TR, Brown ED, Brashear RE: Pulmonary infiltrates following butane "fire-breathing." Arch Intern Med 143:2007, 1983.

25. Baur X, Behr J, Dewair M, et al: Humidifier lung and humidifier fever. Lung 166:113, 1988.

26. McCormack D, Morgan WK: Fansidar hypersensitivity pneumonitis. Br J Dis Chest 81:194, 1987.

27. Eisenbud M: Commentary and update: chemical pneumonia in workers extracting beryllium oxide. Cleve Clin Q 51:441, 1984.

28. Arnon R, Raz I, Chajek-Shaul T, et al: Amiodarone pulmonary toxicity presenting as a solitary lung mass. Chest 93:425, 1988.

29. Kissner DG, Lawrence WD, Selis JE, Flint A: Crack lung: pulmonary disease caused by cocaine abuse. Am Rev Respir Dis 136:1250, 1987.

30. Chastre J, Brun P, Soler P, et al: Acute and latent pneumonitis after subcutaneous injections of silicone in transsexual men. Am Rev Respir Dis 135:236, 1987.

31. Israel HL, Patchefsky AS, Saldana MJ: Wegener's granulomatosis, lymphomatoid granulomatosis, and benign lymphocytic angiitis and granulomatosis of lung. Recognition and treatment. Ann Intern Med 87:691, 1977.

32. Bosken CH, Myers JL, Greenberger PA, Katzenstein AL: Pathologic features of allergic bronchopulmonary aspergillosis. Am J Surg Pathol 12:216, 1988.

33. Wallaert B, Bonniere P, Prin L, et al: Primary biliary cirrhosis. Subclinical inflammatory alveolitis in patients with normal chest roentgenograms. Chest 90:842, 1986.

34. Adickman M, Tuthill TM: Pulmonary infiltrates and eosinophilia associated with drug reactions and parasitic infections. Postgrad Med 60(3):143, 1976.

35. Lakhanpal S, Duffy J, Engel AG: Eosinophilia associated with perimyositis and pneumonitis. Mayo Clin Proc 63:37, 1988.

36. Prin L, Capron M, Gosset P, et al: Eosinophilic lung disease: immunological studies of blood and alveolar eosinophils. Clin Exp Immunol 63:249, 1986.

37. Jederlinic PJ, Sicilian L, Gaensler EA: Chronic eosinophilic pneumonia. A report of 19 cases and a review of the literature. Medicine 67:154, 1988.

38. Symposium: Interstitial lung disease. Eur J Respir Dis 64(S-126):61, 1983.
39. Staples CA, Muller NL, Vedal S, et al: Usual interstitial pneumonia: correlation of CT with clinical, functional, and radiologic findings. Radiology 162:377, 1987.
40. Lipworth B, Woodcock A, Addis B, Turner-Warwick M: Late relapse of desquamative interstitial pneumonia. Am Rev Respir Dis 136:1253, 1987.
41. Bisson G, Lamoureux G, Begin R: Quantitative gallium 67 lung scan to assess the inflammatory activity in the pneumoconioses. Semin Nucl Med 17:72, 1987.
42. Caplan A: Rheumatoid disease and pneumoconiosis. (Caplan's syndrome). Proc R Soc Med 52:1111, 1959.
43. Rosen JM, Braman SS, Hasan FM, Teplitz C: Nontraumatic fat embolization. A rare cause of new pulmonary infiltrates in an immunocompromised patient. Am Rev Respir Dis 134:805, 1986.
44. Brasington RD, Furst DE: Pulmonary disease in systemic lupus erythematosus. Clin Exp Rheumatol 3:269, 1985.
45. Owens GR, Paradis IL, Gryzan S, et al: Role of inflammation in the lung disease of systemic sclerosis: comparison with idiopathic pulmonary fibrosis. J Lab Clin Med 107:253, 1986.
46. Papathanasiou MP, Constantopoulos SH, Tsampoulas C, et al: Reappraisal of respiratory abnormalities in primary and secondary Sjögren's syndrome. A controlled study. Chest 90:370, 1986.
47. Costabel U: The alveolitis of hypersensitivity pneumonitis. Eur Respir J 1:5, 1988.
48. Basset F, Ferrans VJ, Soler P, et al: Intraluminal fibrosis in interstitial lung disorders. Am J Pathol 122:443, 1986.
49. Epler GR, Colby TV, McLoud TC, et al: Bronchiolitis obliterans organizing pneumonia. N Engl J Med 312:152, 1985.
50. Guerry-Force ML, Muller NL, Wright JL, et al: A comparison of bronchiolitis obliterans with organizing pneumonia, usual interstitial pneumonia, and small airways disease. Am Rev Respir Dis 135:705, 1987.
51. Nidus BD, Matalon R, Cantacuzino D, et al: Uremic pleuritis—a clinicopathological entity. N Engl J Med 281:255, 1969.
52. Kohen JA, Opsahl JA, Kjellstrand CM: Deceptive patterns of uremic pulmonary edema. Am J Kidney Dis 7:456, 1986.
53. Heidland A, Heine H, Heidbreder E, et al: Uremic pneumonitis. Evidence for participation of proteolytic enzymes. Contrib Nephrol 41:352, 1984.
54. Rosen SH, Castleman B, Liebow AA, et al: Pulmonary alveolar proteinosis. N Engl J Med 258:1123, 1958.
55. Prakash UB, Barham SS, Carpenter HA, et al: Pulmonary alveolar phospholipoproteinosis: experience with 34 cases and a review. Mayo Clin Proc 62:499, 1987.
56. Ovil Y, Schachner A, Schujman E, et al: Benign endobronchial lipoma masquerading as recurrent pneumonia. Eur J Respir Dis 63:481, 1982.
57. Eastridge CE, Young JM, Steplock AL: Endobronchial lipoma. South Med J 77:759, 1984.
58. Vevaina JR, Mark EJ: Thoracic hemangiomatosis mas-

querading as interstitial lung disease. Chest 93:657, 1988.

59. Bartter T, Irwin RS, Phillips DA, et al: Pulmonary artery pseudoaneurysm. A potential complication of pulmonary artery catheterization. Arch Intern Med 148:471, 1988.

Selected Readings

Fein AM, Feinsilver SH, Niederman MS, et al: When the pneumonia doesn't get better. Clin Chest Med 8:529, 1987.
A clinical review of the approach to nonresolving pneumonia, that should precipitate consideration of less common infectious and noninfectious disorders presenting as pneumonia.

Tobin MJ: Diagnosis of pneumonia: techniques and problems. Clin Chest Med 8:513, 1987.
State-of-the-art review of the usefulness and limitations of diagnostic techniques for evaluating causes of pneumonia.

Warner DO, Warner MA, Divertie MB: Open lung biopsy in patients with diffuse pulmonary infiltrates and acute respiratory failure. Am Rev Respir Dis 137:90, 1988.
Usefulness of open lung biopsy in patients with diffuse pulmonary infiltrates and acute respiratory failure was evaluated in 80 patients over an 11-year period. Biopsy provided an etiologic diagnosis in 53 patients (66%).

See also Selected Readings in Chapter 17 of this section.

19
The Solitary Pulmonary Nodule: Common and Less Common Causes

A solitary pulmonary nodule (coin lesion) is a radiographic finding of a circumscribed mass in the lung that is usually 6 cm or smaller.[1] The most important question is whether the lesion is benign or malignant; experience suggests that this question cannot be solved by radiographic characteristics of the lesion, such as size, calcification, or cavitation; nor is it reasonable to rely on repeated radiographic studies.

Malignant tumors may maintain their form and size for years, and benign lesions may undergo malignant degeneration.[2] Although symptoms are rarely characteristic, some clinical features are helpful in weighing diagnostic probabilities. For example, in patients older than 60 years of age, more than 60% of coin lesions are malignant, with bronchogenic carcinoma the most frequently diagnosed lesion.[2] In the Orient, echinococcus cysts are not uncommon causes of solitary nodules; in the midwestern and southwestern United States, a fungal infection is a frequent cause of a solitary nodule. However, even with recent technologic improvements in radiographic diagnosis, such as CT and MRI, a tissue diagnosis is almost always indicated.[3-5]

Most Common Malignant Causes of Solitary Pulmonary Nodule

Bronchogenic carcinoma: highest incidence in smokers, and most frequent neoplasm presenting as a solitary nodule[6-8]

Metastatic lesions: frequent and sometimes calcified metastases originate from colon, breast, ovary, thyroid, and osteogenic sarcoma.[9-11]

Bronchial adenoma: generally occurs in a younger age group than bronchogenic carcinoma[12]

Bronchiolar-alveolar carcinoma: often associated with prolonged asymptomatic periods[13]

Trophoblastic disease: lung most common site of metastases[14]

Most Common Nonmalignant Causes of Solitary Pulmonary Nodules

Granulomas: granulomas due to fungal infection are the most common cause of benign solitary nodules in endemic areas for histoplasmosis and coccidioidomycosis.

Tuberculosis: tuberculomas are more commonly seen in the institutionalized elderly, HIV-infected patients, and those at risk for HIV infection, particularly intravenous drug abusers.[15-20]

Histoplasmosis: endemic in midwestern United States

Coccidioidomycosis: endemic in southwestern United States[21-23]

Cryptococcus neoformans[24]

Brucellosis

Pulmonary abscesses: postsurgical and immunocompromised patients are at higher risk; CT and MRI may help find suspected pulmonary abscesses in

patients with negative chest radiographs.[25,26]
Hamartomas[27,28]

Less Common Causes of Solitary Pulmonary Nodules

Vascular lesions
  Arteriovenous malformations: hemorrhagic telangiectases[29]
  Hematomas: usually associated with trauma
  Pulmonary infarct: can occur with known or unsuspected pulmonary embolism
  Hematogenous abscesses: usually multiple
  Innominate artery buckling[30]
  Carotid pseudoaneurysm[31]
Sequestration and inflammation
  Focal pneumonitis
  Broncholithiasis: most often associated with pulmonary infections, such as tuberculosis and histoplasmosis[32]
  Bronchopulmonary sequestration: extralobar sequestration is usually congenital.[33]
  Infected bullae[34]
  Bronchiolectasis[34]
  Intrathoracic endometriosis[35]
Foreign bodies and pulmonary malformations
  Intrapulmonary cysts: bronchogenic, infectious
  Enlarged pulmonary arteries
  Intrapulmonary enlarged lymph nodes: see Section X: Hematology, Chapter 112: Lymphadenopathy.
  Amyloidosis[36–38]
Granulomas
  Sarcoidosis: can sometimes be difficult to distinguish from mycobacterium-caused tuberculomas or carcinomas[39–41]
  Parasitic infection: dirofilariasis, ascaris, treponema, viscaral larva migrans, *Ecchinococcus*[42,43]
  Cytomegalovirus[44]
  Larvae of horsefly *Gastrophilus*[45]
  Plasma cell granuloma (inflammatory pseudotumor)[46]
Neoplasms
  Chondromas: CT may be helpful.[47]
  Non-Hodgkin's lymphoma[48]
  Chemodectoma: minute meningothelial-like nodules with an unclear pathologic relationship to pulmonary meningiomas[49]
  Lymphatoid granulomatosis[50]
  Epithelioid hemangioendotheliomas[51]

Smooth muscle tumors: leiomyoma, leiomyosarcoma[52]

Granulocytic sarcoma[53]

Rare infections

Pneumocystis carinii pneumonia: rare radiographic presentation seen in patients with HIV infection[54,55]

Sporotrichosis[56]

Melioidosis[57]

Drug- and toxin-induced

Crack lung: associated with cocaine inhalation[58]

Chemotherapy[59]

References

1. Meyer TJ: The solitary pulmonary nodule: an aggressive workup. Postgrad Med 73(3):66, 1983.
2. Toomes H, Delphendahl A, Manke HG, et al: The coin lesion of the lung. A review of 955 resected coin lesions. Cancer 51:534, 1983.
3. Zerhouni EA, Stitik FP: Controversies in computed tomography of the thorax: the pulmonary nodule-lung cancer staging. Radiol Clin North Am 23:407, 1985.
4. Müller NL, Gamsu G, Webb WR: Pulmonary nodules: detection using magnetic resonance and computed tomography. Radiology 155:687, 1985.
5. Newell JD: Evaluation of pulmonary and mediastinal masses. Med Clin North Am 68:1463, 1984.
6. Gross BH, Glazer GM, Orringer MB, et al: Bronchogenic carcinoma metastatic to normal-sized lymph nodes: frequency and significance. Radiology 166:71, 1988.
7. Pearlberg JL, Sandler MA, Lewis JW Jr, et al: Small-cell bronchogenic carcinoma: CT evaluation. AJR 150:265, 1988.
8. Staples CA, Müller NL, Miller RR, et al: Mediastinal nodes in bronchogenic carcinoma: comparison between CT and mediastinoscopy. Radiology 167:367, 1988.
9. Casey JJ, Stempel BG, Scanlon EF, Fry WA: The solitary pulmonary nodule in the patient with breast cancer. Surgery 96:801, 1984.
10. Peuchot M, Libshitz HI: Pulmonary metastatic disease: radiologic-surgical correlation. Radiology 164:719, 1987.
11. Kagan AR, Steckel RJ: Radiologic contributions to cancer management. Lung metastases. AJR 147:473, 1986.
12. Tischer W, Reddemann H, Herzog P, et al: Experience in surgical treatment of pulmonary and bronchial tumors in childhood. Prog Pediatr Surg 21:118, 1987.
13. Edwards CW: Alveolar carcinoma: a review. Thorax 39:166, 1984.
14. Kumar J, Ilancheran A, Ratnam SS: Pulmonary metastases in gestational trophoblastic disease: a review of 97 cases. Br J Obstet Gynaecol 95:70, 1988.
15. Tenholder MF, Moser RJ III, Tellis CJ: Mycobacteria other than tuberculosis. Pulmonary involvement in pa-

tients with acquired immunodeficiency syndrome. Arch Intern Med 148:953, 1988.

16. Fournier AM, Dickinson GM, Erdfrocht IR, et al: Tuberculosis and nontuberculous mycobacteriosis in patients with AIDS. Chest 93:772, 1988.

17. Creditor MC, Smith EC, Gallai JB, et al: Tuberculosis, tuberculin reactivity, and delayed cutaneous hypersensitivity in nursing home residents. J Gerontol 43:M97, 1988.

18. O'Donnell AE, Pappas LS: Pulmonary complications of intravenous drug abuse. Experience at an inner-city hospital. Chest 94:251, 1988.

19. Barnes PF, Verdegem TD, Vachon LA, et al: Chest roentgenogram in pulmonary tuberculosis. New data on an old test. Chest 94:316, 1988.

20. Wasser LS, Shaw GW, Talavera W: Endobronchial tuberculosis in the acquired immunodeficiency syndrome. Chest 94:1240, 1988.

21. Forseth J, Rohwedder JJ, Levine BE, Saubolle MA: Experience with needle biopsy for coccidioidal lung nodules. Arch Intern Med 146:319, 1986.

22. Winn RE: Solitary pulmonary nodule in the southwest. coccidioidoma or carcinoma? Arch Intern Med 146:250, 1986.

23. Freedman SI, Ang EP, Haley RS: Identification of coccidioidomycosis of the lung by fine needle aspiration biopsy. Acta Cytol 30:420, 1986.

24. Kahn FW, England DM, Jones JM: Solitary pulmonary nodule due to *Cryptococcus neoformans* and *Mycobacterium tuberculosis*. Am J Med 78:677, 1985.

25. Johnson JF, Shiels WE, White CB, Williams BD: Concealed pulmonary abscess: diagnosis by computed tomography. Pediatrics 78:283, 1986.

26. Steyer BJ, Sobonya RE: *Pasteurella multocida* lung abscess. A case report and review of the literature. Arch Intern Med 144:1081, 1984.

27. Siegelman SS, Khouri NF, Scott WW Jr, et al: Pulmonary hamartoma: CT findings. Radiology 160:313, 1986.

28. Steen-Hansen E: The diagnostic value of chest x-ray combined with fine-needle aspiration biopsy in patients suspected for pulmonary hamartomas. Rontgenblatter 40:321, 1987.

29. Teragaki M, Akioka K, Yasuda M, et al: Hereditary hemorrhagic telangiectasia with growing pulmonary arteriovenous fistulas followed for 24 years. Am J Med Sci 295:545, 1988.

30. Tamaki M, Tanabe M, Kamiuchi H, et al: Buckling of the distal innominate artery simulating a nodular lung mass. Chest 83:829, 1983.

31. Rong SH: Carotid pseudoaneurysm simulating pancoast tumor. AJR 142:495, 1984.

32. Haines JD Jr: Coughing up a stone. What to do about broncholithiasis. Postgrad Med 83(3):83, 1988.

33. Stocker JT: Sequestrations of the lung. Semin Diagn Pathol 3:106, 1986.

34. Murata K, Khan A, Herman PG: Pulmonary parenchymal disease: evaluation with high-resolution CT. Radiology 170:629, 1989.

35. Chagares R: Intrathoracic endometriosis: a women's health issue. Heart Lung 16:183, 1987.

36. Vaara J, Tukiainen H, Syrjanen K, Terho EO: Solitary amyloid tumor of the lung: a rare manifestation of primary amyloidosis. Eur J Respir Dis 67:385, 1985.
37. Gibney RT, Connolly TP: Pulmonary amyloid nodules simulating pancoast tumor. J Can Assoc Radiol 35:90, 1984.
38. Hui AN, Koss MN, Hochholzer L, Wehunt WD: Amyloidosis presenting in the lower respiratory tract. Clinicopathologic, radiologic, immunohistochemical, and histochemical studies on 48 cases. Arch Pathol Lab Med 110:212, 1986.
39. Levy H, Feldman C, Wadee AA, Rabson AR: Differentiation of sarcoidosis from tuberculosis using an enzyme-linked immunosorbent assay for the detection of antibodies against *Mycobacterium tuberculosis*. Chest 94:1254, 1988.
40. Rubinstein I, Baum GL, Lieberman Y, Bubis JJ: Asymptomatic pulmonary nodule in sarcoidosis. Eur J Respir Dis 66:74, 1985.
41. Savino A, Ostrovsky PD, Sanders A, Daly SM: Coexistence of sarcoidosis and carcinoma in a solitary pulmonary nodule. NY State J Med 86:648, 1986.
42. Smith LS, Schillaci RF: Pulmonary dirofilariasis in humans—pneumonitis that evolved to a lung nodule. West J Med 145:516, 1986.
43. Masuda Y, Kishimoto T, Ito H, Tsuji M: Visceral larva migrans caused by *Trichuris vulpis* presenting as a pulmonary mass. Thorax 42:990, 1987.
44. Ravin CE, Walker Smith G, Ahern MJ, et al: Cytomegaloviral infection presenting as a solitary pulmonary nodule. Chest 71:220, 1977.
45. Ahmed MJ, Miller A: Pulmonary coin lesion containing a horse bot, *Gasterophilus*. Am J Clin Pathol 52:414, 1969.
46. Fassina AS, Rugge M, Scapinello A, et al: Plasma cell granuloma of the lung (inflammatory pseudotumor). Tumori 72:529, 1986.
47. McGahan JP: Carney syndrome: usefulness of computed tomography in demonstrating pulmonary chondromas. J Comput Assist Tomogr 7:137, 1983.
48. Reverter JC, Coca A, Font J, Ingelmo M: Erythema nodosum and pulmonary solitary nodule as the first manifestations of a non-Hodgkin's lymphoma. Br J Dis Chest 81:397, 1987.
49. Gaffey MJ, Mills SE, Askin FB: Minute pulmonary meningothelial-like nodules. A clinicopathologic study of so-called minute pulmonary chemodectoma. Am J Surg Pathol 12:167, 1988.
50. Paramsothy Y, Ilchyshyn A, Sidky K, Byrne JP: Lymphomatoid granulomatosis mimicking bronchial carcinoma. Postgrad Med J 63:381, 1987.
51. Yousem SA, Hochholzer L: Unusual thoracic manifestations of epithelioid hemangioendothelioma. Arch Pathol Lab Med 111:459, 1987.
52. Yellin A, Rosenman Y, Lieberman Y: Review of smooth muscle tumours of the lower respiratory tract. Br J Dis Chest 78:337, 1984.
53. Callahan M, Wall S, Askin F, et al: Granulocytic sarcoma presenting as pulmonary nodules and lymphadenopathy. Cancer 60:1902, 1987.

54. Barrio JL, Suarez M, Rodriguez JL, et al: *Pneumocystis carinii* pneumonia presenting as cavitating and noncavitating solitary pulmonary nodules in patients with the acquired immunodeficiency syndrome. Am Rev Respir Dis 134:1094, 1986.
55. Hartz JW, Geisinger KR, Scharyj M, Muss HB: Granulomatous pneumocystosis presenting as a solitary pulmonary nodule. Arch Pathol Lab Med 109:466, 1985.
56. England DM, Hochholzer L: Primary pulmonary sporotrichosis. Report of eight cases with clinicopathologic review. Am J Surg Pathol 9:193, 1985.
57. Morrison RE, Lamb AS, Craig DB, Johnson WM: Melioidosis: a reminder. Am J Med 84:965, 1988.
58. Kissner DG, Lawrence WD, Selis JE, Flint A: Crack lung: pulmonary disease caused by cocaine abuse. Am Rev Respir Dis 136:1250, 1987.
59. Talcott JA, Garnick MB, Stomper PC, et al: Cavitary lung nodules associated with combination chemotherapy containing bleomycin. J Urol 138:619, 1987.

Selected Readings

Chaffey MH: The role of percutaneous lung biopsy in the workup of a solitary pulmonary nodule. West J Med 148:176, 1988.
Clinical and well-referenced review.

Cummings SR, Lillington GA, Richard RJ: Estimating the probability of malignancy in solitary pulmonary nodules. A Bayesian approach. Am Rev Respir Dis 134:449, 1986.
Authors applied Bayes' theorem to the decision-making process involved in estimating the likelihood that a nodule is malignant. Variables included nodule size, age of patient, cigarette smoking history, and date of overall prevalence of malignancy in solitary nodules. Authors suggest their method may improve the accuracy of estimating the possible malignancy of solitary nodules.

Cummings SR, Lillington GA, Richard RJ: Managing solitary pulmonary nodules. The choice of strategy is a "close call." Am Rev Respir Dis 134:453, 1986.
Controversies of the initial management of solitary pulmonary nodules are reviewed. Using decision analysis authors compared average life expectancy produced by alternative strategies for managing the patient with a solitary pulmonary nodule. Among strategies discussed were immediate thoracotomy, needle aspiration biopsy, or bronchoscopy followed by either thoracotomy or extended observation.

Eells TP, Pratt DS, Coppolo DP, et al: An improved method of cell recovery following bronchial brushing. Chest 93:727, 1988.
An improved method of cell recovery from bronchial brushing, the Saccamanno brush wash, which appears superior to standard methods of handling bronchial brush specimens, is described.

Fiastro JF, Newell JD: Quantitative computed tomography evaluation of benign solitary pulmonary nodules. J Comput Tomogr 11:103, 1987.
A retrospective study of computed tomography (GE 8800 CT scanner) of 14 patients with stable nodules for at least 24 months and no evidence of calcification within the nodule by plain radiography. Using the phantom quantitative assessment for presence of calcium was found helpful in identifying nodules that proved benign.

Fraser RG, Barnes GT, Hickey N, et al: Potential value of digital radiography. Preliminary observations on the use of dual-energy subtraction in the evaluation of pulmonary nodules. Chest 89(Suppl 4):2498, 1986.

Clinical observations of a dual-energy subtraction method using scanned projection digital radiography to demonstrate calcification in solitary pulmonary nodules.

Fraser RG, Hickey NM, Niklason LT, et al: Calcification in pulmonary nodules: detection with dual-energy digital radiography. Radiology 160:595, 1986.

A clinical study to determine the accuracy of dual-energy digital radiography in revealing nodule calcification was undertaken over a 6-month period. The study included 61 patients with pulmonary nodules. Authors present data suggesting that dual-energy radiography is a highly accurate method of assessing the presence or absence of calcification in pulmonary nodules.

Gamsu G, de Geer G, Cann C, et al: A preliminary study of MRI quantification of simulated calcified pulmonary nodules. Invest Radiol 22:853, 1987.

The potential of MRI quantification of calcium in the evaluation of pulmonary nodules was investigated in simulated nodules. The degree of the T1 and T2 effects was related to particle size, indicating a hydrophilic surface effect. Authors conclude that MRI quantification of calcium within pulmonary nodules will relate to precise composition of calcium salt and to particle size.

Hickey NM, Niklason LT, Sabbagh E, et al: Dual-energy digital radiographic quantification of calcium in simulated pulmonary nodules. AJR 148:19, 1987.

Based on the premise that the presence or absence of calcium in solitary pulmonary nodules may indicate whether the nodule is benign or malignant, a study was carried out to assess the capability of dual-energy digital chest radiography to identify and quantify calcium content of simulated pulmonary nodules. From their data, authors conclude that dual-energy digital radiography is a simple and accurate method of measuring calcium content in solitary pulmonary nodules.

Howe MA, Gross BH: CT evaluation of the equivocal pulmonary nodule. Comput Radiol 11:61, 1987.

Fifty consecutive patients referred to CT for a possible pulmonary nodule were reviewed. Authors reviewed radiographic characteristics of suspected nodules and found that out of a total of 56 questionable nodules on conventional radiograph CT identified no abnormality in 21 cases; parenchymal nodules in 16 cases; scarring, atelectasis or infiltrates in 11 cases; and normal structural variants in 8 cases.

Huston J III, Muhm JR: Solitary pulmonary opacities: plain tomography. Radiology 163:481, 1987.

Five hundred two patients with solitary pulmonary opacities were evaluated with plain tomographic procedures. Repeat chest radiographs in 64 patients and tomograms in 115 patients showed that the opacities were not nodules, but pneumonitis, rib lesions, thickened pleura, or other benign findings. In this series, the plain tomographic procedure, including fluoroscopy and repeat chest radiography, allowed an accurate diagnosis in 67% of the solitary pulmonary nodules studied.

Im JG, Gamsu G, Gordon D, et al: CT densitometry of pulmonary nodules in a frozen human thorax. AJR 150:61, 1988.

Variables of calcium concentration, exposure technique, recon-

struction algorithm, nodule size, and nodule location on CT attenuation values (CT density) of pulmonary nodules were examined in
frozen human thorax. Authors conclude that two major variables in
CT densitometry for pulmonary nodules, kiloelectron voltage of the
x-ray beam, and the reconstruction algorithm used should be standardized with a high kilovoltage and high-resolution algorithm fa-
vored on the GE CT 9800 scanner.

Inouye SK, Sox HC Jr: Standard and computed tomography in the evaluation of neoplasms of the chest. A
comparative efficacy assessment. Ann Intern Med 105:906,
1986.
*A study comparing CT and standard tomography in evaluating
chest neoplasms. Using a Bayesian analysis, authors developed
guidelines for choosing between computed and standard tomography
in patients with lung neoplasms and suspected metastases.*

Khouri NF, Meziane MA, Zerhouni EA, et al: The solitary
pulmonary nodule. Assessment, diagnosis, and management. Chest 91:128, 1987.
*A brief overview of an approach to evaluation of patients with
solitary pulmonary nodules. Authors suggest that with the proper
use of CT densitometry or needle biopsy, such techniques may avoid
the need for thoracotomy in a significant number of patients.*

Levine MS, Weiss JM, Harrell JH, et al: Transthoracic
needle aspiration biopsy following negative fiberoptic bronchoscopy in solitary pulmonary nodules. Chest 93:1152,
1988.
*The utility of transthoracic needle aspiration biopsy following neg-
ative fiberoptic bronchoscopy in patients with solitary pulmonary
nodules was reviewed from records of 262 patients. Fifty-eight patients met the criteria for inclusion in this study. Twenty-five (43%)
were diagnosed by transthoracic needle aspiration, 24 had malignant
lesions, and 1 had M. tuberculosis. Of the remaining 33 patients,
18 went on to surgery or repeat procedures, and 9 of these patients
had a malignancy.*

Mitchell DM, Shah SH, Edwards D, et al: Incidence of
pulmonary nodules detected by computed tomography in
patients with bronchial carcinoma. Clin Radiol 37:151, 1986.
*CT is more sensitive in detecting pulmonary nodules than con-
ventional radiography. Incidences of finding pulmonary nodules in
thoracic CT scans that were not visible on chest radiographs were
27% in patients with small-cell carcinoma and 28% in patients with
nonsmall-cell carcinoma.*

Naidich DP, Sussman R, Kutcher WL, et al: Solitary
pulmonary nodules. CT-bronchoscopic correlation. Chest
93:595, 1988.
*A retrospective study of CT contributions in the management of
solitary pulmonary nodules or masses was conducted in 65 patients
undergoing fiberoptic bronchoscopy. Authors point out the usefulness
of the "positive bronchus sign," that is, the presence in CT cross-
section of a bronchus leading to or contained within the nodule or
mass.*

Penketh AR, Robinson AA, Barker V, Flower CD: Use of
percutaneous needle biopsy in the investigation of solitary
pulmonary nodules. Thorax 42:967, 1987.
*Percutaneous needle biopsies were performed on 683 patients with
solitary pulmonary nodules. Cytologic diagnoses were reviewed from
first biopsies in 473 patients (69%), and from second biopsies in
43 patients. From the second biopsy, a diagnosis of malignancy was*

made in 16 more cases (37%). Authors emphasize that a cytology report indicating no evidence of malignancy, but not diagnostic of a specific benign condition, does not reliably rule out a malignant lesion.

Peuchot M, Libshitz HI: Pulmonary metastatic disease: radiologic–surgical correlation. Radiology 164:719, 1987.

Radiologic–surgical correlative studies were performed in 100 lungs of 84 patients with new pulmonary parenchymal nodules with previously treated extrathoracic malignancies. Of 65 nodules detected as solitary nodules on chest radiography, only 35 (54%) proved to be truly solitary, whereas, 35 of 44 (80%) nodules detected with CT were truly solitary.

Rohwedder JJ: The solitary pulmonary nodule. A new diagnostic agenda. Chest 93:1124, 1988.

Current concepts of evaluation and management reviewed within recent technologic changes and new possibilities of differential diagnosis in certain risk groups.

Sagel SS: The solitary pulmonary nodule: role of CT. AJR 147:26, 1986.

General review of the usefulness of CT in the evaluation of the solitary pulmonary nodule.

Sherrier RH, Chiles C, Johnson GA, Ravin CE: Differentiation of benign from malignant pulmonary nodules with digitized chest radiographs. Radiology 162:645, 1987.

Digital techniques were applied in a retrospective study of 68 patients with proven solitary nodules. Conventional chest radiographs for each patient were digitized and nodules analyzed. Striking differences were noted between 26 malignant nodules and 21 calcified granulomas.

Siegleman SS, Khouri NF, Leo FP, et al: Solitary pulmonary nodules: CT assessment. Radiology 160:307, 1986.

CT evaluation of 634 solitary pulmonary nodules was assessed with each lesion judged by CT criteria to be benign or indeterminate. A total of 176 (63%) benign nodules were correctly predicted to be benign by CT. CT evaluation found more calcification in nodules than was assessed by conventional tomography.

Stoller JK, Ahmad M, Rice TW: Solitary pulmonary nodule. Cleve Clin J Med 55:68, 1988.

State-of-the-art review of current clinical recommendations for the evaluation and management of the solitary pulmonary nodule from the Cleveland Clinic.

Wang X, Itoh S, Ishigaki T, et al: Thin slice CT study of solitary pulmonary nodules with emphasis on the relation to vasculatures. Radiat Med 4:75, 1986.

Thin- (2 mm) and thick-slice (10 mm) CT scanning was performed in 49 and 31 patients respectively to evaluate morphology of solitary pulmonary nodules or masses to determine relationship between tumor and surrounding vasculature. Authors present interesting observations of pulmonary vein and pulmonary artery relationships to tumor or masses and suggest this type of CT evaluation may increase diagnostic accuracy of primary lung cancer.

Zerhouni EA, Stitik FP, Siegelman SS, et al: CT of the pulmonary nodule: a cooperative study. Radiology 160:319, 1986.

A study evaluating the role of CT in the investigation of pulmonary nodules included a special reference phantom that included CT densitometric measurements independent of variations between scanners and patients. A total of 384 nodules considered not calcified by conventional methods were examined. One hundred eighteen (31%) proved to be benign, and in 65 (55%) of them, unsuspected calcification was demonstrated.

20
Hemoptysis: Common and Less Common Causes

A patient's first episode of hemoptysis can be a terrifying experience, whether it is coughing up blood-tinged sputum or a significant amount of blood. Hemoptysis, or coughing up blood, implies that the blood originates below the larynx.[1] When confronted with this clinical picture, the nasopharynx and the gastrointestinal tract should first be excluded as the source of blood. Massive hemoptysis is life-threatening, and management and evaluation are performed on an emergency basis.[2] However, even modest amounts of hemoptysis must be seriously evaluated since hemoptysis can be the initial manifestation of underlying carcinoma or a pulmonary embolism. The most common cause of hemoptysis in the United States is bronchitic infection, which often occurs in the same group of patients at risk for lung cancer. Other infections, such as tuberculosis in the institutionalized elderly and HIV-associated pulmonary infections in otherwise healthy people, not uncommonly present clinically as hemoptysis.[1] If neoplasm and infection are unlikely, there are a myriad of less common causes of hemoptysis to consider, such as certain cardiovascular disorders, trauma, pulmonary-vascular anomalies, diffuse pulmonary disease, systemic disorders, and even certain blood dyscrasias.[3,4]

Infection

Chronic bronchitis: patients with bronchogenic carcinoma often have chronic bronchitis.[1]
Tracheitis: viral[5]

Mycobacterial pneumonia: institutionalized elderly and patients with HIV infection have a higher incidence of pulmonary tuberculosis; *Mycobacterium avium-intracellulare* is increasingly seen in patients with HIV infection.[6-8]

Bacterial pneumonias: klebsiella, pneumococcus, pseudomonas, Friedländer's pneumonia[9]

Lung abscess[10]

Mycetomas: aspergillomas, particularly prevalent in HIV-infected patients; mucormycosis, histoplasmosis[11-17]

Parasitic infections: common in certain immigrant populations; *Paragonimus westermani*, amoebic abscesses, hookworm, hydatid cysts, strongyloidiasis[18]

Bronchiectasis: often postinfectious, particularly following recurrent pneumonia or old tuberculosis infection

Neoplasm

Carcinoma of the lung: primary and metastatic

Endobronchial tumors: often highly vascular tumors

Metastatic disease: bleeding rarer in metastatic than in primary lung carcinoma

Benign hamartoma[19]

Endobronchial polyps

Angiosarcoma: rare tumors and rarely located in the lung[20]

Cystic teratoma[21]

Cardiac histiocytoma[22]

Cardiovascular Disorders

Pulmonary embolism: hemoptysis presumed secondary to associated pulmonary infarction[23]

Mitral stenosis[24]

Secondary pulmonary hypertension

Coronary artery disease[25]

Congestive heart failure: pulmonary edema

Aortic aneurysm: associated with aortobronchopulmonary fistula[26]

Mitral valve regurgitation[27]

Ventricular pseudoaneurysm[28]

Postictal pulmonary edema[29]

Pulmonary Vascular and Other Anomalies

Primary pulmonary hypertension[30]

Arteriovenous malformations: endobronchial telangiectases[31]

Pulmonary artery stenosis[32]

Osler-Weber-Rendu disease

Pulmonary artery agenesis[33,34]
Unilateral absent pulmonary artery[35]
Bronchial artery aneurysm[36]
Tracheocarotid fistula[37]

Traumatic Conditions

Airway injuries: laryngotracheal trauma[38,39]
Lung contusion
Fractured bronchus
Foreign body aspiration: denture fragments, miscellaneous adult and child-related aspirations[40–43]
Penetrating rib fractures
Fat embolism syndrome[44]
Hydrocarbon poisoning[45]
Other toxic inhalants

Systemic Disorders

Systemic lupus erythematosus[46]
Hemorrhagic disorders: von Willebrand's coagulopathy, hemophilia, miscellaneous blood dyscrasias[47]
Wegener's granulomatosis[48,49]
Goodpasture's syndrome[50,51]
Pulmonary alveolar proteinosis
Broncholithiasis: often associated with a history of pulmonary infections, such as tuberculosis or histoplasmosis.[17]
Sarcoidosis: usually occurs in advanced sarcoidosis with cystic or cavitated lesions; rarely can be presenting manifestation of sarcoidosis[52–55]
Cystic fibrosis[56]
Amyloidosis[57]
Histiocytosis[58]
Behçet's syndrome: hemoptysis usually associated with pyrexia, chest pain, and dyspnea[59,60]
Scleroderma[61]
Diffuse pulmonary or alveolar hemorrhagic syndromes[62,63]
Rheumatoid arthritis[64]
Pulmonary endometriosis[65,66]

Iatrogenic Causes

Anticoagulation therapy
Pulmonary irradiation[67]
Factitious hemoptysis[68]
Catheter-induced pulmonary artery hemorrhage[69,70]
Needle biopsy
Swan-Ganz catheterization[71]
Endotracheal intubation

Blalock-Taussig shunt false aneurysm formation[72]

References

1. Israel RH, Poe RH: Hemoptysis. Clin Chest Med 8:197, 1987.
2. Noseworthy TW, Anderson BJ: Massive hemoptysis. Can Med Assoc J 135:1097, 1986.
3. Howard WJ, Rosario EJ, Calhoon SL: Hemoptysis. Causes and a practical management approach. Postgrad Med 77(8):53, 1985.
4. Boren HG, Busey J, Corpe RF, et al: The management of hemoptysis. Am Rev Respir Dis 93:471, 1966.
5. Lewis M, Kallenbach J, Kark P, et al: Severe hemoptysis associated with viral tracheitis. Thorax 37:869, 1982.
6. Teklu B, Felleke G: Massive hemoptysis in tuberculosis. Tubercle 63:213, 1982.
7. Muthuswamy PP, Akbik F, Franklin C, et al: Management of major or massive hemoptysis in active pulmonary tuberculosis by bronchial arterial embolization. Chest 92:77, 1987.
8. Katz PR, Reichman W, Dube D, Feather J: Clinical features of pulmonary tuberculosis in young and old veterans. J Am Geriatr Soc 35:512, 1987.
9. Manfredi F, Daly WJ, Behnke RH: Clinical observations of acute Friedlander pneumonia. Ann Intern Med 58:642, 1963.
10. Rizk N, Duncan SR, Raffin TA: Hemoptysis, large lung "abscess" in alcoholic man with bad teeth. Hosp Pract 22:70, 1987.
11. Lombardo GT, Anandarao N, Lin CS, et al: Fatal hemoptysis in a patient with AIDS-related complex and pulmonary aspergilloma. NY State J Med 87:306, 1987.
12. Glimp RA, Bayer AS: Pulmonary aspergilloma. Diagnostic and therapeutic considerations. Arch Intern Med 143:303, 1983.
13. Kibbler CC, Milkins SR, Bhamra A, et al: Apparent pulmonary mycetoma following invasive aspergillosis in neutropenic patients. Thorax 43:108, 1988.
14. Watts WJ: Bronchopleural fistula followed by massive fatal hemoptysis in a patient with pulmonary mucormycosis. Arch Intern Med 143:1029, 1983.
15. Passamonte PM, Dix JD: Nosocomial pulmonary mucormycosis with fatal massive hemoptysis. Am J Med Sci 289:65, 1985.
16. Zeiss J, Woldenberg LS, Morgan R, Davis JT: Pulmonary histoplasmoma presenting as massive hemoptysis. Pediatr Infect Dis J 6:689, 1987.
17. Haines JD Jr: Coughing up a stone. What to do about broncholithiasis. Postgrad Med 83(3):83, 1988.
18. Singh TS, Mutum SS, Razaque MA: Pulmonary paragonimiasis: clinical features, diagnosis, and treatment of 39 cases in Manipur. Trans R Soc Trop Med Hyg 80:967, 1986.
19. Kleinman J, Zirkin H, Beuchtwanger MM, et al: Benign hamartoma of the lung presenting as massive hemoptysis. J Surg Oncol 33:38, 1986.
20. Palvio DH, Paulsen SM, Henneberg EW: Primary an-

giosarcoma of the lung presenting as intractable hemoptysis. Thorac Cardiovasc Surg 35:105, 1987.
21. Steier KJ: Benign cystic teratoma of the lung. Postgrad Med 83(4):85, 1988.
22. DiNardo-Ekery D, Lau KY, Spicer MJ, Ascherl MV: Malignant fibrous histiocytoma of the heart presenting as hemoptysis. Association with pseudothrombocytopenia. Chest 93:1099, 1988.
23. Sasahara AA, Hyers TM, Cole CM, et al (eds): The urokinase pulmonary embolism trial. A national cooperative study. Circulation 47 (Suppl II):1, 1973.
24. Scarlat A, Bodner G, Liron M: Massive hemoptysis as the presenting symptom in mitral stenosis. Thorax 41:413, 1986.
25. Bansal S, Day JA Jr, Braman SS: Hemoptysis during sexual intercourse. Unusual manifestation of coronary artery disease. Chest 93:891, 1988.
26. Coblentz CL, Sallee DS, Chiles C: Aortobronchopulmonary fistula complicating aortic aneurysm: diagnosis in four cases. AJR 150:535, 1988.
27. Case records of the Massachusetts General Hospital. Weekly clinicopathological exercises. Case 7-1981. N Engl J Med 304:409, 1981.
28. Jain A, Strickman NE, Hall RJ, Ott DA: An unusual complication of left ventricular pseudoaneurysm: hemoptysis. Chest 93:429, 1988.
29. Pacht ER: Postictal pulmonary edema and hemoptysis. J Natl Med Assoc 80:337, 1988.
30. Koerner SK: Pulmonary hypertension: etiology and clinical evaluation. J Thorac Imaging 3:25, 1988.
31. Burke CM, Safai C, Nelson DP, et al: Pulmonary arteriovenous malformations: a critical update. Am Rev Respir Dis 134:334, 1986.
32. Matsumoto AH, Delany DJ, Parker LA, Ney KA: Massive hemoptysis associated with isolated peripheral pulmonary artery stenosis. Cathet Cardiovasc Diagn 13:313, 1987.
33. Cogswell TL, Singh S: Agenesis of the left pulmonary artery as a cause of hemoptysis. Angiology 37:154, 1986.
34. Mehta AC, Livingston DR, Kawalek W, et al: Pulmonary artery agenesis presenting as massive hemoptysis—a case report. Angiology 38:67, 1987.
35. Taguchi T, Ikeda K, Kume K, et al: Isolated unilateral absence of left pulmonary artery with peribronchial arteriovenous malformation showing recurrent hemoptysis. Pediatr Radiol 17:316, 1987.
36. Osada H, Kawada T, Ashida H, et al: Bronchial artery aneurysm. Ann Thorac Surg 41:440, 1986.
37. Dellinger RP, Savage PJ, Carruth C, et al: Tracheocarotid fistula secondary to laryngeal carcinoma presenting as massive hemoptysis. Chest 84:222, 1983.
38. Edwards WH Jr, Morris JA Jr, DeLozier JB III, Adkins RB Jr: Airway injuries. The first priority in trauma. Am Surg 53:192, 1987.
39. Mace SE: Blunt laryngotracheal trauma. Ann Emerg Med 15:836, 1986.
40. Rees JR: Massive hemoptysis associated with foreign body removal. Chest 88:475, 1985.

41. Vander-Salm TJ, Ellis N: Blowgun dart aspiration. J Thorac Cardiovasc Surg 91:930, 1986.
42. Poukkula A, Ruotsalainen EM, Jokinen K, et al: Long-term presence of a denture fragment in the airway (a report of two cases). J Laryngol Otol 102:190, 1988.
43. Pattison CW, Leaming AJ, Townsend ER: Hidden foreign body as a cause of recurrent hemoptysis in a teenage girl. Ann Thorac Surg 45:330, 1988.
44. Williams AG Jr, Mettler FA Jr, Christie JH, Gordon RE: Fat embolism syndrome. Clin Nucl Med 11:495, 1986.
45. Klein BL, Simon JE: Hydrocarbon poisonings. Pediatr Clin North Am 33:411, 1986.
46. Carette S, Macher AM, Nussbaum A, Plotz PH: Severe, acute pulmonary disease in patients with systemic lupus erythematosus: ten years of experience at the National Institutes of Health. Semin Arthritis Rheum 14:52, 1984.
47. Milman N, Rossel K: Recurrent hemoptysis and pulmonary hemosiderosis associated with granulomatous lung disease and von Willebrand's coagulopathy. Eur J Respir Dis 69:192, 1986.
48. Haworth SJ, Savage CO, Carr D, et al: Pulmonary hemorrhage complicating Wegener's granulomatosis and microscopic polyarteritis. Br Med J [Clin Res] 290:1775, 1985.
49. Woodworth TG, Abuelo JG, Austin HA III, Esparza A: Severe glomerulonephritis with late emergence of classic Wegener's granulomatosis. Report of 4 cases and review of the literature. Medicine 66:181, 1987.
50. Mehler PS, Brunvand MW, Hutt MP, Anderson RJ: Chronic recurrent Goodpasture's syndrome. Am J Med 82:833, 1987.
51. Holdsworth S, Boyce N, Thomson NM, Atkins RC: The clinical spectrum of acute glomerulonephritis and lung hemorrhage (Goodpasture's syndrome). Q J Med 55:75, 1985.
52. McLeod DT, Hilton AM, Large DM: Pulmonary sarcoidosis presenting with large hemoptysis. Br J Dis Chest 78:292, 1984.
53. Chang JC, Driver AG, Townsend CA, Kataria YP: Hemoptysis in sarcoidosis. Sarcoidosis 4:49, 1987.
54. Rubinstein I, Baum GL, Hiss Y, Solomon A: Hemoptysis in sarcoidosis. Eur J Respir Dis 66:302, 1985.
55. Burke M, Hallak A, Almog C: Sarcoidosis presenting with acute pleurisy, hemoptysis, pruritus, and eosinophilia. Respiration 51:248, 1987.
56. Murphy S: Cystic fibrosis in adults: diagnosis and management. Clin Chest Med 8:695, 1987.
57. Road JD, Jacques J, Sparling JR: Diffuse alveolar septal amyloidosis presenting with recurrent hemoptysis and medial dissection of pulmonary arteries. Am Rev Respir Dis 132:1368, 1985.
58. Doyle T: Hemoptysis for investigation. Chest 83:551, 1983.
59. Efthimiou J, Johnston C, Spiro SG, Turner-Warwick M: Pulmonary disease in Behçet's syndrome. Q J Med 58:259, 1986.
60. Barberis M, Casadio C, Borghini U: Massive hemoptysis

in Behçet syndrome: case report. Respiration 52:303, 1987.

61. Kim JH, Follett JV, Rice JR, Hampson NB: Endobronchial telangiectasias and hemoptysis in scleroderma. Am J Med 84:173, 1988.
62. Leatherman JW, Davies SF, Hoidal JR: Alveolar hemorrhage syndromes: diffuse microvascular lung hemorrhage in immune and idiopathic disorders. Medicine 63:343, 1984.
63. Albelda SM, Gefter WB, Epstein DM, Miller WT: Diffuse pulmonary hemorrhage: a review and classification. Radiology 154:289, 1985.
64. Bonafede RP, Benatar SR: Bronchocentric granulomatosis and rheumatoid arthritis. Br J Dis Chest 81:197, 1987.
65. Chagares R: Intrathoracic endometriosis: a women's health issue. Heart Lung 16:183, 1987.
66. Hertzanu Y, Heimer D, Hirsch M: Computed tomography of pulmonary endometriosis. Comput Radiol 11:81, 1987.
67. Isaacs RD, Wattie WJ, Wells AU, et al: Massive hemoptysis as a late consequence of pulmonary irradiation. Thorax 42:77, 1987.
68. Feinsilver SJ, Raffin TA, Kornei MC, et al: Factitious hemoptysis. The case of the red towel. Arch Intern Med 143:567, 1983.
69. Thomas R, Siproudhis L, Laurent JF, et al: Massive hemoptysis from iatrogenic balloon catheter rupture of pulmonary artery: successful early management by balloon tamponade. Crit Care Med 15:272, 1987.
70. Carlson TA, Goldenberg IF, Murray PD, et al: Catheter-induced delayed recurrent pulmonary artery hemorrhage. JAMA 261:1943, 1989.
71. Dieden JD, Friloux LA III, Renner JW: Pulmonary artery false aneurysms secondary to Swan-Ganz pulmonary artery catheters. AJR 149:901, 1987.
72. Sethia B, Pollock JC: False aneurysm formation: a complication following the modified Blalock-Taussig shunt. Ann Thorac Surg 41:667, 1986.

Selected Readings

Adelman M, Haponik EF, Bleecker ER, Britt EJ: Cryptogenic hemoptysis. Clinical features, bronchoscopic findings, and natural history in 67 patients. Ann Intern Med 102:829, 1985.
The clinical outcome of 67 patients with hemoptysis and normal or nonlocalizing chest radiographs, as well as a nondiagnostic fiberoptic bronchoscopic examination was reviewed. During an initial follow-up period, 57 (85%) patients remained well without evidence of pulmonary infection or malignancy. Nine patients died of nonpulmonary conditions. Bronchogenic carcinoma was found in 1 patient 20 months after the initial bronchoscopy.

Conlan AA, Hurwitz SS, Krige L, et al: Massive hemoptysis. Review of 123 cases. J Thorac Cardiovasc Surg 85:120, 1983.
Active pulmonary tuberculosis and bronchiectasis were the most common causes of massive hemoptysis in this series.

Corey R, Hla KM: Major and massive hemoptysis: reassessment of conservative management. Am J Med Sci 294:301, 1987.

A retrospective case study and literature review to evaluate current approaches to major and massive hemoptysis was undertaken, including 59 consecutive patients with major hemoptysis, 26 of whom had massive hemoptysis. Outcome was strongly influenced by etiologic factors, operability, and bleeding rate. The mortality rate in patients with hemoptysis caused by carcinoma was 59%; however, good clinical outcome was experienced in patients with other causes of hemoptysis, such as bronchitis, bronchiectasis, tuberculosis, or anticoagulation therapy.

Flower CD: Fiberoptic bronchoscopy in thoracic diagnosis. J Thorac Imaging 2:61, 1987.

State of the art review of uses and limitations of fiberoptic bronchoscopy and the relevance to management and diagnosis of pulmonary lesions first identified by radiographic techniques, such as CT and conventional chest radiographs.

Haponik EF, Britt EJ, Smith PL, Bleecker ER: Computed chest tomography in the evaluation of hemoptysis. Impact on diagnosis and treatment. Chest 91:80, 1987.

Results of computed chest tomograms (CT) and chest roentgenograms (CR) in 32 patients who presented with hemoptysis were compared. Data support a significant augmentation of initial diagnostic data provided by CT information. However, since bronchoscopy was still necessary for diagnosis and management, authors felt that the effect of the information offered by CT did not affect the clinical outcome enough to consider CT evaluation of hemoptysis a routine imaging procedure.

Haponik EF, Rothfeld B, Britt EJ, et al: Radionuclide localization of massive pulmonary hemorrhage. Chest 86:208, 1984.

Authors suggest that selected patients with pulmonary hemorrhage may benefit from radionuclide scanning.

Howard WJ, Rosario EJ, Calhoon SL: Hemoptysis: causes and a practical management approach. Postgrad Med 77(8):53, 1985.

This article reviews the causes of hemoptysis and outlines a systematic approach to diagnosis.

Imgrund SP, Goldberg SK, Walkenstein MD, et al: Clinical diagnosis of massive hemoptysis using the fiberoptic bronchoscope. Crit Care Med 13:438, 1985.

A clinical study reviewing the etiology of massive hemoptysis and the usefulness of flexible bronchoscopy.

Jackson CV, Savage PJ, Quinn DL: Role of fiberoptic bronchoscopy in patients with hemoptysis and a normal chest roentgenogram. Chest 87:142, 1985.

Authors conclude that in patients with hemoptysis and normal chest radiographic findings, routine fiberoptic bronchoscopy may not always be indicated to rule out malignancy.

Katch O, Yamada H, Hiura K, et al: Bronchoscopic and angiographic comparison of bronchial arterial lesions in patients with hemoptysis. Chest 91:486, 1987.

Bronchial arterial lesions that may have caused hemorrhage in seven patients with nonmalignant disease are reviewed. The arterial lesions were examined with bronchoscopy and arteriography. Bulging lesions observed with bronchoscopy corresponded to either an aneurysm or a hypervascular area in the bronchial arteriogram.

Mass lesions corresponded to a hypervacular area or focal dilation in the bronchial arteriogram.

Keller FS, Rosch J, Loflin TG, et al: Nonbronchial systemic collateral arteries: significance in percutaneous embolotherapy for hemoptysis. Radiology 164:687, 1987.

Twenty patients with significant hemoptysis who were treated with percutaneous embolotherapy were reviewed. A variety of malignant, benign, and infectious lesions were identified. Bronchial arteries were embolized in all but one patient. In nine (45%) patients, nonbronchial systemic collateral arteries significantly contributed to the arterial supply of pathologic tissue. Authors stress the importance of recognition and occlusion of nonbronchial systemic collaterals in patients with hypervascular pulmonary lesions.

Poe RH, Israel RH, Marin MG, et al: Utility of fiberoptic bronchoscopy in patients with hemoptysis and a nonlocalizing chest roentgenogram. Chest 93:70, 1988.

A clinical study to determine the indications for fiberoptic bronchoscopy in a patient with hemoptysis and a normal or nonlocalizing chest roentgenogram was undertaken. Authors attempted to develop criteria that would help predict patients most likely to benefit from fiberoptic bronchoscopy in this setting. Factors studied included age, sex, smoking, nonspecific roentgenographic findings, as well as the volume, duration, and recurrence of hemoptysis. By univariate and discriminant analyses, authors found that the presence of two of the three following factors best predicted a diagnosis of malignancy: age of 50 years or more, male sex, and smoking the equivalent of 1 pack a day for 40 years.

Rudzinski JP, del Castillo J: Massive hemoptysis (clinical conference). Ann Emerg Med 16:561, 1987.

Review of management of massive hemoptysis. Loss of a minimum of 600 ml of blood within 48 hours is associated with a high mortality. Initial stabilization management and evaluation maneuvers are outlined.

Strickland B: Investigating hemoptysis. Br J Hosp Med 35:242, 1986.

Clinical review of current approaches to investigating causes of hemoptysis.

Wilson RF, Scullier GW, Wiencek RG: Hemoptysis in trauma. J Trauma 27:1123, 1987.

A retrospective review of 344 patients undergoing thoracotomy for a variety of causes of pulmonary trauma, including traumatic injuries of the trachea, main-stem bronchi, and lungs was undertaken to study the pathophysiology of moderate-to-severe hemoptysis in this clinical situation. Experimental animal studies supplemented this combined clinical and experimental study.

21
Spontaneous Pneumothorax: Common and Uncommon Causes

A pneumothorax occurs when air enters the space between the parietal and visceral pleural space, which results in partial or total lung collapse. Any condition that creates a visceral-pleural tear can cause a pneumothorax. Most pneumothoraces occur spontaneously in young, tall, thin, previously healthy males who usually present with an abrupt onset of sharp, constant chest pain that increases with breathing.[1] Another common clinical setting for spontaneously occurring pneumothorax is the patient with known emphysema or other pulmonary disorders with cystic or cavitary lesions. Although traumatic and iatrogenic causes of pneumothorax are usually obvious, spontaneous pneumothorax in patients without known pulmonary trauma or disease can be obscure. Current epidemiology suggests conditions associated with HIV infection, such as *Penumocystis carinii* pneumonia and certain fungal infections, should be considered as causes of pneumothorax in those patients with known risk factors for HIV infection.[2]

Benign spontaneous pneumothorax: occurs most commonly in thin, previously healthy men between the ages of 20 and 40 years[3,4]

Chronic obstructive pulmonary disease: particularly emphysema with bulla formation[5]

Status asthmaticus: can be complicated by mucous plugging of large and small bronchi[6]

Thoracic trauma[7]

Abdominal trauma[8]

Radiation therapy[9]

Artificial ventilation[10]

Postthoracic or abdominal surgery

Lung carcinoma: primary or metastatic[11–13]

Other neoplasms: lymphoma, rhabdomyosarcoma, mesotheliomas[14–16]

Pulmonary infarction: pulmonary embolus, traumatic, congenital anomaly[17]

Pregnancy: pneumomediastinum, a rare complication of pregnancy, occurs most commonly during the second stage of labor.[18,19]

Bronchiectasis

Endometriosis: may cause some cases of catamenial pneumothorax[20]

Necrotizing pneumonia: staphylococcus, tuberculosis, pseudomonas, klebsiella or anaerobic bacteria[7]

Cystic fibrosis[21,22]

Diffuse interstitial diseases: histiocytosis X, sarcoidosis[23–25]

Catamenial pneumothorax: occurs in young women within 72 hours of menstruation and is usually right-sided with a tendency to recur[20,26–29]

Mycetomas and fungal infections: coccidioidomycosis, aspergillosis[30]

Drug abuse[31]

Parasitic infections: hydatid cysts[32]

Wegener's granulomatosis[33]

Rheumatoid lung disease[34]

Marfan syndrome[35]

von Recklinghausen's disease[36]

Legionnaire's disease[37]

Pneumocystis carinii pneumonia: usually associated with HIV infection[38,39]

Mesenchymal cystic hamartoma of the lung[40]

Desquamative interstitial pneumonia: pneumoconioses.

Familial spontaneous pneumothorax[41]

Cryptogenic fibrosing alveolitis[42]

References

1. Melton LJ III, Hepper NGG, Offord KP: Influence of height on the risk of spontaneous pneumothorax. Mayo Clin Proc 56:678, 1981.
2. Sherman M, Levin D, Breidbart D: *Pneumocystis carinii* pneumonia with spontaneous pneumothorax. A report of three cases. Chest 90:609, 1986.
3. Hyde L: Benign spontaneous pneumothorax. Ann Intern Med 56:746, 1962.
4. Kawakami Y, Irie T, Kamishima K: Stature, lung height, and spontaneous pneumothorax. Respiration 43:35, 1982.
5. Videm V, Pillgram-Larsen J, Ellingsen O, et al: Spontaneous pneumothorax in chronic obstructive pulmonary disease: complications, treatment and recurrences. Eur J Respir Dis 71:365, 1987.
6. Lewis M, Kallenbach J, Zaltzman M, et al: Acute re-

spiratory failure in a young asthmatic patient. Chest 84:733, 1983.

7. Jenkinson SG: Pneumothorax. Clin Chest Med 6:153, 1985.

8. Wall SD, Federle MP, Jeffrey RB, et al: CT diagnosis of unsuspected pneumothorax after blunt abdominal trauma. AJR 141:919, 1983.

9. Rowinsky EK, Abeloff MD, Wharam MD: Spontaneous pneumothorax following thoracic irradiation. Chest 88:703, 1985.

10. Greenough A, Greenall F: Observation of spontaneous respiratory interaction with artificial ventilation. Arch Dis Child 63:168, 1988.

11. Laurens RG Jr, Pine JR, Honig EG: Spontaneous pneumothorax in primary cavitating lung carcinoma. Radiology 146:295, 1983.

12. Kader HA, Bolger JJ, Goepel JR: Bilateral pneumothorax secondary to metastatic angiosarcoma of the breast. Clin Radiol 38:201, 1987.

13. Steinhäuslin CA, Cuttat JF: Spontaneous pneumothorax: a complication of lung cancer? Chest 88:709, 1985.

14. Yellin A, Benfield JR: Pneumothorax associated with lymphoma. Am Rev Respir Dis 134:590, 1986.

15. Mengeot PM, Gailly C: Spontaneous detachment of benign mesothelioma into the pleural space and removal during pleuroscopy. Eur J Respir Dis 68:141, 1986.

16. Allan BT, Day DL, Dehner LP: Primary pulmonary rhabdomyosarcoma of the lung in children. Report of two cases presenting with spontaneous pneumothorax. Cancer 59:1005, 1987.

17. Stocker JT, McGill LC, Orsini EN: Post-infarction peripheral cysts of the lung in pediatric patients: a possible cause of idiopathic spontaneous pneumothorax. Pediatr Pulmonol 1:7, 1985.

18. Karson EM, Saltzman D, Davis MR: Pneumomediastinum in pregnancy: two case reports and a review of the literature, pathophysiology, and management. Obstet Gynecol 64:39S, 1984.

19. Dhalla SS, Teskey JM: Surgical management of recurrent spontaneous pneumothorax during pregnancy. Chest 88:301, 1985.

20. Schoenfeld A, Ziv E, Zeelel Y, et al: Catamenial pneumothorax—a literature review and report of an unusual case. Obstet Gynecol Surv 41:20, 1986.

21. Tomashefski JF Jr, Dahms B, Bruce M: Pleura in pneumothorax. Comparison of patients with cystic fibrosis and idiopathic spontaneous pneumothorax. Arch Pathol Lab Med 109:910, 1985.

22. Tomashefski JF Jr, Bruce M, Stern RC, et al: Pulmonary air cysts in cystic fibrosis: relation of pathologic features to radiologic findings and history of pneumothorax. Hum Pathol 16:253, 1985.

23. Pareek SS, Hawass N el D: An unusual presentation of histiocytosis X. Int J Dermatol 24:126, 1985.

24. Ross RJM, Empey DW: Bilateral spontaneous pneumothorax in sarcoidosis. Postgrad Med J 59:106, 1983.

25. Sharma SK, Pande JN, Mukhopadhay AK, et al: Bilateral recurrent spontaneous pneumothorax in sarcoidosis. Jpn J Med 26:69, 1987.

26. Gray R, Cormier M, Yedlicka J, Moncada R: Catamenial pneumothorax: case report and literature review. J Thorac Imaging 2:72, 1987.
27. Grevy C, Andersen HJ, Hansen LG, Bloch AV: Catamenial pneumothorax. Thorac Cardiovasc Surg 35:238, 1987.
28. Nakamura H, Konishiike J, Sugamura A, et al: Epidemiology of spontaneous pneumothorax in women. Chest 89:378, 1986.
29. Smith SB, Andersen CA: Spontaneous pneumothorax. Am Surg 49:245, 1983.
30. Edelstein G, Levitt RG: Cavitary coccidioidomycosis presenting as spontaneous pneumothorax. AJR 141:533, 1983.
31. Bell C, Borak J, Loeffler JR: Pneumothorax in drug abusers: a complication of internal jugular venous injections. Ann Emerg Med 12:167, 1983.
32. Hadley MD: Occult hydatid disease presenting as a spontaneous pneumothorax. Br J Radiol 58:770, 1985.
33. Jaspan T, Davison AM, Walker WC: Spontaneous pneumothorax in Wegener's granulomatosis. Thorax 37:774, 1982.
34. Ayzenberg O, Reiff DB, Levin L: Bilateral pneumothoraces and pleural effusions complicating rheumatoid lung disease. Thorax 38;159, 1983.
35. Hall JR, Pyeritz RE, Dudgeon DL, et al: Pneumothorax in the Marfan syndrome: prevalence and therapy. Ann Thorac Surg 37:500, 1984.
36. Torrington KG, Ashbaugh DG, Stackle EG: Recklinghausen's disease. Occurrence with intrathoracic vagal neurofibroma and contralateral spontaneous pneumothorax. Arch Intern Med 143:568, 1983.
37. Sundkvist T, Carlsson MG: Legionnaires' disease: unusual presentation with pneumothorax. Scand J Infect Dis 15:127, 1983.
38. Goodman PC, Daley C, Minagi H: Spontaneous pneumothorax in AIDS patients with *Pneumocystis carinii* pneumonia. AJR 147:29, 1986.
39. DeLorenzo LJ, Huang CT, Maguire GP, Stone DJ: Roentgenographic patterns of *Pneumocystis carinii* pneumonia in 104 patients with AIDS. Chest 91:323, 1987.
40. Mark EJ: Mesenchymal cystic hamartoma of the lung. N Engl J Med 315:1255, 1986.
41. Sugiyama Y, Maeda H, Yotsumoto H, Takaku F: Familial spontaneous pneumothorax. Thorax 41:969, 1986.
42. Picado C, Gomez de Almeida R, Xaubet A, et al: Spontaneous pneumothorax in cryptogenic fibrosing alveolitis. Respiration 48:77, 1985.

Selected Readings

Bense L, Eklund G, Wiman LG: Smoking and the increased risk of contracting spontaneous pneumothorax. Chest 92:1009, 1987.
The relationship between smoking and occurrence of spontaneous pneumothorax was studied in a Swedish population of 138 consecutive, mostly urban patients hospitalized for their first spontaneous pneumothorax. Data suggest that smoking increases the relative risk

of spontaneous pneumothorax approximately ninefold in women and twenty-two-fold in men.

Bense SL, Wiman LG, Hedenstierna G: Onset of symptoms in spontaneous pneumothorax: correlations to physical activity. Eur J Respir Dis 71:181, 1987.

The relationship of physical activity at onset of spontaneous pneumothorax was evaluated retrospectively in 219 patients who were predominantly smokers. More than 87% were inactive at the onset of symptoms; moderate exertion was observed in about 2%. Authors suggest their data support a lack of relationship to muscle effort at the time of onset of symptoms of spontaneous pneumothorax.

Fleisher AG, McElvaney G, Lawson L, et al: Surgical management of spontaneous pneumothorax in patients with acquired immunodeficiency syndrome. Ann Thorac Surg 45:21, 1988.

Spontaneous pneumothorax is reported with increasing frequency in patients with AIDS and Pneumocystis carinii *pneumonia. Authors review current recommendations of management, such as closed tube thoracostomy as the initial treatment in symptomatic patients and pleurectomy for air leaks that persist longer than 7 days.*

Granke K, Fischer CR, Gago O, et al: The efficacy and timing of operative intervention for spontaneous pneumothorax. Ann Thorac Surg. 42:540, 1986.

This study assesses the role and timing of operative intervention for spontaneous pneumothorax by reviewing 119 patients retrospectively to compare recurrences, complications, and hospital stays. The study did not find a significant difference in morbidity between patients who were surgically treated. Authors conclude that, considering excellent results with operative pleurodesis and the total hospital days accrued with nonoperative therapy, operative pleurodesis should be considered if an active leak persists more than 3 days after the initial episode of spontaneous pneumothorax.

Guyton SW, Paull DL, Anderson RP: Introducer insertion of mini-thoracostomy tubes. Am J Surg 155:693, 1988.

Outpatient management of spontaneous pneumothorax with small caliber chest tubes is described. Authors suggest this technique is well tolerated and risk of injury to lung and other viscera is minimal.

Hagen RH, Reed W, Solheim K: Spontaneous pneumothorax. Scand J Thorac Cardiovasc Surg 21:183, 1987.

A series of 201 patients withh spontaneous pneumothorax is reviewed with a comparison of various conservative and surgical approaches. Authors include a discussion of special problems of management in elderly patients.

Keller N, Szaff M, Sykulski R: Electrocardiographic changes in spontaneous left pneumothorax. Acta Med Scand 221:499, 1987.

A case report of ECG changes suggestive of anterior myocardial infarction in a young man with a left-sided pneumothorax. Authors point out that, taken in a supine position, the ECG can be misleading in the clinical setting of a pneumothorax or mediastinal emphysema and suggest that, by performing the ECG with the patient in an erect position, these misleading ECG findings may be avoided.

Kounis NG, Mallioris CN, Karavias D, et al: Unusual electrocardiographic changes in intrathoracic conditions. Acta Cardiol 42:179, 1987.

ECG, roentgenographic, and clinical findings are reviewed from five patients with a variety of intrathoracic conditions. Interesting clinical observations include variations associated with intrathoracic anatomy.

Krasnik M, Christensen B, Halkier E, et al: Pleurodesis in spontaneous pneumothorax by means of tetracycline. Follow-up evaluation of a method. Scand J Thorac Cardiovasc Surg 21:181, 1987.

Current recommendations and review of the value and limitations of tetracycline pleurodesis in the treatment of spontaneous pneumothorax.

Robinson CL: Autologous blood for pleurodesis in recurrent and chronic spontaneous pneumothorax. Can J Surg 30:428, 1987.

A series of patients treated with autologous blood for pleurodesis for treatment of recurrent and chronic spontaneous pneumothorax is reviewed. Authors found this procedure successful in 21 (85%) of 25 patients with difficult, chronic, or recurrent pneumothoraces.

Tsutsumi T, Kato T, Osada H, et al: Vectorcardiographic QRS loop in spontaneous pneumothorax. J Electrocardiol 20:375, 1987.

A vector analysis of the often confusing QRS finding on ECG in the setting of spontaneous pneumothorax. Authors suggest that their study supports extracardiac reasons for the described alterations of the QRS loop observed in patients with spontaneous pneumothorax.

GASTROENTEROLOGY

22
Nausea and Vomiting: Common Causes and Associated Disorders

Many functional and organic disorders cause nausea and vomiting; gastroenteritis and drug effects are the most common organic causes. Nausea and vomiting can herald an acute abdominal emergency, reflect systemic illness, metabolic-endocrine dysfunction, chronic or acute gastrointestinal disorders, and occasionally neurologic illness. When there is no known underlying illness, chronic nausea and vomiting are frequently psychogenic. Serious complications of protracted vomiting include hypovolemia, acid-base disorders, aspiration pneumonitis, mucosal tears at the gastroesophageal junction (Mallory-Weiss syndrome) and rupture of the esophagus (Boerhaave's syndrome).[1]

Gastrointestinal Causes

Inflammation, congestion, or ischemia of intra-abdominal and pelvic structures can cause nausea and vomiting.

Gastroenteritis: infectious, drug-induced
Food poisoning: particularly preformed toxins
Gastrointestinal obstruction[2]: mechanical or paralytic. Vomiting occurs more frequently with higher obstructions, i.e., pyloric obstruction.[3]
Acute appendicitis[4]
Acute hepatic injury: viral hepatitis
Reye's syndrome: generally in children and young adults, but can occur in adults[5]
Cholecystitis
Pancreatitis: acute and chronic
Pancreatic carcinoma[6]
Superior mesenteric artery syndrome: risk factors include prolonged bed rest, recent significant weight loss, malnutrition, and body casts[7,8]
Peritonitis[9,10]

Food allergies[11]
Gastric paresis: diabetes,[12,13] postvagotomy gastric tachyarrhythmias, or tachygastria[14]
Achalasia
Intestinal and gastric neoplasia[15]
Esophageal or pharyngeal (Zenker's) diverticula
Tracheoesophageal fistula

Drug Effects

Almost any medication can be associated with nausea or vomiting. Common causes of drug-induced vomiting include the following:

Ethanol
Opioids (usual doses)
Iron preparations
Cancer chemotherapy: particularly cisplatin and anthracyclines[16,17]
Birth control pills
Amphotericin B
Dopamine agonists: levodopa, apomorphine, bromocriptine
Salicylates
Digitalis[18]
Theophylline[19]
Anesthesia[20,21]
Nonsteroidal anti-inflammatory drugs[22]

Psychogenic Causes

Nonspecific stress[23,24]
Bulimia[25-27]
Anorexia nervosa[28]
Rumination: generally considered a psychosomatic disorder, it is associated with anatomic upper gastrointestinal tract abnormalities.[29,30]

Neurologic Causes

Labyrinthitis: infection, idiopathic, Meniere's disease, motion sickness[31]
Vestibulitis[32]
Migraine headaches[33]
Cerebral tumors: particularly posterior fossa lesions can present with intractable vomiting[34-36]
Nontumor causes of increased intracranial pressure: trauma, stroke,[37] and infection or secondary to diffuse swelling of metabolic, infectious, and hypertensive encephalopathies

Miscellaneous

Pregnancy: hydatidiform mole[38,39]
Uremia
Metabolic-endocrine dysfunction: diabetic ketoaci-
dosis, adrenal insufficiency, hyperparathyroidism,
hyponatremia, acid-base abnormalities, hypokale-
mia,[40] hypothyroidism, and hyperthyroidism
Radiotherapy[41]
Myocardial infarction[42,43]
Systemic illness: acute and chronic febrile, pulmo-
nary, cardiac, renal, and gastrointestinal disorders
Pain: any visceral painful condition
Jamaican vomiting illness: hypoglycin A from unripe
akee fruit ingestion[44]
Heimlich maneuver[45]
Asthma[46]

References

1. Singh GS, Slovis CM: "Occult" Boerhaave's syndrome.
   J Emerg Med 6:13, 1988.
2. Thompson DG, Malagelada JR: Vomiting and the small
   intestine. Dig Dis Sci 27:1121, 1982.
3. Abbot FK, Mack M, Wolf S: The relation of sustained
   contraction of the duodenum to nausea and vomiting.
   Gastroenterology 20:238, 1952.
4. Alvarado A: A practical score for the early diagnosis of
   acute appendicitis. Ann Emerg Med 15:557, 1986.
5. Meythaler JM, Varma RR: Reye's syndrome in adults.
   Diagnostic considerations. Arch Intern Med 147:61,
   1987.
6. Barkin JS, Goldberg RI, Sfakianakis GN, Levi J: Pancreatic carcinoma is associated with delayed gastric
   emptying. Dig Dis Sci 31:265, 1986.
7. Rosenburg SA, Sampson A: The syndrome of mesenteric vascular compression of the duodenum. Report of
   eleven cases with operative correction. Arch Surg
   73:296, 1956.
8. Jones PA, Wastell C: Superior mesenteric artery syndrome. Postgrad Med J 59(692):376, 1983.
9. Walton FE, Moore RM, Graham EA: The nerve pathways in the vomiting of peritonitis. Arch Surg 22:829,
   1931.
10. Rimland D, Hand WL: Spontaneous peritonitis: a reap-
    praisal. Am J Med Sci 293:285, 1987.
11. Walker-Smith JA, Ford RP, Phillips AD: The spectrum
    of gastrointestinal allergies to food. Ann Allergy 53:629,
    1984.
12. Loo FD, Palmer DW, Soergel KH, et al: Gastric emp-
    tying in patients with diabetes mellitus. Gastroenterol-
    ogy 86:485, 1984.
13. Mearin F, Camilleri M, Malagelada JR: Pyloric dys-
    function in diabetics with recurrent nausea and vomit-
    ing. Gastroenterology 90:1919, 1986.
14. You CH, Lee KY, Chey WY, et al: Electrogastrographic
    study of patients with unexplained nausea, bloating,
    and vomiting. Gastroenterology 79:311, 1980.

15. Zollinger RM Jr: Primary neoplasms of the small intestine. Am J Surg 151:654, 1986.
16. Durant JR: The problem of nausea and vomiting in modern cancer chemotherapy. CA 34:2, 1984.
17. OBrien ME, Cullen MH: Therapeutic progress—review XXVIII. Are we making progress in the management of cytotoxic drug-induced nausea and vomiting? J Clin Pharm Ther 13:19, 1988.
18. Moorman JR: Digitalis toxicity at Duke Hospital, 1973 to 1984. South Med J 78:561, 1985.
19. Amitai Y, Lovejoy FH Jr: Characteristics of vomiting associated with acute sustained release theopylline poisoning: implications for management with oral activated charcoal. J Toxicol Clin Toxicol 25:539, 1987.
20. Palazzo MGA, Strunin L: Anesthesia and emesis. I. Etiology. Can Anaesth Soc J 31:178, 1984.
21. Boucher BA, Witt WO, Foster TS: The postoperative adverse effects of inhalational anesthetics. Heart Lung 15:63, 1986.
22. Vale JA, Meredith TJ: Acute poisoning due to non-steroidal anti-inflammatory drugs. Clinical features and management. Med Toxicol 1:12, 1986.
23. Wruble LD, Rosenthal RH, Webb WL Jr: Psychogenic vomiting: a review. Am J Gastroenterol 77:318, 1982.
24. Clouse RE, Alpers DH: The relationship of psychiatric disorder to gastrointestinal illness. Annu Rev Med 37:283, 1986.
25. Fairburn CG, Cooper PJ: Self-induced vomiting and bulimia nervosa: an undetected problem. Br Med J 284:1153, 1982.
26. Humphries LL: Bulimia: diagnosis and treatment. Compr Ther 13:12, 1987.
27. Mitchell JE, Seim HC, Colon E, Pomeroy C: Medical complications and medical management of bulimia. Ann Intern Med 107:71, 1987.
28. Garfinkel PE, Kaplan AS, Garner DM, et al: The differentiation of vomiting/weight loss as a conversion disorder from anorexia nervosa. Am J Psychiatr 140:1019, 1983.
29. Brown WR: Rumination in the adult. A study of two cases. Gastroenterology 54:933, 1968.
30. Amarnath RP, Abell TL, Malagelada JR: The rumination syndrome in adults. A characteristic manometric pattern. Ann Intern Med 105:513, 1986.
31. Mauro CA, Smith DE: A statistical analysis of motion sickness incidence data. Aviat Space Environ Med 54:253, 1983.
32. Miller AD, Wilson VJ: Vestibular-induced vomiting after vestibulocerebellar lesions. Brain Behav Evol 23:26, 1983.
33. Lanzi G, Balottin U, Ottolini A, et al: Cyclic vomiting and recurrent abdominal pains as migraine or epileptic equivalents. Cephalalgia 3:115, 1983
34. Baker PC, Bernat JL: The neuroanatomy of vomiting in man: association of projectile vomiting with a solitary metastasis in the lateral tegmentum of the pons and the middle cerebellar peduncle. J Neurol Neurosurg Psychiatry 48:1165, 1985.
35. Torrealba G, Del Villar S, Arriagada P: Protracted

vomiting as the presenting sign of posterior fossa mass lesions. J Neurol Neurosurg Psychiatry 50:1539, 1987.

36. Diamond S, Singleton R: Sudden respiratory arrest following headache. Postgrad Med 74(2):103, 1983.

37. Sherman DG, Easton JD: Cerebral edema in stroke. A common, often fatal complication. Postgrad Med 68(1):107, 1980.

38. Jarnfelt-Samsioe A: Nausea and vomiting in pregnancy: a review. Obstet Gynecol Surv 42:422, 1987.

39. Fardy HJ: Vomiting in late pregnancy due to diaphragmatic hernia. Case report. Br J Obstet Gynecol 91:390, 1984.

40. Richardson RM, Forbath N, Karanicolas S: Hypokalemic metabolic alkalosis caused by surreptitious vomiting: report of four cases. Can Med Assoc J 129:142, 1983.

41. Westbrook C, Glaholm J, Barrett A: Vomiting associated with whole body irradiation. Clin Radiol 38:263, 1987.

42. Sleight P: Cardiac vomiting. Br Heart J 46:5, 1981.

43. Herlihy T, McIvor ME, Cummings CC, et al: Nausea and vomiting during acute myocardial infarction and its relation to infarct size and location. Am J Cardiol 60:20, 1987.

44. Tanaka K, Kean EA, Johnson B: Jamaican vomiting sickness. Biochemical investigation of two cases. N Engl J Med 295:461, 1976.

45. Orlowski JP: Vomiting as a complication of the Heimlich maneuver. JAMA 258:512, 1987.

46. Schreier L, Cutler RM, Saigal V: Vomiting as a dominant symptom of asthma. Ann Allergy 58:118, 1987.

Selected Readings

Baker PCH, Bernat JL: The neuroanatomy of vomiting in man: association of projectile vomiting with a solitary metastasis in the lateral tegmentum of the pons and the middle cerebellar peduncle. J Neurol Neurosurg Psychiatry 48:1165, 1985.
Interesting case report and discussion of the neuroanatomy of vomiting.

Geldof H, Van Der Schee EJ, Van Blankenstein M, et al: Electrogastrographic study of gastric myoelectrical activity in patients with unexplained nausea and vomiting. Gut 27:799, 1986.
A study that relates abnormal myoelectrical activity to symptoms of otherwise unexplained nausea and vomiting.

Hanson JS, McCallum RW: The diagnosis and management of nausea and vomiting. A review. Am J Gastroenterol 80:210, 1985.
Review that includes the differential diagnosis for nausea and vomiting.

Kinzel T: Symptom control in geriatric patients with terminal cancer: pain, nausea, and vomiting. Geriatrics 43(6):83, 1988.
Useful review of current treatment choices available to significantly relieve symptoms of pain, nausea, and vomiting with an emphasis on the geriatric patient.

Malagelada JR, Camilleri M: Unexplained vomiting: a diagnostic challenge. Ann Intern Med 101:211, 1984.

Well-referenced discussion of unexplained vomiting, including an algorithmic approach for patient management.

Menkes JH, Ament ME: Neurologic disorders of gastroesophageal function. Adv Neurol 49:409, 1988.

This paper reviews current concepts of pathophysiology of certain problems, including gastroesophageal reflux, cyclic vomiting, achalasia, and rumination. Current concepts of pertinent neurophysiology are reviewed.

Talley NJ, Phillips SF: Non-ulcer dyspepsia: potential causes and pathophysiology. Ann Intern Med 108:865, 1988.

Current concepts of dyspepsia defined as chronic or recurrent upper abdominal pain or nausea that stresses the heterogeneity of patients with nonulcer dyspepsia. Authors recommend empiric trials of treatment based on their experience and review of controlled treatment trials.

23
Dysphagia: Esophageal, Oropharyngeal, and Neurologic Causes

Dysphagia is the sensation described when there is a hesitation or pause in the normal process of swallowing, generally described as food "sticking" or "not going down right." Multiple esophageal and oropharyngeal disorders can cause dysphagia. Obstruction and esophageal motor dysfunction are the most common mechanisms causing difficulty in swallowing. In older adults, particularly smokers and alcoholics, the presence of dysphagia will generally require evaluation of the esophagus by upper endoscopy to rule out an esophageal malignancy.

Causes of Esophageal Obstruction

Tumors, benign or malignant: dysphagia is often the presenting symptom of esophageal carcinoma.[1-3]
Strictures: reflux esophagitis is the most common

cause of benign esophageal strictures[4,5]; other causes include peptic strictures, idiopathic,[6] malignant, and following caustic injury.[7]

Esophageal webs and rings, including the Plummer-Vinson syndrome: upper esophageal eccentric web of squamous epithelium, iron deficiency anemia and dysphagia, a premalignant condition[8] and the Schatzki's ring[9]

Extrinsic compression or local extension: mediastinal or gastric tumors, aortic aneurysm or tortuous nonaneurysmal atherosclerotic aorta, left atrial hypertrophy, or aberrant subclavian artery[10–13]

Hypertrophic cervical osteophytes: Forestier's syndrome, cervical spine surgery[14–17]

Barrett's esophagus (or columnar-lined esophagus): often associated with esophagitis, ulceration, or strictures[18,19]

Aortoesophageal fistula: chest pain, dysphagia, and intermittent hematemesis may herald significant gastrointestinal bleeding.[20]

Causes of Oropharyngeal Obstruction

Macroglossia: inflammation, trauma, amyloidosis, hypothyroidism

Pharyngitis: viral, diphtheria

Oropharyngeal neoplasms: lymphoma,[21,22] Kaposi's sarcoma,[23,24] and squamous cell carcinomas of the oral cavity and tonsils

Tonsillar inflammation: tonsillitis, tonsillar abscess, tonsillar cyst[25,26]

Iatrogenic: postsurgical, postirradiation

Thyroid enlargement

Hypopharyngeal ulceration[27]

Causes of Esophageal Motor Dysfunction

The three most common esophageal motility disorders that cause dysphagia are achalasia, scleroderma, and diffuse esophageal spasm.[28]

Diffuse esophageal spasm: can mimic pain of angina pectoris[29]

Achalasia: nocturnal regurgitation may cause aspiration.[30–31]

Connective tissue disease[32]: especially in the presence of Raynaud's phenomenon; scleroderma,[33] CREST syndrome,[34] Behçet's disease,[35] systemic lupus erythematosus, Sjögren's syndrome,[36] polymyositis, and dermatomyositis.[37]

Drug-induced esophageal injury[38]: tetracyclines,[39] clindamycin, acetylsalicylic acid, indomethacin, phenylbutazone, chemotherapy, potassium supplements,[40] cimetidine, ferrous sulfate,[41] ascorbic acid, quinidine,[42] doxycycline,[43] ergonovine,[44] neuroleptics,[45] alcohol,[46] and cocaine abuse

Myxedema[47]

Diabetes mellitus[48,49]

Pernicious anemia[50]

Postirradiation[51]

Amyloidosis[52]

Dysautonomic syndromes[53]

Idiopathic

Causes of Oropharyngeal Neuromuscular Dysfunction

Oropharyngeal dysfunction can cause choking and subsequent aspiration. Greater difficulty swallowing fluids than solids suggests a neurologic etiology, that could be secondary to central, peripheral (cranial nerves), or neuromuscular dysfunction.

Disorders Causing Bulbar Muscle Dysfunction

Myasthenia gravis[54]

Head and neck cancer surgery or radiotherapy[55]

Motor neuron disease: progressive bulbar palsy[56,57]

Brain stem tumors

Syringobulbia: syringomyelia of the cervical cord[58]

Muscular dystrophy[59-61]

Hyperthyroidism[62]

Cervical spine disease[63,64]

Eaton-Lambert syndrome: myasthenic syndrome sometimes associated with oat cell carcinoma and other neoplastic disorders

Botulism[65]

Tetanus: associated with trismus[66,67]

Curare poisoning

Multiple sclerosis[68]

Meigs syndrome[69]

Stiff-man syndrome[70]

Oculopharyngeal myopathy[71]

Myotonic dystrophica[72]

Postpolio[73]

Disorders That Can Cause Cranial Nerve Weakness

Brain stem infarction (bilateral)

Brain stem and nasopharyngeal tumors

Postvagotomy syndromes[74]

Sarcoidosis: basilar granulomatous meningitis that infiltrates and compresses cranial nerves[75]

Infection: poliomyelitis, diphtheria, tuberculosis,[76] fungal, cephalic tetanus
Cranial polyneuritis
Carcinomatosis
Iatrogenic: trigeminal nerve anesthesia[77]
Paget's disease: osteophytic impingement on cranial nerves[78]
Polyneuropathy: Guillain-Barré variant[79,80]

Central Nervous System Disorders Causing Bulbar Weakness

Cerebrovascular infarction[81-83]
Head trauma[84,85]
Huntington's disease[86]
Parkinson's disease
Cocaine abuse: can precipitate cardiovascular accident[87]

References

1. Pope CE II: Tumors. P. 479. In Sleisenger MH, Fordtran JS (eds): Gastrointestinal Disease, 3rd Ed. WB Saunders Philadelphia, 1983.
2. Brindley GV Jr, Hayward RH, Korompai FL, Knight WL: Carcinoma of the esophagus. Surg Clin North Am 66:673, 1986.
3. Goldberg RI, Rams H, Stone B, Barkin JS: Dysphagia as the presenting symptom of recurrent breast carcinoma. Cancer 60:1085, 1987.
4. Ahtaridis G, Snape WJ Jr, Cohen S: Clinical and manometric findings in benign peptic strictures of the esophagus. Dig Dis Sci 24:858, 1979.
5. Waterfall WE, Craven MA, Allen CJ: Gastroesophageal reflux: clinical presentations, diagnosis, and management. Can Med Assoc J 135:1101, 1986.
6. Mukhopadhyay AK: Idiopathic lower esophageal sphincter incompetence and esophageal stricture. Arch Intern Med 140:1493, 1980.
7. Kozarek RA, Sanowski RA: Caustic cicatrization of the pharynx associated with dysphagia and premalignant mucosal changes. Am J Gastroenterol 77:5, 1982.
8. Chisholm M: The association between webs, iron, and postcricoid carcinoma. Postgrad Med J 50:215, 1974.
9. Arvanitakis C: Lower esophageal ring: endoscopic and therapeutic aspects. Gastrointest Endosc 24:17, 1977.
10. Mittal RK, Siskind BN, Hongo M, et al: Dysphagia aortica. Clinical, radiological, and manometric findings. Dig Dis Sci 31:379, 1986.
11. Johnson CE, Wardman AG, McMahon MJ, et al: Dysphagia complicating malignant mesothelioma. Thorax 38:635, 1983.
12. Roark GD, Schoppe LE: Painful dysphagia from infiltrating oat cell carcinoma. J Clin Gastroenterol 5:331, 1983.
13. Hansen HA II, Haun CL, Mansour KA: Bronchogenic carcinoma masquerading as primary esophageal disease. Am Surg 48:175, 1982.

14. Brandenberg G, Leibrock LG: Dysphagia and dysphonia secondary to anterior cervical osteophytes. Neurosurgery 18:90, 1986.
15. Eviatar E, Harell M: Diffuse idiopathic skeletal hyperostosis with dysphagia (a review). J Laryngol Otol 101:627, 1987.
16. Deutsch EC, Schild JA, Mafee MF: Dysphagia and Forestier's disease. Arch Otolaryngol 111:400, 1985.
17. Welsh LW, Welsh JJ, Chinnici JC: Dysphagia due to cervical spine surgery. Ann Otol Rhinol Laryngol 96:112, 1987.
18. Cooper BT, Barbezat GO: Barrett's oesophagus: a clinical study of 52 patients. Q J Med 62:97, 1987.
19. Katzka DA, Reynolds JC, Saul SH, et al: Barrett's metaplasia and adenocarcinoma of the esophagus in scleroderma. Am J Med 82:46, 1987.
20. Khawaja FI, Varindani MK: Aortoesophageal fistula. Review of clinical, radiographic, and endoscopic features. J Clin Gastroenterol 9:342, 1987.
21. Saul SH, Kapadia SB: Primary lymphoma of Waldeyer's ring. Clinicopathologic study of 68 cases. Cancer 56:157, 1985.
22. Okerbloom JA, Armitage JO, Zetterman R, Linder J: Esophageal involvement by non-Hodgkin's lymphoma. Am J Med 77:359, 1984.
23. Patow CA, Stark TW, Findlay PA, et al: Pharyngeal obstruction by Kaposi's sarcoma in a homosexual male with acquired immune deficiency syndrome. Otolaryngol Head Neck Surg 92:713, 1984.
24. Emery CD, Wall SD, Federle MP, Sooy CD: Pharyngeal Kaposi's sarcoma in patients with AIDS. AJR 147:919, 1986.
25. Twigg HL, Kinnison ML, Smirniotopoulos JG: Radiographic diagnosis of tonsillar cyst presenting as dysphagia. Gastrointest Radiol 6:305, 1981.
26. Fitzgerald P, OConnell D: Massive hypertrophy of the lingual tonsils: an unusual cause of dysphagia. Br J Radiol 60:505, 1987.
27. Harrison DF: Idiopathic ulceration of the hypopharynx. Laryngoscope 95:292, 1985.
28. Castell DO, Knuff TE, Brown FC, et al: Dysphagia. Gastroenterology 76:1015, 1979.
29. Benjamin SB, Gerhardt DC, Castell DO: High amplitude peristaltic esophageal contractions associated with chest pain and/or dysphagia. Gastroenterology 77:478, 1979.
30. Vantrappen G, Janssens J, Hellemans J, et al: Achalasia, diffuse esophageal spasm, and related motility disorders. Gastroenterology 76:450, 1979.
31. Bianco A, Cagossi M, Scrimieri D, Greco AV: Appearance of esophageal peristalsis in treated idiopathic achalasia. Dig Dis Sci 31:40, 1986.
32. Turner R, Rittenberg G, Lipshutz W, et al: Esophageal dysfunction in collagen disease. Am J Med Sci 265:191, 1973.
33. Zamost BJ, Hirschberg J, Ippoliti AF, et al: Esophagitis in scleroderma. Prevalence and risk factors. Gastroenterology 92:421, 1987.
34. Lovy MR, Levine JS, Steigerwald JC: Lower esophageal

rings as a cause of dysphagia in progressive systemic sclerosis—coincidence or consequence? Dig Dis Sci 28:780, 1983.

35. Brookes GB: Pharyngeal stenosis in Behçet's syndrome. The first reported case. Arch Otolaryngol 109:338, 1983.
36. Kjellen G, Fransson SG, Lindstrom F, et al: Esophageal function, radiography, and dysphagia in Sjögren's syndrome. Dig Dis Sci 31:225, 1986.
37. de Merieux P, Verity MA, Clements PJ, et al: Esophageal abnormalities and dysphagia in polymyositis and dermatomyositis. Clinical, radiographic, and pathologic features. Arthritis Rheum 26:961, 1983.
38. Collins FJ, Matthews HR, Baker SE, et al: Drug-induced esophageal injury. Br Med J 1:1673, 1979.
39. Crowson TD, Head LH, Ferrante WA: Esophageal ulcers associated with tetracycline therapy. JAMA 235:2747, 1976.
40. Lubbe WF, Cadogan ES, Kannemeyer AHR: Esophageal ulceration due to slow-release potassium in the presence of left atrial enlargement. NZ Med J 90:377, 1979.
41. Abbarah TR, Fredell JE, Ellenz GB: Ulceration by oral ferrous sulfate. JAMA 236:2320, 1976.
42. Bohane TD, Perrault J, Fowler RS: Esophagitis and esophageal obstruction from quinidine tablets in association with left atrial enlargement: a case report. Aust Paediatr J 14:191, 1978.
43. Amendola MA, Spera TD: Doxycycline-induced esophagitis. JAMA 253:1009, 1985.
44. Lieberman DA, Jendrezejewski JW, McAnulty JH: Ergonovine-provoked esophageal spasm during coronary angiography. West J Med 140:403, 1984.
45. Moss HB, Green A: Neuroleptic-associated dysphagia confirmed by esophageal manometry. Am J Psychiatry 139:515, 1982.
46. Hogan WJ, Viegas de Andrade SR, Winship DH: Ethanol-induced acute esophageal motor dysfunction. J Appl Physiol 32:755, 1972.
47. Wright RA, Penner DB: Myxedema and upper esophageal dysmotility. Dig Dis Sci 26:376, 1981.
48. Ippoliti A: Esophageal disorders in diabetes mellitus. Yale J Biol Med 56:267, 1983.
49. Keshavarzian A, Iber FL, Nasrallah S: Radionuclide esophageal emptying and manometric studies in diabetes mellitus. Am J Gastroenterol 82:625, 1987.
50. Farrell RL, Nebel OT, McGuire AT, et al: The abnormal lower esophageal sphincter in pernicious anemia. Gut 14:767, 1973.
51. O'Rourke IC, Tiver K, Bull C, et al: Swallowing performance after radiation therapy for carcinoma of the esophagus. Cancer 61:2022, 1988.
52. Lavergne A, Galian A, Defrance R, et al: Amyloidosis revealed by monosymptomatic dysphagia. Report of one case. Hepatogastroenterology 29:72, 1982.
53. Sparberg M, Knudsen KB, Frank ST: Dysautonomia and dysphagia. Neurology 18:504, 1968.
54. Huang MH, King KL, Chien KY: Esophageal manometric studies in patients with myasthenia gravis. J Thorac Cardiovasc Surg 95:281, 1988.

55. Welch RW, Luckmann K, Ricks PM, et al: Manometry of the normal upper esophageal sphincter and its alterations in laryngectomy. J Clin Invest 63:1036, 1979.
56. Smith AWM, Mulder DW, Code CF: Esophageal motility in amyotrophic lateral sclerosis. Mayo Clin Proc 32:438, 1957.
57. Janzen VD, Rae RE, Hudson AJ: Otolaryngologic manifestations of amyotrophic lateral sclerosis. J Otolaryngol 17:41, 1988.
58. Bleck TP, Shannon KM: Disordered swallowing due to a syrinx: correction by shunting. Neurology (Cleveland) 34:1497, 1984.
59. Duranceau AC, Beauchamp G, Jamieson GG, et al: Oropharyngeal dysphagia and oculopharyngeal muscular dystrophy. Surg Clin North Am 63:825, 1983.
60. Dobrowski JM, Zajtchuk JT, LaPiana FG, Hensley SD Jr: Oculopharyngeal muscular dystrophy: clinical and histopathologic correlations. Otolaryngol Head Neck Surg 95:131, 1986.
61. Kiel DP: Oculopharyngeal muscular dystrophy as a cause of dysphagia in the elderly. J Am Geriatr Soc 34:144, 1986.
62. Branski D, Levy J, Globus M, et al: Dysphagia as a primary manifestation of hyperthyroidism. J Clin Gastroenterol 6:437, 1984.
63. Lambert JR, Tepperman PS, Jimenez J, et al: Cervical spine disease and dysphagia. Am J Gastroenterol 76:35, 1981.
64. Hirano H, Suzuki H, Sakakibara T, et al: Dysphagia due to hypertrophic cervical osteophytes. Clin Orthop 167:168, 1982.
65. Hughes JM, Blumenthal JR, Merson MH, et al: Clinical features of types A and B food-borne botulism. Ann Intern Med 95:442, 1981.
66. Weinstein L: Tetanus. N Engl J Med 289:1293, 1973.
67. Wang L, Karmody CS: Dysphagia as the presenting symptom of tetanus. Arch Otolaryngol 111:342, 1985.
68. Daly DD, Code CF, Andersen HA: Disturbances of swallowing and esophageal motility in patients with multiple sclerosis. Neurology 12:250, 1962.
69. Kakigi R, Shibasaki H, Kuroda Y, et al: Miege's syndrome associated with spasmodic dysphagia (letter). J Neurol Neurosurg Psychiatry 46:589, 1983.
70. Sulway MJ, Baume PE, Davis E: Stiff-man syndrome presenting with complete esophageal obstruction. Am J Dig Dis 15:79, 1970.
71. Bender MD: Esophageal manometry in oculopharyngeal dystrophy. Am J Gastroenterol 65:215, 1976.
72. Siegel CL, Hendrix TR, Harvey JC: The swallowing disorder in myotonic dystrophica. Gastroenterology 50:541, 1966.
73. Buchholz D: Dysphagia in post-polio patients. Birth Defects 23:55, 1987.
74. Greatorex RA, Thorpe JAC: Achalasia-like disturbance of esophageal motility following truncal-vagotomy and atrectomy. Postgrad Med J 59:100, 1983.
75. Delaney P: Neurologic manifestations in sarcoidosis. Review of the literature, with a report of 23 cases. Ann Intern Med 87:336, 1977.

76. Savage PE, Grundy A: Esophageal tuberculosis: an unusual cause of dysphagia. Br J Radiol 57:1153, 1984.
77. Lawrence WH, Partyka EK: Chronic dysphagia and trigeminal anesthesia after trichloroethylene exposure. Ann Intern Med 95:710, 1981.
78. Frank MS, Brandt LJ, Kaufman DM, et al: Oropharyngeal dysphagia in Paget's disease of bone (osteitis deformans): response to calcitonin. Am J Gastroenterol 77:450, 1982.
79. Smith JL, Walsh FB: Syndrome of external ophthalmoplegia, ataxia, and areflexia (Fisher). Arch Ophthalmol 58:109, 1957.
80. Donaghy M, Earl CJ: Ocular palsy preceding chronic relapsing polyneuropathy by several weeks. Ann Neurol 17:49, 1985.
81. Butcher RB II: Treatment of chronic aspiration as a complication of cerebrovascular accident. Laryngoscope 92:681, 1982.
82. Gordon C, Hewer RL, Wade DT: Dysphagia in acute stroke. Br Med J 295:411, 1987.
83. Veis SL, Logemann JA: Swallowing disorders in persons with cerebrovascular accident. Arch Phys Med Rehabil 66:372, 1985.
84. Winstein CJ: Neurogenic dysphagia: frequency, progression, and outcome in adults following head injury. Phys Ther 63:1992, 1983.
85. Lazarus C, Logemann JA: Swallowing disorders in closed head trauma patients. Arch Phys Med Rehabil 68:79, 1987.
86. Leopold NA, Kagel MC: Dysphagia in Huntington's disease. Arch Neurol 42:57, 1985.
87. DeVore RA, Tucker HM: Dysphagia and dysarthria as a result of cocaine abuse. Otolaryngol Head Neck Surg 98:174, 1988.

Selected Readings

Bancewicz J, Osugi H, Marples M: Clinical implications of abnormal esophageal motility. Br J Surg 74:416, 1987.

The usefulness of esophageal manometry in 202 patients investigated for esophageal symptoms was studied. Detection and treatment of gastroesophageal reflex was found to be the most useful component of clinical management.

Bott S, Prakash C, McCallum RW: Medication-induced esophageal injury: survey of the literature. Am J Gastroenterol 82:758, 1987.

One hundred twenty-seven cases of drug-induced esophagitis are reported. Drugs most commonly implicated included emepronium bromide, tetracycline, potassium chloride, and quinidine. Endoscopy was considered the diagnostic study of choice.

Duranceau A, Lafontaine ER, Taillefer R, Jamieson GG: Oropharyngeal dysphagia and operations on the upper esophageal sphincter. Surg Annu 19:317, 1987.

Oropharyngeal dysphagia is difficult to evaluate because of the wide spectrum of conditions causing symptoms. A comprehensive discussion of pathophysiology, including discussion of neurogenic, myogenic, structural, iatrogenic, and mechanical causes of oropharyngeal dysphagia, is presented, as well as current concepts of evaluation, including use of cineroentogenography, videoroentgen-

ography, radionuclide studies, motility studies, and endoscopy. Well referenced.

Ekberg O, Wahlgren L: Dysfunction of pharyngeal swallowing. A cineradiographic investigation in 854 dysphagia patients. Acta Radiol 26:389, 1985.
Cineradiography of pharyngeal swallowing in 854 patients with dysphagia was analyzed for pharyngeal function. Findings in decreased frequency included defective closure of laryngeal vestibule, cricopharyngeal muscle dysfunction, epiglottic dysmotility, pharyngeal constrictor paresis, pharyngeal webs, and diverticulae. Age and sex differences were noted.

Gupta SD, Petrus LV, Gibbins FJ, Dellipiani AW: Endoscopic evaluation of dysphagia in the elderly. Age Ageing 16:159, 1987.
A clinical study of 100 consecutive endoscopies on elderly patients with suspected obstructive dysphagia found lesions in 78 patients. Benign strictures and malignancy were the most common findings. Authors conclude that upper gastrointestinal endoscopy is safe and valuable in elderly patients with dysphagia.

Herrington JP, Burns TW, Balart LA: Chest pain and dysphagia patients with prolonged peristaltic contractile duration of the esophagus. Dig Dis Sci 29:134, 1984.
Description of a subgroup of patients complaining of dysphagia and chest pain characterized by prolonged peristaltic contractile duration and normal contractile amplitude.

Humphreys B, Mathog R, Rosen R, et al: Videofluoroscopic and scintigraphic analysis of dysphagia in the head and neck cancer patient. Laryngoscope 97:25, 1987.
Two advances in the evaluation of swallowing function in the patient afflicted with head and neck cancer are reviewed: videofluoroscopy improved by computer-assisted image analysis and radionuclide scintigraphy, a complementary technique that measures transit time and the degree of aspiration.

Jones B, Donner MW: Examination of the patient with dysphagia. Radiology 167:319, 1988.
A clinical review of swallowing problems, with an emphasis on radiologic techniques and evaluation of the elderly population.

Katz PO, Castell DO: Review: esophageal motility disorders. Am J Med Sci 290:61, 1985.
Well-referenced state-of-the-art review with an emphasis on diagnostic modalities.

Katz PO, Dalton CB, Richter JE, et al: Esophageal testing of patients with noncardiac chest pain or dysphagia. Results of three years' experience with 1161 patients. Ann Intern Med 106:593, 1987.
Manometric findings in a large study of patients referred for esophageal manometry with complaints of noncardiac chest pain and dysphagia were compared. The nutcracker esophagus was found to be a manometric marker of noncardiac chest pain, whereas manometric findings of achalasia and nonspecific esophageal motility were commonly associated with dysphagia.

Keenan DJM, Hamilton JRL, Gibbons J, et al: Surgery for benign esophageal stricture. J Thorac Cardiovasc Surg 88:182, 1984.
Discussion of the pros and cons of surgical antireflux procedures.

Little AG, Skinner DB, Chen WH, et al: Physiologic evaluation of esophageal function in patients with achalasia and diffuse esophageal spasm. Ann Surg 203:500, 1986.

Current concepts of the evaluation of esophageal function in patients with achalasia and diffuse esophageal spasm.

Llamas-Elvira JM, Martinez-Parades M, Sopena-Monforte R, et al: Value of radionuclide esophageal transit in studies of functional dysphagia. Br J Radiol 59:1073, 1986.

Radionuclide esophageal transit time was evaluated in 70 individuals and separated into three categories: Normal patients, those with nonorganic dysphagia, and patients with primary esophageal motility disorders showed a significant decrease in residual activity after treatment with perendoscopic forced-pneumatic dilation.

Logemann JA: Dysphagia in movement disorders. Adv Neurol 49:307, 1988.

This paper reviews direct and indirect effects of various movement disorders, such as Parkinson's disease, chorea, and dystonia, on the swallowing process. Neuromuscular and mechanical-postural mechanisms are discussed.

Merlo A, Cohen S: Swallowing disorders. Annu Rev Med 39:17, 1988.

Clinical review of current concepts in evaluation of swallowing disorders. A differential diagnosis is organized under categories of obstructive lesions and motility disorders.

Ott DJ, Gelfand DW, Wu WC, Chen YM: Radiological evaluation of dysphagia. JAMA 256:2718, 1986.

A review of current techniques available for esophageal evaluation in patients with dysphagia, including clinical history, endoscopy, and esophageal manometry, with an emphasis on effective integration of radiologic techniques.

Price GJ, Jones CJ, Charlton RA, Allen CM: A combined approach to the assessment of neurological dysphagia. Clin Otolaryngol 12:197, 1987.

A review of techniques focused on evaluation of dysphagia in patients with neurologic disorders. New approaches to the assessment and management of acquired neurologic dysphagia are presented.

Richter JE, Castell DO: Diffuse esophageal spasm: a reappraisal. Ann Intern Med 100:242, 1984.

Reappraisal of manometry and a proposed manometric criteria for diffuse esophageal spasm.

Richter JE, Johns DN, Wu WC, et al: Are esophageal motility abnormalities produced during the intraesophageal acid perfusion test? JAMA 253:1914, 1985.

Study indicating that acid-induced motor abnormalities are not a common accompaniment and are not necessary for the production of acid-induced pain in the esophagus.

Wheeler RR, Peacock JE Jr, Cruz JM, Richter JE: Esophagitis in the immunocompromised host: role of esophagoscopy in diagnosis. Rev Infect Dis 9:88, 1987.

A review of 30 episodes of presumed infectious esophagitis in immunocompromised patients evaluated by esophagoscopy. Esophagoscopy resulted in specific infectious diagnosis in 57% of the episodes. Indications for evaluation of esophageal symptoms in this patient population are discussed.

24
Constipation: Common and Uncommon Associations

The complaint of constipation arises when a patient's normal frequency of defecation is slowed. Stool bulk is decreased or stools are hard or painful to expel. Most normal adults pass at least three stools per week ranging in weight from 35 to 225 g, but the definition of normal bowel habits is difficult since a substantial number of people with "normal" stool habits complain of symptoms compatible with irritable bowel syndrome. Most causes of constipation affect one of three major requirements for normal defecation: (1) fecal material with appropriate bulk and consistency, (2) an unobstructed passage, and (3) an intact gastrointestinal neuromuscular system. Constipation is a frequent and occasionally serious problem in the elderly and needs to be addressed during any hospitalization that will result in a prolonged period of inactivity.

Causes of Inadequate Fecal Material

Normal stools not meeting patient's expectations[1]
Low fiber diet[2,3]
Inadequate fluid intake

Mechanical Obstruction of Intestinal Lumen

Fecal impaction[4,5]
Neoplasms: extrinsic and intrinsic, benign and malignant[6]
Volvulus: acute or chronic[7]
Adhesions[8]
Painful anorectal lesions: thrombosed hemorrhoids, fissures, abscesses, rectal prolapse, or rectocele
Malformations, especially in children: anterior ectopic anus,[9] diaphragmatic hernia[10,11]

**Drugs and Disorders
Affecting
Neuromuscular
Transport**

Drugs: laxative abuse,[12] nonabsorbable calcium, bismuth and aluminum-containing antacids,[13] anticholinergics, antidepressants,[14] opiates,[15] anesthetic agents, anticonvulsants, barium sulfate, ferrous sulfate, benzodiazepines, phenothiazines, hypolipidemic agents,[16] calcium channel blockers[17]

Irritable bowel syndrome[18-20]

Diverticulosis[21]

Endocrine dysfunction: hypothyroidism, hyperparathyroidism, diabetes[22,23]

Electrolyte abnormalities: hypokalemia,[24] hypercalcemia, uremia

Pregnancy

Long-term debilitating illness[25,26]

Heavy metals: lead, arsenic, mercury, phosphorus

Food allergies[27]

Spinal cord lesions: trauma, neoplasms, infection

Tabes dorsalis

Multiple sclerosis[28]

Hirschsprung's disease (aganglionic megacolon)[29]

Parkinsonism

Chronic idiopathic pseudo-obstruction[30]

Idiopathic megacolon or megarectum[31,32]

Botulism[33]

References

1. Moore-Gillon V: Constipation: what does the patient mean? J R Soc Med 77:108, 1984.
2. Graham DY, Moser SE, Estes MK: The effect of bran on bowel function in constipation. Am J Gastroenterol 77:599, 1982.
3. Jenkins DJ, Jenkins AL, Wolever TM, et al: Fiber and starchy foods: gut function and implications in disease. Am J Gastroenterol 81:920, 1986.
4. Klein H: Constipation and fecal impaction. Med Clin North Am 66:1135, 1982.
5. Read NW, Abouzekry L, Read MG, et al: Anorectal function in elderly patients with fecal impaction. Gastroenterology 89:959, 1985.
6. Echenique J, Graham SD Jr: Pelvic fibrous mesothelioma with obstructive symptoms. Urology 31:142, 1988.
7. Fanning J, Cross CB: Post-cesarean section cecal volvulus. Am J Obstet Gynecol 158:1200, 1988.
8. Agrawal NW, Akdamar K, Litwin MS: Postoperative adhesions causing colon obstruction. Am Surg 50:479, 1984.
9. Upadhyaya P: Mid-anal sphincteric malformation, cause of constipation in anterior perineal anus. J Pediatr Surg 19:183, 1984.
10. Nehme AE: Constipation. An uncommon etiology. Dis Colon Rectum 27:819, 1984.
11. Likongo Y, Devroede G, Schang JC, et al: Hindgut

dysgenesis as a cause of constipation with delayed colonic transit. Dig Dis Sci 31:993, 1986.

12. Binder HJ: Use of laxatives in clinical medicine. Pharmacology 36(Suppl 1):226, 1988.

13. Saunders D, Sillery J, Chapman R: Effect of calcium carbonate and aluminum hydroxide on human intestinal function. Dig Dis Sci 33:409, 1988.

14. Pollack MH, Rosenbaum JF: Management of antidepressant-induced side effects: a practical guide for the clinician. J Clin Psychiatry 48:3, 1987.

15. Kaufman PN, Krevsky B, Malmud LS, et al: Role of opiate receptors in the regulation of colonic transit. Gastroenterology 94:1351, 1988.

16. Knodel LC, Talbert RL: Adverse effects of hypolipidaemic drugs. Med Toxicol 2:10, 1987.

17. Russell RP: Side effects of calcium channel blockers. Hypertension 11:1142, 1988.

18. Tucker H, Schuster MM: Irritable bowel syndrome: newer pathophysiologic concepts. Adv Intern Med 27:183, 1982.

19. Krag E: Irritable bowel syndrome: current concepts and future trends. Scand J Gastroenterol 109 (Suppl):107, 1985.

20. Marcus SN, Heaton KW: Irritable bowel-type symptoms in spontaneous and induced constipation. Gut 28:156, 1987.

21. Eastwood MA, Smith AN, Brydon WG, et al: Colonic function in patients with diverticular disease. Lancet 1:1181, 1978.

22. Battle WM, Cohen JD, Snape WF Jr: Disorders of colonic motility in patients with diabetes mellitus. Yale J Biol Med 56:277, 1983.

23. Feldman M, Schiller LR: Disorders of gastrointestinal motility associated with diabetes mellitus. Ann Intern Med 98:378, 1983.

24. Cohen PG: The hypokalemic, bowel, bladder, headache relationship. Med Hypotheses 15:135, 1984.

25. Bulmash JM: Confronting the three most common medical problems of long-term illness. Geriatrics 36(12):79, 1981.

26. Watier A, Devroede GT, Duranceau A, et al: Constipation with colonic inertia. A manifestation of systemic disease? Dig Dis Sci 28:1025, 1983.

27. Chin KC, Tarlow MJ, Allfree AJ: Allergy to cows' milk presenting as chronic constipation. Br Med J 287:1593, 1983.

28. Glick ME, Meshkinpour H, Haldeman S, et al: Colonic dysfunction in multiple sclerosis. Gastroenterology 83:1002, 1982.

29. Rich AJ, Lennard TWJ, Wilsdon JB: Hirschsprung's disease as a cause of chronic constipation in the elderly. Br Med J 287:1777, 1983.

30. Stanghellini V, Camilleri M, Malagelada JR: Chronic idiopathic intestinal pseudo-obstruction: clinical and intestinal manometric findings. Gut 28:5, 1987.

31. Lane RHS, Todd IP: Idiopathic megacolon: a review of 42 cases. Br J Surg 64:305, 1977.

32. Preston DM, Lennard-Jones JE, Thomas BM: Towards a radiologic definition of idiopathic megacolon. Gastrointest Radiol 10:167, 1985.

33. Lecour H, Ramos H, Almeida B, Barbosa R: Food-borne botulism. A review of 13 outbreaks. Arch Intern Med 148:578, 1988.

Selected Readings

Beck DE, Jagelman DG, Fazio VW: The surgery of idiopathic constipation. Gastroenterol Clin North Am 16:143, 1987.
This paper describes methods of patient evaluation and treatment developed at the Cleveland Clinic Foundation for patients with idiopathic constipation.

Brocklehurst JC: Colonic disease in the elderly. Clin Gastroenterol 14:725, 1985.
Clinical review that addresses constipation in the elderly. Completely referenced and comprehensive. Topics covered include aging and bowel habits, fecal impaction, megacolon and sigmoid volvulus, laxatives, colorectal cancer, inflammatory bowel disease, and colonic angiodysplasia. Valuable clinical reference.

Bueno L, Frexinos J, Fioramonti J: Role of motility in pathogenesis of constipation and diarrhea. Pharmacology 36(Suppl):15, 1988.
Disturbances of colonic motility are categorized and discussed with a focus on concepts, particularly relevant to symptoms of diarrhea and constipation.

Corazziari E, Materia E, Bausano G, et al: Laxative consumption in chronic nonorganic constipation. J Clin Gastroenterol 9:427, 1987.
A clinical study that evaluated laxative consumption and its relationship to bowel habits, total gastrointestinal transit time, and symptoms in patients with chronic nonorganic constipation. Laxative intake appeared to increase with age and duration of constipation.

Ewe K: Intestinal transport in constipation and diarrhoea. Pharmacology 36(Suppl):73, 1988.
Current concepts of intestinal transport with a focus on the pathophysiology of constipation and diarrhea. Useful clinical correlations.

Hill JC: Selection of elderly patients for barium enema examination with respect to significant bowel pathology especially carcinoma of the colon and rectum: the results of a retrospective study. Age Ageing 17:134, 1988.
A retrospective study of barium enemas in 123 consecutive patients over 65 years suggests the following criteria for significant bowel pathology in the elderly: weight loss, mass, obstruction, blood loss, iron deficiency anemia, pain, constipation, diarrhea, and change of bowel habits.

Huizinga JD: Electrophysiology of human colon motility in health and disease. Clin Gastroenterol 15:879, 1986.
A review of current concepts of electrophysiology measurement and evaluation of colon motility. Certain patterns of electrical activity are related to symptoms of irritable bowel syndrome, diarrhea, and constipation.

Kallman H: Constipation in the elderly. Am Fam Physician 27(1):179, 1983.
Recommendations for correcting constipation in the elderly.

Koch TR, Carney JA, Go L, Go VL: Idiopathic chronic constipation is associated with decreased colonic vasoactive intestinal peptide. Gastroenterology 94:300, 1988.

This study measured six neuropeptides, including vasoactive intestinal peptide, peptide histidine-methionine, and substance P, in four patients with chronic idiopathic constipation to investigate the reported association between idiopathic chronic constipation and morphologic abnormalities of enteric nerves. Authors suggest that decreased colinic concentrations of vasoactive intestinal peptide may be associated with diminution of inhibitory innervation of colonic smooth muscle in some patients.

Lennard-Jones JE: Symposium II-Constipation: Pathophysiology of constipation. Br J Surg (Suppl):S7, 1985.
Concise discussion of the pathophysiology of constipation concludes that fiber deficiency is the most common cause of mild constipation in the western world.

MacDonald L, Freeling P: Bowels: beliefs and behaviour. Fam Pract 3(2):80, 1986.
A questionnaire about knowledge, beliefs, and experiences of bowel function was generated by 171 patients aged 55 years and over from a group of general practitioners in London. Suggestions are made to reduce the delay in diagnosis of colorectal cancer.

Meerof JC: Approach to the patient with constipation. Hosp Pract 20(1):148, 1985.
An algorithmic approach to patients with constipation.

Melkersson M, Andersson H, Bosaeus I, et al: Intestinal transit time in constipated and nonconstipated geriatric patients. Scand J Gastroenterol 18:593, 1983.
Results of a study comparing intestinal transit time of elderly patients with young healthy subjects suggest that old age does not necessarily imply an increased transit time.

Portenoy RK: Constipation in the cancer patient: causes and management. Med Clin North Am 71:303, 1987.
Useful clinical discussion of bowel physiology and laxative pharmacology with an emphasis on constipation symptoms in the cancer patient.

Read NW, Timms JM: Defecation and the pathophysiology of constipation. Clin Gastroenterol 15:937, 1986.
Valuable comprehensive clinical reference covering all aspects of constipation with detailed clinical descriptions of symptoms, current concepts of pathophysiology, differential diagnosis, and management. Impressively referenced.

Reynolds JC, Ouyang A, Lee CA, et al: Chronic severe constipation. Prospective motility studies in 25 consecutive patients. Gastroenterology 92:414, 1987.
This study attempted to determine patterns of gastrointestinal and anal sphincter motility in 25 consecutive patients with severe constipation. Three patterns of abnormal motility emerged: isolated anal sphincter dysfunction, generalized gastrointestinal dysmotility, and retrosigmoid dysfunction.

Sasaki D, Kido A, Yoshida Y: An endoscopic method to study the relationship between bowel habit and motility of the ascending and sigmoid colon. Gastrointest Endosc 32:185, 1986.
Authors describe a new method of rapidly accessing the entire colon for pressure sensors with endoscopic retrograde bowel insertion. Findings in patients with irritable bowel syndrome and right-sided diverticular disease of the colon suggest that mechanisms of altered bowel habits in these groups are quite different.

Shouler P, Keighley MRB: Changes in colorectal function

in severe idiopathic chronic constipation. Gastroenterology 90:414, 1986.

Physiologic studies of colorectal and anal function in patients with severe idiopathic long-standing constipation suggest that there is often a motor abnormality of the pelvic floor and the colon.

Turnbull GK, Bartram CI, Lennard-Jones JE: Radiologic studies of rectal evacuation in adults with idiopathic constipation. Dis Colon Rectum 31:190, 1988.

A series of 58 consecutive patients with idiopathic constipation were studied with evacuation proctography and compared with 20 controls. Varying degrees of defecatory impairment was established among many patients with constipation.

Varma JS, Bradnock J, Smith RG, Smith AN: Constipation in the elderly. A physiologic study. Dis Colon Rectum 31:111, 1988.

Colorectal motility was studied in 25 elderly patients with chronic constipation and compared with a control group. Significant impairment of rectal sensory threshold and prolonged transit time were found in constipated patients. Authors suggest that neurogenic deficits of the sacral spinal cord may play a role in rectal motor and sensory dysfunction in the elderly.

Vela AR, Rosenberg AJ: Anorectal manometry: a new simplified technique. Am J Gastroenterol 77:486, 1982.

Discussion of a simplified technique for assessing anal sphincter function.

Yazbeck S, Schick E, O'Regan S: Relevance of constipation to enuresis, urinary tract infection, and reflux. A review. Eur Urol 13:318, 1987.

A review of the relationship of urinary symptoms to constipation. Authors suggest that constipation may cause uninhibited bladder contractions that cause urinary tract infection, enuresis, and vesicoureteral reflux.

25
Pancreatitis

Causes of Acute and Chronic Pancreatitis

Since the etiology and pathophysiology of pancreatitis are poorly understood, both the diagnosis and causes of pancreatitis can be difficult to establish. Acute and chronic pancreatitis present with variable clinical pictures. Chronic pancreatitis can present in the outpatient setting with mild to severe intermittent epigastric pain, perhaps simulating gastritis. A more dramatic, not uncommon form of acute pancreatitis is the severe abdominal pain with shock, which can mimic the surgical abdomen. An elevation of serum amylase is the most specific laboratory marker. However, amylase elevations are also variable and can be transient, as well as occasionally normal, even during acute pancreatitis. Since the clinical and laboratory criteria for the diagnosis of pancreatitis are so variable, it is important to consider this diagnosis in patients with risk factors for acute and chronic pancreatitis. By far the most common causes of acute pancreatitis are alcoholism and gallstones. The most common causes of chronic pancreatitis are alcoholism, hyperlipidemia, hyperparathyroidism, drugs, and pancreatic duct obstructions. Rarer associations include several congenital and familial forms.[1]

Idiopathic
Alcoholism[2–4]
Biliary tract disease[5,6]: gallstones,[7–9] biliary tract surgery[10]
Drugs[11]
    Diuretics: thiazides, furosemide, ethacrynic acid[12]
    Antibiotics: isoniazid, tetracycline,[13,14] rifampin
    Anti-inflammatory agents: corticosteroids,[15] azathioprine, sulfasalazine,[16,17] indomethacin
    Oral contraceptives[18,19]
    Phenformin[20]
    Chemotherapy: L-asparaginase, 6-mercaptopurine[21]
    Valproic acid[22,23]
    Pentamidine[24,25]
    Analgesics: propoxyphene, acetaminophen, opiates
    Antihypertensive agents: methyldopa, diazoxide
    Ergotamine[26]
    Disodium azodisalicylate[27]
    Isotretinoin[28]
Pancreatic outflow obstruction[29]: pancreas divisum,[30] annular pancreas,[31] duodenal Crohn's disease, diverticula, primary or metastatic carcinoma,[32–35] afferent loop obstruction after Billroth II gastrojejunostomy, congenital pancreatic duct strictures

and anomalies,[36-39] carcinoma of ampulla of Vater[40,41]

Hypercalcemia

Hyperparathyroidism: pancreas sometimes calcified[42-44]

Cystic fibrosis: especially in children

Hyperlipidemia: types I, IV, and V[45]

Penetrating duodenal ulcer[46]

Infections: mumps,[47] coxsackievirus,[48] echovirus, cytomegalovirus, *Legionella*[49]

Trauma: blunt abdominal trauma, i.e., steering wheel or bicycle handle-bar injury, postoperative injury, spinal cord trauma[50]

Parasitic infestations: ascariasis,[51] hydatid cysts, *Clonorchis sinensis*

Hepatic injury: Reye's syndrome, fulminant hepatitis

Pancreatic duct injections: endoscopic retrograde cholangiopancreatography (ERCP),[52] T-tube cholangiography

Pregnancy: 90% associated with gallstones[53]

Hereditary[54,55]

Severe malnutrition

Systemic lupus erythematosus[56-58] and other vasculitities

Ischemic: shock, emboli

Scorpion bites

Occupational chemicals[59]

Kawasaki disease[60]

Inflammatory bowel disease: ulcerative colitis,[61] Crohn's disease[62,63]

Peritoneal dialysis[64,65]

Cardiac and cardiopulmonary transplantation[66]

Surgical Conditions That Can Mimic Acute Pancreatitis

Surgically correctable intra-abdominal disorders need to be excluded before the diagnosis of acute pancreatitis is made; pain and elevated amylase can occur in some of the following surgically correctable conditions[67]:

Perforated peptic ulcer (duodenal)

Acute intestinal obstruction

Mesenteric vascular occlusion[68]
Dissecting or ruptured aortic aneurysm
Peritonitis
Acute cholecystitis
Appendicitis[69]
Common bile duct obstruction

References

1. Balart LA, Ferrante WA: Pathophysiology of acute and chronic pancreatitis. Arch Intern Med 142:113, 1982.
2. Geokas MC: Ethanol and the pancreas. Med Clin North Am 68:57, 1984.
3. Sarles H, Laugier R: Alcoholic pancreatitis. Clin Gastroenterol 10:401, 1981.
4. Malagelada JR: The pathophysiology of alcoholic pancreatitis. Pancreas 1:270, 1986.
5. Van Gossum A, Seferian V, Rodzynek JJ, et al: Early detection of biliary pancreatitis. Dig Dis Sci 29:97, 1984.
6. Lillemor KD, Pitt HA, Cameron JL: Sclerosing cholangitis. Adv Surg 21:65, 1987.
7. Mayer AD, McMahon MJ: Biochemical identification of patients with gallstones associated with acute pancreatitis on the day of admission to hospital. Ann Surg 201:68, 1985.
8. Moreau JA, Zinsmeister AR, Melton LJ III, DiMagno EP: Gallstone pancreatitis and the effect of cholecystectomy: a population-based cohort study. Mayo Clin Proc 63:466, 1988.
9. Carter DC: Pancreatitis and the biliary tree: the continuing problem. Am J Surg 155:10, 1988.
10. Vernava A, Andrus C, Herrmann VM, Kaminski DL: Pancreatitis after biliary tract surgery. Arch Surg 122:575, 1987.
11. Mallory A, Kern F Jr: Drug-induced pancreatitis: a critical review. Gastroenterology 78:813, 1980.
12. Eckhauser ML, Dokler M, Imbembo AL: Diuretic-associated pancreatitis: a collective review and illustrative cases. Am J Gastroenterol 82:865, 1987.
13. Elmore MF, Rogge JD: Tetracycline-induced pancreatitis. Gastroenterology 81:1134, 1981.
14. Torosis J, Vender R: Tetracycline-induced pancreatitis. J Clin Gastroenterol 9:580, 1987.
15. Nelp WB: Acute pancreatitis associated with steroid therapy. Arch Intern Med 108:102, 1961.
16. Chiba M, Horie Y, Ishida H, et al: A case of salicylazosulfapyridine (Salazopyrin)-induced acute pancreatitis with positive lymphocyte stimulation test (LST). Gastroenterol Jpn 22:228, 1987.
17. Block MB, Genant HK, Kirsner JB: Pancreatitis as an adverse reaction to salicylazosulfapyridine. N Engl J Med 282:380, 1970.
18. Davidoff F, Tishler S, Rosoff C: Marked hyperlipidemia and pancreatitis associated with oral contraceptive therapy. N Engl J Med 289:552, 1973.
19. Metabolic effects of oral contraceptives. A panel discussion. J Reprod Med 31(Suppl 6):569, 1986.

20. Chase HS Jr, Mogan GR: Phenformin-associated pancreatitis. Ann Intern Med 87:314, 1977.
21. Socinski MA, Garnick MB: Acute pancreatitis associated with chemotherapy for germ cell tumors in two patients. Ann Intern Med 108:567, 1988.
22. Wyllie E, Wyllie R, Cruse RP, et al: Pancreatitis associated with valproic acid therapy. Am J Dis Child 138:912, 1984.
23. Dickinson RG, Bassett ML, Searle J, et al: Valproate hepatotoxicity: a review and report of two instances in adults. Clin Exp Neurol 21:79, 1985.
24. Murphey SA, Josephs AS: Acute pancreatitis associated with pentamidine therapy. Arch Intern Med 141:56, 1981.
25. Zuger A, Wolf BA, el-Sadr W, et al: Pentamidine-associated fatal acute pancreatitis. JAMA 256:2383, 1986.
26. Deviere J, Reuse C, Askenasi R: Ischemic pancreatitis and hepatitis secondary to ergotamine poisoning. J Clin Gastroenterol 9:350, 1987.
27. Poldermans D, van Blankenstein M: Pancreatitis induced by disodium azodisalicylate. Am J Gastroenterol 83:578, 1988.
28. Flynn WJ, Freeman PG, Wickboldt LG: Pancreatitis associated with isotretinoin-induced hypertriglyceridemia. Ann Intern Med 107:63, 1987.
29. Drewnisk SJ, Gerzof SG, Langevin RE, Banks PA: Delayed common bile duct obstruction in acute pancreatitis. Int J Pancreatol 3:129, 1988.
30. Warshaw AL, Schapiro RH: Pancreas divisum and pancreatitis. Surg Annu 20:101, 1988.
31. Gilinsky NH, Lewis JW, Flueck JA, Fried AM: Annular pancreas associated with diffuse chronic pancreatitis. Am J Gastroenterol 82:681, 1987.
32. Gudjonsson B, Livstone EM, Spiro HM: Cancer of the pancreas. Diagnostic accuracy and survival statistics. Cancer 42:2494, 1978.
33. Kohler H, Lankisch PG: Acute pancreatitis and hyperamylasemia in pancreatic carcinoma. Pancreas 2:117, 1987.
34. Noseda A, Gangji D, Cremer M: Acute pancreatitis as presenting symptom and sole manifestation of small cell lung carcinoma. Dig Dis Sci 32:327, 1987.
35. Anderson JH, Morran CG, Anderson JR, Carter DC: Acute pancreatitis and non-Hodgkin's lymphoma. Postgrad Med J 63(736):137, 1987.
36. Turner LJ: Chronic pancreatitis and congenital strictures of the pancreatic duct. Am J Surg 145:582, 1983.
37. Agha FP, Williams KD: Pancreas divisum: incidence, detection, and clinical significance. Am J Gastroenterol 82:315, 1987.
38. Stelling T, von Rooij WJ, Tio TL, et al: Pancreatitis associated with congenital duodenal duplication cyst in an adult. Endoscopy 19:171, 1987.
39. Feller ER: Stenosis of the main pancreatic duct in acute pancreatitis of unknown etiology. Gastrointest Endosc 34:131, 1988.
40. Hayes DH, Bolton JS, Willis GW, Bowen JC: Carcinoma of the ampulla of Vater. Ann Surg 206:572, 1987.

41. Robertson JF, Imrie CW: Acute pancreatitis associated with carcinoma of the ampulla of Vater. Br J Surg 74:395, 1987.
42. Mixter CG Jr, Keynes WM, Chir M, et al: Further experience with pancreatitis as a diagnostic clue to hyperparathyroidism. N Engl J Med 266:265, 1962.
43. Sitges Serra A, Alonso M, de Lecea C, et al: Pancreatitis and hyperparathyroidism. Br J Surg 75:158, 1988.
44. Shearer MG, Imrie CW: Parathyroid hormone levels, hyperparathyroidism, and acute pancreatitis. Br J Surg 73:282, 1986.
45. Farmer RG, Winkelman EI, Brown HB, et al: Hyperlipoproteinemia and pancreatitis. Am J Med 54:161, 1973.
46. Vantini I, Piubello W, Scuro LA, et al: Duodenal ulcer in chronic relapsing pancreatitis. Digestion 24:23, 1982.
47. Becker Y: Complications after mumps result from damage to the pancreas. Med Hypotheses 18:187, 1985.
48. Shanmugam J, Balakrishnan V, George M, Shenoy KT: Study of Coxsackie B viral infections in chronic pancreatitis patients from Kerala. J Postgrad Med 33:29, 1987.
49. Krige JE, Lewis G, Bornman PC: Recurrent pancreatitis caused by a calcified ascaris in the duct of Wirsung. Am J Gastroenterol 82:256, 1987.
50. Eitrem R, Forsgren A, Nilsson C: Pneumonia and acute pancreatitis most probably caused by a *Legionella longbeachae* infection. Scand J Infect Dis 19:381, 1987.
51. Leppaniemi A, Haapiainen R, Kiviluoto T, Lempinen M: Pancreatic trauma: acute and late manifestations. Br J Surg 75:165, 1988.
52. Hamilton I, Lintott DJ, Rothwell J, et al: Acute pancreatitis following endoscopic retrograde cholangiopancreatography. Clin Radiol 34:543, 1983.
53. Young MKR; Acute pancreatitis in pregnancy: two case reports. Obstet Gynecol 60:653, 1982.
54. Haynes JH Jr, Martin JC, Kurzweg FT: Hereditary pancreatitis. Am Fam Physician 25(5):153, 1982.
55. Rao SS, Riley SA, Foster PN, et al: Hereditary pancreatitis presenting with ascites. Postgrad Med J 62:873, 1986.
56. Reynolds JC, Inman RD, Kimberly RP, et al: Acute pancreatitis in systemic lupus erythematosus: report of twenty cases and a review of the literature. Medicine 61:25, 1982.
57. Bruijn JA, van Albada-Kuipers GA, Smit VT, Eulderink F: Acute pancreatitis in systemic lupus erythematosus. Scand J Rheumatol 15:363, 1986.
58. Wolman R, de Gara C, Isenberg D: Acute pancreatitis in systemic lupus erythematosus: report of a case unrelated to drug therapy. Ann Rheum Dis 47:77, 1988.
59. Braganza JM, Jolley JE, Lee WR: Occupational chemicals and pancreatitis: a link? Int J Pancreatol 1:9, 1986.
60. Stoler J, Biller JA, Grand RJ: Pancreatitis in Kawasaki disease. Am J Dis Child 141:306, 1987.
61. Forbes D, Scott RB, Trevensen C, et al: Chronic pancreatitis associated with ulcerative colitis. Clin Invest Med 10:321, 1987.
62. Altman HS, Phillips G, Bank S, Klotz H: Pancreatitis

associated with duodenal Crohn's disease. Am J Gastroenterol 78:174, 1983.
63. Meyers S, Greenspan J, Greenstein AJ, et al: Pancreatitis coincident with Crohn's ileocolitis. Report of a case and review of the literature. Dis Colon Rectum 30:119, 1987.
64. Singh S, Wadhwa N: Peritonitis, pancreatitis, and infected pseudocyst in a continuous ambulatory peritoneal dialysis patient. Am J Kidney Dis 9:84, 1987.
65. Caruana RJ, Wolfman NT, Karstaedt N, Wilson DJ: Pancreatitis: an important cause of abdominal symptoms in patients on peritoneal dialysis. Am J Kidney Dis 7:135, 1986.
66. Aziz S, Bergdahl L, Baldwin JC, et al: Pancreatitis after cardiac and cardiopulmonary transplantation. Surgery 97:653, 1985.
67. Salt WB II, Schenker S: Amylase—its clinical significance: a review of the literature. Medicine 55:269, 1976.
68. Goldofsky E, Cohen BA, Greenstein AJ: Acute septic pancreatitis presenting as colonic necrosis. Am J Gastroenterol 79:548, 1984.
69. Swensson EE, Maull KI: Clinical significance of elevated serum and urine amylase levels in patients with appendicitis. Am J Surg 142:667, 1981.

Selected Readings

Baker RJ, Duarte B: The current status of recognition and treatment of severe necrotizing pancreatitis. Surg Annu 18:129, 1986.
This paper reviews the controversial and difficult diagnosis and management decisions involved in the care of patients with severe necrotizing pancreatitis. Early surgical management of the nonalcoholic patient yields the most satisfying results.

Bank S: Chronic pancreatitis: clinical features and medical management. Am J Gastroenterol 81:153, 1986.
A clinical review of current concepts of chronic pancreatitis. Pathophysiology, classification, clinical features, complications, and management are well discussed. Fully referenced.

Barkin JS, Garrido J: Acute pancreatitis and its complications: diagnostic and therapeutic strategies. Postgrad Med 79(4):241, 1986.
Useful clinical discussion.

Basran GS, Ramasubramanian R, Verma R: Intrathoracic complications of acute pancreatitis. Br J Dis Chest 81:326, 1987.
Authors review major intrathoracic complications of acute pancreatitis, including pleural effusions, acute pulmonary dysfunction, hypoxemia without pulmonary infiltrates, and adult respiratory distress syndrome (ARDS). Authors point out that intrathoracic complications are a significant cause of death in this patient population.

Block S, Buchler M, Bittner R, Beger HG: Sepsis indicators in acute pancreatitis. Pancreas 2:499, 1987.
An analysis of 21 routine clinical and laboratory data in 161 patients with necrotizing pancreatitis undergoing surgical treatment attempted to identify clinical markers of infection. Three criteria were considered highly predictive of infection: rectal temperature greater

than 38.5°C, base excess greater than − 4 mmol/L, and a hematocrit less than 35%.

Bockman DE, Buchler M, Malfertheiner P, Beger HG: Analysis of nerves in chronic pancreatitis. Gastroenterology 94:1459, 1988.

An interesting study that attempts to characterize the histopathology of pancreatic nerves in chronic pancreatitis. The pancreatic nerves appeared preferentially preserved with an increased mean diameter. Authors suggest these findings argue against fibrotic constriction of pancreatic nerves as the cause of pancreatic pain.

Bovo P, Mirakian R, Merigo F, et al: HLA molecule expression on chronic pancreatitis specimens: is there a role for autoimmunity? A preliminary study. Pancreas 2:350, 1987.

This study prospectively assessed the possibility of an aberrant expression of HLA-DR molecules in the pathogenesis of chronic pancreatitis. Findings were similar to those in immune diseases such as thyroiditis and primary biliary cirrhosis.

Brady PG: Endoscopic retrograde cholangiopancreatography: its role in diagnosis and therapy of pancreatitis. Postgrad Med 79(4):253, 1986.

Indications for endoscopic cholangiopancreatography in the evaluation of pancreatitis.

Clavien PA, Hauser H, Meyer P, Robner A: Value of contrast-enhanced computerized tomography in the early diagnosis and prognosis of acute pancreatitis. A prospective study of 202 patients. Am J Surg 155:457, 1988.

Two hundred two patients admitted with the clinical suspicion of acute pancreatitis were studied with computerized tomography scanning within 36 hours of admission. Authors found a high diagnostic and prognostic yield.

Crist DW, Cameron JL: The current management of acute pancreatitis. Adv Surg 20:69, 1987.

Well-referenced, comprehensive discussion of current concepts of pathophysiology, etiology, and management of acute pancreatitis. Excellent clinical reference out of the Johns Hopkins Department of Surgery.

Davidson BR, Neoptolemos JP, Leese T, Carr-Locke DL: Biochemical prediction of gallstones in acute pancreatitis: a prospective study of three systems. Br J Surg 75:213, 1988.

Three clinicobiochemical systems proposed for predicting gallstones in acute pancreatitis were studied: (1) serum transaminase alone; (2) alkaline phosphatase, bilirubin, and serum transaminase; and (3) female gender, age, amylase, alkaline phosphatase, and transaminase. The first two systems were considered marginally better.

Dreiling DA, Robert J, Toledano AE: Vascular pancreatitis. A clinical entity of growing importance. J Clin Gastroenterol 10:3, 1988.

An editorial discussion of vascular causes of acute pancreatitis suggests that vascular etiologies should be considered more often. Among vascular etiologies discussed are diabetes, Ortner's syndrome, vasculitis, aged vessels, post-transplantation, and shock syndromes.

Dubick MA, Mar G, Mayer AD, et al: Digestive enzymes and protease inhibitors in plasma from patients with acute pancreatitis. Pancreas 2:187, 1987.

Plasma levels of certain digestive enzymes and protease inhibitors were determined in 40 patients with alcoholic, gallstone, and id-

iopathic acute pancreatitis. Plasma levels of pancreatic digestive enzymes appeared to reflect clinical severity and clinical features, such as the presence of concomitant ascites, pancreatic pseudocyst, or abscesses.

Dubick MA, Mayer AD, Majumdar AP, et al: Biochemical studies in peritoneal fluid from patients with acute pancreatitis. Relationship to etiology. Dig Dis Sci 32:305, 1987.
Pancreatic digestive enzymes, lysosomal hydrolases, and protease inhibitors were measured in ascites fluid from 24 patients with alcoholic, gallstone-induced, and idiopathic acute pancreatitis. Enzyme levels in ascites from idiopathic pancreatitis were higher than in alcoholic and gallstone acute pancreatitis.

Garrison R: Amylase. Emerg Med Clin North Am 4:315, 1986.
A clinical review of the usefulness and cost effectiveness of serum and urine amylase determinations from an emergency room perspective. The meaning of depressed and elevated amylase levels is discussed.

Geokas MC, Baltaxe HA, Banks PA, et al: Acute pancreatitis. Ann Intern Med 103:86, 1985.
Well-referenced review of acute pancreatitis from the Interdepartmental Dean's Conference, University of California, Davis.

Greenstein RJ, Krakoff LR, Felton K: Activation of the renin system in acute pancreatitis. Am J Med 82:401, 1987.
Renin-angiotensin activity was assessed in groups of patients with acute pancreatitis, normal patients, and in those with abdominal pain without pancreatitis. Active plasma renin values were nearly 500% higher than in nonacute pancreatitis groups.

Hacker JF, Chobanian SJ: Pain of chronic pancreatitis: etiology, natural history, therapy. Dig Dis 5:41, 1987.
This paper reviews concepts of the pathogenesis of pain in chronic pancreatitis. Newer treatment modalities, such as pancreatic enzyme therapy and celiac plexus blocks, are discussed.

Hiatt JR, Calabria RP, Passaro E Jr, Wilson SE: The amylase profile: a discriminant in biliary and pancreatic disease. Am J Surg 154:490, 1987.
Serial serum amylase determinations in 85 consecutive patients with alcoholic and biliary tract pancreatitis were analyzed. Distinct amylase profiles emerged that appeared to separate alcoholic from biliary tract pancreatitis. Patients with biliary tract disease appeared to have initially higher amylase values and lower final values when compared with alcoholic pancreatitis.

Little JM: Alcohol abuse and chronic pancreatitis. Surgery 101:357, 1987.
A study of 28 alcoholics with pancreatitis emphasizes the importance of abstinence from alcohol. Authors discuss problems of potential narcotic abuse within this patient population and recommend nonsurgical approaches to treatment in patients with a history of significant narcotic abuse.

Miyake H, Harada H, Kunichika K, et al: Clinical course and prognosis of chronic pancreatitis. Pancreas 2:378, 1987.
The course of 125 patients with chronic pancreatitis was followed from 1 to 20 years. An increased incidence of chronic pancreatitis was attributed to alcoholic and idiopathic chronic pancreatitis appearing in the elderly. Major complications included peptic ulcer disease, pancreatic pseudocyst, and bile duct stenosis. Morbidity was significantly related to malignant neoplasms, diabetes, and continued alcohol abuse.

Moossa AR: Diagnostic tests and procedures in acute pancreatitis. N Engl J Med 311:639, 1984.
Procedures and tests for diagnosing acute pancreatitis are reviewed.

Moreau JA, Zinsmeister AR, Melton LJ III, DiMagno EP: Gallstone pancreatitis and the effect of cholecystectomy: a population-based cohort study. Mayo Clin Proc 63:466, 1988.
This study assesses the risk of acute pancreatitis in patients with gallstones and the effect of cholecystectomy on the risk. From a review of 2,583 medical records, authors found a considerably increased relative risk for acute pancreatitis in patients with gallstones. They also found that cholecystectomy reduces the risk to almost the same as the general population. However, because of the overall low incidence of pancreatitis, recommendations for cholecystectomy were limited to those patients in whom acute pancreatitis had occurred.

Niederau C, Grendell JH: Diagnosis of chronic pancreatitis. Gastroenterology 88:1973, 1985.
Well-referenced state-of-the-art review.

Nuutinen P, Kivisaari L, Schroder T: Contrast-enhanced computed tomography and microangiography of the pancreas in acute human hemorrhagic/necrotizing pancreatitis. Pancreas 3:53, 1988.
A study of 5 patients with severe acute pancreatitis who had low contrast enhancement of the pancreas in CT and underwent subtotal pancreatectomy. Histopathologic and radiographic correlations suggest that one can define necrotic and edematous pancreatic tissue in this clinical setting by noninvasive means.

Park J, Fromkes J, Cooperman M: Acute pancreatitis in elderly patients. Pathogenesis and outcome. Am J Surg 152:638, 1986.
A study of 40 patients over 70 years of age with acute pancreatitis found biliary tract disease the most common cause. The mortality rate was 20%; multisystem failure was the major cause of death. Authors recommend aggressive evaluation for biliary tract disease and cholecystectomy to prevent recurrent attacks.

Potts JR III: Acute pancreatitis. Surg Clin North Am 68:281, 1988.
A state-of-the-art clinical review from a surgical perspective of the problems of acute pancreatitis in the setting of the acute abdomen. CT was considered the single most useful diagnostic modality.

Rocca G, Gaia E, Iuliano R, et al: Increased incidence of cancer in chronic pancreatitis. J Clin Gastroenterol 9:175, 1987.
In a study of a population of 172 consecutive patients with chronic pancreatitis, an increased incidence of cancer was found. The incidence of cancer appeared to increase significantly with age, but not with smoking, alcohol use, or diabetes.

Sarles H: Etiopathogenesis and definition of chronic pancreatitis. Dig Dis Sci 31:91S, 1986.
Critical review of papers published on definition, classification, etiology, and pathogenesis of chronic pancreatitis from 1981 to 1985.

Shaff MI, Tarr RW, Partain CL, James AE Jr: Computed tomography and magnetic resonance imaging of the acute abdomen. Surg Clin North Am 68:233, 1988.
A state-of-the-art review of the two major noninvasive modes of imaging the acute abdomen: CT and MRI.

Srensen EV: Subcutaneous fat necrosis in pancreatic disease. A review and two new case reports. J Clin Gastroenterol 10:71, 1988.

A review and two case report descriptions of subcutaneous fat necrosis, the rare cutaneous manifestation of pancreatic disease. Findings of painful erythematous nodules, often on the legs, coupled with histopathologic findings are pathognomonic.

Steer ML, Meldolesi J: Pathogenesis of acute pancreatitis. Annu Rev Med 39:95, 1988.

A review of selected current concepts of the pathophysiology of acute pancreatitis derived from animal models.

Thomson SR, Hendry WS, McFarlane GA, Davidson AI: Epidemiology and outcome of acute pancreatitis. Br J Surg 74:398, 1987.

Acute pancreatitis in Scotland from January 1983 to December 1985 was evaluated. A serum amylase greater than 1,000 U/L, laparotomy, or postmortem criteria were used. Biliary tract disease was the most common cause, followed by alcohol. Complications included pseudocyst, pancreatic abscesses, respiratory failure, renal failure, and disseminated intravascular coagulation.

Warshaw AL, Hawboldt MM: Puzzling persistent hyperamylasemia, probably neither pancreatic nor pathologic. Am J Surg 155:453, 1988.

One hundred seventeen consecutive patients with abnormally high serum amylase levels for 3 to 48 weeks were studied. Clinical and radiographic evaluations failed to explain the elevated amylase levels. In 79% of the patients, nonpancreatic causes for hyperamylasemia were found.

26
Malabsorption and Indigestion: Diseases Causing Malabsorption and Indigestion*

Early signs of malabsorption or maldigestion are generally nonspecific, such as vague constitutional symptoms or subtle, slight changes in bowel habits.

*(Adapted from Gray,[1] with permission.)

Therefore, malabsorption is usually suspected only after major clinical manifestations have developed, such as anemia or glossitis secondary to specific deficiencies, bulky diarrhea secondary to unabsorbed fat and fatty acids, or unexplained weight loss. Subtle, early symptoms may consist of complaints of fatigue, weakness, abdominal bloating, or intermittent diarrhea. More obvious signs, such as foul-smelling, bulky stools and anorexia, occur later in the clinical course. Major causes of malabsorption and maldigestion are grouped under three major phases of the digestive process: (1) an intraluminal phase during which chemical and physical disturbances alter nutrients preventing normal absorption; (2) an absorptive or mucosal phase during which chemical, anatomic, and cellular abnormalities prevent normal absorption; and (3) a transit phase during which absorbed materials may be misdirected by aberrant intestinal anatomy, lymphatics, or vascular flow.

Deficient Intraluminal Pancreatic Enzymes	Chronic pancreatitis[2] Pancreatic resection Pancreatic carcinoma Cystic fibrosis of pancreas[3-5]
Deficient Bile Acids	Biliary obstruction with and without jaundice: gallstone disease Jejunal bacterial overgrowth Ileal resection[6] Ileitis: Crohn's disease
Small Intestinal Disease	Disaccharidase deficiencies[7] Massive resection[8] Radiation enteritis Intestinal ischemia Celiac sprue Tropical sprue Whipple's disease Primary intestinal lymphoma[9] Lymphangiectasia Hypogammaglobulinemia[10,11] Dermatitis herpetiformis Eosinophilic gastroenteritis Food allergy Amyloidosis

Parasitoses[12]: schistosomiasis[13]
Graft-versus-host disease
Acquired immune deficiency syndrome (AIDS) associated enteropathy[14]: Kaposi's sarcoma[15]
Nonmalignant immunoproliferative small intestinal disease[16]
Primary bile acid malabsorption[17]
Mastocytosis[18]
Somatostatinoma[19]

Defects of Multiple Stages of Digestion–Absorption

Postgastrectomy[20]
Diabetes mellitus
Endocrinopathies
Scleroderma
Postjejunoileal bypass[21]

Drugs Producing Maldigestion and Malabsorption

Cholestyramine[22]
Cathartics
Colchicine
Neomycin

References

1. Gray GM: Maldigestion and malabsorption: clinical manifestations and specific diagnosis. p. 240. In Sleisenger MH, Fordtran JS (eds): Gastrointestinal Disease. 3rd Ed. WB Saunders, Philadelphia, 1983.
2. Neff CC, Ferrucci JT Jr: Pancreatitis. Surg Clin North Am 64:23, 1984.
3. Park RW, Grand RJ: Gastrointestinal manifestations of cystic fibrosis: a review. Gastroenterology 81:1143, 1981.
4. Penny DJ, Ingall CB, Boulton P, et al: Intestinal malabsorption in cystic fibrosis. Arch Dis Child 61:1127, 1986.
5. Sitrin MD, Lieberman F, Jensen WE, et al: Vitamin E deficiency and neurologic disease in adults with cystic fibrosis. Ann Intern Med 107:51, 1987.
6. Aldini R, Roda A, Festi D, et al: Bile acid malabsorption and bile acid diarrhea in intestinal resection. Dig Dis Sci 27:495, 1982.
7. Rumessen JJ, Gudmand-Hyer E: Malabsorption of fructose-sorbitol mixtures. Interactions causing abdominal distress. Scand J Gastroenterol 22:431, 1987.
8. Gray DS: Short bowel syndrome. Am Fam Physician 30(3):227, 1984.
9. Rosenfelt F, Rosenberg SA: Diffuse histiocytic lymphoma presenting with gastrointestinal tract lesions. Cancer 45:2188, 1980.
10. Cunningham-Rundles C: Clinical and immunologic

analyses of 103 patients with common variable immunodeficiency. J Clin Immunol 9:22, 1989.

11. Aguilar FP, Alfonso V, Rivas S, et al: Jejunal malignant lymphoma in a patient with adult-onset hypo-gammaglobulinemia and nodular lymphoid hyperplasia of the small bowel. Am J Gastroenterol 82:472, 1987.

12. Brasitus TA: Parasites and malabsorption. Clin Gastroenterol 12:495, 1983.

13. Kiire CF, Gwavava N: Protein losing enteropathy: an unusual presentation of intestinal schistosomiasis. Gut 28:616, 1987.

14. Gillin JS, Shike M, Alcock N, et al: Malabsorption and mucosal abnormalities in the acquired immunodeficiency syndrome. Ann Intern Med 102:619, 1985.

15. Colman N, Grossman F: Nutritional factors in epidemic Kaposi's sarcoma. Semin Oncol 14(Suppl 3):54, 1987.

16. Manousos O, Economidou J, Papademetriou C, et al: Malabsorption associated with nonmalignant immunoproliferative small intestinal disease. Digestion 36:182, 1987.

17. Popovic OS, Kostic KM, Milovic VB, et al: Primary bile acid malabsorption. Histologic and immunologic study in three patients. Gastroenterology 92:1851, 1987.

18. Reisberg IR, Oyakawa S: Mastocytosis with malabsorption, myelofibrosis, and massive ascites. Am J Gastroenterol 82:54, 1987.

19. Harris GJ, Tio F, Cruz AB Jr: Somatostatinoma: a case report and review of the literature. J Surg Oncol 36:8, 1987.

20. Ladas SD, Isaacs PET, Quereshi Y, et al: Role of the small intestine in postvagotomy diarrhea. Gastroenterology 85:1088, 1983.

21. Halverson JD: Vitamin and mineral deficiencies following obesity surgery. Gastroenterol Clin North Am 16:307, 1987.

22. Knodel LC, Talbert RL: Adverse effects of hypolipidemic drugs. Med Toxicol 2:10, 1987.

Selected Readings

Beck IT: Laboratory assessment of inflammatory bowel disease. Dig Dis Sci 32(Suppl 12):26S, 1987.

A review of current laboratory modalities helpful in the evaluation of inflammatory bowel disease. Of particular importance are tests to exclude infectious agents and to assess the absorptive capacity of the terminal ileum.

Black DA: Malabsorption: common causes and their practical diagnosis. Geriatrics 43(1):65, 1988.

A helpful, clinical review of practical, nonmajor medical center approaches to the evaluation of malabsorption syndromes in the elderly. The usefulness of plain abdominal radiographs, endoscopy with duodenal biopsy, and small bowel meals in this setting is reviewed.

Corazza GR, Strocchi A, Rossi R, et al: Sorbitol malabsorption in normal volunteers and in patients with coeliac disease. Gut 29:44, 1988.

Previous studies have invoked sorbitol ingestion as a cause of nonspecific gastrointestinal distress. This study compared sorbitol malabsorption in 30 patients with 7 untreated patients with celiac disease and 9 patients with celiac disease on a gluten-free diet. Symptoms in all groups were dose dependent. Authors suggest that malabsorption and intolerance of sorbitol may occur in doses or concentrations found in commonly used foods and drugs and may be an underestimated cause of gastrointestinal symptoms.

Heitlinger LA, Lebenthal E: Disorders of carbohydrate digestion and absorption. Pediatr Clin North Am 35:239, 1988.

A clinical review of the carbohydrate malabsorptive syndromes with a focus on young adults and children. Authors point out that adult type hypolactasia and lactose intolerance following rotavirus infection are recognized with increasing frequency in the primary care setting.

Kastrup W, Mobacken H, Stockbrugger R, et al: Malabsorption of vitamin B_{12} in dermatitis herpetiformis and its association with pernicious anaemia. Acta Med Scand 220:261, 1986.

Serum vitamin B_{12} levels and pentagastrin tests were performed in patients with dermatitis herpetiformis. Low serum vitamin B_{12} levels and achlorhydria were found in a significant number of patients who were then further investigated for hematologic and gastrointestinal dysfunction. Morphologic or functional involvement of the small intestine was found in almost all patients with vitamin B_{12} deficiency.

Mathias JR, Clench MH: Review: pathophysiology of diarrhea caused by bacterial overgrowth of the small intestine. Am J Med Sci 289:243, 1985.

Well-referenced review.

Montgomery RD, Haboubi NY, Mike NH, et al: Causes of malabsorption in the elderly. Age Ageing 15:235, 1986.

The causes of malabsorption in 70 patients who presented over the age of 65 years were evaluated. Major causes include pancreatic insufficiency secondary to alcoholism and gallstone disease, postgastrectomy syndromes, small bowel diverticulosis, celiac disease, and gastric atrophy.

Pedersen NT, Halgreen H: Simultaneous assessment of fat maldigestion and fat malabsorption by a double-isotope method using fecal radioactivity. Gastroenterology 88:47, 1985.

A discussion of a test that may be a useful alternative to fecal fat measurement.

Pedersen NT, Halgreen H, Worning H: Estimation of the 3-day fecal fat excretion and fat concentration as a differential test of malabsorption and maldigestion. Scand J Gastroenterol 22:91, 1987.

A prospective study of 87 consecutive patients was conducted to estimate the diagnostic efficiency of the fecal fat excretion and fecal fat concentration in uncontrolled 3-day collections. Authors conclude that the 1-day fecal fat concentration appears useful as the first screening test in suspected malabsorption.

Roberts IM: Workup of the patient with malabsorption. Postgrad Med 81(7):32, 1987.

Practical clinical review of the workup of malabsorption. Author declares that the quantitative determination of fecal fat is still the gold standard test. Following a Sudan black B fat stain screening test and fecal fat quantitation, a decision tree is outlined to determine the source: intestinal disease or abnormality, pancreatic disease, or bacterial overgrowth.

Roe DA: Drug-nutrient interactions in the elderly. Geriatrics 41(3):57, 1986.

Drug metabolism and efficacy may be affected simply by changing the diet of an elderly patient.

Stamp GW, Evans DJ: Accumulation of ceroid in smooth muscle indicates severe malabsorption and vitamin E deficiency. J Clin Pathol 40:798, 1987.

Four patients with ceroid in smooth muscle (lipofuscinosis) and vitamin E deficiency in three of the four patients are described. Authors suggest that studies of smooth muscle function are indicated in patients with histopathologic findings of ceroid accumulation.

Targan SR, Kagnoff MF, Brogan MD, Shanahan F: Immunologic mechanisms in intestinal diseases. Ann Intern Med 106:853, 1987.

A review of current concepts of genetic and immune mechanisms involved in the pathophysiology of celiac disease and inflammatory bowel disease.

Thompson WG, Babitz L, Cassino C, et al: Evaluation of current criteria used to measure vitamin B_{12} levels. Am J Med 82:291, 1987.

Recent improvements in the serum vitamin B_{12} assay require a reassessment of previous literature and prior assay methods used in measuring B_{12} levels. Authors suggest the use of an mean corpuscular volume (MCV) below 95 fl and a B_{12} level below 100 pg/ml as abnormal values may not detect some clinically important B_{12} deficiencies.

Worning H: Exocrine pancreatic function in dyspepsia. Digestion, 37(Suppl 1):3, 1987.

Authors suggest that one-third of patients with chronic pancreatitis present with exocrine pancreatic insufficiency. Their data suggest the prevalence of chronic pancreatitis in the Western world to be around 70 per 100,000.

27

Flatulence: Conditions and Foods Associated with Excessive Flatulence

Intestinal gas, or flatulence, is primarily comprised of carbon dioxide, hydrogen, oxygen, nitrogen, and methane.[1] Average diets in normals produce from 400 to 1,600 ml of flatus daily.[2] Most patients who complain of excessive flatulence excrete large amounts of hydrogen, which is produced by bacteria normally located in the colon.[2] Major causes of increased flatulence include (1) certain foods, such as legumes and lactulose, (2) conditions such as small bowel malabsorption, that allow excessive carbohydrates to reach the colon; and (3) increased air swallowing or aerophagia.

Foods Associated with Flatulence

Certain foods such as legumes, milk products, and wheat products are more likely to produce flatulence. Since carbohydrates provide substrate to hydrogen-producing colonic flora, patients with carbohydrate intolerance, such as lactase deficiency, are at higher risk for producing flatulence.[3]

Milk products: lactose
Legumes: baked beans[4]
Wheat products
Carbonated beverages
Bulk sweeteners: sorbitol in chewing gum

Conditions Associated with Increased Aerophagia

Air swallowing is a habit of which the patient is usually not aware. It may be associated with thoracic or abdominal disorders or be idiopathic or psychogenic. Disorders commonly associated with aerophagia include the following:

Esophageal disease: reflux, achalasia, obstructing lesions, gas-bloating syndrome following hernia repair[5]
Gastric disease: gastritis, gastric ulcer, carcinoma
Biliary tract disease: cholecystitis or cholelithiasis
Abnormal intestinal motility: diabetes, scleroderma, autonomic dysfunction, postvagotomy state, irritable bowel syndrome

Conditions Associated with Malabsorption of Protein or Carbohydrates

Analysis of rectal gas can determine whether excessive flatus is due to air swallowing (N_2 and O_2) or intraluminal gas production (H_2, CO_2, NH_4). Unabsorbed carbohydrates and proteins can be fermented by colonic bacteria to form gas.[6]

Pancreatic enzyme deficiencies
Bile acid deficiencies
Small intestinal disaccharidase deficiency

Small intestinal structural disease

Bacterial overgrowth states: postgastrectomy, diverticulae, neoplasms, fistulae, strictures, postradiation[7]

Drug-induced malabsorption: antibiotics

Irritable bowel syndrome[8,9]

References

1. Kirk E: The quantity and composition of human colonic flatus. Gastroenterology 12:782, 1949.
2. Levitt MD: Volume and composition of human intestinal gas determined by means of an intestinal washout technic. N Engl J Med 284:1394, 1971.
3. Levitt MD: Intestinal gas production—recent advances in flatology (editorial). N Engl J Med 302:1474, 1980.
4. O'Donnell AU, Fleming SE: Influence of frequent and long-term consumption of legume seeds on excretion of intestinal gases. Am J Clin Nutr 40:48, 1984.
5. Woodward ER, Thomas HF, McAlhany JC: Comparison of crural repair and Nissen fundoplication in the treatment of esophageal hiatus hernia with peptic esophagitis. Ann Surg 173:782, 1971.
6. Olsen WA: A pathophysiologic approach to diagnosis of malabsorption. Am J Med 67:1007, 1979.
7. Drude RB Jr, Hines C Jr: The pathophysiology of intestinal bacterial overgrowth syndromes. Arch Intern Med 140:1349, 1980.
8. Atoba MA: Irritable bowel syndrome in Nigerians. Dig Dis Sci 33:414, 1988.
9. Thompson WG, Patel DG: Clinical picture of diverticular disease of the colon. Clin Gastroenterol 15:903, 1986.

Selected Readings

Altman F: Downwind update—a discourse on matters gaseous (clinical conference). West J Med 145:502, 1986.
A definite read for those interested in this subject. Genesis of intestinal gases and clinical effects are cogently discussed.

Brydon WG, McKay LF, Eastwood MA: Intestinal gas formation and the use of breath measurements to monitor the influence of diet and disease. Dig Dis 4:1, 1986.
A review of techniques of intestinal gas analysis that may help understand the influence of diet on intestinal gas production and identifying causes of malabsorption.

Levitt MD: Excessive gas: patient perception vs reality. Hosp Pract 20(11):143, 1985.
Clinically useful article that separates out many symptoms sometimes mistakenly attributed to excessive bowel gas. Author begins his clinical evaluation by categorizing patients as belchers, bloaters, and gas-passers.

Read NW: Mechanisms of flatulence and diarrhoea. Br J Surg 72:S5, 1985.
Concise discussion of pathophysiology.

Stone-Dorshow T, Levitt MD: Gaseous response to ingestion of a poorly absorbed fructo-oligosaccharide sweetener. Am J Clin Nutr 46:61, 1987.

An interesting study comparing absorption and subsequent hydrogen production after ingesting lactulose and a poorly absorbed fructo-oligosaccharide concludes that adaptation of colonic bacteria to carbohydrate malabsorption is variable and depends on quantity or nature of the carbohydrate.

Van Ness MM, Cattau EL Jr: Flatulence: pathophysiology and treatment. Am Fam Physician 31(4):198, 1985.

Helpful clinical approach combining pathophysiology and management suggestions.

28

Gastrointestinal Bleeding: Common and Less Common Causes of Gastrointestinal Bleeding

Upper and lower gastrointestinal bleeding can be acute or chronic, with a wide range of clinical manifestations. Acute gastrointestinal bleeding is often unexpected and life-threatening. In contrast, chronic gastrointestinal bleeding can be intermittent, occult, or relentless, often presenting with an anemia as the first sign of blood loss. Acute upper gastrointestinal bleeding is most commonly caused by peptic ulcers, varices, and esophagitis.[1] Although hemorrhoids are probably the most common source of lower gastrointestinal bleeding, patients who require angiography or colonoscopy for diagnosis of a significant lower gastrointestinal bleed most often have diverticular disease or angiodysplasia.

Most Common Causes of Upper Gastrointestinal Bleeding

Peptic ulcers: duodenal and gastric
Esophageal varices[2,3]
Acute gastritis
Esophagitis[4]

Mallory-Weiss tear
Gastric neoplasms[5]

Most Common Causes of Lower Gastrointestinal Bleeding

Hemorrhoids
Diverticular disease[6,7]
Angiodysplasia: vascular ectasia of the right colon is an important cause of bleeding in the elderly[8,9]
Polyps: neoplastic and benign
Carcinoma of the colon
Ischemic bowel disease: superior mesenteric artery disease
Inflammatory bowel disease: Crohn's disease[10,11]
Meckel's diverticulum[12,13]

Less Common Causes of Gastrointestinal Bleeding

Most common causes of gastrointestinal bleeding are detected with early use of conventional diagnostic techniques; however, some less common causes of gastrointestinal bleeding can be missed despite adequate sigmoidoscopy, panendoscopy, and barium contrast studies of upper and lower gastrointestinal tracts.[14] Underlying bleeding disorders and epistaxis should be excluded before the following less common causes of gastrointestinal bleeding are considered.[15]

Drug-induced: alcohol, aspirin,[16] methotrexate,[17] indomethacin, anticoagulants, antibiotics,[18] laxative abuse,[19] non-narcotic analgesics,[20] nonsteroidal anti-inflammatory drugs,[21-25]
Esophageal disease: neoplasms, caustic injury, ulcer
Anal fissure
Infection: *Salmonella typhi*,[26] cytomegalovirus[27]
Less common idiopathic gastrointestinal ulcerations: esophagus, ileum,[28] large bowel, rectum[29]
Less common gastrointestinal varices: duodenum,[30] ileum[31]
Arteriovenous malformations[32]: vascular ectasia of the colon or duodenum,[33] hereditary hemorrhagic telangiectasia, blue rubber bleb syndrome, CREST syndrome, hemangiomas,[34] mesenteric venous occlusion,[35,36] arterial fibrodysplasia[37]
Aortoenteric fistulae: esophageal,[38,39] duodenal, hiatal hernia,[40] enteric,[41] grafts,[42] shunts,[43] gastritis cystica polyposa[44]
Aneurysms: traumatic, atherosclerotic[37]
Neoplasms: primary carcinoma,[5] leiomyoma, sar-

coma,[45] lymphoma, extramedullary hematopoiesis, leukemia,[46] metastatic[47,48]

Vasculitis: collagen vascular disease, polyarteritis nodosa, Henoch-Schönlein purpura

Radiation-induced proctitis[49]

Uncommon diverticulae: duodenal, jejunal[50]

Intussusception

Amyloidosis[51,52]

Chronic renal disease: cecal ulcers

Hemodialysis[53]

Hemobilia: vascular communication with the biliary tract, usually caused by trauma,[54] invading cancer, hepatic abscess, hepatic artery aneurysm, choledocholithiasis[55]

Pancreatitis[56]: tuberculosis of the pancreas[57]

Long distance running[58-60]

Pseudoxanthoma elasticum[61,62]

Ehlers-Danlos syndrome

Neurofibromatosis: intestinal neurofibromas and leiomyomas[63,64]

Ménétrier's disease

Blood dyscrasias: von Willebrand's disease,[65] hemophilia[66]

Postcardiac transplant[67]

References

1. Wara P: Incidence, diagnosis, and natural course of upper gastrointestinal hemorrhage. Prognostic value of clinical factors and endoscopy. Scand J Gastroenterol 137(Suppl):26, 1987.
2. Sutton FM: Upper gastrointestinal bleeding in patients with esophageal varices. What is the most common source? Am J Med 83:273, 1987.
3. Tabibian N, Graham DY: Source of upper gastrointestinal bleeding in patients with esophageal varices seen at endoscopy. J Clin Gastroenterol 9:279, 1987.
4. Cooper BT, Barbezat GO: Barrett's esophagus: a clinical study of 52 patients. Q J Med 62:97, 1987.
5. Moreno-Otero R, Rodriguez S, Carbo J, et al: Acute upper gastrointestinal bleeding as primary symptom of gastric carcinoma. J Surg Oncol 36:130, 1987.
6. Almy T, Howell DA: Diverticular disease of the colon. N Engl J Med 302:324, 1980.
7. Bingley LJ Jr, Iung E: Colonic diverticular disease. Its spectrum in a community hospital. Postgrad Med 81(5):79, 1987.
8. Levine DS: Intestinal vascular ectasia. Improving diagnostic capability poses therapeutic dilemma. Am J Med 76:1151, 1984.
9. Tung KT, Millar AB: Gastric angiodysplasia—a missed cause of gastrointestinal bleeding. Postgrad Med J 63:865, 1987.

10. Mesleh G, Lemons J: Massive lower gastrointestinal hemorrhage in Crohn's disease. IMJ 164:182, 1983.
11. McGarrity TJ, Manasse JS, Koch KL, Weidner WA: Crohn's disease and massive lower gastrointestinal bleeding: angiographic appearance and two case reports. Am J Gastroenterol 82:1096, 1987.
12. Maglinte DDT, Jordan LG, Van Hove ED, et al: Chronic gastrointestinal bleeding from Meckel's diverticulum: radiological considerations. J Clin Gastroenterol 3:47, 1981.
13. Brown CK, Olshaker JS: Meckel's diverticulum. Am J Emerg Med 6:157, 1988.
14. Spechler SJ, Schimmel EM: Gastrointestinal tract bleeding of unknown origin. Arch Intern Med 142:236, 1982.
15. Hutchison SM, Finlayson ND: Epistaxis as a cause of hematemesis and melena. J Clin Gastroenterol 9:283, 1987.
16. Graham DY, Smith JL: Aspirin and the stomach. Ann Intern Med 104:390, 1986.
17. Gispen JG, Alarcon GS, Johnson JJ, et al: Toxicity of methotrexate in rheumatoid arthritis. J Rheumatol 14:74, 1987.
18. Gould PC, Khawaja FI, Rosenthal WS: Antibiotic-associated hemorrhagic colitis. Am J Gastroenterol 77:491, 1982.
19. Weiss BD, Wood GA: Laxative abuse causing gastrointestinal bleeding. J Fam Pract 15:177, 1982.
20. Ivey KJ: Gastrointestinal intolerance and bleeding with nonnarcotic analgesics. Drugs 32(Suppl 4):71, 1986.
21. Tenenbaum J: Non-steroidal anti-inflammatory drugs (NSAIDs) cause gastrointestinal intolerance and major bleeding—or do they? Clin Invest Med 10:246, 1987.
22. Eliakim R, Ophir M, Rachmilewitz D: Duodenal mucosal injury with nonsteroidal antiinflammatory drugs. J Clin Gastroenterol 9:395, 1987.
23. Langman MJ: Ulcer complications and nonsteroidal anti-inflammatory drugs. Am J Med 84:15, 1988.
24. Giercksky KE: Piroxicam and gastrointestinal bleeding. Am J Med 81:2, 1986.
25. Graham DY: Prevention of gastroduodenal injury induced by chronic nonsteroidal antiinflammatory drug therapy. Gastroenterology 96(Suppl):675, 1989.
26. Reyes E, Hernandez J, Gonzalez A: Typhoid colitis with massive lower gastrointestinal bleeding. An unexpected behavior of *Salmonella typhi*. Dis Colon Rectum 29:511, 1986.
27. Ng JW, Chan AY: Severe hemorrhage from cytomegalovirus rectal ulcers in a burned adult. Am J Gastroenterol 82:695, 1987.
28. Stevens JM, Northover JMA, Raphael JMA, et al: The localization of bleeding small bowel lesions for conservative resection: a simple radiographic technique. Br J Radiol 54:909, 1981.
29. Haycock CE, Suryanarayan G, Spillert CR, et al: Massive hemorrhage from benign solitary ulcer of the rectum. Am J Gastroenterol 78:83, 1983.
30. Khouqeer F, Morrow C, Jordan P: Duodenal varices as a cause of massive upper gastrointestinal bleeding. Surgery 102:548, 1987.

31. Falchuk KR, Aiello MR, Trey C, et al: Recurrent gastrointestinal bleeding from ileal varices associated with intraabdominal adhesions: case report and review of the literature. Am J Gastroenterol 77:859, 1982.
32. Trudel JL, Fazio VW, Sivak MV: Colonoscopic diagnosis and treatment of arteriovenous malformations in chronic lower gastrointestinal bleeding. Clinical accuracy and efficacy. Dis Colon Rectum 31:107, 1988.
33. Tai DI, Chou FF, Lee TY, Lin CC: Vascular ectasia of the duodenum detected by duodenoscopy. Am J Gastroenterol 82:1071, 1987.
34. Sutton D, Murfitt J, Howarth F: Gastrointestinal bleeding from large angiomas. Clin Radiol 32:629, 1981.
35. Soper NJ, Rikkers LF, Miller FJ: Gastrointestinal hemorrhage associated with chronic mesenteric venous occlusion. Gastroenterology 88:1964, 1985.
36. Miyaki CT, Park YS, Gopalswamy N: Upper gastrointestinal bleeding in acute mesenteric thrombosis. J Clin Gastroenterol 10:84, 1988.
37. den Butter G, van Bockel JH, Aarts JC: Arterial fibrodysplasia: rapid progression complicated by rupture of a visceral aneurysm into the gastrointestinal tract. J Vasc Surg 7:449, 1988.
38. Patel NM, Sangchantr C, Sangchantr WS: Aortoesophageal fistula and sentinel hemorrhage. IMJ 167:58, 1985.
39. Khawaja FI, Varindani MK: Aortoesophageal fistula. Review of clinical, radiographic, and endoscopic features. J Clin Gastroenterol 9:342, 1987.
40. Kielhofner MA, Schnell G, Schubert TT, Kebede-Daniels D: Aortogastric fistula from hiatal hernia ulcer. A cause of massive upper gastrointestinal bleeding. J Clin Gastroenterol 9:697, 1987.
41. Banai J, Salfay G, Szeleczky M, et al: An uncommon endoscopic finding: bleeding secondary aortoenteric fistula. Endoscopy 14:185, 1982.
42. Yeager RA, Sasaki TM, McConnell DB, Vetto RM: Clinical spectrum of patients with infrarenal aortic grafts and gastrointestinal bleeding. Am J Surg 153:459, 1987.
43. Attias E, Smadja C, Vons C, et al: Bleeding from intestinal varices after a Warren shunt. J Clin Gastroenterol 9:585, 1987.
44. Ozenc AM, Ruacan S, Aran O: Gastritis cystica polyposa. Arch Surg 123:372, 1988.
45. McGrath PC, Neifeld JP, Lawrence W Jr, et al: Gastrointestinal sarcomas. Analysis of prognostic factors. Ann Surg 206:706, 1987.
46. Tucker J, Cachia PG: Gastrointestinal bleeding due to large bowel infiltration by chronic lymphocytic leukaemia. Postgrad Med J 62(723):45, 1986.
47. Lynch-Nyhan A, Fishman EK, Kadir S: Diagnosis and management of massive gastrointestinal bleeding owing to duodenal metastasis from renal cell carcinoma. J Urol 138:611, 1987.
48. Yang PM, Sheu JC, Yang TH, et al: Metastasis of hepatocellular carcinoma to the proximal jejunum manifested by occult gastrointestinal bleeding. Am J Gastroenterol 82:165, 1987.

49. Taverner D, Talbot IC, Carr-Locke DL, et al: Massive bleeding from the ileum: a late complication of pelvic radiotherapy. Am J Gastroenterol 77:29, 1982.
50. Wilcox RD, Shatney CH: Massive rectal bleeding from jejunal diverticula. Surg Gynecol Obstet 165:425, 1987.
51. Yood RA, Skinner M, Rubinow A, et al: Bleeding manifestations in 100 patients with amyloidosis. JAMA 249:1322, 1983.
52. Weinrauch LA, Desautels RE, Christlieb AR, et al: Amyloid deposition in serosal membranes. Its occurrence with cardiac tamponade, bilateral obstruction, and gastrointestinal bleeding. Arch Intern Med 144:630, 1984.
53. Zuckerman GR, Cornette GL, Clouse RE, et al: Upper gastrointestinal bleeding in patients with chronic renal failure. Ann Intern Med 102:588, 1985.
54. Bismuth H: Hemobilia. N Engl J Med 288:617, 1973.
55. Lutter DR, Berger ML: Diagnosis of nontraumatic hematobilia by computerized tomography of the abdomen. Am J Gastroenterol 83:329, 1988.
56. Hall RI, Lavelle MI, Venables CW: Chronic pancreatitis as a cause of gastrointestinal bleeding. Gut 23:250, 1982.
57. Fan ST, Yan KW, Lau WY, Wong KK: Tuberculosis of the pancreas: a rare cause of massive gastrointestinal bleeding. Br J Surg 73:373, 1986.
58. Buckman MT: Gastrointestinal bleeding in long-distance runners (editorial). Ann Intern Med 101:127, 1984.
59. Chillag SA: Endurance athletes: physiologic changes and nonorthopedic problems. South Med J 79:1264, 1986.
60. Robertson JD, Maughan RJ, Davidson RJ: Fecal blood loss in response to exercise. Br Med J (Clin Res) 295:303, 1987.
61. Morgan AA: Recurrent gastrointestinal hemorrhage: an unusual cause. Am J Gastroenterol 77:925, 1982.
62. Lebwohl M, Phelps RG, Yannuzzi L, et al: Diagnosis of pseudoxanthoma elasticum by scar biopsy in patients without characteristic skin lesions. N Engl J Med 317:347, 1987.
63. Devereux RB, Koblenz LW, Cipriano P, et al: Gastrointestinal hemorrhage—an unusual manifestation of neurofibromatosis. Am J Med 58:135, 1975.
64. Petersen JM, Ferguson DR: Gastrointestinal neurofibromatosis. J Clin Gastroenterol 6:529, 1984.
65. Bush RW, Huff JW: Von Willebrand's disease and severe gastrointestinal bleeding. Report of a kindred. West J Med 140:781, 1984.
66. Mittal R, Spero JA, Lewis JH, et al: Patterns of gastrointestinal hemorrhage in hemophilia. Gastroenterology 88:515, 1985.
67. Colon R, Frazier OH, Kahan BD, et al: Complications in cardiac transplant patients requiring general surgery. Surgery 103:32, 1988.

Selected Readings

Adkins RB Jr, DeLozier JB, McKnight WG, Waterhouse G: Carcinoma of the colon in patients 35 years of age and younger. Am Surg 53:141, 1987.

A review of 705 patients with carcinoma of the colon who were 35 years of age or younger. Average age was 29.3 years. Presenting symptoms in order of decreasing frequency were pain, change in bowel habits, and gastrointestinal bleeding. Major poor prognostic factors of carcinoma in the young include the usually unfavorable tumor histology and the advanced disease at the time of presentation.

Ahlquist DA, McGill DB, Schwartz S, et al: Fecal blood levels in health and disease. N Engl J Med 312:1422, 1985.

Authors conclude that HemoQuant is a more sensitive measure of gastrointestinal bleeding than Hemoccult.

Bansal SK, Gautam PC, Sahi SP, et al: Upper gastrointestinal hemorrhage in the elderly: a record of 92 patients in a joint geriatric/surgical unit. Age Ageing 16:279, 1987.

Ninety-two consecutive elderly patients with acute gastrointestinal bleeding were studied over a 3-year period. Conservative management and joint care between geriatricians and surgeons are major factors in the overall low mortality of 5.4% in this patient series.

Booker JA, Johnston M, Booker CI, et al: Prognostic factors for continued or rebleeding and death from gastrointestinal hemorrhage in the elderly. Age Ageing 16:208, 1987.

One hundred three episodes of upper gastrointestinal bleeding in 88 elderly patients were reviewed to determine which clinical and laboratory findings on admission were most predictive of continued bleeding, rebleeding, and mortality. Most predictive variables included size of the bleed, prolonged prothrombin time, elevated serum creatinine, and premorbid condition of the patient.

Brandt LJ: Managing GI disorders of aging: noncardiac chest pain and rectal bleeding. Geriatrics 41(7):20, 1986.

Author feels that esophageal manometry is crucial in the evaluation of patients suspected of having angina pectoris without discernible evidence of cardiac disease.

Clouse RE, Costigan DJ, Mills BA, et al: Angiodysplasia as a cause of upper gastrointestinal bleeding. Arch Intern Med 145:458, 1985.

This study concludes that angiodysplasia, although uncommon, should be considered in the differential diagnosis of both occult and overt upper GI bleeding.

Gupta S, Walker DL, Keshavarzian A, Hodgson HJ: Upper endoscopy for occult bleeding in renal failure. J Clin Gastroenterol 9:43, 1987.

Forty-one patients with renal failure were prospectively studied to assess the value of upper gastrointestinal endoscopy in detecting occult bleeding. Although mucosal abnormalities of the upper gastrointestinal tract were common, authors felt that clinically inapparent gastrointestinal bleeding was only rarely responsible for sudden drops in hemoglobin in this patient group.

Hemingway AP, Allison DJ: Complications of embolization: analysis of 410 procedures. Radiology 166:669, 1988.

A 10-year study of 284 patients who underwent 410 embolization procedures for treatment of various tumors, gastrointestinal bleeding, or systemic or pulmonary arteriovenous malformations. Major complications and mortality occurred in patients with serious underlying abnormalities in whom no alternative treatment was available.

Jacques PF, Fitch DD: Anal verge and low rectal bleeding. A diagnostic problem. J Clin Gastroenterol 8:38, 1986.

Five patients with lower gastrointestinal bleeding and negative endoscopy are described who subsequently proved to have bleeding sources in the rectum near the anal verge. Failure of endoscopic diagnosis was attributed to endoscopic geometry within the rectum, inadequate colonic preparation, and low clinical suspicion for distal lesions.

King RM, Pluth JR, Giuliani ER: The association of unexplained gastrointestinal bleeding with calcific aortic stenosis. Ann Thorac Surg 44:514, 1987.

An interesting review of the problemmatic association of chronic gastrointestinal bleeding in patients with aortic stenosis. Ninety-one patients aged 38 to 80 years of age are reviewed. In this series, gastrointestinal surgery was successful in only 5%; aortic valve replacement was effective in 93%. Authors suggest that aortic valve replacement be considered in such cases of aortic stenosis and unexplained gastrointestinal bleeding.

Laine L, Weinstein WM: Histology of alcoholic hemorrhagic "gastritis": a prospective evaluation. Gastroenterology 94:1254, 1988.

Hemorrhagic gastritis in alcoholics usually refers to endoscopic findings of subepithelial hemorrhages. To better define this entity, 125 actively drinking alcoholics were prospectively screened with upper endoscopy. Biopsy findings of gastric subepithelial hemorrhages in 20 patients included localized hemorrhage and edema but were without prominent inflammatory cell infiltrates. In the absence of inflammatory changes, authors suggest that the term "subepithelial hemorrhages" more adequately describes such findings than the more commonly used term "hemorrhagic gastritis."

Lau WY, Fan ST, Wong SH, et al: Preoperative and intraoperative localization of gastrointestinal bleeding of obscure origin. Gut 28:869, 1987.

The following techniques were successfully used to localize bleeding lesions preoperatively in 36 of 37 patients with obscure gastrointestinal bleeding: endoscopy, barium meal and follow through, small bowel enema, 99mTc pertechnetate scan, 99mTc-labeled red blood cell scan, and selective coelic and mesenteric angiography.

Lewis BS, Waye JD: Chronic gastrointestinal bleeding of obscure origin: role of small bowel enteroscopy. Gastroenterology 94:1117, 1988.

Authors site 5% of patients with chronic gastrointestinal bleeding in whom the source of bleeding remains undetermined. A new technique of small bowel enteroscopy was used in 60 patients referred with obscure etiologies of chronic gastrointestinal bleeding. Thirty-three percent of patients had the source of blood loss identified within the small bowel by this technique.

Lutter DR, Berger ML: Diagnosis of nontraumatic hematobilia by computerized tomography of the abdomen. Am J Gastroenterol 83:329, 1988.

A case report of a 73-year-old man with recurrent abdominal pain and episodic hematochezia in whom upper and lower gastrointestinal tract endoscopy failed to identify the source of bleeding. Computed tomography, however, demonstrated a thickened gall bladder filled with blood-density material. The diagnostic evaluation of hematobilia is reviewed.

Manzione NC, Das KM, Wolkoff AW, Carnevale N: Unusual sites of upper gastrointestinal variceal bleeding. J Clin Gastroenterol 9:40, 1987.

Usual sites for varices causing portal hypertension are in the *esophagus and gastric fundus; however, varices can develop else-where. Authors report two such patients and review the literature.*

Meeroff JC: Management of massive gastrointestinal bleeding. Hosp Pract 121(5):154A, 1985.
Discussion of management of complications of massive gastrointestinal bleeding as well as location of bleeding sources and etiologic diagnosis.

Pingleton SK: Recognition and management of upper gastrointestinal hemorrhage. Am J Med 83:41, 1987.
A clinical review of current concepts of diagnosis and management of upper gastrointestinal hemorrhage.

Provenzale D, Sandler RS, Wood DR, et al: Development of a scoring system to predict mortality from upper gastrointestinal bleeding. Am J Med Sci 294:26, 1987.
Authors developed and validated a scoring system based on prognostic indicators of increased mortality to select high-risk upper gastrointestinal bleeding in patients who might benefit most from aggressive management and therapeutic endoscopy.

Richards WO, Grove-Mahoney D, Williams LF: Hemorrhage from a Dieulafoy type ulcer of the colon: a new cause of lower gastrointestinal bleeding. Am Surg 54:121, 1988.
A case report describing massive bleeding from Dieulafoy's ulcer or exulceratio simplex, which is a submucosal artery and small mucosal erosion, a condition originally described in the stomach. Authors describe angiographic and pathologic confirmation of such lesions in the colon of one patient and cite three other reports of similar lesions.

Rutgeerts P, Vantrappen G: The benefits of endoscopy in upper gastrointestinal bleeding. Endoscopy 18(Suppl 2):15, 1986.
Review of indications, usefulness, and limitations of endoscopy in upper gastrointestinal bleeding. Authors discuss effective methods available for endoscopic hemostasis of bleeding ulcers and bleeding varices.

Santangelo WC, Krejs GJ: Gastrointestinal manifestations of the acquired immunodeficiency syndrome. Am J Med Sci 292:328, 1986.
A necessary review of gastrointestinal manifestations in patients with HIV infection. The gastrointestinal tract is involved in approximately 50% of patients with acquired immune deficiency syndrome. Common problems include diarrhea, malabsorption, and weight loss. Gastrointestinal bleeding can be a presenting manifestation or one of many symptoms that occurs during the period of debilitation.

Schaffner J: Acute gastrointestinal bleeding. Med Clin North Am 70:1055, 1986.
A review of the pathophysiology and consequences of acute gastrointestinal bleeding.

Snook JA, Holdstock GE, Bamforth J: Value of a simple biochemical ratio in distinguishing upper and lower sites of gastrointestinal hemorrhage. Lancet 1:1064, 1986.
Authors suggest that this simple ratio may be valuable in determining the sequence of investigations in patients with an unidentified source of gastrointestinal hemorrhage.

Steer ML, Silen W: Diagnostic procedures in gastrointestinal hemorrhage. N Engl J Med 309:646, 1983.
Current concepts in diagnosing the cause and locating the site of gastrointestinal hemorrhage.

Thompson JN, Salem RR, Hemingway AP, et al: Specialist investigation of obscure gastrointestinal bleeding. Gut 28:47, 1987.

A review of investigation and treatment of 131 patients with obscure gastrointestinal bleeding. Presenting symptoms in order of decreasing frequency were melena, anemia, rectal bleeding, hematemesis, and ileostomy bleeding. Diagnoses in order of decreasing frequency were colonic angiodysplasia, small bowel vascular anomalies, Meckel's diverticular disease, and miscellaneous lesions. No lesions were found in 21 patients.

Trudal JL, Fazio VW, Sivak MV: Colonoscopic diagnosis and treatment of arteriovenous malformations in chronic lower gastrointestinal bleeding. Clinical accuracy and efficacy. Dis Colon Rectum 31:107, 1988.

A review of diagnosis and treatment of lower gastrointestinal bleeding from colonic arteriovenous malformations.

29

Hepatic Failure: Causes of Fulminant Hepatic Failure

Fulminant hepatic failure is defined as an acute hepatic injury that leads to encephalopathy within 8 weeks of onset of symptoms in a patient without preexisting evidence of liver disease. Although a relatively rare condition, it is associated with an 80 to 90% mortality rate. Its prognosis is directly related to the depth of coma at the time of presentation. Its most serious complications include encephalopathy and cerebral edema; coagulopathy and gastrointestinal bleeding; cardiorespiratory and renal failure; susceptibility to infections; hypoglycemia, and electrolyte and acid-base disorders.

In children and young adults, viral hepatitis and drug or toxin ingestions are frequently the etiologic agents. In older adults or hospitalized patients, acute hemodynamic failure becomes an important cause of this syndrome. Treatment consists of withdrawal of any offending agents and support by aggressive treatment of metabolic, hemodynamic, or infectious complications. The role of liver transplantation is yet to be defined.

Infectious Causes

Hepatitis B: especially with a superimposed or simultaneous infection with hepatitis delta[1]

Non-A, non-B hepatitis: in the United States, it is most often identified following blood transfusions, but it may occur as a water-borne, epidemic illness in tropical regions.[2-4]

Hepatitis A

Cytomegalovirus[5]

Epstein-Barr virus[6]

Reye's syndrome: a postinfectious syndrome of children and young adults classically presenting as severe nausea following a flulike illness. The use of aspirin during the preceding illness has been associated with a higher incidence of this frequently fatal complication.[7]

Exotic viral infections and zoonoses: yellow fever, Rift Valley fever, Marburg virus, Ebola virus[8]

Coxiella burnetii (Q fever)

Amebic hepatic abscess[9]

Plasmodium falciparum[10]

Meningococcus[11]

Drugs and Toxins

Acetaminophen: alcoholics may be more prone to injury with acetaminophen.[12-16]

Halothane and other halogenated hydrocarbon anesthetic agents[17]

Ethanol: usually there is evidence of preexisting liver disease, and criteria for fulminant hepatic failure is not met.[18]

Antibiotics: particularly isoniazid (where it is seen most often in patients older than 35 years)[19] and tetracycline; rarely nitrofurantoin and sulfonamides

Mushroom poisoning: *Amanita phalloides* in Europe, *Amanita verna* in North America. A late summer or fall disease, generally affecting a family or group of wild mushroom pickers, with a greater than 30% mortality rate[20]

Antidepressants; especially MAO inhibitors, iproniazid, tricyclics[21]

Nonsteroidal anti-inflammatory agents: particularly aspirin, phenylbutazone and gold salts

Methyldopa

Anticonvulsants: sodium valproate,[22] dantrolene, and phenytoin; the latter has a distinctive clinical syndrome with fever, lymphadenopathy and eosinophilia[23]

Occupational poisons: carbon tetrachloride, trichloroethylene, 2-nitropropane,[24] and other industrial poisons.

Allopurinol

Yellow phosphorus

Copper or iron poisoning

Perhexiline maleate

Oral hypoglycemic agents: particularly acetohexamide

Propylthiouracil

Drugs: chlorzoxazone,[25] progabide,[26] pyrimethamine-sulfadoxine[27]

Hemodynamic Insults

Heat stroke: described in extreme environmental stress situations, such as marathon runners and South African mine workers[28,29]

Acute circulatory failure[30]

Congestive heart failure[31]

Trauma[32]

Inherited Metabolic Disorders

Wilson's disease: serum copper levels will discriminate between Wilson's disease and other causes[33,34]

Galactosemia

Hereditary fructose intolerance

Hereditary tyrosinemia

Niemann-Pick disease[35]

Protoporphyria[36]

Miscellaneous

Morbid obesity: almost exclusively from fatty liver after a jejunoileal bypass[37,38]

Pregnancy-related: acute fatty liver of pregnancy or toxemia of pregnancy[39,40]

Replacement of liver by primary or metastatic carcinoma[41–43] hepatocellular carcinoma[44,45]

Renal transplant population: associated infection[46,47]

Amyloidosis[48]

Idiopathic hemochromatosis[49]
Budd-Chiari syndrome[50,51]

References

1. Smedile A, Farci P, Verma G, et al: Influence of delta infection on the severity of hepatitis B. Lancet 2:945, 1982.
2. Dienstag JL: Non-A, non-B hepatitis. I. Recognition, epidemiologic and clinical features. Gastroenterology 85:439, 1983.
3. Ramalingaswami V, Purcell RH: Waterborne non-A, non-B hepatitis. Lancet 1:571, 1988.
4. Wejstal R, Lindberg J, Lundin P, Norkrans G: Chronic non-A, non-B hepatitis. A long-term follow-up study in 49 patients. Scand J Gastroenterol 22:1115, 1987.
5. Shusterman NH, Frauenhoffer C, Kinsey MD: Fatal massive hepatic necrosis in cytomegalovirus mononucleosis. Ann Intern Med 88:810, 1978.
6. Shaw NJ, Evans JH: Liver failure and Epstein-Barr virus infection. Arch Dis Child 63:432, 1988.
7. Heubi JE, Daugherty CC, Partin JS, et al: Grade I Reye's syndrome—outcome and predictors of progression to deeper coma grades. N Engl J Med 311:1539, 1984.
8. Ishak KG, Walker DH, Coetzer JAW, et al: Viral hemorrhagic fevers with hepatic involvement: pathologic aspects with clinical correlations. Prog Liver Dis 7:495, 1982.
9. Saltzman DA, Smithline N, Davis JR: Fulminant hepatic failure secondary to amebic abscesses. Dig Dis Sci 23:561, 1978.
10. Joshi YK, Tandon BN, Acharya SK, et al: Acute hepatic failure due to *Plasmodium falciparum* liver injury. Liver 6:357, 1986.
11. Ellison RT III, Mason SR, Kohler PF, et al: Meningococcemia and acquired complement deficiency. Association in patients with hepatic failure. Arch Intern Med 146:1539, 1986.
12. Black M: Acetaminophen hepatotoxicity. Gastroenterology 78:382, 1980.
13. Baeg NJ, Bodenheimer HC Jr, Burchard K: Long-term sequelae of acetaminophen-associated fulminant hepatic failure: relevance of early histology. Am J Gastroenterol 83:569, 1988.
14. Mitchell JR: Acetaminophen toxicity. N Engl J Med 319:1601, 1988.
15. Meredith TJ, Vale JA: Non-narcotic analgesics. Problems of overdosage. Drugs 32(Suppl 4):177, 1986.
16. Prescott LF: Liver damage with non-narcotic analgesics. Med Toxicol 1(Suppl 1):44, 1986.
17. Kenna JG, Neuberger J, Mieli-Vergani G, et al: Halothane hepatitis in children. Br Med J (Clin Res) 294:1209, 1987.
18. Bigatello LM, Broitman SA, Fattori L, et al: Endotoxemia, encephalopathy, and mortality in cirrhotic patients. Am J Gastroenterol 82:11, 1987.
19. Mitchell JR, Zimmerman HJ, Ishak KG, et al: Isoniazid

liver injury: clinical spectrum, pathology, and probable pathogenesis. Ann Intern Med 84:181, 1976.

20. Mitchel DH: *Amanita* mushroom poisoning. Annu Rev Med 31:51, 1980.

21. Larrey D, Rueff B, Pessayre D, et al: Cross hepatotoxicity between tricyclic antidepressants. Gut 27:726, 1986.

22. Laub MC, Paetzke-Brunner I, Jaeger G: Serum carnitine during valproic acid therapy. Epilepsia 27:559, 1986.

23. Lee TJ, Carney CN, Lapis JL, et al: Diphenylhydantoin-induced hepatic necrosis. Gastroenterology 70:422, 1976.

24. Harrison R, Letz G, Pasternak G, Blanc P: Fulminant hepatic failure after occupational exposure to 2-nitropropane. Ann Intern Med 107:466, 1987.

25. Powers BJ, Cattau EL Jr, Zimmerman HJ: Chlorzoxazone hepatotoxic reactions. An analysis of 21 identified or presumed cases. Arch Intern Med 146:1183, 1986.

26. Munoz SJ, Fariello R, Maddrey WC: Submassive hepatic necrosis associated with the use of progabide: a GABA receptor agonist. Dig Dis Sci 33:375, 1988.

27. Zitelli BJ, Alexander J, Taylor S, et al: Fatal hepatic necrosis due to pyrimethamine-sulfadoxine (Fansidar). Ann Intern Med 106:393, 1987.

28. Kew M, Bersohn I, Seftel H, et al: Liver damage in heatstroke. Am J Med 49:192, 1970.

29. Yaqub BA, Al-Harthi SS, Al-Orainey IO, et al: Heat stroke at the Mekkah pilgrimage: clinical characteristics and course of 30 patients. Q J Med 59:523, 1986.

30. Nouel O, Henrion J, Bernuau J, et al: Fulminant hepatic failure due to transient circulatory failure in patients with chronic heart disease. Dig Dis Sci 25:49, 1980.

31. Kaymakcalan H, Dourdourekas D, Szanto PB, et al: Congestive heart failure as a cause of fulminant hepatic failure. Am J Med 65:384, 1978.

32. Negre J, Teerenhovi O, Autio V: Hepatic coma resulting from diaphragmatic rupture and hepatic herniation. Arch Surg 121:950, 1986.

33. Rakela J, Lange SM, Ludwig J, et al: Fulminant hepatitis: Mayo Clinic experience with 34 cases. Mayo Clin Proc 60:289, 1985.

34. Hartleb M, Zahorska-Markiewicz B, Ciesielski A: Wilson's disease presenting in sisters as fulminant hepatitis with hemolytic episodes. Am J Gastroenterol 82:549, 1987.

35. Wilson JA, Raufman JP: Hepatic failure in adult Niemann-Pick disease. Am J Med Sci 292:168, 1986.

36. Morton KO, Schneider F, Weimer MK, et al: Hepatic and bile porphyrins in patients with protoporphyria and liver failure. Gastroenterology 94:1488, 1988.

37. Halverson JD, Wise L, Wazna MF, et al: Jejunoileal bypass for morbid obesity. Am J Med 64:461, 1978.

38. Cairns SR, Kark AE, Peters TJ: Raised hepatic free fatty acids in a patient with acute fatty liver after gastric surgery for morbid obesity. J Clin Pathol 39:647, 1986.

39. Kaplan MM: Acute fatty liver of pregnancy. N Engl J Med 313:367, 1985.

40. Himelman RB: Fulminant hepatic failure six weeks postpartum. Hosp Pract 21(7):105, 1986.

41. Harrison HB, Middleton HM III, Crosby JH, et al: Fulminant hepatic failure: an unusual presentation of metastatic liver disease. Gastroenterology 80:820, 1981.
42. Bouloux PM, Scott RJ, Goligher JE, Kindell C: Fulminant hepatic failure secondary to diffuse liver infiltration by melanoma. J R Soc Med 79:302, 1986.
43. Bozzetti F, Doci R, Bignami P, et al: Patterns of failure following surgical resection of colorectal cancer liver metastases. Rationale for a multimodal approach. Ann Surg 205:264, 1987.
44. Levy LJ, Swinburne LM, Boulton RP, Losowsky MS: Primary hepatocellular carcinoma presenting as fulminant hepatic failure in a young woman. Postgrad Med J 62:1135, 1986.
45. Hsu HC, Wu TT, Wu MZ, et al: Tumor invasiveness and prognosis in resected hepatocellular carcinoma. Clinical and pathogenetic implications. Cancer 61:2095, 1988.
46. Boyce NW, Holdsworth SR, Hooke D, et al: Nonhepatitis B-associated liver disease in a renal transplant population. Am J Kidney Dis 11:307, 1988.
47. Rao KV, Andersen RC: Long-term results and complications in renal transplant recipients. Observations in the second decade. Transplantation 45:45, 1988.
48. Case records of the Massachusetts General Hospital. Weekly clinicopathological exercises. Case 50-1987. A 43-year-old woman with hepatic failure after renal transplantation because of amyloidosis. N Engl J Med 317:1520, 1987.
49. Stankoski JA, Roth JA, Gillin JS: Chronic active hepatitis and hepatic failure in the setting of idiopathic hemochromatosis. Am J Gastroenterol 82:61, 1987.
50. Gupta S, Blumgart LH, Hodgson HJ: Budd-Chiari syndrome: long-term survival and factors affecting mortality. Q J Med 60:781, 1986.
51. Powell-Jackson PR, Ede RJ, Williams R: Budd-Chiari syndrome presenting as fulminant hepatic failure. Gut 27:1101, 1986.

Selected Readings

Bihari DJ, Gimson AE, Williams R: Cardiovascular, pulmonary, and renal complications of fulminant hepatic failure. Semin Liver Dis 6:119, 1986.

The common occurrence of cardiovascular, pulmonary, and renal complications during hepatic failure is reviewed, with an emphasis on the pathogenesis of the hemodynamic abnormalities in fulminant hepatic failure and its relation to the development of tissue hypoxia. Management is outlined and well referenced.

Cerra FB: Hypermetabolism, organ failure, and metabolic support. Surgery 101:1, 1987.

Concepts of isolated organ failure are changing to organ failure seen as part of a systemic response to injury and repair. Hypermetabolism associated with organ failure and subsequent malnutrition are now recognized as significant factors affecting morbidity and mortality in the surgical intensive care setting.

Chang TM: Experimental artificial liver support with emphasis on fulminant hepatic failure: concepts and review. Semin Liver Dis 6:148, 1986.

Current concepts of artificial liver support based on a review of clinical trials and animal studies.

Gimson AE, O'Grady J, Ede RJ, et al: Late onset hepatic failure: clinical, serological, and histological features. Hepatology 6:288, 1986.
Forty-seven patients with late onset hepatic failure were reviewed for clinical, laboratory, and histologic features. Histopathologic features of lobular inflammatory infiltrates, bridging necrosis, and multilobular collapse were present in the acute stage of both survivors and fatal cases. No significant improvement in survival was seen in patients given corticosteroids. Hepatic transplantation was successful in one patient.

Guarner F, Hughes RD, Gimson AE, Williams R: Renal function in fulminant hepatic failure: hemodynamics and renal prostaglandins. Gut 28:1643, 1987.
Eighteen patients with fulminant liver failure were studied with attention to renal dysfunction. Marked renal vasconstriction, with increased plasma renin activity and reduced renal prostaglandin excretion, was found.

Iwatsuki S, Esquivel CO, Gordon RD, et al: Liver transplantation for fulminant hepatic failure. Semin Liver Dis 5:325, 1985.
An initial report on this approach from the largest liver transplantation center.

Jones EA, Schafer DF: Fulminant hepatic failure. p. 415. In Zakim D, Boyer TD (eds): Hepatology, A Textbook of Liver Disease. WB Saunders, Philadelphia, 1982.
An in-depth and well-written review of the subject.

Komori H, Hirasa M, Takakuwa H, et al: Concept of the clinical stages of acute hepatic failure. Am J Gastroenterol 81:544, 1986.
Serial diagnostic imagings were performed on 15 patients with acute hepatic failure to assess liver size and correlate findings with the clinical picture. Authors found a poorer survival rate in patients who presented with hepatic atrophy.

Myslobodsky MS: gamma-Aminobutyric acid (GABA) and hepatic encephalopathy: testing the validity of electroencephalographic evidence of the GABA hypothesis. Hepatogastroenterology 34:58, 1987.
A review of recent advances in understanding GABAergic mechanisms involved in the encephalopathy and electrographic correlates of hepatic encephalopathy.

O'Brien CJ, Wise RJ, O'Grady JG, Williams R: Neurological sequelae in patients recovered from fulminant hepatic failure. Gut 28:93, 1987.
Two case reports of young adults who recovered from fulminant hepatic failure, grade 4 encephalopathy, and clinical signs of cerebral edema. Both patients suffered permanent neurologic sequelae. Authors discuss current concepts of management of cerebral edema associated with increased intracranial pressure.

O'Grady JG, Langley PG, Isola LM, et al: Coagulopathy of fulminant hepatic failure. Semin Liver Dis 6:159, 1986.
Since the liver plays a central role in hemostasis, the problems with coagulopathy in hepatic failure are complex. This article identifies and reviews specific coagulation abnormalities in hepatic failure and outlines suggestions for management.

Pappas SC: Fulminant hepatic failure and the need for artificial liver support. Mayo Clin Proc 63:198, 1988.

Editorial statement of the current clinical experience, limitations, and indications for artificial liver support in the setting of acute failure of liver function occurring in patients with no known antecedent liver disease and hepatic encephalopathy supervening within 8 weeks of onset of clinical symptoms.

Payne JA: Fulminant liver failure. Med Clin North Am 70:1067, 1986.
A clinical review of causes, pathogenesis, sequelae, and management of fulminant liver failure.

Rakela J, Kurtz SB, McCarthy JT, et al: Postdilution hemofiltration in the management of acute hepatic failure: a pilot study. Mayo Clin Proc 63:113, 1988.
A pilot study was conducted to assess the feasibility and efficacy of postdilution hemofiltration in the management of seven consecutive patients with acute hepatic failure. The hemodynamic status of two patients precluded treatment. However, in four of five treated patients, hepatic encephalopathy was ameliorated. Thrombocytopenia and bleeding were the major complications. The role for this temporary artificial liver support system is discussed.

Tygstrup N, Ranek L: Assessment of prognosis in fulminant hepatic failure. Semin Liver Dis 6:129, 1986.
Authors identify clinical and laboratory factors that may be potentially helpful in predicting outcome of hepatic failure. Major clinical factors included age and grade of coma, which reflected degree of hepatic failure. Major laboratory factors included alpha-1-fetoprotein, bile acid conjugation, tolerance tests that reflected hepatic metabolic capacity, and biopsy assessment of hepatocyte volume.

30

Diarrhea in AIDS: Common Enteropathic Agents and Other Causes

Diarrhea sometimes can be the initial manifestation of infection in an immune compromised host, particularly in patients considered at high risk for human immunodeficiency virus (HIV) infection. Sometimes the isolation of certain enteric pathogens in patients with diarrhea can be the first clue leading to the diagnosis of concomitant HIV infection.[1] Evaluation of diarrhea in known HIV-infected patients should include the search for the same common bacterial and viral enteric pathogens that inflict diarrhea in otherwise healthy persons. However, several studies in patients with diarrhea who were also considered at high risk for HIV infection or seropositive for HIV infection, have consistently found certain enteric pathogens that are less common in other patient populations. Neoplasia and an ill-defined enteropathy can also cause diarrhea in this population.[2]

Cryptosporidium: most commonly reported pathogen associated with diarrhea in AIDS patients[3-8]

Shigellae[9]

Salmonellae: especially *S. typhimurium*

Campylobacter jejuni[10-13]

Giardia lamblia[14]

Entamoeba histolytica[15]

Neisseria gonorrhoeae

Herpes simplex

Chlamydia trachomatis[16]

Allergic proctitis: lubricants,[17] perfumes

Cytomegalovirus: colitis is a common presentation.[18-20]

Gastric tuberculosis[21]

Mycobacterium avium: can present with clinical and histologic picture mimicking Whipple's disease[22-24]

Tumors: lymphoma, Kaposi's sarcoma

Idiopathic AIDS enteropathy: possibly due to HIV virus[25]

Other intestinal parasites: *Endolimax nana, Entamoeba coli, Entamoeba hartmanni, Dientamoeba fragilis, Iodamoeba buetschlii, Chilomastix mesnili,* and *Isospora belli*[26,27]

References

1. Peters CS, Kathpalia SB, Chittom-Swiatlo AL, et al: *Isospora belli* and *Cryptosporidium* sp. from a patient not suspected of having acquired immunodeficiency syndrome. Diagn Microbiol Infect Dis 8:197, 1987.
2. Santangelo WC, Krejs GJ: Gastrointestinal manifestations of the acquired immunodeficiency syndrome. Am J Med Sci 292:328, 1986.
3. Centers for Disease Control: Update: treatment of cryptosporidiosis in patients with acquired immunodeficiency syndrome (AIDS). MMWR 33:117, 1984.
4. Laughon BE, Druckman DA, Vernon A, et al: Prevalence of enteric pathogens in homosexual men with and without acquired immunodeficiency syndrome. Gastroenterology 94:984, 1988.

5. Soave R, Armstrong D: Cryptosporidium and cryptosporidiosis. Rev Infect Dis 8:1012, 1986.
6. Fischer MC, Agger WA: Cryptosporidiosis. Am Fam Physician 36(4):201, 1987.
7. Connolly GM, Dryden MS, Shanson DC, Gazzard BG: Cryptosporidial diarrhoea in AIDS and its treatment. Gut 29:593, 1988.
8. Tzipori S: Cryptosporidiosis in perspective. Adv Parasitol 27:63, 1988.
9. Nelson JD, Kusmiesz H, Jackson LH, et al: Trimethoprim-sulfamethoxazole therapy for shigellosis. JAMA 235:1239, 1976.
10. Laughon BE, Vernon AA, Druckman DA, et al: Recovery of *Campylobacter* species from homosexual men. J Infect Dis 158:464, 1988.
11. Edmonds P, Patton CM, Griffin PM, et al: *Campylobacter hyointestinalis* associated with human gastrointestinal disease in the United States. J Clin Microbiol 25:685, 1987.
12. Tee W, Anderson BN, Ross BC, Dwyer B: Atypical campylobacters associated with gastroenteritis. J Clin Microbiol 25:1248, 1987.
13. Dworkin B, Wormser GP, Abdoo RA, et al: Persistence of multiple antibiotic-resistant *Campylobacter jejuni* in a patient with the acquired immune deficiency syndrome. Am J Med 80:965, 1986.
14. Janoff EN, Smith PD, Blaser MJ: Acute antibody responses to *Giardia lamblia* are depressed in patients with AIDS. J Infect Dis 157:798, 1988.
15. Allason-Jones E, Mindel A, Sargeaunt P, et al: *Entamoeba histolytica* as a commensal intestinal parasite in homosexual men. N Engl J Med 315:353, 1986.
16. Jones RB, Rabinovitch RA, Katz BP, et al: *Chlamydia trachomatis* in the pharynx and rectum of heterosexual patients at risk for genital infection. Ann Intern Med 102:757, 1985.
17. Fisher AA, Brancaccio RR: Allergic contact sensitivity to propylene glycol in a lubricant jelly. Arch Dermatol 115:1451, 1979.
18. Meiselman MS, Cello JP, Margaretten W: Cytomegalovirus colitis. Gastroenterology 88:171, 1985.
19. Rene E, Marche C, Chevalier T, et al: Cytomegalovirus colitis in patients with acquired immunodeficiency syndrome. Dig Dis Sci 33:741, 1988.
20. Weber JN, Thom S, Barrison J, et al: Cytomegalovirus colitis and esophageal ulceration in the context of AIDS: clinical manifestations and preliminary report of treatment with Foscarnet (phosphonoformate). Gut 28:482, 1987.
21. Brody JM, Miller DK, Zeman RK, et al: Gastric tuberculosis: a manifestation of acquired immunodeficiency syndrome. Radiology 159:347, 1986.
22. Gillin JS, Urmacher C, West R, et al: Disseminated *Mycobacterium avium-intracellulare* infection in acquired immunodeficiency syndrome mimicking Whipple's disease. Gastroenterology 85:1187, 1983.
23. Rotterdam H: Tissue diagnosis of selected AIDS-related opportunistic infections. Am J Surg Pathol 11(Suppl 1):3, 1987.
24. Wallace JM, Hannah JB: *Mycobacterium avium* complex

infection in patients with the acquired immunodeficiency syndrome. A clinicopathologic study. Chest 93:926, 1988.

25. Gillin JS, Shike M, Alcock N, et al: Malabsorption and mucosal abnormalities of the small intestine in the acquired immunodeficiency syndrome. Ann Intern Med 102:619, 1985.

26. Peters CS, Sable R, Janda WM, et al: Prevalence of enteric parasites in homosexual patients attending an outpatient clinic. J Clin Microbiol 24:684, 1986.

27. DeHovitz JA, Pape JW, Boncy M, Johnson WD Jr: Clinical manifestations and therapy of *Isospora belli* infection in patients with the acquired immunodeficiency syndrome. N Engl J Med 315:87, 1986.

Selected Readings

Arbo A, Santos JI: Diarrheal diseases in the immunocompromised host. Pediatr Infect Dis 6:894, 1987.

Review of disorders, infections, and other causes of diarrhea in various immunocompromised hosts. Immune dysfunction, such as humoral type (B cell) immunodeficiency, T and B cell disorders, neoplasia-related immune dysfunction, and immunosuppression, are reviewed with relevant pathophysiology and most likely pathogens to cause diarrhea. Extensively referenced.

Bush RA Jr, Owen WF Jr: Trauma and other noninfectious problems in homosexual men. Med Clin North Am 70:549, 1986.

A review of trauma and other noninfectious problems associated with anal-receptive intercourse.

Colebunders R, Francis H, Mann JM, et al: Persistent diarrhea, strongly associated with HIV infection in Kinshasa, Zaire. Am J Gastroenterol 82:859, 1987.

A clinical study from central Africa that attempted to define further the relationship between patients presenting with persistent diarrhea and the presence of HIV infection. One hundred twenty-eight consecutive patients presenting at Mama Yemo Hospital with diarrhea were tested for HIV antibodies. Eighty-four percent of the 128 patients with diarrhea for longer than 1 month were HIV seropositive.

Gelb A, Miller S: AIDS and gastroenterology. Am J Gastroenterol 81:619, 1986.

Concise review covering most common infections and neoplasms involving the liver and gastrointestinal tract.

Jones MJ, Miller JN, George WL: Microbiological and biochemical characterization of spirochetes isolated from the feces of homosexual males. J Clin Microbiol 24:1071, 1986.

Spirochetes were isolated from feces of 11 homosexual males. Based on biochemical tests, preformed enzyme patterns and volatile fatty-acid production, authors suggest that these spirochetes represent a heterogenous group of spirochetes that can exist in the human colon. Further study of their taxonomy and virulence may be warranted.

Owen WF Jr: Sexually transmitted diseases and traumatic problems in homosexual men. Ann Intern Med 92:805, 1980.

Well-referenced discussion of the conditions transmitted by male homosexual contact including amebiasis, giardiasis, and shigellosis.

Phillips SC, Mildvan D, William DC, et al: Sexual transmission of enteric protozoa and helminths in a venereal-disease-clinic population. N Engl J Med 305:603, 1981.
Study showing a high incidence of infections with E. histolytica or G. lamblia in homosexual men and an approach for prevention.

Quinn TC, Corey L, Chaffee RG, et al: The etiology of anorectal infections in homosexual men. Am J Med 71:395, 1981.
A presentation and review of the different etiologic forms of anorectal infections in homosexual men. Well referenced.

Siegel D, Cohen PT, Neighbor M, et al: Predictive value of stool examination in acute diarrhea. Arch Pathol Lab Med 111:715, 1987.
A prospective evaluation of the value of fecal blood and fecal leukocytes in predicting whether acute diarrhea in adults is associated with a positive stool culture for a bacterial pathogen was carried out on 113 patients with diarrhea. The patient population included women, heterosexual men, and homosexual men. Forty-seven percent of all patients had positive stool cultures with the presence of both fecal leukocytes and fecal blood in the culture. C. jejuni was the most common organism in the entire cohort; Shigella species was the most common organism found in homosexual men.

Smith PD, Lane HC, Gill VJ, et al: Intestinal infections in patients with the acquired immunodeficiency syndrome (AIDS). Etiology and response to therapy. Ann Intern Med 108:328, 1988.
A prospective, consecutive sample study to determine the frequency of pathogenic gastrointestinal microorganisms in patients with AIDS and diarrhea was conducted in a referral-based clinic and ward of the National Institute of Health. Pathogen identification, treatment, and clinical outcome are discussed.

Weller IV: ABC of AIDS. Gastrointestinal and hepatic manifestations. Br Med J 294:1474, 1987.
Pithy, illustrated review of clinical signs and symptoms related to gastrointestinal and hepatic disorders frequently seen in AIDS patients.

31
Traveler's Diarrhea: Major Etiologic Agents

Diarrhea is the most common disease affecting international travelers.[1] Travelers at highest risk are those from the United States or northern Europe traveling to Latin America, Africa, Asia, and the Middle East. Traveler's diarrhea is caused by infectious agents that stimulate intact intestinal cells with toxins that stimulate enzymatic processes which release liquid and ions.[2] Toxigenic *Escherichia coli* and *Shigellae*, ingested in fecally contaminated food or water, are the most common pathogens to produce a syndrome characterized by about 5 days of nausea, cramps, and watery diarrhea.[3-5] Other infectious agents, such as viruses, bacteria, and protozoa, as well as occasional noninfectious agents, such as drugs, can produce similar symptoms. Occasionally, more chronic symptoms may reflect the unmasking of a preexisting diarrheal condition.[6]

Most Common Etiologic Agents

Enterotoxigenic *E. coli*[7,8]
Shigella[9,10]
Plesiomonas shigelloides[11]
Campylobacter jejuni
Salmonella[12]
Giardia lamblia[13,14]
Entamoeba histolytica[15]
Vibrio parahaemolyticus
Cryptosporidium[16,17]

Common Etiologic Agents

Antibiotic-associated diarrhea[18]
Clostridium difficile
Vibrios: V. parahaemolyticus, V. cholerae, V. fluvialis
Yersinia enterocolitica
Aeromonas hydrophila
Plesiomonas shigelloides
Viruses: rotavrius,[19] Norwalk-like agents[20]
Dientamoeba fragilis
Isospora belli

Balantidium coli
Strongyloides stercoralis
Schistosomiasis[21]
Heterophyes heterophyes: intestinal fluke that can be
eaten in sushi[22]

References

1. Turner AC: Traveller's diarrhea: a survey of symptoms,
   occurrence, and possible prophylaxis. Br Med J 4:653,
   1967.
2. Kean BH: Travelers' diarrhea: an overview. Rev Infect
   Dis 8(Suppl 2):S111, 1986.
3. Brown KR, Phillips SM: Tropical diseases of importance
   to the traveler. Adv Intern Med 29:59, 1984.
4. Shore EG, Dean AG, Holik KJ, et al: Enterotoxin-
   producing *Escherichia coli* and diarrheal disease in adult
   travelers: a prospective study. J Infect Dis 129:577,
   1974.
5. MacDonald KL, Cohen ML: Epidemiology of travelers'
   diarrhea: current perspectives. Rev Infect Dis 8(Suppl
   2):S117, 1986.
6. Giannella RA: Chronic diarrhea in travelers: diagnostic
   and therapeutic considerations. Rev Infect Dis 8(Suppl
   2):S223, 1986.
7. Powell DW: Enterotoxigenic diarrhea: mechanisms and
   prospects for therapy. Pharmacol Ther 23:407, 1984.
8. Oprandy JJ, Thornton SA, Gardiner CH, et al: Alkaline
   phosphatase-conjugated oligonucleotide probes for enterotoxigenic *Escherichia coli* in travelers to South America and West Africa. J Clin Microbiol 26:92, 1988.
9. Keusch GT, Donohue-Rolfe A, Jacewicz M: Shigella
   toxin(s): description and role in diarrhea and dysentery.
   Pharmacol Ther 15:403, 1982.
10. Spika JS, Dabis F, Hargrett-Bean N, et al: Shigellosis at
    a Caribbean resort. Hamburger and North American
    origin as risk factors. Am J Epidemiol 126:1173, 1987.
11. Holmberg SD, Wachsmuth IK, Hickman-Brenner FW,
    et al: *Plesiomonas* enteric infections in the United States.
    Ann Intern Med 105:690, 1986.
12. Morbidity and Mortality Weekly Report: Salmonellosis
    at a resort hotel—Puerto Rico. MMWR 35:766, 1986.
13. Osterholm MT, Forfang JC, Ristinen TL, et al: An
    outbreak of foodborne giardiasis. N Engl J Med 304:24,
    1981.
14. Holtan NR: Giardiasis. A crimp in the life-style of
    campers, travelers, and others. Postgrad Med 83(5):54,
    1988.
15. Pherson PO: Amoebiasis in a non-endemic country.
    Scand J Infect Dis 15:207, 1983.
16. Elsser KA, Moricz M, Proctor EM: *Cryptosporidium* in-
    fections: a laboratory review. Can Med Assoc J 135:211,
    1986.
17. Tzipori S: Cryptosporidiosis in perspective. Adv Par-
    asitol 27:63, 1988.
18. Stergachis A, Perera DR, Schnell MM, et al: Antibiotic-
    associated colitis. West J Med 140:217, 1984.

19. Hrdy DB: Epidemiology of rotaviral infection in adults. Rev Infect Dis 9:461, 1987.
20. Blacklow NR, Cukor G: Viral gastroenteritis. N Engl J Med 304:397, 1981.
21. Doehring E: Schistosomiasis in childhood. Eur J Pediatr 147:2, 1988.
22. Adams KO, Jungkind DL, Bergguist EJ, Wirts CW: Intestinal fluke infection as a result of eating sushi. Am J Clin Pathol 86:688, 1986.

Selected Readings

Adler PM: Stool examination: culture versus Gram stain. Ann Emerg Med 15:337, 1986.
Guidelines for the emergency room evaluation of stool in infectious diarrhea.

Black RE: Pathogens that cause travelers' diarrhea in Latin America and Africa. Rev Infect Dis 8(Suppl 2):S131, 1986.
Studies of travelers to Latin America and Africa suggest that approximately 50% develop diarrhea. One-third of these cases are associated with E. coli. Other important infectious agents include rotavirus, Norwalk virus, Shigella, Salmonella, G. lamblia, and E. histolytica.

Blaser MJ: Environmental interventions for the prevention of traveler's diarrhea. Rev Infect Dis 8(Suppl 2):S142, 1986.
A review of environmental methods to minimize exposure to infectious agents causing traveler's diarrhea. Common infectious sources of food and water are discussed, as well as acceptable methods for disinfecting potentially contaminated sources.

Cantey JR: Infectious diarrhea. Pathogenesis and risk factors. Am J Med 68(S6B):65, 1985.
Update of etiologic agents, mechanisms, and pathogenesis of infectious diarrhea.

DuPont HL, Ericsson CD, Robinson A, Johnson PC: Current problems in antimicrobial therapy for bacterial enteric infection. Am J Med 82:324, 1987.
This study evaluated the problem of resistant strains of bacterial enteropathogens to trimethoprim-sulfamethoxazole in a clinical trial involving a United States student population in Mexico. Although trimethoprim-sulfamethoxazole is the current treatment of choice for shigellosis and severe traveler's diarrhea, it is less effective against resistant strains of C. jejuni strains and other bacterial enteropathogens. Alternative choices of treatment are suggested.

Edelman R: Prevention and treatment of infectious diarrhea. Speculation on the next 10 years. Am J Med 68(S6B):99, 1985.
Discussion of advances in genetic engineering including enteric vaccines against cholera, E. coli, Shigella, typhoid fever, and rotavirus.

Ericsson CD, DuPont HL, Mathewson JJ, et al: Test-of-cure stool cultures for traveler's diarrhea. J Clin Microbiol 26:1047, 1988.
The persistence or eradication of enteropathogens in stool cultures was compared with the duration of symptoms in 251 patients with traveler's diarrhea. The durations of diarrhea were similar within

the antimicrobial agent-treated and placebo-treated groups. Authors suggest that test-of-cure stool cultures may be useful in study of treatment failures and in asymptomatic carriage of enteropathogens after treatment, but may not help assess clinical efficacy of treatment.

Ericsson CD, Patterson TF, Dupont HL: Clinical presentations as a guide to therapy for traveler's diarrhea. Am J Med Sci 294:91, 1987.

Clinical features of infectious traveler's diarrhea in United States travelers in Mexico were studied to determine indications for empirical antimicrobial therapy. Fever, stool mucus, blood, and fecal leukocytes were significantly more common in patients with shigellosis. Withholding therapy from patients with mild presentations resulted in 48% of these patients continuing to have symptoms up to 48 hours. Authors recommend empiric use of antimicrobial agents in travelers with diarrhea associated with fever, bloody stools, or fecal leukocytes and for travelers with moderate to severe diarrhea.

Farrar WE: Antibiotic resistance in developing countries. J Infect Dis 152:1103, 1985.

Important and disturbing review of multiresistant strains of enteric bacterial pathogens reported in increasing frequency over the last 15 years. Antibiotic resistance is a part of diarrheal disease due to enteric pathogens in large areas of the world.

Kimmey M: Infectious diarrhea. Emerg Med Clin North Am 3:127, 1985.

Article focusing on the clinical approach to the patient with diarrhea presenting to the emergency room.

Lange WR, Kreider S: Traveler's diarrhea. Controversy and consensus. Postgrad Med 77(4):255, 1985.

A review of controversies regarding prevention and treatment of traveler's diarrhea.

Mathewson JJ, Johnson PC, DuPont HL, et al: A newly recognized cause of traveler's diarrhea: enteroadherent *Escherichia coli.* J Infect Dis 151:471, 1985.

Study showing that enteroadherent E. coli (EAEC) are associated with diarrhea in travelers to Mexico and may explain the effect of antibiotics in the prevention of traveler's diarrhea in patients with no recognized bacterial enteropathogens.

NIH Consensus Development Conference: Travelers' diarrhea. JAMA 253:2700, 1985.

Consensus regarding the epidemiology, causes, prevention, and treatment of traveler's diarrhea.

Oprandy JJ, Thornton SA, Gardiner CH, et al: Alkaline phosphatase-conjugated oligonucleotide probes for enterotoxigenic *Escherichia coli* in travelers to South America and West Africa. J Clin Microbiol 26:92, 1988.

Interesting discussion of a new enzyme-labeled oligonucleotide probes that may be a significant advance in laboratory techniques available to identify enterotoxigenic E. coli-associated diarrheal disease.

Peate WF, Pust RE: Health precautions for travelers to Mexico. South Med J 78:335, 1985.

A useful summarization of potential health hazards to travelers to Mexico with an outline for health advice for patients.

Quinn TC, Bender BS, Bartlett JG: New developments in infectious diarrhea. DM 32:165, 1986.

Clinical update including the current concepts of infectious diarrhea in AIDS patients.

Steffen R: Epidemiologic studies of traveler's diarrhea,

severe gastrointestinal infections, and cholera. Rev Infect Dis 8(Suppl 2):S122, 1986.

A retrospective study based on interviews between 1975 and 1984 with 20,000 European tourists again identifies traveler's diarrhea as the most frequent health problem that travelers encounter in the tropics. Giardiasis, amebiasis, typhoid fever, and cholera were associated with gastrointestinal infections of greater severity.

Steffen R, Mathewson JJ, Ericsson CD, et al: Traveler's diarrhea in West Africa and Mexico: fecal transport systems and liquid bismuth subsalicylate for self-therapy. J Infect Dis 157:1008, 1988.

This study attempted to compare the etiology of traveler's diarrhea in West Africa and Mexico, to evaluate two fecal transport systems for recovery of enteropathogens, and to verify the clinical efficacy of bismuth subsalicylate. A two-vial system of Enteric Plus medium and polyvinyl alcohol system was considered slightly superior for identifying enteric pathogens. Bismuth subsalicylate significantly shortened disease duration.

Strum WB: Update on traveler's diarrhea. Postgrad Med 84(1):163, 1988.

Current concepts of traveler's diarrhea continue to emphasize avoidance of high risk food and water. Prophylactic medications are discussed.

Svanteson B, Thoren A, Castor B, et al: Acute diarrhea in adults: etiology, clinical appearance and therapeutic aspects. Scand J Infect Dis 20:303, 1988.

A prospective 15-month study from Sweden of acute diarrhea included 731 patients, 240 controls, and a cluster of travelers. Forty-three percent were infected abroad. Pathogens found in decreasing frequency included Campylobacter, *enterotoxigenic* E. coli, Salmonella *spp.,* rotavirus, Y. enterocolitica, G. lamblia, Shigella *spp.,* C. difficile, *enteroviruses, and* E. histolytica. *More than 90% of bacterial or parasitic enteropathogens were found in the first stool sample.*

Taylor DN, Echeverria P: Etiology and epidemiology of traveler's diarrhea in Asia. Rev Infect Dis 8(Suppl 2):S136, 1986.

Traveler's diarrhea in Asia was studied among Peace Corps volunteers in Thailand, Japanese travelers, and foreign residents in Bangladesh. Infectious agents identified in decreasing frequency included enterotoxigenic E. coli, Salmonella, Shigella, Campylobacter, *and* V. parahaemolyticus. *Multiple pathogens were identified in 9 to 22% of diarrheal episodes studied.*

Taylor DN, Houston R, Shlim DR, et al: Etiology of diarrhea among travelers and foreign residents in Nepal. JAMA 260:1245, 1988.

A study of bacterial pathogens causing diarrhea in Nepal reviewed pathogens isolated from 47% of 328 expatriate patients with diarrhea in Nepal. Although a wide variety of enteropathogens was detected, the most frequently isolated pathogens were enterotoxigenic E. coli, Shigella, *and* Campylobacter *species. Patients with prolonged symptoms were more likely to be infected with Giardia.*

Wanger AR, Murray BE, Echeverria P, et al: Enteroinvasive *Escherichia coli* in travelers with diarrhea. J Infect Dis 158:640, 1988.

The enteric pathogen enteroinvasive E. coli *can cause symptoms that mimic* Shigella *infection. In this study of diarrhea in students traveling to Mexico, enteroinvasive* E. coli *was detected by using total plasmid content (TPC). Authors suggest this pathogen may be underdiagnosed because the organism may a lactose jermenter and misdiagnosed or overlooked as a nonpathogenic* E. coli.

IV

ENDOCRINOLOGY

32
Hypoglycemia: Common and Less Common Causes

Hypoglycemia triggers adrenergic symptoms of hunger, anxiety, tremulousness, and palpitations. Such nonspecific and common symptoms are frequently the basis for the self-diagnosis of hypoglycemia. However, based on the diagnostic triad of Whipple (hypoglycemia symptoms, low plasma glucose, and response to glucose ingestion), the diagnosis is rare.[1] Symptoms of hypoglycemia usually fall either into a postprandial (reactive) pattern or a fasting hypoglycemia. Major causes of reactive or postprandial hypoglycemia include gastric surgery, endocrinopathies, and functional hypoglycemia. Fasting hypoglycemia is rarer and may be associated with a serious medical disorder, particularly if symptoms are associated with hypoglycemia below 50 mg/dl. The three most common drug-induced causes of hypoglycemia leading to hospitalization are insulin, the sulfonylureas, and alcohol.[2]

Medical Disorders Most Commonly Associated with Hypoglycemia

The three most common serious medical disorders associated with hypoglycemia are hepatic failure, renal insufficiency, and sepsis.

Hepatic failure: cirrhosis,[3] hepatocellular carcinoma
Renal insufficiency[4]
Sepsis[5]
Postoperative alimentary hypoglycemia
Starvation
Pregnancy: frequently associated with concomitant pituitary deficiency[6]
Hypopituitarism
Addison's disease
Immune disorders with counter-regulatory hormones and insulin receptor antibodies[7]
Glycogen storage disease
Hereditary fructose intolerance

Malaria[8]
Glucagon deficiency
Isolated growth hormone deficiency

Exogenous Agents Causing Hypoglycemia

Insulin: hyperinsulinism is the most common cause of fasting hypoglycemia in adults.[9]
Ethanol[10]
Sulfonylureas[11]
Miscellaneous drugs: aspirin,[12] propanolol hydrochloride, disopyramide,[13] diazoxide, pentamidine, lithium, acetaminophen, phenothiazines, amphetamines, sulfa drugs, quinine
Miscellaneous toxins: hypoglycin in akee fruit, some bush teas

Tumors Associated with Hypoglycemia

Excess insulin or insulin-like factor can often be identified with pancreatic tumors causing hypoglycemia. An insulin-like growth factor (IGF-like material) has been identified with some nonpancreatic tumors associated with hypoglycemia.[14]

Insulinomas: pancreatic islet cell tumors, 90% benign, 10% multiple[15]
Beta-cell hypertrophy[16]
Mesenchymal tumors within the abdomen or thorax: most common extrapancreatic tumors associated with hypoglycemia[17]
Adrenocortical carcinoma: IGF-like material
Hepatic carcinoma: primary and metastatic
Pheochromocytoma: although hyperglycemia is a more common association, hypoglycemia has been associated with IGF-like material and pheochromocytomas.[18]
Lymphomas
Other tumors sometimes associated with IGF-like material: hemangiopericytoma, fibrosarcoma, neurilemmoma, mesothelioma, leiomyosarcoma[18]
Neurofibrosarcoma[19]
Carcinoid tumors[20]
Paraneoplastic endocrine syndromes[21]

Causes of Spurious Hypoglycemia

Leukocytosis: autoglycolysis can cause a spurious hypoglycemia with leukocytosis of any cause.[22]
Leukemia: chronic myelogenous leukemia[23]
Polycythemia vera[24]

Munchausen syndrome or factitious hypoglycemia: associated with insulin or sulfonylurea

References

1. Nelson RL: Hypoglycemia: fact or fiction? Mayo Clin Proc 60:844, 1985.
2. Betteridge DJ: Reactive hypoglycemia. Br Med J (Clin Res) 295:286, 1987.
3. Nouel O, Bernuau J, Rueff B, et al: Hypoglycemia. A common complication of septicemia in cirrhosis. Arch Intern Med 141:1477, 1981.
4. Rutsky EA, McDaniel HG, Tharpe DL, et al: Spontaneous hypoglycemia in chronic renal failure. Arch Intern Med 138:1364, 1978.
5. Miller SI, Wallace RJ Jr, Musher DM, et al: Hypoglycemia as a manifestation of sepsis. Am J Med 68:649, 1980.
6. Smallridge RC, Corrigan DF, Thomason AM, et al: Hypoglycemia in pregnancy. Arch Intern Med 140:564, 1980.
7. Taylor SI, Grunberger G, Marcus-Samuels B, et al: Hypoglycemia associated with antibodies to the insulin receptor. N Engl J Med 307:1422, 1982.
8. White NJ, Warrell DA, Chanthavanich P, et al: Severe hypoglycemia and hyperinsulinemia in falciparum malaria. N Engl J Med 309:61, 1983.
9. Santiago JV, Pereira MB, Avioli LV: Fasting hypoglycemia in adults. Arch Intern Med 142:455, 1982.
10. Williams HE: Alcoholic hypoglycemia and ketoacidosis. Med Clin North Am 68:33, 1984.
11. Jordan RM, Kammer H, Riddle MR: Sulfonylurea-induced factitious hypoglycemia. Arch Intern Med 137:390, 1977.
12. Torella R, Giugliano D, Siniscalchio N, et al: Influence of acetylsalicylic acid on plasma glucose, insulin, glucagon, and growth hormone levels following tolbutamide stimulation in man. Metabolism 28:887, 1979.
13. Nappi JM, Dhanani S, Lovejoy JR, et al: Severe hypoglycemia associated with disopyramide. West J Med 138:95, 1983.
14. Merimee TJ: Insulin-like growth factors in patients with nonislet cell tumors and hypoglycemia. Metabolism 35:360, 1986.
15. Service FJ, Dale AJD, Elveback LR, et al: Insulinoma. Mayo Clin Proc 51:417, 1976.
16. Weinstock G, Margulies P, Kahn E, et al: Islet cell hyperplasia: an unusual cause of hypoglycemia in an adult. Metabolism 35:110, 1986.
17. Lowbeer L: Hypoglycemia-producing extrapancreatic neoplasms. A review. Am J Clin Pathol 35:233, 1961.
18. Gorden P, Hendricks CM, Kahn CR, et al: Hypoglycemia associated with non-islet-cell tumor and insulin-like growth factors. N Engl J Med 305:1452, 1981.
19. Lyall SS, Marieb NJ, Wise JK, et al: Hyperinsulinemic hypoglycemia associated with a neurofibrosarcoma. Arch Intern Med 135:865, 1975.
20. Modhi G, Nicolis G: Hypoglycemia associated with carcinoid tumors. Cancer 53:1804, 1984.

21. Ariyoshi Y: Paraneoplastic endocrine syndromes. Gan To Kagaku Ryoho 13:2023, 1986.
22. Goodenow TJ, Malarkey WB: Leukocytosis and artifactual hypoglycemia. JAMA 237:1961, 1977.
23. Field JB, Williams HE: Artifactual hypoglycemia associated with leukemia. N Engl J Med 265:946, 1961.
24. Billington CJ, Casciato DA, Choquette DL, et al: Artifactual hypoglycemia associated with polycythemia vera. JAMA 249:774, 1983.

Selected Readings

Auer RN: Progress review: hypoglycemic brain damage. Stroke 17:699, 1986.
Interesting review distinguishing pathogenic mechanisms involved in anoxic brain damage from those operating during hypoglycemic brain damage. Endogenous excitotoxins produced during hypoglycemia may correlate with increased frequency of seizure activity observed in hypoglycemic patients.

Bauman WA, Yalow RS: Hyperinsulinemic hypoglycemia. JAMA 252:2730, 1984.
Current methods of radioimmunoassays to distinguish exogenous from endogenous secretion of insulin.

Crapo PA, Olefsky JM: Food fallacies and blood sugar (editorial). N Engl J Med 309:44, 1983.
A review of recent studies reporting a spectrum of blood-glucose curve responses to different complex and simple carbohydrates.

Fischer KF, Lees JA, Newman JH: Hypoglycemia in hospitalized patients. Causes and outcomes. N Engl J Med 315:1245, 1986.
A study analyzing 137 episodes of hypoglycemia in 94 adult hospitalized patients concluded that hypoglycemia is common in hospitalized patients with renal insufficiency and is usually iatrogenic.

Fish HR, Chernow B, O'Brian JT: Endocrine and neurophysiologic responses of the pituitary to insulin-induced hypoglycemia: a review. Metabolism 35:763, 1986.
Well-referenced state-of-the-art review.

Gastineau CF: Is reactive hypoglycemia a clinical entity? (editorial). Mayo Clin Proc 58:545, 1983.
A concise review of current concepts of reactive hypoglycemia.

Harris MD, Davidson MB: Idiopathic fasting hypoglycemia in an adult. Am J Med 82:303, 1987.
Interesting case report of a 73-year-old man with a 22-year history of extensively studied symptoms of fasting hypoglycemia reported as the first known case of idiopathic fasting hypoglycemia in an adult.

Kaplan EL, Arganini M, Kang SJ: Diagnosis and treatment of hypoglycemic disorders. Surg Clin North Am 67:395, 1987.
A surgical review of the evaluation of hypoglycemia, with an emphasis on the diagnosis and localization of islet cell tumors.

Kitabchi AE, Goodman RC: Hypoglycemia. Pathophysiology and diagnosis. Hosp Pract 22(11A):45, 1987.
Useful review for the clinician faced with the frequent challenge of the patient with symptoms suggesting hypoglycemia.

Malouf R, Brust JCM: Hypoglycemia: causes, neurological manifestations, and outcome. Ann Neurol 17:421, 1985.

Clinical study of neurologic manifestations and sequelae of hypoglycemia.

Nelson RL: Hypoglycemia: fact or fiction? Mayo Clin Proc 60:844, 1985.
This review defines requirements necessary for glucose homeostasis and organic hypoglycemia and offers a logical approach to diagnosis and treatment.

Nelson RL: Oral glucose tolerance test: indications and limitations. Mayo Clin Proc 63:263, 1988.
The clinical uses and limitations of the oral glucose tolerance test are reviewed. The test should not be used to evaluate reactive hypoglycemia. Recommendations are made for use in pregnancy.

Uhde TW, Vittone BJ, Post RM: Glucose tolerance testing in panic disorder. Am J Psychiatry 141:1461, 1984.
This study reports a poor correlation between hypoglycemia and panic attacks in nine patients with panic disorders.

33

Diabetes Mellitus and Glucose Intolerance: Clinical Classification

Diabetes mellitus is characterized by hyperglycemia caused by an absolute or relative insulin deficiency. Current concepts of the pathogenesis and pathophysiology of diabetes mellitus define diabetes mellitus as a clinically heterogeneous disorder. The classification of diabetes mellitus and other categories of glucose intolerance as published by the National Diabetes Data Group reflect this diversity of clinical subgroups.[1,2] Two major categories of diabetes remain: (1) insulin-dependent, ketosis-prone diabetes, formerly termed juvenile diabetes; and (2) noninsulin-dependent, nonketosis-prone diabetes, formerly termed adult or maturity onset diabetes. Other categories of diabetes include gestational diabetes and types of diabetes caused by or associated with certain disorders. Categories of impaired glucose intolerance and other statistical risk categories complete the clinical classifications. This classification can lead to a more individualized and rational therapy for the various types of diabetes mellitus and glucose intolerance.[3]

Insulin-dependent Diabetes Mellitus, Type I

Patients with insulin-dependent diabetes mellitus (IDDM) are insulinopenic, ketosis-prone, and require insulin to sustain life. IDDM usually presents abruptly in a young person with polyuria, polydipsia, and polyphagia; however, it can begin at any age. Heterogeneous genetics, particularly certain histocompatibility antigens (HLA) on chromosome 6, environmental factors, and abnormal immune responses are all proposed etiologic factors of this heterogeneous disorder.[4–12]

Noninsulin-dependent Diabetes Mellitus, Type II

Patients with noninsulin-dependent diabetes mellitus (NIDDM) can have normal, decreased, or even increased insulin with a variety of insulin responses to glucose. Characteristically, patients with NIDDM have long asymptomatic periods and manifest slowly progressive stages, which include the classic vascular and neurologic complications of diabetes mellitus. Although usually noninsulin dependent, patients with NIDDM may become insulin dependent when stressed, particularly with infection or trauma. Although multiple etiologic factors are suggested, most NIDDM is probably the result of combined genetic susceptibility and environmental factors.[13–16]

Nonobese NIDDM: since obesity is considered a significant etiologic factor in NIDDM, patients who are not obese may be considered a clinical subcategory.[1]

Obese NIDDM: excessive caloric intake resulting in weight gain, obesity, and disordered carbohydrate metabolism is considered an important cause of NIDDM, particularly in patients with genetic susceptibility possibly combined with certain environmental factors.[17–22]

Other Types of Diabetes and Diabetes Associated with Certain Disorders

Pancreatic disease: pancreatic viral infection, a variety of familial, inflammatory, neoplastic, infectious, and postsurgical pancreatic disorders have been linked with diabetes[23–26]

Hormonal-induced diabetes: endocrinopathies such as acromegaly, Cushing's syndrome, glucagonomas, pheochromocytoma, and mineralocorticoid excess have all been associated with diabetes.[27-32]

Insulin-receptor abnormalities: multiple insulin-receptor abnormalities and insulin-receptor blocking antibodies have been causally linked to diabetes.[33-35]

Genetic syndromes: a variety of diabetogenic mechanisms have been postulated within this group, such as inborn errors of metabolism and insulin resistance.[36,37]

Drug and chemical-induced diabetes: diuretics, antihypertensive agents, exogenous hormones, psychoactive drugs, and many miscellaneous drugs have been associated with diabetes and impaired glucose tolerance.[1]

Impaired glucose tolerance (IGT): a degree of glucose intolerance between normal and diabetic may identify patients at risk for IDDM or NIDDM.[38-40]

Gestational diabetes: gestational diabetes begins with glucose intolerance or diabetes mellitus during pregnancy. This heterogeneous disorder is important to identify because of increased obstetric and perinatal risk.[41-43]

References

1. National Diabetes Data Group: Classification and diagnosis of diabetes mellitus and other categories of glucose intolerance. Diabetes 28:1039, 1979.
2. Sanz N, Karam JH: The molecular genetics of diabetes mellitus. Ciba Found Symp 130:167, 1987.
3. Craig JW: Clinical implications of the new diabetes classification. Postgrad Med 68(4):122, 1980.
4. Chaplin DD, Kemp ME: The major histocompatibility complex and autoimmunity. Year Immunol 3:179, 1986.
5. Drash AL: The epidemiology of insulin-dependent diabetes mellitus. Clin Invest Med 10:432, 1987.
6. Nerup J, Mandrup-Poulsen T, Mlvig J: The HLA-IDDM association: implications for etiology and pathogenesis of IDDM. Diabetes Metab Rev 3:779, 1987.
7. Orchard TJ, Dorman JS, LaPorte RE, et al: Host and environmental interactions in diabetes mellitus. J Chronic Dis 39:979, 1986.
8. Boitard C, Debray-Sachs M, Bach JF: Autoimmune disorders in diabetes. Adv Nephrol 15:281, 1986.
9. Vadheim CM, Rotter JI, Maclaren NK, et al: Preferential transmission of diabetic alleles within the HLA gene complex. N Engl J Med 315:1314, 1986.
10. Srikanta S, Ricker AT, McCulloch DK, et al: Autoim-

munity to insulin, beta cell dysfunction, and development of insulin-dependent diabetes mellitus. Diabetes 35:139, 1986.

11. Rubinstein P, Walker M, Ginsberg-Fellner F: Excess of DR3/4 in type I diabetes. What does it portend? Diabetes 35:985, 1986.

12. Johnston C, Raghu P, McCulloch DK, et al: Beta-cell function and insulin sensitivity in nondiabetic HLA-identical siblings of insulin-dependent diabetics. Diabetes 36:829, 1987.

13. O'Rahilly S, Spivey RS, Holman RR, et al: Type II diabetes of early onset: a distinct clinical and genetic syndrome? Br Med J (Clin Res) 294:923, 1987.

14. Davidson MB: Pathogenesis of type 2 diabetes mellitus: an interpretation of current data. Am J Med Sci 292:35, 1986.

15. Goldberg AP, Coon PJ: Non-insulin-dependent diabetes mellitus in the elderly. Influence of obesity and physical inactivity. Endocrinol Metab Clin North Am 16:843, 1987.

16. Swislocki AL, Donner CC, Fraze E, et al: Can insulin resistance exist as a primary defect in noninsulin-dependent diabetes mellitus? J Clin Endocrinol Metab 64:778, 1987.

17. Sinha MK, Taylor LG, Pories WJ, et al: Long-term effect of insulin on glucose transport and insulin binding in cultured adipocytes from normal and obese humans with and without noninsulin-dependent diabetes. J Clin Invest 80:1073, 1987.

18. Ravussin E, Zawadzki JK: Thermic effect of glucose in obese subjects with non-insulin-dependent diabetes mellitus. Diabetes 36:1441, 1987.

19. Bolinder J, Lithell H, Skarfors E, Arner P: Effects of obesity, hyperinsulinemia, and glucose intolerance on insulin action in adipose tissue of sixty-year-old men. Diabetes 35:282, 1986.

20. Lillioja S, Mott DM, Zawadzki JK, et al: Glucose storage is a major determinant of in vivo "insulin resistance" in subjects with normal glucose tolerance. J Clin Endocrinol Metab 62:922, 1986.

21. Wilson PW, Anderson KM, Kannel WB: Epidemiology of diabetes mellitus in the elderly. The Framingham Study. Am J Med 80:3, 1986.

22. Abbott WG, Lillioja S, Young AA, et al: Relationships between plasma lipoprotein concentrations and insulin action in an obese hyperinsulinemic population. Diabetes 36:897, 1987.

23. Irvine WJ: Classification of idiopathic diabetes. Lancet 1:638, 1977.

24. O'Rahilly SP, Nugent Z, Rudenski AS, et al: Beta-cell dysfunction, rather than insulin insensitivity, is the primary defect in familial type 2 diabetes. Lancet 2:360, 1986.

25. Groop LC, Bottazzo GF, Doniach D: Islet cell antibodies identify latent type I diabetes in patients aged 35–75 years at diagnosis. Diabetes 35:237, 1986.

26. Stutchfield PR, O'Halloran S, Teale JD, et al: Glycosylated hemoglobin and glucose intolerance in cystic fibrosis. Arch Dis Child 62:805, 1987.

27. Matsuoka LY, Goldman J, Wortsman J, et al: Antibodies against the insulin receptor in paraneoplastic acanthosis nigricans. Am J Med 82:1253, 1987.
28. Thesleff P, Benoni C, Martensson H, et al: A mixed endocrine adrenal tumour causing steatorrhoea. Gut 28:1298, 1987.
29. Bauer G: Pheochromocytoma as an unexpected anesthesia complication. Anaesthesist 35:628, 1986.
30. Bloom SR, Polak JM: Glucagonoma syndrome. Am J Med 82:25, 1987.
31. Roth KA, Wilson DM, Eberwine J, et al: Acromegaly and pheochromocytoma: a multiple endocrine syndrome caused by a plurihormonal adrenal medullary tumor. J Clin Endocrinol Metab 63:1421, 1986.
32. Reaven GM, Chen YD, Golay A, et al: Documentation of hyperglucagonemia throughout the day in nonobese and obese patients with noninsulin-dependent diabetes mellitus. J Clin Endocrinol Metab 64:106, 1987.
33. Ludwig SM, Faiman C, Dean HJ: Insulin and insulin-receptor autoantibodies in children with newly diagnosed IDDM before insulin therapy. Diabetes 36:420, 1987.
34. Caro JF, Sinha MK, Raju SM, et al: Insulin receptor kinase in human skeletal muscle from obese subjects with and without noninsulin dependent diabetes. J Clin Invest 79:1330, 1987.
35. Sinha MK, Pories WJ, Flickinger EG, et al: Insulin-receptor kinase activity of adipose tissue from morbidly obese humans with and without NIDDM. Diabetes 36:620, 1987.
36. National Diabetes Data Group: Classification and diagnosis of diabetes mellitus and other categories of glucose intolerance. Diabetes 28:1045 (Table 3), 1979.
37. Morrell D, Chase CL, Kupper LL, Swift M: Diabetes mellitus in ataxia-telangiectasia, Fanconi anemia, xeroderma pigmentosum, common variable immune deficiency, and severe combined immune deficiency families. Diabetes 35:143, 1986.
38. Hitchcock CL, Riley WJ, Alamo A, et al: Lymphocyte subsets and activation in prediabetes. Diabetes 35:1416, 1986.
39. Jackson RA, Hawa MI, Roshania RD, et al: Influence of aging on hepatic and peripheral glucose metabolism in humans. Diabetes 37:119, 1988.
40. Harris MI, Hadden WC, Knowler WC, Bennett PH: Prevalence of diabetes and impaired glucose tolerance and plasma glucose levels in U.S. population aged 20–74 yr. Diabetes 36:523, 1987.
41. Gabbe SG: Definition, detection, and management of gestational diabetes. Obstet Gynecol 67:121, 1986.
42. Sacks DA, Abu-Fadil S, Karten GJ, et al: Screening for gestational diabetes with the one-hour 50-g glucose test. Obstet Gynecol 70:89, 1987.
43. Efendic S, Hanson U, Persson B, et al: Glucose tolerance, insulin release, and insulin sensitivity in normal-weight women with previous gestational diabetes mellitus. Diabetes 36:413, 1987.

Selected Readings

Atkinson MA, Maclaren NK, Riley WJ, et al: Are insulin autoantibodies markers for insulin-dependent diabetes mellitus? Diabetes 35:894, 1986.
Insulin autoantibodies occur in patients with newly diagnosed insulin-dependent diabetes mellitus (IDDM) before insulin treatment. This study tested and supports the hypothesis that insulin autoantibodies, such as islet cell antibodies, reflect ongoing beta-cell destruction.

Davidson MB: Pathogenesis of type 2 diabetes mellitus: an interpretation of current data. Am J Med Sci 292:35, 1986.
Discussion of the pathogenesis of noninsulin-dependent diabetes mellitus (NIDDM) that focuses on currently held possible etiologic receptor mechanisms.

Harris MI, Hadden WC, Knowler WC, Bennett PH: Prevalence of diabetes and impaired glucose tolerance and plasma glucose levels in U.S. population aged 20–74 yr. Diabetes 36:523, 1987.
A study of the prevalence of physician-diagnosed diabetes and of undiagnosed diabetes and impaired glucose tolerance is presented, including estimates for the U.S. population aged 20 to 74 years from 1976 to 1980. Interesting epidemiologic data.

Johnson SR, Kolberg BH, Varner MW, Railsback LD: Maternal obesity and pregnancy. Surg Gynecol Obstet 164:431, 1987.
Authors examined the risk of maternal obesity in 588 pregnant women weighing at least 113.6 kg (250 pounds) during pregnancy. They report a significantly increased risk compared to controls for gestational diabetes, hypertension, therapeutic induction, prolonged labor, shoulder dystocia, and infants weighting more than 4,000 g. Certain operative complications are also discussed.

Klatt EC, Meyer PR: Geriatric autopsy pathology in centenarians. Arch Pathol Lab Med 111:367, 1987.
An autopsy study of pathologic findings in 32 patients aged 100 or older found that atherosclerosis, neoplasia, and bronchopneumonia were common; but diabetes mellitus, obesity, hypertension, and cerebrovascular accidents were absent to rare.

Kreisberg RA: Aging, glucose metabolism, and diabetes: current concepts. Geriatrics 42:67, 1987.
An informative review of current concepts of glucose metabolism, diabetes mellitus, and impaired glucose tolerance in the elderly.

Kuglin B, Gries FA, Kolb H: Evidence of IgG autoantibodies against human proinsulin in patients with IDDM before insulin treatment. Diabetes 37:130, 1988.
IgG proinsulin autoantibodies have been identified in sera of some patients with newly diagnosed IDDM before insulin treatment. Authors suggest precursors of insulin are part of the immune process of IDDM.

Lehrer JF, Poole DC, Seaman M, et al: Identification and treatment of metabolic abnormalities in patients with vertigo. Arch Intern Med 146:1497, 1986.
One hundred patients with vertigo in an otolaryngology practice were studied to determine the significance of hyperinsulinism, impaired glucose tolerance, and hypertriglyceridemia in order to identify patients who might respond to dietary therapy. Authors suggest

that reactive hypoglycemia may be overdiagnosed as a cause of vertigo and that insulin resistance, particularly in overweight patients, was the basic abnormality associated with vertigo in their series of patients.

O'Hare JA: The enigma of insulin resistance and hypertension. Insulin resistance, blood pressure, and the circulation. Am J Med 84:505, 1988.

An interesting update of concepts of insulin resistance and its significance in the link between obesity and hypertension. Multiple conditions are associated with a tendency toward elevated blood pressure and insulin resistance, such as pregnancy, oral contraceptives, acromegaly, and excessive glucocorticoids.

Reaven GM: Abnormal lipoprotein metabolism in non-insulin-dependent diabetes mellitus. Pathogenesis and treatment. Am J Med 83:31, 1987.

A review of current concepts and pathogenesis of lipoprotein abnormalities in diabetes mellitus. These concepts are particularly important in NIDDM because of the significant contribution of lipid abnormalities to increased morbidity and mortality from coronary artery disease in patients with NIDDM.

Sims EA, Weed LB: 1987 Herman award lecture. A plea for an integrated approach to characterization and management of obesity, type II diabetes, hyperlipidemias, and hypertension: a role for the personal computer? Am J Clin Nutr 46:726, 1987.

Interesting paper for computer users discussing computer programs developed to facilitate an integrated clinical and investigative approach to integrate problems in obesity, type II diabetes, hyperlipidemias, and hypertension.

Tarn AC, Thomas JM, Dean BM, et al: Predicting insulin-dependent diabetes. Lancet 1:845, 1988.

Seven hundred nineteen first-degree relatives of diabetic children were followed to assess the predictive value of HLA haplotype sharing and of islet-cell antibodies for prediction of insulin-dependent diabetes antibodies. Within a maximum of 8 years, 16 unaffected relatives including 5 parents and 11 siblings became insulin dependent.

34
Obesity: Associated Metabolic–Endocrine and Inherited Disorders

Obesity is defined as body fat that can be measured by using the body-mass index (BMI), i.e., by dividing weight (kg) by height (meters squared). Morbidity and mortality increase in the Western population when the BMI exceeds 30.[1] Overeating is the primary cause of obesity. Physicians are frequently asked to evaluate the endocrine status of obese patients with the hope of finding a treatable endocrinologic disorder that has caused unwanted weight gain. However, most endocrine abnormalities associated with obesity, such as increased cortisol production and insulin resistance, are secondary to obesity rather than primary causes.[2] Recent evidence suggests that genetics plays a major role in determining body weight and familial obesity.[3] Some interesting and less common causes of obesity include the following:

Genetically-determined, impaired adaptive thermogenesis[4]

Hyperinsulinemia of noninsulin-dependent diabetes mellitus

Hypothyroidism

Polycystic ovary syndrome

Cushing's disease (see Ch. 41 under Disorders that can Mimic Cushing's Syndrome).

Psychotropic drugs: studies and clinical experience indicate that neuroleptic drugs, tricyclic and monoamine oxidase inhibitor antidepressants, and lithium can stimulate carbohydrate craving, causing weight gain.[5]

Hypothalamic lesions: destruction of the satiety center leads to hyperphagia and obesity.[6,7]

Laurence-Moon-Biedl syndrome: retinitis pigmentosa, microcephaly, hypogonadism, polydactyly

Alström's syndrome: retinitis pigmentosa and nerve deafness

Prader-Labhart-Willi syndrome: short stature, hypotonia, mental retardation, glucose intolerance[8]

Idiopathic adiposogenital dystrophy: early childhood obesity and genital hypoplasia

Fröhlich's syndrome: obesity, retarded growth, and genital hypoplasia associated with a hypothalamic tumor

Lipodystrophy: regional lipid deposits, particularly on the legs, sometimes sparing face and trunk

References

1. Boisaubin EV: Approach to obese patients. West J Med 140:794, 1984.
2. Jung R: Endocrinological aspects of obesity. Clin Endocrinol Metab 13:597, 1984.
3. Bogardus C, Lillioja S, Ravussin E, et al: Familial dependence of the resting metabolic rate. N Engl J Med 315:96, 1986.
4. Himms-Hagen J: Thermogenesis in brown adipose tissue as an energy buffer: implications for obesity. N Engl J Med 311:1549, 1984.
5. Bernstein JG: Induction of obesity by psychotropic drugs. Ann NY Acad Sci 499:203, 1987.
6. Bray GA, Gallagher TF Jr: Manifestations of hypothalamic obesity in man: a comprehensive investigation of eight patients and a review of the literature. Medicine 54:301, 1975.
7. De Luca B, Monda M, Pellicano MP, Zenga A: Cortical control of thermogenesis induced by lateral hypothalamic lesion and overeating. Am J Physiol 253:R626, 1987.
8. Burke CM, Kousseff BG, Gleeson M, et al: Familial Prader-Willi syndrome. Arch Intern Med 147:673, 1987.

Selected Readings

Danforth E Jr, Burger A: The role of thyroid hormones in the control of energy expenditure: Clin Endocrinol Metab 13:581, 1984.
Current concepts of thyroid control of energy expenditure.

Herzog DB, Copeland PM: Eating disorders. N Engl J Med 313:295, 1985.
Well-referenced discussion of bulimia and anorexia nervosa.

Kopelman PG: Clinical complications of obesity. Clin Endocrinol Metab 13:613, 1984.
Discussion of respiratory and hypertensive complications of obesity.

Peiris A, Kissebah A: Endocrine abnormalities in morbid obesity. Gastroenterol Clin North Am 16:389, 1987.
A useful review of hormonal changes known to accompany morbid obesity. Understanding these changes can prevent inappropriate investigations and help provide rational approaches to reducing the morbidity and mortality of obesity.

Simopoulos AP, Van Itallie TB: Body weight, health, and longevity. Ann Intern Med 100:285, 1984.

An analytic review of recent studies of the effect of obesity on mortality.

Stunkard AJ, Foch TT, Hrubec Z: A twin study of human obesity. JAMA 256:51, 1986.
Evidence presented to suggest that human fatness is genetically controlled.

Van Itallie TB: Bad news and good news about obesity (editorial). N Engl J Med 314:239, 1986.
Pithy editorial discussion.

Welle SL, Seaton TB, Campbell RG: Some metabolic effects of overeating in man. Am J Clin Nutr 44:718, 1986.
Interesting data from a study evaluating metabolic responses to 20 days of overeating in 5 volunteers. A variable increase in basal metabolic rate was found, but no change in metabolic rate was found during light excercise.

35
Hyperthyroidism: Common and Less Common Causes

Hyperthyroidism is due to excess thyroid hormone and is most commonly caused by Graves' disease (diffuse toxic goiter).[1] Clinical manifestations are usually obvious and reflect hyperadrenergic and hypermetabolic states, classically expressed as heat intolerance, excessive sweating, palpitations, increased appetite, weight loss, and an enlarged thyroid. Symptoms of hyperthyroidism in the elderly[2] and in those patients with less common underlying disorders can be less obvious, such as the transient hyperthyroid symptoms seen in patients with thyroiditis.[3]

Grave's disease: most common cause of hyperthyroidism in younger age groups; a systemic condition that may occasionally present with ophthalmopathy, dermopathy, and thyroid acropachy, sometimes without clinical hyperthyroidism[4]

Plummer's disease: toxic multinodular goiter; a subgroup of patients with clinically defined toxic multinodular goiter, probably have autoimmune hyperthyroidism[5]

Thyroid adenoma[6]

Thyroiditis: Hashimoto's thyroiditis, subacute granulomatous thyroiditis, subacute lymphocytic thyroiditis, suppurative thyroiditis, Riedel's struma, and other autoimmune phenomena[7,8]

Thyroid carcinoma: usually metastatic undifferentiated[9-11]

Choriocarcinoma[12]

Struma ovarii: metastatic thyroid carcinoma[13,14]; in females with unexplained hyperthyroidism and low ^{131}I uptake by the cervical thyroid, consider imaging the pelvis.[15]

Factitious hyperthyroidism[16]

TSH-secreting pituitary tumor[17]

Exogenous iodide induced: Basedow goiter syndrome[18]

Pituitary insensitivity to TSH[19,20]

References

1. Dorfman SG: Hyperthyroidism: usual and unusual causes (editorial). Arch Intern Med 137:995, 1977.
2. Tibaldi JM, Barzel US, Albin J, Surks M: Thyrotoxicosis in the very old. Am J Med 81:619, 1986.
3. Hay ID: Thyroiditis: a clinical update. Mayo Clin Proc 60:836, 1985.
4. Spaulding SW, Lippes H: Hyperthyroidism: causes, clinical features, and diagnosis. Med Clin North Am 69:937, 1985.
5. Kraiem Z, Glaser B, Yigla M, et al: Toxic multinodular goiter: a variant of autoimmune hyperthyroidism: J Clin Endocrinol Metab 65:659, 1987.
6. Hamburger JI: Solitary autonomously functioning thyroid lesions. Am J Med 58:740, 1975.
7. Dorfman SG, Cooperman MT, Nelson RL, et al: Painless thyroiditis and transient hyperthyroidism without goiter. Ann Intern Med 86:24, 1977.
8. Hamburger JI: The various presentations of thyroiditis. Ann Intern Med 104:219, 1986.
9. Federman DD: Hyperthyroidism due to functioning metastatic carcinoma of the thyroid. Medicine 43:267, 1964.
10. Bowden WD, Jones RE: Thyrotoxicosis associated with distant metastatic follicular carcinoma of the thyroid. South Med J 79:483, 1986.
11. Ober KP, Cowan RJ, Sevier RE, Poole GJ: Thyrotoxicosis caused by functioning metastatic thyroid carcinoma. A rare and elusive cause of hyperthyroidism with low radioactive iodine uptake. Clin Nucl Med 12:345, 1987.

12. Morley JE, Jacobson RJ, Melamed J, et al: Choriocarcinoma as a cause of thyrotoxicosis. Am J Med 60:1036, 1976.
13. Judd ES, Buie LA Jr: Hyperthyroidism associated with struma ovarii. Arch Surg 84:692, 1962.
14. Willemse PH, Oosterhuis JW, Aalders JG, et al: Malignant struma ovarii treated by ovariectomy, thyroidectomy, and ^{131}I administration. Cancer 60:178, 1987.
15. March DE, Desai AG, Park CH, et al: Struma ovarii: hyperthyroidism in a postmenopausal woman. J Nucl Med 29:263, 1988.
16. Gorman CA, Wahner HW, Tauxe WN: Metabolic malingerers. Am J Med 48:708, 1970.
17. Spitz IM, Sheinfeld M, Glasser B, et al: Hyperthyroidism due to inappropriate TSH secretion with associated hyperprolactinemia—a case report and review of the literature. Postgrad Med J 60:328, 1984.
18. Fradkin JE, Wolff J: Iodide-induced thyrotoxicosis. Medicine 62:1, 1983.
19. Weintraub BD, Gershengorn MC, Kourides IA, et al: Inappropriate secretion of thyroid-stimulating hormone. Ann Intern Med 95:339, 1981.
20. Clore JN, Sharpe AR, Sahni KS, et al: Thyrotropin-induced hyperthyroidism: evidence for a common progenitor stem cell. Am J Med Sci 295:3, 1988.

Selected Readings

Cobb WE, Lamberton RP, Jackson IMD: Use of a rapid, sensitive immunoradiometric assay for thyrotropin to distinguish normal from hyperthyroid subjects. Clin Chem 30:1558, 1984.
Highly sensitive rapid assay to distinguish hyperthyroidism.

Fatourechi V, Gharib H: Hyperthyroidism following hypothyroidism. Data on six cases. Arch Intern Med 148:976, 1988.
Six cases of spontaneous hyperthyroidism following hypothyroidism. Authors stress that this phenomenon is probably more common than recognized.

Felicetta JV: Thyroid disease in the elderly. Special features, changes in management. Postgrad Med 83(3):145, 1988.
Thyroid physiology and manifestations of thyroid disease are different in the elderly; symptoms of thyroid dysfunction can be subtle. This paper outlines an approach toward evaluating thyroid disease in the elderly.

Hamburger JI: The various presentations of thyroiditis. Ann Intern Med 104:219, 1986.
A comprehensive review of clinical and diagnostic considerations of thyroiditis. Well referenced.

Mazzaferri EL: Thyrotoxicosis: clinical syndromes and laboratory diagnosis. Postgrad Med 73(4):85, 1983.
A review of thyrotoxicosis and conditions that can mask or mimic hyperthyroidism.

Melliere D, Etienne G, Becquemin JP: Operation for hyperthyroidism. Methods and rationale. Am J Surg 155:395, 1988.

A review of 500 patients operated on for hyperthyroidism. Seventy-two percent of patients who presented with atrial fibrillation returned to normal sinus rhythm postoperatively.

Salata R, Klein I: Effects of lithium on the endocrine system: a review. J Lab Clin Med 110:130, 1987.

Lithium has been known to cause hypothyroidism and goiter, as well as hypercalcemia, diabetes insipidus, and altered carbohydrate metabolism. Hyperthyroidism is a rare but reported side effect of lithium.

Schlumberger M, Travagli JP, Fragu P, et al: Follow-up of patients with differentiated thyroid carcinoma. Experience at Institut Gustave-Roussy, Villejuif. Eur J Cancer Clin Oncol 24:345, 1988.

The combined use of serum thyroglobulin and ^{131}I total body scan is recommended to detect relapses when radiographs are still normal.

Settipane GA, Hamolsky MW: Status asthmaticus associated with hyperthyroidism. New Engl Reg Allergy Proc 8:323, 1987.

Hyperthyroidism presenting in patients with status asthmaticus may be iodide-induced, especially in those patients with diffuse or nodule thyroid goiter. Authors stress that this combination may be more common than currently recognized.

Thomas CG Jr, Croom RD III: Current management of the patient with autonomously functioning nodular goiter. Surg Clin North Am 67:315, 1987.

The decision to treat a solitary nodule depends on age, nodule size, and amount of nodular function. Radioiodine therapy and long-term antithyroid drugs are alternatives for patients who are poor surgical risks.

Utiger RD: Thyrotropin-releasing hormone and thyrotropin secretion. J Lab Clin Med 109:327, 1987.

Current concepts of physiology of thyrotropin-releasing hormone and thyrotropin secretion in a well-referenced state-of-the-art review.

Wing SS, Fantus IG: Adverse immunologic effects of antithyroid drugs. Can Med Assoc J 136:121, 1987.

A report of two cases and a review of the literature studying adverse effects of antithyroid drugs, propylthiouracil, and methimazole.

36
Hypothyroidism: Unusual Presentations

Classic clinical features of hypothyroidism, such as cold intolerance, fatigability, dry skin, and alopecia, can be masked by less common, but often dramatic and sometimes life-threatening, effects of thyroid deficiency. Since thyroid hormone affects virtually all organ systems, there are many less commonly recognized manifestations involving hematologic, muscular, cardiac, and rheumatologic systems, all responsive to thyroid hormone replacement.[1] Hypothyroidism is a common adult disorder and, particularly in the elderly, can present with signs and symptoms easily mistaken for disorders common to old age, such as congestive heart failure, constipation, lethargy, and cold intolerance.[2] Some unusual and atypical presentations of hypothyroidism are listed as follows:

Loss of taste[3]
Loss of smell[3]
Somnolence
Psychosis: depression or mania, "myxedema madness"[4,5]
Cerebellar ataxia
Polyneuropathy[6]
Muscle stiffness[7]: pseudomyotonia
Hyponatremia: consider hypothyroidism, particularly in the elderly hyponatremic patient who does not respond to treatment for syndrome of inappropriate antidiuretic hormone (SIADH).[8]
Carpal tunnel syndrome
Joint effusions
Arthralgias: myxedema[9]
Sleep apnea[10]
Pituitary enlargement: usually due to reactive hyperplasia and correlates with degree of thyroid-stimulating hormone (TSH) elevation,[11,12] which can present with amenorrhea, decreased libido, or galactorrhea[13]
Hematologic abnormalities: serious hematologic dis-

orders are usually secondary to more than an endocrinopathy.[14]

Decreased platelet adhesiveness[15]

Factor VIII dysfunction[16]

Anemia: can be normocytic, microcytic, or macrocytic anemia[17]

Iron deficiency anemia

Megaloblastic anemia and associated folate and/or B_{12} deficiency[18]

Pericardial effusion[19]

Pleural effusion[20]

Pseudotumor cerebri[21]

Hypertension[22]

Polymyositis[23]

Intestinal pseudo-obstruction[24]

Postpartum hypothyroidism: may be an early manifestation of Hashimoto's disease[25]

Cerebellar calcifications[26]

References

1. Klein I, Levey GS: Unusual manifestations of hypothyroidism. Arch Intern Med 144:123, 1984.
2. Gambert SR: Atypical presentation of thyroid disease in the elderly. Geriatrics 40(2):63, 1985.
3. McConnell RJ, Menendez CE, Smith FR, et al: Defects of taste and smell in patients with hypothyroidism. Am J Med 59:354, 1975.
4. Gold MS, Pottash ALC, Extein I: Hypothyroidism and depression. JAMA 245:1919, 1981.
5. Fava GA, Sonino N, Morphy MA: Major depression associated with endocrine disease. Psychiatr Dev 5:321, 1987.
6. Nickel SN, Frame B, Bebin J, et al: Myxedema neuropathy and myopathy. Neurology 11:125, 1961.
7. Klein I, Parker M, Shebert R, et al: Hypothyroidism presenting as muscle stiffness and pseudohypertrophy: Hoffmann's syndrome. Am J Med 70:891, 1981.
8. Macaron C, Famuyiwa O: Hyponatremia of hypothyroidism. Appropriate suppression of antidiuretic hormone levels. Arch Intern Med 138:820, 1978.
9. Bland JH, Frymoyer JW: Rheumatic syndromes of myxedema. N Engl J Med 282:1171, 1970.
10. Millman RP, Bevilacqua J, Peterson DD, et al: Central sleep apnea in hypothyroidism. Am Rev Respir Dis 127:504, 1983.
11. Chanson P: Thyrotropic pituitary adenoma. Clinical aspects, course and treatment. Presse Med 16:1644, 1987.
12. Smallridge RC: Thyrotropin-secreting pituitary tumors. Endocrinol Metab Clin North Am 16:765, 1987.
13. Onishi T, Miyai K, Aono T, et al: Primary hypothyroidism and galactorrhea. Am J Med 63:373, 1977.
14. Orwoll ES, Orwoll RL: Hematologic abnormalities in

patients with endocrine and metabolic disorders. Hematol Oncol Clin North Am 1:261, 1987.
15. Edson JR, Fecher DR, Doe RP: Low platelet adhesiveness and other hemostatic abnormalities in hypothyroidism. Ann Intern Med 82:342, 1975.
16. Rogers JS II, Shane SR, Jencks FS: Factor VIII activity and thyroid function. Ann Intern Med 97:713, 1982.
17. Tudhope GR, Wilson GM: Anemia in hypothyroidism. Q J Med 29:513, 1960.
18. Caplan RH, Davis K, Bengston B, et al: Serum folate and vitamin B_{12} levels in hypothyroid and hyperthyroid patients. Arch Intern Med 135:701, 1975.
19. Zimmerman J, Yahalom J, Bar-On H: Clinical spectrum of pericardial effusion as the presenting feature of hypothyroidism. Am Heart J 106:770, 1983.
20. Brown SD, Brashear RE, Schnute RB: Pleural effusion in a young woman with myxedema. Arch Intern Med 143:1458, 1983.
21. Press OW, Ladenson PW: Pseudotumor cerebri and hypothyroidism. Arch Intern Med 143:167, 1983.
22. Saito I, Ito K, Saruta T: Hypothyroidism as a cause of hypertension. Hypertension 5:112, 1983.
23. Cabili S, Pines A, Kaplinsky N, et al: Hypothyroidism masquerading as polymyositis. Postgrad Med J 58:545, 1982.
24. Tachman ML, Guthrie GP Jr: Hypothyroidism: diversity of presentation. Endocr Rev 5:456, 1984.
25. Pryds O, Lervang HH, Kristensen HP, et al: HLA-DR factors associated with postpartum hypothyroidism: an early manifestation of Hashimoto's thyroiditis? Tissue Antigens 30:34, 1987.
26. Burke JW, Williamson BR, Hurst RW: "Idiopathic" cerebellar calcifications: association with hypothyroidism? Radiology 167:533, 1988.

Selected Readings

Drinka PJ, Nolten WE: Subclinical hypothyroidism in the elderly: to treat or not to treat? Am J Med Sci 295:125, 1988.
Helpful discussion of evaluation and treatment of hypothyroidism in the elderly, with an emphasis on the subclinical manifestations of hypothyroidism and indications for thyroid replacement.

Fatourechi V, Gharib H: Hyperthyroidism following hypothyroidism. Data on six cases. Arch Intern Med 148:976, 1988.
Data on 6 patients with hyperthyroidism for 2 to 20 years who then became hypothyroid is presented. An autoimmune mechanism is suggested.

Feingold KR, Elias PM: Endocrine-skin interactions. Cutaneous manifestations of pituitary disease, thyroid disease, calcium disorders, and diabetes. J Am Acad Dermatol 17:921, 1987.
Interesting review of cutaneous manifestations of endocrinologic disorders. Occasionally, such cutaneous manifestations can be the initial or most prominent symptom.

Gavin LA: The diagnostic dilemmas of hyperthyroxinemia and hypothyroxinemia. Adv Intern Med 33:185, 1988.

Important current review of clinical features and thyroid function tests used in evaluating thyrotoxicosis and hypothyroidism.

Hamburger JI: The various presentations of thyroiditis. Diagnostic considerations. Ann Intern Med 104:219, 1986.

Hypothyroidism may be a transient or permanent manifestation of thyroiditis. This article presents a current review of syndromes of thyroiditis including Hashimoto's thyroiditis, the most common thyroiditis, usually presenting with goiter and hypothyroidism. Other syndromes include subacute granulomatous thyroiditis, subacute lymphocytic thyroiditis, acute suppurative thyroiditis, and Riedel's struma.

Nicoloff JT: Thyroid storm and myxedema coma. Med Clin North Am 69:1005, 1985.

A helpful clinical discussion reminding clinicians that signs and symptoms of myxedema coma are often masked by concurrent illnesses.

Tachman ML, Guthrie GP Jr: Hypothyroidism: diversity of presentation. Endocr Rev 5:456, 1984.

Interesting clinical review of selected manifestations of hypothyroidism.

37
Cold Thyroid Nodules: Common and Less Common Causes

The evaluation and management of thyroid nodules continue to be problematic. Traditionally, nodules have been classified as cold (nonfunctioning) or warm (hyperfunctioning), based on the fraction of ingested radioactive iodine absorbed by thyroid tissue. Although most cold nodules prove benign, a cold thyroid nodule remains the most common clinical presentation of thyroid carcinoma.[1] Newer techniques, such as fine-needle aspiration biopsy, new radionuclide scanning agents, and ultrasonography, vary in reliability and sometimes discover impalpable thyroid nodules of uncertain clinical significance.[2] Risk factors for thyroid cancer include prior exposure to ionizing radiation, advanced age, and certain areas of increased prevalence of thyroid cancer. Although symptoms, such as obstruction and hoarseness, occur most frequently with malignant tissue invasion, similar symptoms can occur with benign goiters and even with thyroid cysts.[3] Nonthyroid masses, such as parathyroid cysts or anterior cervical lipomas, can mimic cold thyroid nodules.

Thyroid adenomas: multinodular goiter[4] and cystic lesions

Thyroid cysts: usually benign[5]; may be adenomatous, benign, or malignant

Chronic lymphocytic thyroiditis[6]

Subacute thyroiditis or de Quervain's thyroiditis: can present as a cold nodule in the early stages[7]

Papillary carcinoma: highly curable form of thyroid cancer in patients younger than 40 years of age[8]

Follicular carcinoma: Hürthle cell[9,10]

Anaplastic carcinoma: aggressive carcinoma that frequently presents as a rapidly growing thyroid mass in a preexisting goiter[11]

Medullary carcinoma: tumor of parafollicular or C cells that may secrete calcitonin, be familial, or be part of a multiple endocrine neoplasia type IIa syndrome.[12,13]

Clear cell variant: clear cells in thyroid neoplasms can reflect a nonspecific change or represent a variant of thyroid carcinoma.[14]

Metastatic nonthyroid carcinoma: suspect metastatic carcinoma in cold nodules of cancer patients with a nonthyroid primary[15]

Nonthyroid Cervical Nodules and Cysts

Parathyroid cysts and nodules

Thyroglossal duct cysts

Cystic hygromas

Branchial cysts

Lymph node lesions: infectious, inflammatory, and neoplastic

Lymph node metastases: most common nonthyroid neck mass in Nigerians over 30 years of age[16]

Tuberculosis: most common nonthyroid neck mass in Nigerians under 30 years of age[16]

Primary lymphoma

Cervical lipomas: anterior cervical lipomas[17]

Osseous choristoma[18]

Tortuous carotid artery[19]

Hydatid cyst[20,21]

References

1. Bartold KP, Abghari R, Sangi VB: Uncommon presentations of thyroid carcinoma. Clin Nucl Med 11:786, 1986.
2. Rojeski MT, Gharib H: Nodular thyroid disease. N Engl J Med 313:428, 1985.
3. Morrison JM: Simple thyroid cyst: cause of acute bilateral recurrent laryngeal nerve palsy. Br Med J 294:1128, 1987.
4. Kraiem Z, Glaser B, Yigla M, et al: Toxic multinodular goiter: a variant of autoimmune hyperthyroidism. J Clin Endocrinol Metab 65:659, 1987.
5. Clark OH, Okerlund MD, Cavalieri RR, et al: Diagnosis and treatment of thyroid, parathyroid, and thyroglossal duct cysts. J Clin Endocrinol Metab 48:983, 1979.
6. Ott RA, Calandra DB, McCall A, et al: The incidence of thyroid carcinoma in patients with Hashimoto's thyroiditis and solitary cold nodules. Surgery 98:1202, 1985.
7. Bartels PC, Boer RO: Subacute thyroiditis (de Quervain) presenting as a painless "cold" nodule. J Nucl Med 28:1488, 1987.
8. Rossi RL, Nieroda C, Cady B, et al: Malignancies of the thyroid gland. Surg Clin North Am 65:211, 1985.
9. Watson RG, Brennan MD, Goellner JR, et al: Invasive Hurthle cell carcinoma of the thyroid: natural history and management. Mayo Clin Proc 59:851, 1984.
10. Rosen IB, Luk S, Katz I: Hurthle cell tumor behavior: dilemma and resolution. Surgery 98:777, 1985.
11. Nel CJC, van Heerden JA, Goellner JR, et al: Anaplastic carcinoma of the thyroid: a clinicopathologic study of 82 cases. Mayo Clin Proc 60:51, 1985.
12. Saad MF, Ordonez NG, Rashid RK, et al: Medullary carcinoma of the thyroid. Medicine 63:319, 1984.
13. Wells SA Jr, Dilley WG, Farndon JA, et al: Early diagnosis and treatment of medullary thyroid carcinoma. Arch Intern Med 145:1248, 1985.
14. Civantos F, Nadji M, Albores-Saavedra J, et al: Clear cell variant of thyroid carcinoma. Am J Surg Pathol 8:187, 1984.
15. McCabe DP, Farrar WB, Petkov TM, et al: Clinical and pathologic correlations in disease metastatic to the thyroid gland. Am J Surg 150:519, 1985.
16. Onuoro VC: Non-thyroid neck masses in tropical Africans. Trop Geogr Med 39:256, 1987.
17. Leonidas JR, Goldman JM, Wheeler MF: Cervical lipomas masquerading as thyroid nodules. JAMA 253:1436, 1985.
18. Banerjee SN, Ananthakrishnan N, Veliath AJ, Ratnakar C: Osseous choristoma presenting as a cold solitary thyroid nodule. Postgrad Med J 62:1035, 1986.
19. Buck RT, Siddiqui AR: Thyroid abnormality secondary to tortuous carotid artery. Eur J Nucl Med 12:51, 1986.
20. Gurses N, Baysal K, Gurses N: Hydatic cyst in the thyroid and submandibular salivary glands in a child. Z Kinderchir 41:362, 1986.
21. Dotzenrath C, Burring KF, Goretzki PE: Echinococcus cyst of the thyroid gland. A case report. Chirurg 59:106, 1988.

Selected Readings

Al-Sayer HM, Krukowski ZH, Williams VMM, et al: Fine needle aspiration cytology in isolated thyroid swellings: a prospective two year evaluation. Br Med J 290:1490, 1985.
The study presents data in favor of using this outpatient diagnostic technique as a screen for selecting surgical management.

Bell RM: Thyroid carcinoma. Surg Clin North Am 66:13, 1986.
Useful clinical review of concepts and controversies in surgical management of thyroid neoplasms.

Ichiya Y, Nakashima T, Gunasekera R, et al: Coexistence of a nonfunctioning thyroid nodule in Plummer's disease demonstrated by thallium-201 imaging. Clin Nucl Med 13:117, 1988.
An interesting case report of a patient with Plummer's disease in whom thallium-201 imaging demonstrated a coexisting nonfunctioning nodule.

Laing MR, Mclay KA: Ectopic thyroid malignancy in the midline of the neck (a case report and literature review). J Laryngol Otol 102:93, 1988.
An interesting case report of a midline neck mass initially thought to be a thyroglossal cyst, but proved pathologically to be a mixed papillary-follicular carcinoma of the thyroid without cystic elements. Pertinent literature is reviewed.

McCall A, Jarosz H, Lawrence AM, Paloyan E: The incidence of thyroid carcinoma in solitary cold nodules and in multinodular goiters. Surgery 100:1128, 1986.
A retrospective study found that, once risk factors such as radiation exposure and thyroiditis were eliminated, there was no significant difference in the incidence of carcinoma in patients with multinodular goiters compared with patients with a solitary cold nodule.

Mountz JM, Glazer GM, Dmuchowski C, Sisson JC: MR imaging of the thyroid: comparison with scintigraphy in the normal and diseased gland. J Comput Assist Tomogr 11:612, 1987.
This study found that spin-echo MRI of the thyroid gland could not reliably distinguish benign from malignant tumors.

Panza N, Lombardi G, De Rosa M, et al: High serum thyroglobulin levels. Diagnostic indicators in patients with metastases from unknown primary sites. Cancer 60:2233, 1987.
Thyroglobulin measurement in patients with cold thyroid nodules and metastases from an unknown primary site can help determine if a metastatic lesion is of thyroid origin.

Poston RN, Sidhu YS: Diagnosing tumours on routine surgical sections by immunohistochemistry: use of cytokeratin, common leucocyte, and other markers. J Clin Pathol 39:514, 1986.
This study discusses the importance of immunohistochemistry in determining tumor type.

Rojeski MT, Gharib H: Nodular thyroid disease. N Engl J Med 313:428, 1985.
Comprehensive, well-referenced update.

Ron E, Griffel B, Liban E, et al: Histopathologic reproducibility of thyroid disease in an epidemiologic study. Cancer 57:1056, 1986.

A study that reexamines the long-term effects of childhood scalp irradiation on the risk of developing thyroid tumors.

Rossi RL, Nieroda C, Cady B, et al: Malignancies of the thyroid gland. Surg Clin North Am 65:211, 1985.
A review of a large experience in diagnosis and management of thyroid malignancies.

Sarda AK, Bal S, Dutta Gupta S, Kapur MM: Diagnosis and treatment of cystic disease of the thyroid by aspiration. Surgery 103:593, 1988.
This study of 141 cases of euthyroid solitary cold nodules that were evaluated and treated with aspiration suggests certain clinical factors that may point toward a greater probability of malignancy. Clinical factors present in patients selected for surgery included recurrent cyst formation after aspiration, nodules larger than 3 cm in diameter, and palpable tissue after aspiration.

Tindall H, Griffiths AP, Penn ND: Is the current use of thyroid scintigraphy rational? Postgrad Med J 63:869, 1987.
Authors reviewed 131 consecutive requests for thyroid scintigraphy and analyzed the diagnostic contribution to subsequent medical management. They conclude that the primary role of thyroid scintigraphy lies in the investigation of the solitary nodule and in detecting toxic nodules in thyrotoxic patients without evidence of Graves disease.

38

Aberrant Thyroid Functions in Euthyroid Patients: Common and Uncommon Causes

Thyroid function tests are increasingly used for routine evaluation of medical disorders, particularly when symptoms include neurologic and psychiatric manifestations. When abnormal thyroid functions do not correlate with the clinical picture, it is important to remember that not all patients with depressed thyroid functions are hypothyroid and not all patients with increased T_4 levels are hyperthyroid. Major causes of abnormal thyroid functions in euthyroid patients include increased thyroid hormone binding by acquired or inherited binding protein abnormalities, peripheral resistance to thyroid hormone, and multiple drug and toxin effects.[1] A wide spectrum of clinical situations has been associated with aberrant thyroid functions in euthyroid patients. Awareness of potential spurious results occurring in these situations may avoid error in diagnosis and treatment.

Hyperthyroxinemia of acute illness[2]

Hypothyroxinemia due to chronic and serious illnesses

Pregnancy: thyroid functions that increase include radioactive iodine uptake, response to thyrotropin-releasing hormone, thyroxine-binding globulin, total thyroxine and triiodothyronine chorionic thyrotropin, and thyroid-stimulating hormone (TSH).[3]

Birth control pills: estrogen effect[4]

Liver disease

Porphyria[5]

Hydatidiform mole[6]

Drug addicts[7]

Congenital thyroid-binding globulin deficiency[8]

Inherited or acquired peripheral insensitivity to T_4: mimics Graves disease, i.e., "inappropriate TSH" is present, and patient is euthyroid[9]

Familial hyperthyroxinemia syndromes: pituitary and peripheral resistance to thyroid hormone[10,11]

Drugs: multiple drugs including dicumarol, phenytoin, heparin, lithium, phenothiazines, salicylates, sulfonamides, corticosteroids, iopanoic acid, ipodate, amiodarone,[12] beta-blockers

Hyperthyroxinemia in acute psychosis[13]

Malnutrition and cancer cachexia: low T_3 syndrome[14]

Systemic lupus erythematosus (SLE): although abnormal thyroid functions are common in hospitalized SLE patients, patients with SLE are at risk for incipient true primary hypothyroidism.[15]

Hepatocellular carcinoma[16]

References

1. Hay ID: Euthyroid hyperthyroxinemia (editorial). Mayo Clin Proc 60:61, 1985.
2. Gavin LA, Rosenthal M, Cavalieri RR: The diagnostic dilemma of isolated hyperthyroxinemia in acute illness. JAMA 242:251, 1979.
3. Burrow GN: Hyperthyroidism during pregnancy. N Engl J Med 298:150, 1978.

4. Winikoff D, Taylor K: Oral contraceptives and thyroid function tests. Med J Aust 2:108, 1966.
5. Hellman ES, Tschudy DP, Robbins J, et al: Elevation of the serum protein-bound iodine in acute intermittent porphyria. J Clin Endocrinol Metab 23:1185, 1963.
6. Galton VA, Ingbar SH, Jimenez-Fonseca J, et al: Alterations in thyroid hormone economy in patients with hydatidiform mole. J Clin Invest 50:1345, 1971.
7. Webster JB, Coupal JJ, Cushman P Jr: Increased serum thyroxine levels in euthyroid narcotic addicts. J Clin Endocrinol Metab 37:928, 1973.
8. Silverberg JDH, Premachandra BN: Familial hyperthyroxinemia due to abnormal thyroid hormone binding. Ann Intern Med 96:183, 1982.
9. Kaplan MM, Swartz SL, Larsen PR: Partial peripheral resistance to thyroid hormone. Am J Med 70:1115, 1981.
10. Gharib H, Klee GG: Familial euthyroid hyperthyroxinemia secondary to pituitary and peripheral resistance to thyroid hormones. Mayo Clin Proc 60:9, 1985.
11. Ruiz M, Rajatanavin R, Young RA, et al: Familial dysalbuminemic hyperthyroxinemia. N Engl J Med 306:635, 1982.
12. Fragu P, Schlumberger M, Davy JM, et al: Effects of amiodarone therapy of thyroid iodine content as measured by x-ray fluorescence. J Clin Endocrinol Metab 66:762, 1988.
13. Spratt DI, Pont A, Miller MB, et al: Hyperthyroxinemia in patients with acute psychiatric disorders. Am J Med 73:41, 1982.
14. Persson H, Bennegärd K, Lundberg P, et al: Thyroid hormones in conditions of chronic malnutrition. Ann Surg 201:45, 1985.
15. Miller FW, Moore GF, Weintraub BD, Steinberg AD: Prevalence of thyroid disease and abnormal thyroid function test results in patients with systemic lupus erythematosus. Arthritis Rheum 30:1124, 1987.
16. Alexopoulos A, Hutchinson W, Bari A, et al: Hyperthyroxinemia in hepatocellular carcinoma: relation to thyroid binding globulin in the clinical and preclinical stages of the disease. Br J Cancer 57:313, 1988.

Selected Readings

Borst GC, Eil C, Burman KD: Euthyroid hyperthyroxinemia. Ann Intern Med 98:366, 1983.
A review of recently recognized syndromes associated with hyperthyroxinemia without thyrotoxicosis. Well referenced.

Chen JJ, Ladenson PW: Euthyroid pretibial myxedema. Am J Med 82:318, 1987.
Interesting case report of a clinically euthyroid patient who presented with biopsy-proven pretibial myxedema without the common manifestations expected in Graves disease.

de Nayer P, Lambot MP, Desmons MC, et al: Sex hormone-binding protein in hyperthyroxinemic patients: a discriminator for thyroid status in thyroid hormone resistance and familial dysalbuminemic hyperthyroxinemia. J Clin Endocrinol Metab 62:1309, 1986.

Interesting study evaluating hepatic interactions of thyroid hormone resistance, familial dysalbuminemic hyperthyroxinemia, and free T_4 and analyzing how these interactions relate to the clinical picture in patients with familial dysalbuminemic hyperthyroxinemia.

Kabadi UM, Rosman PM: Thyroid hormone indices in adult healthy subjects: no influence of aging. J Am Geriatr Soc 36:312, 1988.

Certain aspects of aging thyroid hormone metabolism are considered controversial. This study evaluated thyroid hormone metabolism in 152 euthyroid, healthy adult subjects and concluded concurrent, underlying disorders, rather than age per se, may account for the abnormalities previously postulated to be due to age alone.

Kahn BB, Weintraub BD, Csako G, Zweig MH: Factitious evaluation of thyrotropin in a new ultrasensitive assay: implications for the use of monoclonal antibodies in "sandwich" immunoassay. J Clin Endocrinol Metab 66:526, 1988.

A report of three patients who received treatment based on falsely elevated TSH concentrations in a mouse monoclonal immunoradiometric assay. Authors discuss potential antibody interference in assays and offer suggestions to avoid false results.

Kaplan MM: Clinical and laboratory assessment of thyroid abnormalities. Med Clin North Am 69:863, 1985.

A discussion that focuses on optimal use and limitations of current clinical and laboratory thyroid tests.

Sakata S, Nakamura S, Miura K: Autoantibodies against thyroid hormones or iodothyronine. Ann Intern Med 103:579, 1985.

A comprehensive and useful review.

Schultz AL: Thyroid function tests. Postgrad Med 80(2):219, 1986.

A practical discussion that reviews common tests with an emphasis on cost-effective diagnosis.

Silberman H, Eisenberg D, Ryan J, et al: The relation of thyroid indices in the critically ill patient to prognosis and nutritional factors. Surg Gynecol Obstet 166:223, 1988.

A study of 73 critically ill euthyroid patients performed within 48 hours of hospital admission presents data suggesting that thyroid parameters measured early in the acute illness may be a useful clinical prediction of outcome.

Zaloga GP, O'Brian JT: Euthyroid sick syndrome. Am Fam Physician 31(2):236, 1985.

A helpful clinical discussion of the pathophysiology and evaluation of thyroid function tests during illness.

39
Osteopenia: Major Causes and Clinical Associations

Osteopenia is radiographically apparent when up to 10 to 30% of bone mass is lost. Osteoporosis is the most common cause of adult osteopenia, particularly in the elderly. However, it is important to differentiate osteoporosis from other less common causes of osteopenias that have different natural histories, pathophysiology, and treatment, such as osteomalacia, primary hyperparathyroidism, myeloma, and malignant disorders. The identification of certain treatable clinical disorders can reduce the risk of bone fractures and significant disability.[1]

Osteoporosis: Common and Less Common Associations

Osteoporosis or loss of bone mass is usually asymptomatic until far advanced. Suspect coexisting osteomalacia in symptomatic patients who do not have bony fractures to explain their symptoms.

Involutional (senile or postmenopausal) osteoporosis: serum calcium, phosphate, and alkaline phosphatase are usually normal.
Idiopathic osteoporosis: uncommon disorder in young patients
Hyperparathyroidism: often associated with elevated serum calcium, decreased serum phosphate, and renal stones[2]
Hyperthyroidism: both endogenous and exogenous hyperthyroidism can cause osteopenia.[3,4]
Diabetes mellitus
Alcoholism: can occur in relatively young male alcoholics[5]
Chronic renal failure
Chronic liver failure
Cushing's syndrome
Drug-induced: heparin, steroids[6]

Immobilization

Osteogenesis imperfecta: include in differential diagnosis of women with crush fractures of the spine[7]

Turner's syndrome

Calcium deficiency

Lactase deficiency[8]

Hyperprolactinemia[9]

Hypogonadism

Chronic obstructive pulmonary disease

Homocystinuria

Anorexia nervosa: subnormal osteocalcin concentrations and decreased osteoclastic activity noted in these patients[10–12]

Primary biliary cirrhosis[13]

Hemodialysis: an osteoarthropathy associated with hemodialysis in addition to well-known secondary hyperparathyroidism is recognized.[14]

Vertebral osteomyelitis: osteomyelitis should be considered in patients with severe back pain, fever, elevated sedimentation rate, even without an obvious focus of infection.[15]

Amenorrheic running women[16]

Osteomalacia: Common and Less Common Associations

Osteomalacia or inadequate bony mineralization causes bone softening, pain and fractures. Frequently seen serum abnormalities are low phosphate, low calcium, and high alkaline phosphatase. Pathognomonic pseudofractures occur in fewer than 15% of patients.

Vitamin D deficiency: most frequent cause of osteomalacia[17]

Chronic renal disease: serum phosphate is often decreased with osteomalacia caused by chronic renal insufficiency.[18,19]

Hyperparathyroidism: primary and secondary[20,21]

Renal tubular acidosis

Pancreatic insufficiency

Hepatic disease

Postgastrectomy[22]

Small bowel disease: malabsorption

Laxative abuse

Hereditary impaired vitamin D metabolic disorders

Hereditary mineralization defects: hypophosphatasia, hypophosphatemic rickets

Acidosis: renal, tubular, hereditary, secondary

Drug-induced: acetazolamide, outdated tetracycline,

fluorides, diphosphonate, phenytoin,[23] aluminum hydroxide,[24] carbamazepine[25]

Aluminum-related osteodystrophy: occurs in patients with aplastic bone disease and decreased total body aluminum[26]

Fanconi's syndrome[27]

Paget's disease[28]

Reflex sympathetic dystrophy: rare presenting manifestation of underlying osteomalacia and renal tubular acidosis[29]

Plantar fasciitis: rare manifestation of nutritional osteomalacia[30]

Malignancies Associated with Osteopenia

Multiple myeloma

Metastatic bone disease

Tumor osteomalacia[31-33]

Hypophosphatemic osteomalacia: associated with a polymorphic group of mesenchymal tumors[34-36]

References

1. Mundy GR: Osteopenia. DM 33:537, 1987.
2. Kochersberger G, Buckley NJ, Leight GS, et al: What is the clinical significance of bone loss in primary hyperparathyroidism? Arch Intern Med 147:1951, 1987.
3. Fallon MD, Perry HM III, Bergfeld M, et al: Exogenous hyperthyroidism with osteoporosis. Arch Intern Med 143:442, 1983.
4. Ross DS, Neer RM, Ridgway EC, Daniels GH: Subclinical hyperthyroidism and reduced bone density as a possible result of prolonged suppression of the pituitary-thyroid axis with L-thyroxine. Am J Med 82:1167, 1987.
5. Spencer H, Rubio N, Rubio E, et al: Chronic alcoholism: frequently overlooked cause of osteoporosis in men. Am J Med 80:393, 1986.
6. Hajiroussou VJ, Webley M: Prolonged low-dose corticosteroid therapy and osteoporosis in rheumatoid arthritis. Ann Rheum Dis 43:24, 1984.
7. Paterson CR, McAllion S, Stellman JL: Osteogenesis imperfecta after the menopause. N Engl J Med 310:1694, 1984.
8. Newcomer AD, Hodgson SF, McGill DB, et al: Lactase deficiency: prevalence in osteoporosis. Ann Intern Med 89:218, 1978.
9. Klibanski A, Neer RM, Beitins IZ, et al: Decreased bone density in hyperprolactinemic women. N Engl J Med 303:1511, 1980.
10. Szmukler GI, Brown SW, Parsons V, et al: Premature loss of bone in chronic anorexia nervosa. Br Med J 290:26, 1985.
11. Fonseca VA, D'Souza V, Houlder S, et al: Vitamin D

deficiency and low osteocalcin concentrations in anorexia nervosa. J Clin Pathol 41:195, 1988.

12. Treasure JL, Russell GF, Fogelman I, Murby B: Reversible bone loss in anorexia nervosa. Br Med J 295:474, 1987.

13. Mitchison HC, Malcolm AJ, Bassendine MF, James OF: Metabolic bone disease in primary biliary cirrhosis at presentation. Gastroenterology 94:463, 1988.

14. Naidich JB, Karmel MI, Mossey RT, et al: Osteoarthropathy of the hand and wrist in patients undergoing long-term hemodialysis. Radiology 164:205, 1987.

15. McHenry MC, Duchesneau PM, Keys TF, et al: Vertebral osteomyelitis presenting as spinal compression fracture. Six patients with underlying osteoporosis. Arch Intern Med 148:417, 1988.

16. Fisher EC, Nelson ME, Frontera WR, et al: Bone mineral content and levels of gonadotropins and estrogens in amenorrheic running women. J Clin Endocrinol Metab 62:1232, 1986.

17. Lund B, Sørenson OH, Lund B, et al: Vitamin D metabolism and osteomalacia in patients with fractures of the proximal femur. Acta Orthop Scand 53:251, 1982.

18. Andress D, Felsenfeld AJ, Voigts A, et al: Parathyroid hormone response to hypocalcemia in hemodialysis patients with osteomalacia. Kidney Int 24:364, 1983.

19. Cushner HM, Adams ND: Review: renal osteodystrophy—pathogenesis and treatment. Am J Med Sci 291, 264, 1986.

20. Kaplan FS, Soffer SR, Fallon MD, et al: Osteomalacia as a very late manifestation of primary hyperparathyroidism. Clin Orthop 228:26, 1988.

21. Breslau NA: Update on secondary forms of hyperparathyroidism. Am J Med Sci 294:120, 1987.

22. Klein KB, Orwoll ES, Lieberman DA, et al: Metabolic bone disease in asymptomatic men after partial gastrectomy with Billroth II anastomosis. Gastroenterology 92:608, 1987.

23. Christiansen C, Rødbro P, Tjellesen L: Pathophysiology behind anticonvulsant osteomalacia. Acta Neurol Scand S94:21, 1983.

24. Carmichael KA, Fallon MD, Dalinka M, et al: Osteomalacia and osteitits fibrosa in a man ingesting aluminum hydroxide antacid. Am J Med 76:1137, 1984.

25. Tjellesen L, Gotfredsen A, Christiansen C: Effect of vitamin D_2 and D_3 on bone-mineral content in carbamazepine-treated epileptic patients. Acta Neurol Scand 68:424, 1983.

26. Andress DL, Maloney NA, Coburn JW, et al: Osteomalacia and aplastic bone disease in aluminum-related osteodystrophy. J Clin Endocrinol Metab 65:11, 1987.

27. Rao DS, Parfitt AM, Villanueva AR, et al: Hypophosphatemic osteomalacia and adult Fanconi syndrome due to light-chain nephropathy. Another form of oncogenous osteomalacia. Am J Med 82:333, 1987.

28. Gibbs CJ, Aaron JE, Peacock M: Osteomalacia in Paget's disease treated with short term, high dose sodium etidronate. Br Med J 292:1227, 1986.

29. Huaux JP, Malghem J, Maldague B, et al: Reflex

sympathetic dystrophy syndrome: an unusual mode of presentation of osteomalacia. Arthritis Rheum 29:918, 1986.
30. Paice EW, Hoffbrand BI: Nutritional osteomalacia presenting with plantar fasciitis. J Bone Joint Surg (Br) 69:38, 1987.
31. Ryan EA, Reiss E: Oncogenous osteomalacia: review of the world literature of 42 cases and report of two new cases. Am J Med 77:501, 1984.
32. Siris ES, Clemens TL, Dempster DW, et al: Tumor-induced osteomalacia. Kinetics of calcium, phosphorus, and vitamin D metabolism and characteristics of bone histomorphometry. Am J Med 82:307, 1987.
33. McClure J, Smith PS: Oncogenic osteomalacia. J Clin Pathol 40:446, 1987.
34. Weidner N, Santa Cruz D: Phosphaturic mesenchymal tumors. A polymorphous group causing osteomalacia or rickets. Cancer 59:1442, 1987.
35. Gitelis S, Ryan WG, Rosenberg AG, Templeton AC: Adult-onset hypophosphatemic osteomalacia secondary to neoplasm. A case report and review of the pathophysiology. J Bone Joint Surg (Am) 68:134, 1986.
36. Cotton GE, Van Puffelen P: Hypophosphatemic osteomalacia secondary to neoplasia. J Bone Joint Surg (Am) 68:129, 1986.

Selected Readings

Aloia JF, Cohn SH, Vaswani A, et al: Risk factors for postmenopausal osteoporosis. Am J Med 78:95, 1985.
Current concepts of risk factors and choices of replacement therapy.

Bellantoni MF, Blackman MR: Osteoporosis: diagnostic screening and its place in current care (clinical conference). Geriatrics 43(2):63, 69, 1988.
Clinical review of management of age-related bone loss, including a discussion of associated chronic diseases, medications, and an assessment of helpful routine laboratory and radiographic studies.

Consensus Development Conference: Prophylaxis and treatment of osteoporosis. Br Med J 295:914, 1987.
Current recommendations and concepts of bone densitometry.

Cummings SR, Black D: Should perimenopausal women be screened for osteoporosis? Ann Intern Med 104:817, 1986.
A critical look at the use of noninvasive methods of evaluating bone mass in perimenopausal women.

Falch JA, Oftebro H, Haug E: Early postmenopausal bone loss is not associated with a decrease in circulating levels of 25-hydroxyvitamin D, 1,25-dihydroxyvitamin D, or vitamin D-binding protein. J Clin Endocrinol Metab 64:836, 1987.
Interesting study of 19 normal premenopausal women who were evaluated for bone loss before and after menopause with appendicular bone mass measurements, serum estrone, estradiol, and vitamin D metabolites followed serially. Study concludes that changes in vitamin D metabolite levels are not associated with early postmenopausal bone loss.

Lian JB, Gundberg CM: Osteocalcin. Biochemical considerations and clinical applications. Clin Orthop 226:267, 1988.

Current concepts of osteocalcin, a vitamin K-dependent protein of bone, suggest that serum osteocalcin measurements provide a noninvasive specific marker of bone metabolism.

Lindsay R: Prevention of osteoporosis. Clin Orthop 222:44, 1987.

A clinical review of risk factors and management of osteoporosis with an emphasis on prevention.

Martin AD, Houston CS: Osteoporosis, calcium, and physical activity. Can Med Assoc J 136:587, 1987.

This study suggests that weight-bearing activity undertaken in early adult life not only helps increase bone mass but may delay the onset of bone loss, as well as slow the rate of loss of bone mass.

McKenna MJ, Frame B: Hormonal influences on osteoporosis. Am J Med 82:61, 1987.

There may be a particular subset of postmenopausal women particularly susceptible to estrogen deficiency; however, osteoporosis is not the result of a single hormone deficiency. Other hormonal influences are discussed.

Orwoll ES, Weigel RM, Oviatt SK, et al: Serum protein concentrations and bone mineral content in aging normal men. Am J Clin Nutr 46:614, 1987.

Two populations of men were evaluated to examine the relationship of serum protein concentration, protein intake, and bone mineral content. The study concludes that certain alterations of protein metabolism may affect bone mineral content and play a role in the development of senile osteopenia.

Raisz LG: Local and systemic factors in the pathogenesis of osteoporosis. N Engl J Med 318:818, 1988.

Current concepts of pathophysiology of osteoporosis. Well referenced.

Riggs BL, Melton LJ III: Involutional osteoporosis. N Engl J Med 314:1676, 1986.

Comprehensive state-of-the-art review.

Santora AC II: Role of nutrition and exercise in osteoporosis. Am J Med 82:73, 1987.

Current concepts of optimal calcium intake and other nutritional requirements for prevention of osteoporosis. The role of exercise is emphasized.

Silverberg SJ, Lindsay R: Postmenopausal osteoporosis. Med Clin North Am 71:41, 1987.

Review of current concepts of risk factors and evaluation of patients at risk for postmenopausal osteoporosis. Therapeutic options are discussed.

Wahner HW: Assessment of metabolic bone disease: review of new nuclear medicine procedures. Mayo Clin Proc 60:827, 1985.

Bone mineral measurements and bone scintigraphy techniques are discussed as two possible clinically useful and nontraumatic diagnostic procedures.

40
Hyperprolactinemia: Common and Less Common Causes

Elevated serum prolactin has a wide spectrum of clinical significance, ranging from a first clinical sign of pituitary-hypothalamic disease to a hormonal reflection of a benign physiologic state. Hyperprolactinemia is a particularly important finding in patients with clinical signs that could reflect hypothalamic-pituitary disease, such as galactorrhea, anovulation, oligospermia, or impotence, because elevated serum prolactin is the most frequent hormone marker for pituitary tumors.[1] Certain drugs, such as phenothiazines and other dopamine-receptor blocking agents, are well-known, common causes of hyperprolactinemia. Occasionally, elevated prolactin levels can be caused by ectopic prolactin-producing tumors. Sources of physiologic prolactin stimulation, such as exercise and breast feeding, or iatrogenic causes should be ruled out before aggressive evaluation is undertaken.

Pituitary-Hypothalamic Disorders

Any disorder that disrupts normal hypothalamic tonic inhibition of prolactin secretion can cause hyperprolactinemia.[2,3]

Pituitary adenomas: prolactin-secreting pituitary adenoma is a common cause of galactorrhea, amenorrhea, and infertility.[4]

Prolactinomas in multiple endocrine neoplastic syndrome type I: most pituitary tumors with this syndrome are nonfunctional.[5]

Prolactin cell carcinoma of the pituitary: rare tumor[6]

Pituitary tumor associated with von Recklinghausen's disease[7]

Pituicytoma[8]

Hypothalamic granulomas: sarcoidosis, tuberculosis, eosinophilic granuloma, histiocytosis

Hypothalamic gliomas

Craniopharyngioma: most commonly diagnosed in young patients; may occur in older patients[9-11]

Empty-sella syndrome: may mimic an intrasellar tumor, particularly in patients with galactorrhea-amenorrhea[12]

Intrasellar germinoma: rare tumor[13]

Hypothalamic dysfunction following whole-brain irradiation[14]

Sphenoid mucocele[15]

Drugs Associated with Hyperprolactinemia

Dopamine-receptor blocking agents: phenothiazines, butyrophenones, metoclopramide

Catechol-depleting agents: reserpine, alpha-methyl-dopa

Reuptake interference: imipramine hydrochloride, amphetamine

Anesthesia[16]

Thyrotropin-releasing factor (TRF)

Estrogen

Birth control pills[17]: may stimulate growth of existing pituitary tumors[18]

Testosterone[19]

Clinical States Associated with Hyperprolactinemia

Prolactin is elevated in certain physiologic states and, therefore, does not always mean an underlying pathologic state exists.[1] Multiple endocrine and metabolic states have been associated with hyperprolactinemia, as well as rare ectopic prolactin-producing tumors.

Idiopathic hyperprolactinemia: elevated serum prolactin without evidence of pituitary or central nervous system disease[20]

Breast feeding and other chest wall stimulation[21]

Pregnancy[22,23]

Sleep

Exercise[24,25]

Stress: i.e., postsurgical[26]

Postictal: may be a helpful marker in distinguishing patients with complex partial seizures arising from the temporal lobe with behavioral manifestations from those with pseudoseizures[27,28]

Hypothyroidism: thyrotropin-releasing hormone (TRH) may mediate hyperprolactinemia[29-31]

Cushing's disease[32]

Nelson's syndrome: hyperpigmentation and pituitary tumor following bilateral adrenalectomy[32]

Acromegaly[33]

Polycystic ovary syndrome: may have anovulation, hyperandrogenism, obesity, and multicystic ovaries[34,35]

Macroprolactinemia: a large-molecular-weight form of prolactin may cause massive hyperprolactinemia without evidence of a pituitary tumor[36]

Hypoglycemia-induced prolactin release[37]

Uremia and hemodialysis[38]

Ectopic prolactin secretion: renal cell carcinoma,[39] bronchogenic carcinoma

References

1. Kirby RW, Kotchen TA, Rees ED: Hyperprolactinemia—a review of recent clinical advances. Arch Intern Med 139:1415, 1979.
2. Ferrari C, Rampini P, Benco R, et al: Functional characterization of hypothalamic hyperprolactinemia. J Clin Endocrinol Metab 55:897, 1982.
3. Moore TJ: Prolactinomas. Our raised consciousness (editorial). Arch Intern Med 139:1223, 1979.
4. Martin MC, Schriock ED, Jaffe RB: Prolactin-secreting pituitary adenomas. West J Med 139:663, 1983.
5. Hershon KS, Kelly WA, Shaw CM, et al: Prolactinomas as part of the multiple endocrine neoplastic syndrome type I. Am J Med 74:713, 1983.
6. Scheithauer BW, Randall RV, Laws ER Jr, et al: Prolactin cell carcinoma of the pituitary. Cancer 55:598, 1985.
7. Pinnamaneni K, Birge SJ, Avioli LV: Prolactin-secreting pituitary tumor associated with von Recklinghausen's disease. Arch Intern Med 140:397, 1980.
8. Rossi ML, Bevan JS, Esiri MM, et al: Pituicytoma (pilocytic astrocytoma). Case report. J Neurosurg 67:768, 1987.
9. Lederman GS, Recht A, Loeffler JS, et al: Craniopharyngioma in an elderly patient. Cancer 60:1077, 1987.
10. Barral G, Fayol JC, Alloin C, Le Maout F: Craniopharyngioma. A relatively uncommon etiology for an amenorrhea at the age of 45. Apropos of a case. Rev Fr Gynecol Obstet 82:591, 1987.
11. Wheatley T, Clark JD, Stewart S: Craniopharyngioma with hyperprolactinaemia due to a prolactinoma. J Neurol Neurosurg Psychiatry 49:1305, 1986.
12. Gharib H, Frey HM, Laws ER Jr, et al: Coexistent primary empty sella syndrome and hyperprolactinemia. Arch Intern Med 143:1383, 1983.
13. Marcovitz S, Guyda HJ, Finlayson MH, et al: Intrasellar germinoma associated with hyperprolactinemia. Surg Neurol 22:387, 1984.
14. Mechanick JI, Hochberg FH, LaRocque A: Hypothalamic dysfunction following whole-brain irradiation. J Neurosurg 65:490, 1986.

15. Fody EP, Binet EF: Sphenoid mucocele causing hyperprolactinemia: radiologic/pathologic correlation. South Med J 79:1017, 1986.
16. Hempenstall PD, Campbell JP, Bajurnow AT, et al: Cardiovascular, biochemical, and hormonal responses to intravenous sedation with local analgesia versus general anesthesia in patients undergoing oral surgery. J Oral Maxillofac Surg 44:441, 1986.
17. Luciano AA, Sherman BM, Chapler FK, et al: Hyperprolactinemia and contraception: a prospective study. Obstet Gynecol 65:506, 1985.
18. Sherman BM, Harris CE, Schlechte J, et al: Pathogenesis of prolactin-secreting pituitary adenomas. Lancet 2:1019, 1978.
19. Nicoletti I, Filipponi P, Fedeli L, et al: Testosterone-induced hyperprolactinaemia in a patient with a disturbance of hypothalamo-pituitary regulation. Acta Endocrinol 105:167, 1984.
20. Martin TL, Kim M, Malarkey WB: The natural history of idiopathic hyperprolactinemia. J Clin Endocrin Metab 60:855, 1985.
21. Glasier A, McNeilly AS, Howie PW: The prolactin response to suckling. Clin Endocrinol 21:109, 1984.
22. Molitch ME: Pregnancy and the hyperprolactinemic woman. N Engl J Med 312:1364, 1985.
23. Liu JH, Park KH: Gonadotropin and prolactin secretion increases during sleep during the puerperium in nonlactating women. J Clin Endocrinol Metab 66:839, 1988.
24. Yahiro J, Glass AR, Fears WB, et al: Exaggerated gonadotropin response to luteinizing hormone-releasing hormone in amenorrheic runners. Am J Obstet Gynecol 156:586, 1987.
25. Chang FE, Dodds WG, Sullivan M, et al: The acute effects of exercise on prolactin and growth hormone secretion: comparison between sedentary women and women runners with normal and abnormal menstrual cycles. J Clin Endocrinol Metab 62:551, 1986.
26. Delitala G, Tomasi P, Virdis R: Prolactin, growth hormone, and thyrotropin-thyroid hormone secretion during stress states in man. Clin Endocrinol Metab 1:391, 1987.
27. Laxer KD, Mullooly JP, Howell B: Prolactin changes after seizures classified by EEG monitoring. Neurology 35:31, 1985.
28. Dana-Haeri J, Trimble MR, Oxley J: Prolactin and gonadotrophin changes following generalized and partial seizures. J Neurol Neurosurg Psychiatry 46:331, 1983.
29. Honbo KS, Van Herle AJ, Kellett KA: Serum prolactin levels in untreated primary hypothyroidism. Am J Med 64:782, 1978.
30. Grubb MR, Chakeres D, Malarkey WB: Patients with primary hypothyroidism presenting as prolactinomas. Am J Med 83:765, 1987.
31. Fish LH, Mariash CN: Hyperprolactinemia, infertility, and hypothyroidism. A case report and literature review. Arch Intern Med 148:709, 1988.
32. Yamaji T, Ishibashi M, Teramoto A, et al: Hyperprolactinemia in Cushing's disease and Nelson's syndrome. J Clin Endocrinol Metab 58:790, 1984.

33. Losa M, Schopohl J, Konig A, et al: Growth hormone (GH) and prolactin responses to repetitive administration of GH-releasing hormone in acromegaly. J Clin Endocrinol Metab 63:475, 1986.
34. Luciano AA, Chapler FK, Sherman BM: Hyperprolactinemia in polycystic ovary syndrome. Fertil Steril 41:719, 1984.
35. Gindoff PR, Jewelewicz R: Polycystic ovarian disease. Obstet Gynecol Clin North Am 14:931, 1987.
36. Jackson RD, Wortsman J, Malarkey WB: Macroprolactinemia presenting like a pituitary tumor. Am J Med 78:346, 1985.
37. May PB, Burrow GN, Kayne RD, et al: Hypoglycemia-induced prolactin release. Arch Intern Med 138:918, 1978.
38. Mastrogiacomo I, DeBesi L, Serafini E, et al: Hyperprolactinemia and sexual disturbances among uremic women on hemodialysis. Nephron 37:195, 1984.
39. Stanisic TH, Donovan J: Prolactin secreting renal cell carcinoma. J Urol 136:85, 1986.

Selected Readings

Archer DF: Current concepts and treatment of hyperprolactinemia. Obstet Gynecol Clin North Am 14:979, 1987.
Recommendations for evaluating hyperprolactinemia in the female patient include testing pituitary and thyroid function.

Bevan JS, Burke CW, Esiri MM, et al: Misinterpretation of prolactin levels leading to management errors in patients with sellar enlargement. Am J Med 82:29, 1987.
Serum prolactin concentrations and clinical characteristics were correlated with histopathology in 128 surgically diagnosed patients without acromegaly or Cushing's syndrome who were evaluated for pituitary adenoma. Evaluation and management recommendations are made with an emphasis on prolactin serum levels and prognosis.

Brenner SH, Lessing JB, Quagliarello J, et al: Hyperprolactinemia and associated pituitary prolactinomas. Obstet Gynecol 65:661, 1985.
A study that analyzed the association between serum prolactin and the presence of pituitary tumors, as identified with CT scans; a poor correlation with the level of hyperprolactinemia was found.

Drago F: Prolactin and sexual behavior: a review. Neurosci Biobehav Rev 8:433, 1984.
Human sexual behavior correlates are suggested from animal models.

Martin TL, Kim M, Malarkey WB: The natural history of idiopathic hyperprolactinemia. J Clin Endocrin Metab 60:855, 1985.
Data challenging the use of ablative pituitary therapy for idiopathic hyperprolactinemia.

Pereira MC, Sobrinho LG, Afonso AM, et al: Is idiopathic hyperprolactinemia a transitional stage toward prolactinoma? Obstet Gynecol 70:305, 1987.
Serial prolactin levels, prolactin response to thyrotropin-releasing hormone and domperidone, and thyroid-stimulating hormone responses to domperidone were studied in 75 female controls and compared with 44 female patients with moderate hyperprolactinemia.

The study concludes that idiopathic hyperprolactinemia is a heterogeneous entity that includes women with normal secretion, patients with macroprolactinemia, and patients with undiagnosed prolactinomas.

Scoccia B, Schneider AB, Marut EL, Scommegna A: Pathological hyperprolactinemia suppresses hot flashes in menopausal women. J Clin Endocrinol Metab 66:868, 1988.

An interesting study of the effect of hyperprolactinemia in menopausal women, with emphasis on its effect on hot flashes and gonadotropin secretion.

Strebel PM, Zacur HA, Gold EB: Headache, hyperprolactinemia, and prolactinomas. Obstet Gynecol 68:195, 1986.

A study that analyzed prolactin levels in women with headaches and nonpuerperal hyperprolactinemia suggests that headache in women with secondary amenorrhea or galactorrhea may be a clinical indicator of an occult prolactinoma.

41

Cushing's Syndrome: Clinical Associations and Mimics

Clinical hypercortisolism characterizes Cushing's syndrome. Common manifestations of hypercortisolism include hypertension, obesity, diabetes mellitus, hirsuitism, and menstrual irregularities. Cushing's syndrome can be due to hypercortisolism, which is pituitary-dependent or adrenal-dependent, and frequently is iatrogenic when associated with exogenous steroid administration. The three major noniatrogenic causes of Cushing's syndrome are (1) pituitary-dependent processes due to pituitary adenomas or microadenomas causing adrenal hyperplasia; (2) pituitary-independent primary adrenal causes, predominantly unilateral adenomas, and rarely multiple adenomas or adrenal carcinoma; and (3) ectopic sources of adrenocorticotropic hormone (ACTH), which usually reflect an underlying neoplasm.[1]

Rarely, diabetes mellitus or alcoholism can cause a pseudo-Cushing's syndrome.

Exogenous steroid administration: a common cause of Cushing's syndrome[2]
  Oral steroids
  Topical steroids[3]
  Steroid nasal spray[4]
  Betamethasone nasal drops[5]
  Dexamethasone acetate intramuscular treatments[6]
Pituitary-dependent causes: the majority of patients with Cushing's syndrome have a hypothalamic-pituitary disorder.
  ACTH-producing microadenoma: most common cause of hypercortisolism in Cushing's syndrome[7-9]
  Hypothalamic overproduction of corticotropin-releasing factor
  Empty-sella turcica[10]
  Ectopic pituitary adenoma[11]
  Craniopharyngioma: secondary hypothalamic dysfunction may cause Cushing's syndrome.[12]
  Primary multinodular corticotrope hyperplasia[13]
Adrenal-dependent causes
  Adrenal tumors:
    Adenoma
    Carcinoma[14]
  Adrenal hyperplasia:
    Microadenomata
    Hyperplasia secondary to excessive pituitary or ectopic ACTH stimulation
    Bilateral primary pigmented nodular adrenocortical disease[15,16]
    Primary adrenocortical nodular dysplasia[1]
    Primary micronodular adrenocortical dysplasia[17]
Ectopic ACTH-producing tumors
  Lung carcinoma: most frequent carcinoma associated with ectopic ACTH[18]
  Small cell carcinoma
  Pancreatic carcinoma[19,20]
  Thymoma carcinoma
  Bronchial carcinoids[21,22]
  Medullary carcinoma of the thyroid
  Pheochromocytoma[23,24]
  Thymic carcinoid tumor[25]
  Renal oncocytic carcinoid tumor[26]
  Multiple endocrine neoplasia type I[27]
  Gastrinomas: ACTH-like activity is found in about

one-third of gastrinomas in Zollinger-Ellison syndrome.[28]

Disorders That Can Mimic Cushing's Syndrome

Alcohol-induced pseudo-Cushing's syndrome: rare syndrome that may be a centrally mediated defect[29]

Diabetic children with brittle diabetes: seen with frequent Somogyi reactions[30]

Obesity: pseudo-nonsuppressibility

Depression[31]

Factitious Cushing's syndrome[32]

References

1. Larsen JL, Cathey WJ, Odell WD: Primary adrenocortical nodular dysplasia, a distinct subtype of Cushing's syndrome. Case report and review of the literature. Am J Med 80:976, 1986.
2. Cook DM, Kendall JW, Jordan R: Cushing syndrome: current concepts of diagnosis and therapy. West J Med 132:111, 1980.
3. Ruiz-Maldonado R, Zapata G, Tamayo L, et al: Cushing's syndrome after topical application of corticosteroids. Am J Dis Child 136:274, 1982.
4. Champion PK Jr: Cushing syndrome secondary to abuse of dexamethasone nasal spray. Arch Intern Med 134:750, 1974.
5. Stevens DJ: Cushing's syndrome due to the abuse of betamethasone nasal drops. J Laryngol Otol 102:219, 1988.
6. Hughes JM, Hichens M, Booze GW, Thorner MO: Cushing's syndrome from the therapeutic use of intramuscular dexamethasone acetate. Arch Intern Med 146:1848, 1986.
7. Schulte HM, Allolio B, Gunther RW, et al: Bilateral and simultaneous sinus petrosus inferior catheterization in patients with Cushing's syndrome: plasma-immunoreactive-ACTH-concentrations before and after administration of CRF. Horm Metab Res 16(Suppl):66, 1987.
8. Cushing H: The basophil adenomas of the pituitary body and their clinical manifestations (pituitary basophilism). Bull Johns Hopkins Hosp 50:137, 1932.
9. Orth DN, DeBold CR, DeCherney GS, et al: Pituitary microadenomas causing Cushing's disease respond to corticotropin-releasing factor. J Clin Endocrinol Metab 55:1017, 1982.
10. Smith DJ, Kohler PC, Helminiak R, et al: Intermittent Cushing's syndrome with an empty sella turcica. Arch Intern Med 142:2185, 1982.
11. Kammer H, George R: Cushing's disease in a patient with an ectopic pituitary adenoma. JAMA 246:2722, 1981.
12. Ackland FM, Stanhope R, Preece MA: Cushing's disease and craniopharyngioma. Arch Dis Child 62:1077, 1987.
13. Young WF Jr, Scheithauer BW, Gharib H, et al: Cushing's syndrome due to primary multinodular corticotrope hyperplasia. Mayo Clin Proc 63:256, 1988.

14. Grunberg SM: Development of Cushing's syndrome and virilization after presentation of a nonfunctioning adrenocortical carcinoma. Cancer 50:815, 1982.
15. Kaplowitz PB, Carpenter R, Newsome HH Jr, Downs RW Jr: Cushing's syndrome resulting from primary pigmented nodular adrenocortical disease. Am J Dis Child 140:1072, 1986.
16. Grant CS, Carney JA, Carpenter PC, van Heerden JA: Primary pigmented nodular adrenocortical disease: diagnosis and management. Surgery 100:1178, 1986.
17. Hodge BO, Froesch TA: Familial Cushing's syndrome. Micronodular adrenocortical dysplasia. Arch Intern Med 148:1133, 1988.
18. Gold EM: The Cushing syndromes: changing views of diagnosis and treatment. Ann Intern Med 90:829, 1979.
19. Clark ES, Carney JA: Pancreatic islet cell tumor associated with Cushing's syndrome. Am J Surg Pathol 8:917, 1984.
20. Melmed S, Yamashita S, Kovacs K, et al: Cushing's syndrome due to ectopic proopiomelanocortin gene expression by islet cell carcinoma of the pancreas. Cancer 59:772, 1987.
21. Ward PS, Mott MG, Smith J, et al: Cushing's syndrome and bronchial carcinoid tumour. Arch Dis Child 59:375, 1984.
22. Schteingart DE, Lloyd RV, Akil H, et al: Cushing's syndrome secondary to ectopic corticotropin-releasing hormone-adrenocorticotropin secretion. J Clin Endocrinol Metab 63:770, 1986.
23. Lamovec J, Memoli VA, Terzakis JA, et al: Pheochromocytoma producing immunoreactive ACTH with Cushing's syndrome. Ultrastruct Pathol 7:41, 1984.
24. Beaser RS, Guay AT, Lee AK, et al: An adrenocorticotropic hormone-producing pheochromocytoma: diagnostic and immunohistochemical studies. J Urol 135:10, 1986.
25. Estopinan V, Varela C, Riobo P, et al: Ectopic Cushing's syndrome with periodic hormonogenesis—a case suggesting a pathogenetic mechanism. Postgrad Med J 63:887, 1987.
26. Hannah J, Lippe B, Lai-Goldman M, Bhuta S: Oncocytic carcinoid of the kidney associated with periodic Cushing's syndrome. Cancer 61:2136, 1988.
27. Miyagawa K, Ishibashi M, Kasuga M, et al: Multiple endocrine neoplasia type I with Cushing's disease, primary hyperparathyroidism, and insulin-glucagonoma. Cancer 61:1232, 1988.
28. Maton PN, Gardner JD, Jensen RT: Cushing's syndrome in patients with the Zollinger-Ellison syndrome. N Engl J Med 315:1, 1986.
29. Kirkman S, Nelson DH: Alcohol-induced pseudo-Cushing's disease: a study of prevalence with review of the literature. Metabolism 37:390, 1988.
30. Bolli GB, Gottesman IS, Campbell PJ, et al: Glucose counterregulation and waning of insulin in the Somogyi phenomenon (posthypoglycemic hyperglycemia). N Engl J Med 311:1214, 1984.
31. Kelly WF, Checkley SA, Bender DA, et al: Cushing's disease and depression—a prospective study of 26 patients. Br J Psychiatry 142:16, 1983.

32. Cook DM, Meikle AW: Factitious Cushing's syndrome. J Clin Endocrinol Metab 61:385, 1985.

Selected Readings

Aron DC, Tyrrell JB, Fitzgerald PA, et al: Cushing's syndrome: problems in diagnosis. Medicine 60:25, 1981.
The wide spectrum of clinical manifestations and sometimes difficult diagnosis are discussed.

Burch WM: Cushing's disease: a review. Arch Intern Med 145:1106, 1985.
Concise review of clinical features and current concepts of treatment.

Carpenter PC: Cushing's syndrome: update of diagnosis and management. Mayo Clin Proc 61:49, 1986.
Comprehensive, well-referenced update.

Chrousos GP, Schuermeyer TH, Doppman J, et al: Clinical applications of corticotropin-releasing factor. Ann Intern Med 102:344, 1985.
Well-referenced, comprehensive review of the clinical usefulness of this test.

Contreras LN, Hane S, Tyrrell JB: Urinary cortisol in the assessment of pituitary-adrenal function: utility of 24-hour and spot determinations. J Clin Endocrinol Metab 62:965, 1986.
A study assessing diurnal variation of cortisol responses by measuring the active fraction of cortisol in 24-hour and spot urine samples concludes that urinary cortisol in 1-hour samples may provide a practical and simple method of assessing cortisol secretion and an effective screen for Cushing's syndrome and hypoadrenalism.

Dwyer AJ, Frank JA, Doppman JL, et al: Pituitary adenomas in patients with Cushing disease: initial experience with Gd-DTPA-enhanced MR imaging. Radiology 163:421, 1987.
An early study of the usefulness of MRI of pituitary adenomas suggests high sensitivity, particularly with contrast enhancement.

Enzi G, Gasparo M, Biondetti PR, et al: Subcutaneous and visceral fat distribution according to sex, age, and overweight, evaluated by computed tomography. Am J Clin Nutr 44:739, 1986.
An interesting clinical study of fat distribution concludes that the subcutaneous and visceral fat distribution ratio in Cushing's patients at the abdominal level was lower than in age-, sex-, and body mass index-matched controls.

Findling JW, Tyrrell JB: Occult ectopic secretion of corticotropin. Arch Intern Med 146:929, 1986.
This review advocates the use of selective venous sampling for ACTH when ectopic secretion is suspected.

Gold PW, Loriaux DL, Roy A, et al: Responses to corticotropin-releasing hormone in the hypercortisolism of depression and Cushing's disease. N Engl J Med 314:1329, 1986.
This study suggests that the pathophysiologic features of hypercortisolism in depression and Cushing's disease are distinct and that corticotropin-releasing hormone stimulation tests may be helpful in making the distinction.

Guilhaume B, Bertagna X, Thomsen M, et al: Transsphenoidal pituitary surgery for the treatment of Cushing's disease: results in 64 patients and long term follow-up studies. J Clin Endocrinol Metab 66:1056, 1988.
Useful clinical data following patients with transsphenoidal pituitary surgery correlating postoperative pituitary function studies with prognosis.

Hermus AR, Pieters GF, Pesman GJ, et al: The corticotropin-releasing-hormone test versus the high-dose dexamethasone test in the differential diagnosis of Cushing's syndrome. Lancet 2:540, 1986.
A study that compares the corticotropin-releasing-hormone (CRH) test with oral high-dose dexamethasone suppression test in the differential diagnosis of Cushing's syndrome concludes that the diagnostic accuracy of both tests is comparable and that the highest accuracy may be achieved by using both tests.

Hermus AR, Pieters GF, Smals AG, et al: Transition from pituitary-dependent to adrenal-dependent Cushing's syndrome. N Engl J Med 318:966, 1988.
Interesting case report that involves ACTH-dependent hypercortisolism in the presence of ACTH suppression and absence of ACTH response to corticotropin-releasing hormone. The finding of atrophy in the extranodular adrenal cortex further supports the authors' hypothesis that this case represents a transition from pituitary-dependent to adrenal-dependent Cushing's syndrome.

Kapcala LP: Alcohol-induced pseudo-Cushing's syndrome mimicking Cushing's disease in a patient with an adrenal mass. Am J Med 82:849, 1987.
An interesting case report of an alcoholic with alcohol-induced pseudo-Cushing's syndrome in whom an adrenal mass was identified.

Koerten JM, Morales WJ, Washington SR III, Castaldo TW: Cushing's syndrome in pregnancy: a case report and literature review. Am J Obstet Gynecol 154:626, 1986.
The difficult evaluation and management of pregnant patients with Cushing's syndrome is discussed with a literature review of 32 cases.

Laudat MH, Cerdas S, Fournier C, et al: Salivary cortisol measurement: a practical approach to assess pituitary-adrenal function. J Clin Endocrinol Metab 66:343, 1988.
A study that establishes normal and pathologic ranges of salivary cortisol measurement concludes that salivary cortisol measurements provide an alternative and practical approach to assess pituitary-adrenal function.

Pojunas KW, Daniels DL, Williams AL, et al: Pituitary and adrenal CT of Cushing syndrome. AJR 146:1235, 1986.
This study adds to current data cautioning that normal adrenal or pituitary CT scans do not exclude Cushing's syndrome.

Urbanic RC, George JM: Cushing's disease—18 years' experience. Medicine 60:14, 1981.
A study of 46 patients with Cushing's syndrome and Cushing's disease. Well referenced.

Van Cauter E, Refetoff S: Evidence for two subtypes of Cushing's disease based on the analysis of episodic cortisol secretion. N Engl J Med 312:1343, 1985.
Subtypes of Cushing's disease postulated with significant prognostic implications.

V

NEUROLOGY

42

Headache: Current Classification and Major Causes

A severe headache of new onset, particularly if followed by focal neurologic signs, suggests intracranial hemorrhage or infection and should be treated as a neurologic emergency. However, even in the setting of the "worst headache in my life," the evaluation is often frustrated with negative radiographic and cerebrospinal fluid studies. The intensity of pain in headache is not a reliable indicator of the underlying cause. For example, an intracranial mass or impending stroke may cause subacute, moderate, chronic pain, whereas an underlying anxiety state can cause an intense, severe headache.[1] The diagnostic dilemma is that various illnesses, both focal and systemic, cause and exacerbate headaches that meet diagnostic criteria for the more commonly diagnosed headaches.[2] The three most commonly diagnosed headaches are classic migraine, common migraine, and muscle contraction (tension) headaches.[3] The International Headache Society has currently revised the classification and diagnostic criteria for headaches with a fully constructed, coded classification and operational diagnostic criteria published in *Cephalalgia*.[4] Although the following classification and description of headache syndromes will attempt to adhere to the major categories introduced in this recent reclassification,[4] deletions and additions are written from our clinical perspective and current literature.

Migraine

Recurrent headaches may correspond to food sensitivity,[5] menstrual periods,[6] and/or stress.[7]

Migraine without aura: headaches are typically pulsating, unilateral, and associated with nausea and photophobia; may switch from side to side.

267

Migraine with aura: visual phenomena, such as scintillations or scotomas, are the most common auras.

Familial hemiplegic migraine

Basilar migraine: usually occur in young adults[8,9]

Ophthalmoplegic migraine: rare form of migraine with headache and ocular motor cranial nerve paresis

Retinal migraine: diagnosis of exclusion after ocular and retinal pathology have been ruled out.

Childhood periodic syndromes that may be associated with migraine: alternating hemiplegia of childhood, episodic vertigo, amaurosis fugax, abdominal migraine[9–11]

Status migrainosus: migraine lasting more than 72 hours in spite of treatment.

Other migrainous disorders

Tension-type Headache

Characteristically bilateral, described as a bandlike tightening around the head or pressure-pain.[12]

Episodic tension-type headache with disorders of pericranial muscles

Episodic tension-type headache without disorders of pericranial muscles

Chronic tension-type headache with disorders of pericranial muscles

Chronic tension-type headache without disorders of pericranial muscles

Other tension-type headaches

Cluster Headache and Chronic Paroxysmal Hemicrania

Headaches are unilateral, severely painful, and focal and often are associated with autonomic phenomena and a stereotypic tempo of attacks.[13]

Cluster headache: brief episodes of headache that may occur several times a day; occur more frequently in males; headaches frequently awaken patient from sleep with severe pain, which is usually maximal around the orbit[13]

Chronic paroxysmal hemicrania: occurs more frequently in females; headaches can be similar to cluster headaches; however, they may be distinguished by a significant response to indomethacin[14]

Other cluster headaches

Miscellaneous Headaches Unassociated with Structural Lesion

Idiopathic stabbing headache: described as momentary or "ice pick" pain; characterized by brief, sharp, stabbing, or shooting headache pain[15]

External compression headache: secondary to wearing tight bands, such as swim goggles

Cold stimulus headache: can be caused by a cold environment or ingestion of cold substances

Benign cough headache: occurs after coughing[16]

Benign exertional headache: often follows significant exercise[17]

Headache associated with sexual activity: coital cephalgia, an acute headache related to sexual intercourse with maximal symptoms often at orgasm[18,19]

Headache Associated with Head Trauma[20,21]

Acute post-traumatic headache

Chronic post-traumatic headache

Headache Associated with Cerebrovascular Disorders[25]

Acute ischemic cerebrovascular disease: transient ischemic attack (TIA), thromboembolic stroke[22-24]

Subarachnoid hemorrhage: headache and vomiting frequently herald the onset of a subarachnoid hemorrhage or an intraparenchymal hemorrhage.[26-28]

Unruptured vascular malformation: arteriovenous malformation, saccular aneurysm[29,30]

Temporal arteritis: headache, often intense, deep, aching, throbbing; associated with tenderness of the temporal artery. Although an elevated erythrocyte sedimentation rate (ESR) is a diagnostic hallmark, a normal ESR in the appropriate clinical setting should not dissuade one from performing a temporal artery biopsy[31-34]

Carotid or vertebral dissection: headache and neck pain ipsilateral to the dissection[35-37]

Carotidynia: tenderness and swelling overlying the carotid artery, without carotid structural abnormality; usually self-limiting disorder

Venous thrombosis: seizures and headache can herald this syndrome, often idiopathic; pregnant women and post-traumatic patients are amongst those at risk.

Cavernous sinus thrombosis: most commonly follows *Staphylococcus aureus* infections of the face and sinuses[38]

Arterial hypertension: drug-induced, pheochromocytoma, malignant hypertension, preeclampsia[39,40]

Other vascular disorders: infectious and inflammatory arteritis and vasculitis, granulomatous angiitis[41,42]

Headache Associated with Nonvascular Intracranial Disorders

Benign intracranial hypertension or pseudotumor cerebri[43,44]

High pressure hydrocephalus: third ventricle colloid cysts are a rare cause of intermittent hydrocephalus and headache.

Postlumbar puncture headache: prolonged postlumbar headache may be secondary to lumbar puncture-induced cerebrospinal fluid fistula.[45,46]

Hypoliquorrheic headache: idiopathic[47]

Viral encephalitis: can cause explosive, severe headaches mimicking subarachnoid hemorrhage (see Section VII, Infectious Disease; Ch. 71)

Other acute and intracranial infections: bacterial, fungal, abscess, mycobacterial, parasitic[48–52]; consider opportunistic infections in those at high risk for HIV infection

Noninfectious inflammatory intracerebral disorders such as sarcoidosis

Chemical meningitis: dermoid cysts, postcontrast studies

Intracranial neoplasms: headache with a slow-growing tumor or metastases can be mild in early stages.

Headache Associated with Substance Use and Withdrawal

Headache induced by acute substance use or exposure: nitrate/nitrite, monosodium glutamate, carbon monoxide, alcohol[53]

Headache induced by chronic substance use or exposure: ergotamine, analgesic abuse, other substances

Headache from withdrawal of acute substance abuse: alcohol hangover, other substances

Headache from withdrawal of chronic substance use: ergotamine, caffeine, narcotics, other substances

Headaches associated with substance use with uncertain mechanisms: birth control pills or estrogens, other substances

Headache Associated with Noncephalic Infection

Viral infection: focal, systemic

Bacterial infection: focal, systemic

Headache related to other infection

Headache Associated with Metabolic Disorders[56]

Hypoxia: high altitude, sleep apnea, cardiac disorders[54,55]

Hypercapnia

Mixed hypoxia and hypercapnia

Hypoglycemia
Dialysis
Other metabolic abnormalities

Headache or Facial Pain Associated with Disorders of Cranium, Neck, Eyes, Ears, Nose, Sinuses, Teeth, Mouth, or Other Facial Structures[61,62]

Cranial bone disorders: traumatic, osteomyelitis, neo-plasms

Cervical spine disorders: suspect cervical spine involvement in patients with occipital-cervical pain, particularly in patients with rheumatoid arthritis, post-traumatic whiplash, or cervical spondylosis[57–60]

Retropharyngeal disorders

Glaucoma: low tension glaucoma can mimic migraine headaches, particularly in the elderly.[63,64]

Refractive errors: eye strain[62]

Ear disorders: particularly middle ear disorders

Nasal obstruction: can present as a myofacial pain syndrome, usually unilateral with pain in the ear or preauricular area[65]

Other nasal and sinus disorders[66,67]

Teeth, jaws, and related structures[68,69]

Temporomandibular joint disease[70,71]

Cranial Neuralgia, Nerve Trunk Pain, and Deafferentation Pain

Compression or distortion of cranial nerves and second or third cervical roots

Optic neuritis (retrobulbar neuritis): painful eye, usually with visual impairment, such as a visual scotoma

Cranial nerve infarction: diabetic third nerve infarction

Acute herpes zoster: often affects trigeminal ganglion, causing herpetic eruption and facial pain; pain may precede onset of typical rash.

Chronic postherpetic neuralgia[72,73]

Tolosa-Hunt syndrome: orbital pain with cranial nerve paralysis

Neck-tongue syndrome: pain in region of lingual nerve and second cervical nerve, precipitated by sudden turning of the head

Other causes of pain of cranial nerve origin

Trigeminal neuralgia: explosive, intense, unilateral, with trigger points and confined to sensory distribution of the trigeminal nerve[74]

Paratrigeminal Raeder's syndrome: pain in the distribution of the ophthalmic and maxillary divisions of the fifth nerve, often associated with ptosis and miosis[75,76]

Glossopharyngeal neuralgia: paroxysmal, unilateral, severe pain in pharyngeal region precipitated by specific stimuli, such as swallowing or chewing

Nervous intermedius neuralgia: rare disorder with pain in the posterior wall of the auditory canal, often associated with herpes zoster

Superior laryngeal neuralgia: rare pain syndrome in throat with trigger points usually in lateral throat region

Occipital neuralgia: stabbing, aching pain over the occipital nerves; often associated with tenderness to palpation of the occipital nerves

Anesthesia dolorosa

Thalamic pain

Other facial pain: atypical facial pain

Miscellaneous Causes of Headache

Postictal headaches: occur more frequently after major seizures than after minor seizures[77]

Meningeal carcinomatosis[78-80]

Human immunodeficiency virus (HIV)-associated meningitis: can be the first clinical manifestation of HIV infection[81]

References

1. Friedman AP: Clinical approach to the patient with headache. Neurol Clin 1:361, 1983.
2. Caviness VS Jr, O'Brien P: Headache. Current concepts. N Engl J Med 302:446, 1980.
3. Ziegler DK: The headache symptom. How many entities? Arch Neurol 42:273, 1985.
4. Headache Classification Committee of the International Headache Society: Classification and diagnostic criteria for headache disorders, cranial neuralgias and facial pain. Cephalalgia 8(Suppl 7):10, 1988.
5. Diamond S, Prager J, Freitag FG: Diet and headache. Is there a link? Postgrad Med 79(4):279, 1986.
6. Nattero G, Allais G, DeLorenzo C, et al: Menstrual migraine: new biochemical and psychological aspects. Headache 28:103, 1988.
7. Moskowitz MA: The neurobiology of vascular head pain. Ann Neurol 16:157, 1984.
8. Diamond S: Basilar artery migraine. A commonly misdiagnosed disorder. Postgrad Med 81(7):45, 1987.
9. Harker LA, Rassekh CH: Episodic vertigo in basilar artery migraine. Otolaryngol Head Neck Surg 96:239, 1987.
10. Harker LA, Rassekh C: Migraine equivalent as a cause of episodic vertigo. Laryngoscope 98:160, 1988.
11. Appleton R, Farrell K, Buncic JR, Hill A: Amaurosis fugax in teenagers. A migraine variant. Am J Dis Child 142:331, 1988.

12. Riley TL: Muscle-contraction headache. Neurol Clin 1:489, 1983.
13. Kudrow L: Cluster headache: new concepts. Neurol Clin 1:369, 1983.
14. Price RW, Posner JB: Chronic paroxysmal hemicrania: a disabling headache syndrome responding to indomethacin. Ann Neurol 3:183, 1978.
15. O'Donnell L, Martin EA: Cephalgia fugax: a momentary headache. Br Med J 292:663, 1986.
16. Williams B: Cough headache due to craniospinal pressure dissociation. Arch Neurol 37:226, 1980.
17. Thompson JK: Exercise-induced migraine prodrome symptoms. Headache 27:250, 1987.
18. Porter M, Jankovic J: Benign coital cephalalgia. Differential diagnosis and treatment. Arch Neurol 38:710, 1981.
19. Johns DR: Benign sexual headache within a family. Arch Neurol 43:1158, 1986.
20. Scherokman B, Massey W: Post-traumatic headaches. Neurol Clin 1:457, 1983.
21. Edmeads J: Headache and head injury . . . post hoc, or propter hoc? (editorial). Headache 28:228, 1988.
22. Gorelick PB, Hier DB, Caplan LR, et al: Headache in acute cerebrovascular disease. Neurology 36:1445, 1986.
23. Edmeads J: The headaches of ischemic cerebrovascular disease. Headache 19:345, 1979.
24. Portenoy RK, Abissi CJ, Lipton RB, et al: Headache in cerebrovascular disease. Stroke 15:1009, 1984.
25. Edmeads J: Headache in cerebrovascular disease. A common symptom of stroke. Postgrad Med 81(8):191, 1987.
26. Sahs AL, Nishioka H, Torner JC, et al: Cooperative study of intracranial aneurysms and subarachnoid hemorrhage: a long-term prognostic study. Arch Neurol 41:1140, 1984.
27. Scott WR, Miller BR: Intracerebral hemorrhage with rapid recovery. Arch Neurol 42:133, 1985.
28. Godersky JC, Biller J: Diagnosis and treatment of spontaneous intracerebral hemorrhage. Compr Ther 13:22, 1987.
29. Steiger HJ, Tew JM Jr: Hemorrhage and epilepsy in cryptic cerebrovascular malformations. Arch Neurol 41:722, 1984.
30. Testa D, Frediani F, Bussone G: Cluster headache-like syndrome due to arteriovenous malformation. Headache 28:36, 1988.
31. Huston KA, Hunder GG, Lie JT, et al: Temporal arteritis. A 25-year epidemiologic, clinical, and pathologic study. Ann Intern Med 88:162, 1978.
32. Wong RL, Korn JH: Temporal arteritis without an elevated erythrocyte sedimentation rate. Am J Med 80:959, 1986.
33. Solomon S, Cappa KG: The headache of temporal arteritis. J Am Geriatr Soc 35:163, 1987.
34. Ferguson BJ, Allen NB, Farmer JC Jr: Giant cell arteritis and polymyalgia rheumatica. Review for the otolaryngologist. Ann Otol Rhinol Laryngol 96:373, 1987.
35. West TET, Davies RJ, Kelly RE: Horner's syndrome

and headache due to carotid artery disease. Br Med J 1:818, 1976.

36. Kline LB, Vitek JJ, Raymon BC: Painful Horner's syndrome due to spontaneous carotid artery dissection. Ophthalmology 94:226, 1987.
37. Caplan LR, Zarins CK, Hemmati M: Spontaneous dissection of the extracranial vertebral arteries. Stroke 16:1030, 1985.
38. DiNubile MJ: Septic thrombosis of the cavernous sinuses. Arch Neurol 45:567, 1988.
39. Bravo EL, Gifford RW Jr: Pheochromocytoma: diagnosis, localization, and management. N Engl J Med 311:1298, 1984.
40. Krane NK: Clinically unsuspected pheochromocytomas. Experience at Henry Ford Hospital and a review of the literature. Arch Intern Med 146:54, 1986.
41. Bryant GL, Weinblatt ME, Rumbaugh C, Coblyn JS: Cerebral vasculopathy: an analysis of sixteen cases. Semin Arthritis Rheum 15:297, 1986.
42. Calabrese LH, Mallek JA: Primary angiitis of the central nervous system. Report of 8 new cases, review of the literature, and proposal for diagnostic criteria. Medicine 67:20, 1988.
43. Fishman RA: The pathophysiology of pseudotumor cerebri. An unsolved puzzle (editorial). Arch Neurol 41:257, 1984.
44. Hoffman HJ: Controversies in neurology: how is pseudotumor cerebri diagnosed? Arch Neurol 43:167, 1986.
45. Spielman FJ: Post-lumbar puncture headache. Headache 22:280, 1982.
46. Olsen KS: Epidural blood patch in the treatment of post-lumbar puncture headache. Pain 30:293, 1987.
47. Labadie EL, Hamilton RH, Lundell DC, et al: Hypoliquorrheic headache and pneumocephalus caused by thoraco-subarachnoid fistula. Neurology 27:993, 1977.
48. Lyons RW, Andriole VT: Fungal infections of the CNS. Neurol Clin 4:159, 1986.
49. Waterston JA, Gilligan BB: Cryptococcal infections of the central nervous system: a ten year experience. Clin Exp Neurol 23:127, 1987.
50. Chun CH, Johnson JD, Hofstetter M, Raff MJ: Brain abscess. A study of 45 consecutive cases. Medicine 65:415, 1986.
51. Yang SY: Brain abscess: a review of 400 cases. J Neurosurg 55:794, 1981.
52. Earnest MP, Reller LB, Filley CM, Grek AJ: Neurocysticercosis in the United States: 35 cases and a review. Rev Infect Dis 9:961, 1987.
53. Heckerling PS, Leikin JB, Maturen A, Perkins JT: Predictors of occult carbon monoxide poisoning in patients with headache and dizziness. Ann Intern Med 107:174, 1987.
54. Lefkowitz D, Biller J: Bregmatic headache as a manifestation of myocardial ischemia. Arch Neurol 39:130, 1982.
55. Das G: Pacemaker headaches. PACE 7:802, 1984.
56. Metzer WS, Lucy DD: Hypermetabolic disorders presenting as headache with anxiety and depression. Headache 27:571, 1987.

57. Edmeads J: Headaches and head pains associated with diseases of the cervical spine. Med Clin North Am 62:533, 1978.
58. Kankaanpaa U, Santavirta S: Cervical spine involvement in rheumatoid arthritis. Ann Chir Gynaecol 74(Suppl 198):117, 1985.
59. Balla J, Karnaghan J: Whiplash headache. Clin Exp Neurol 23:179, 1987.
60. Iansek R, Heywood J, Karnaghan J, Balla JI: Cervical spondylosis and headaches. Clin Exp Neurol 23:175, 1987.
61. Carter JE: Ophthalmic and neuro-ophthalmic aspects of headache and head pain. Neurol Clin 1:415, 1983.
62. Kohrman BD, Warfield CA: Eye pain: ocular and nonocular causes. Hosp Pract 22(12):33, 1987.
63. Phelps CD, Corbett JJ: Migraine and low-tension glaucoma. A case-control study. Invest Ophthalmol Vis Sci 26:1105, 1985.
64. Eisenberg E, Bental E: Postprandial transient painful amaurosis fugax. J Neurol 233:209, 1986.
65. Schonsted-Madsen U, Stoksted P, Christensen P-H, et al: Chronic headache related to nasal obstruction. J Laryngol Otol 100:165, 1986.
66. Kibblewhite DJ, Cleland J, Mintz DR: Acute sphenoid sinusitis: management strategies. J Otolaryngol 17:159, 1988.
67. Moore GF, Massey JD, Emanuel JM, et al: Head pain secondary to nasal allergies. Ear Nose Throat J 66:502, 1987.
68. Romoli M, Cudia G: Cluster headache due to an impacted superior wisdom tooth: case report. Headache 28:135, 1988.
69. Heir GM: Facial pain of dental origin—a review for physicians. Headache 27:540, 1987.
70. Guralnick W, Kaban LB, Merrill RG: Temporomandibular-joint afflictions. N Engl J Med 299:123, 1978.
71. Turkewitz LJ, Levin M: Acute inflammation of the temporomandibular joint presenting as classical trigeminal neuralgia—case report and hypothesis. Headache 28:24, 1988.
72. Watson PN, Evans RJ: Postherpetic neuralgia. A review. Arch Neurol 43:836, 1986.
73. Diamond S: Postherpetic neuralgia. Prevention and treatment. Postgrad Med 81:321, 1987.
74. Fromm GH, Terrence CF, Maroon JC: Trigeminal neuralgia. Current concepts regarding etiology and pathogenesis. Arch Neurol 41:1204, 1984.
75. Harrington HJ, Mayman CI: Carotid body tumor associated with partial Horner's syndrome and facial pain ("Raeder's syndrome"). Arch Neurol 40:564, 1983.
76. Grimson BS, Thompson HS: Raeder's syndrome. A clinical review. Surv Ophthalmol 24:199, 1980.
77. Schon F, Blau JN: Post-epileptic headache and migraine. J Neurol Neurosurg Psychiatry 50:1148, 1987.
78. Sorensen SC, Eagan RT, Scott M: Meningeal carcinomatosis in patients with primary breast or lung cancer. Mayo Clin Proc 59:91, 1984.
79. Redman BG, Tapazoglou E, Al-Sarraf M: Meningeal carcinomatosis in head and neck cancer. Report of six

cases and review of the literature. Cancer 58:2656, 1986.
80. DeAngelis LM, Payne R: Lymphomatous meningitis presenting as atypical cluster headache. Pain 30:211, 1987.
81. Hollander H, Stringari S: Human immunodeficiency virus-associated meningitis. Clinical course and correlations. Am J Med 83:813, 1987.

Selected Readings

Broderick JP, Swanson JW: Migraine-related strokes. Clinical profile and prognosis in 20 patients. Arch Neurol 44:868, 1987.
Records of 4,874 patients, 50 years and younger with the diagnosis of migraine, migraine equivalent, or vascular headache, were reviewed to evaluate the incidence of cerebral infarction. Twenty patients with migraine-associated brain infarctions are described. Most angiographic abnormalities and infarctions were in the posterior cerebral circulation.

Dalessio DJ: Is there a difference between classic and common migraine? Arch Neurol 42:275, 1985.
A concise review of migraine with a focus on clinical manifestations.

Daroff RB: New headache classification. Neurology 38:1138, 1988.
Pithy editorial comment on the pros and cons of the new headache classification.

Diamond S, Freitag FG, Solomon GD, Millstein E: Migraine headache. Working for the best outcome. Postgrad Med 81(8):174, 1987.
Useful clinical review.

Drinnan AJ: Differential diagnosis of orofacial pain. Dent Clin North Am 31:627, 1987.
Interesting review of conditions that can cause orofacial pain from a dental perspective.

Elkind AH: Muscle contraction headache. Overview and update of a common affliction. Postgrad Med 81(8):203, 1987.
Pharmacologic therapy, biofeedback, and indications for neurologic and/or psychiatric consultation are discussed.

Facchinetti F, Martignoni E, Gallai V, et al: Neuroendocrine evaluation of central opiate activity in primary headache disorders. Pain 34:29, 1988.
Current concepts of central opiate activity and its potential usefulness in the diagnosis and treatment of pain syndromes.

Greve E, Mal J: Cluster headache-like headaches: a symptomatic feature? A report of three patients with intracranial pathologic findings. Cephalalgia 8:79, 1988.
A report of three patients with cluster headache-like symptoms associated with intracranial findings, underscoring the possibility that this clinical syndrome may reflect intracranial pathology.

Hale WE, May FE, Marks RG, et al: Headache in the elderly: an evaluation of risk factors. Headache 27:272, 1987.
A discussion of headache in the elderly based on a study of an ambulatory elderly population with 1,284 participants. Risk factors were evaluated. No relationship between age and reported headache

was found. Frontal headaches were most common. Specific symptoms associated with headache differed in frequency between men and women. Other coexisting conditions were often found to contribute to headaches in the elderly.

Hansotia P: Evaluation and treatment of headache. Practical approach to a common symptom. Postgrad Med 79(6):75, 1986.
A practical approach to patient workup of chronic headaches, including history, physical examination, and diagnostic tests.

Hyman RA, Gorey MT: Imaging strategies for MR of the brain. Radiol Clin North Am 26:471, 1988.
Current recommendations for using imaging modalities of the brain in various clinical situations. CT is considered the imaging modality of choice in patients with acute neurologic deficits, such as stroke and acute onset of severe headaches, and when fine bone detail is needed. MRI is the procedure of choice for imaging the effects of trauma after the acute stage.

Kaplan RD, Solomon GD, Diamond S, Freitag FG: The role of MRI in the evaluation of a migraine population: preliminary data. Headache 27:315, 1987.
A study compared contrast-enhanced CT and MRI in a migraine population. Additional information obtained from cerebral MRI was present in approximately 33% of their patients. Authors conclude that MRI is a necessary adjunct in the detection of intracerebral pathology in this patient population.

Krabbe AA: Cluster headache: a review. Acta Neurol Scand 74:1, 1986.
Clinical features and a variety of diagnostic and management strategies are summarized in this useful review.

Kudo H, Tamaki N, Kim S, et al: Intraspinal tumors associated with hydrocephalus. Neurosurgery 21:726, 1987.
Three case reports of intraspinal tumors associated with hydrocephalus are reported with a review of literature of this relatively rare clinical setting. The review discusses the diagnostic pitfalls associated with intraspinal tumors presenting with hydrocephalus. These tumors are not easily diagnosed, particularly since the chief complaints usually include headache or dementia, but not back pain.

Kumar KL, Cooney TG: Vascular headache. J Gen Intern Med 3:384, 1988.
Useful clinical review written for the internist evaluating and treating vascular headaches. Well referenced.

Lance JW: Headache. Ann Neurol 10:1, 1981.
A well-referenced synopsis of the diagnosis of headache.

Lauritzen M: Cerebral blood flow in migraine and cortical spreading depression. Acta Neurol Scand 113(Suppl):1, 1987.
This review summarizes clinical and experimental studies of two commonly held theories of pathophysiology underlying migraine headaches: (1) the vascular theory, which attributes migraine to cerebral artery spasm that causes local hypoxia and transient focal symptoms followed by neurogenically mediated vasodilation and headache and (2) the more recent theory relating migraine to a paroxysmal, transient depolarization of primarily cortical neurons that causes transient focal symptoms and headache, i.e., migraine as primary disorder of neuronal function.

Lipsitt DR: Pain in the neck, face, and head. Role of the

consultation-liaison psychiatrist. Psychiatr Clin North Am 10:69, 1987.
Current concepts of the psychiatric management and views of psychopathology involved in pain in the neck, face, and head.

Littlewood JT, Gibb C, Glover V, et al: Red wine as a cause of migraine. Lancet 1:558, 1988.
A clinical study that challenged patients with migraine who believed that red wine, but not alcohol in general, provoked their headaches. Vodka and a diluted mixture of equivalent alcohol content, both cold, with disguised colors and flavor, were tested. Red wine with a negligible tyramine content did provoke typical migraine in 9 of 11 such patients in contrast to the absence of attacks in these patients when challenged with vodka or other alcohol.

Mansfield LE: Food allergy and headache. Whom to evaluate and how to treat. Postgrad Med 83(7):46, 1988.
The role of food allergies as a cause of migraine and sinus headaches and management suggestions are discussed, including diet logs, diets, and food challenges.

Masters SJ, McClean PM, Arcarese JS, et al: Skull x-ray examinations after head trauma. Recommendations by a multidisciplinary panel and validation study. N Engl J Med 316:84, 1987.
A management strategy formulated by a multidisciplinary panel assembled to review indications for skull radiography in cases of head trauma. High and low risk groups defined in this article.

McKenna JP: Cluster headaches. Am Fam Physician 37(4):173, 1988.
Cluster headaches are reviewed with an emphasis on the sometimes difficult clinical overlap of migraine or trigeminal neuralgia syndromes. Treatment options for both acute and chronic cluster headaches are well outlined.

McNeil SL, Spruill WA, Langley RL, et al: Multiple subdural hematomas associated with breakdancing. Ann Emerg Med 16:114, 1987.
Interesting case report of a previously healthy 17-year-old male breakdancer who presented with a 3-month history of crescendo headache and was found to have several extracranial lesions, which were surgically diagnosed as subdural hematoma and one probable arachnoid cyst containing a hematoma.

Rubenfeld M, Wirtschafter JD: The role of medical imaging in the practice of neuro-ophthalmology. Radiol Clin North Am 25:863, 1987.
This article presents an overview of pathology and imaging indications from a neuro-ophthalmologist's perspective. The discussion includes common conditions found in the orbit, optic nerve, cavernous sinus, chiasm, posterior visual pathway, cerebral cortex, brain stem, and spinal cord.

Saper JR: Approaches to chronic headache. Hosp Pract 22(5A):21, 1987.
Clinical review of current concepts of diagnosis and management of the chronic headache. Author includes indications for referral.

Shesser R: Headache caused by serious illness. Evaluation in an emergency setting. Postgrad Med 81(3):117, 1987.
Current concepts of the evaluation and use of modern technology

of the severe headache in the emergency room. Authors focus on emergency evaluations of subarachnoid hemorrhage and meningitis.

Shuaib A, Hachinski VC: Migraine and the risks from angiography. Arch Neurol 45:911, 1988.
A retrospective study of 142 patients with migraine, which included 149 angiograms performed for acute headache, new focal symptoms, and other causes. Focal cerebral events occurred in 2.6% of cases compared to a 2.8% rate of complications in a prospective study of 1,002 patients from the same center. Authors conclude that, even though transient focal neurologic symptoms are not infrequent in their migraine population who underwent angiography, angiography during episodes of acute headache is a safe procedure.

Solomon S, Cappa KG, Smith CR: Common migraine: criteria for diagnosis. Headache 28:124, 1988.
To better define diagnostic criteria for common migraine, clinical features of 100 consecutive patients diagnosed as common migraine were compared with 100 cases of chronic daily headaches, considered forms of "tension headaches." Features that occurred significantly more often in patients with common migraine were nausea, vomiting, unilateral site, throbbing quality, photophobia or phonophobia, increase with menstruation, and a family history of migraine.

Standefer JA Jr, Mattox DE: Head and neck manifestations of collagen vascular diseases. Otolaryngol Clin North Am 19:181, 1986.
A useful review for those taking care of patients with collagen vascular disease of various associated head and neck symptoms that occur in this setting.

Tegeler CH, Bell RD: Vascular headache. Otolaryngol Clin North Am 20:65, 1987.
Clinical review of vascular headaches, including current concepts of pathophysiology and management.

Vilming ST, Schrader H, Monstad I: Post-lumbar-puncture headache: the significance of body posture. A controlled study of 300 patients. Cephalalgia 8:75, 1988.
The significance of body posture following lumbar puncture was studied in a single-blind, randomized study of 300 neurologic inpatients. Immediate mobilization was compared to 6 hours of bed rest. This study did not show significant differences between recumbent and ambulant patients when the frequency of post-lumbar-puncture headache was evaluated.

Warner JJ: Headaches in older patients: Ddx and Tx of vascular and inflammatory pain. Geriatrics 40(10):30, 1985.
Author stresses the importance of using caution in diagnosing migraine in the elderly, as cerebrovascular dysfunction or structural lesions can also cause headache.

Warner JJ: Headaches in older patients: Ddx and Tx of common nonvascular causes. Geriatrics 40(11):69, 1985.
Discussion of headaches in the elderly arising from musculoskeletal causes, extracranial and intracranial disorders and visual and dental abnormalities.

Watson CP, Evans RJ: Chronic cluster headache—a review of 60 patients. Headache 27:158, 1987.
Data from treatment of 60 patients with chronic cluster headache and an extended follow-up of 46 patients presents a variety of therapeutic trials. A literature review enhances authors experience.

Wijdicks EF, Kerkhoff H, van Gijn J: Long-term follow-

up of 71 patients with thunderclap headache mimicking
subarachnoid hemorrhage. Lancet 2:68, 1988.

*Seventy-one patients with sudden, severe headache who had nor-
mal CT scans and cerebrospinal fluid (CSF) were followed for an
average of 3.3 years. Cerebral angiography was performed in four
patients after their first attack and in two patients after recurrent
episodes. Angiography was normal in all patients studied. Thirty-
one (44%) of the 71 patients subsequently developed regular episodes
of tension or common migraine headaches. Authors conclude that
angiography may not be indicated in this clinical setting if CT and
CSF studies are normal.*

43
Dizziness and Vertigo: Common and Less Common Causes

Dizziness and vertigo are two of the most common
and frustrating complaints that present to emergency
rooms and outpatient clinics. The most important
clinical question is to distinguish clearly between
dizziness and vertigo. Dizziness can be described by
the patient as giddiness, dysequilibrium, imbalance,
or lightheadedness. Vertigo is described as a sense
of rotation of either patient or the environment and
reflects peripheral or central vestibular dysfunction.
If the patient has nystagmus, certain characteristics
of the nystagmus may help to distinguish peripheral
from central lesions: primary positional nystagmus
without vertigo is usually central in origin, whereas
peripheral jerk-type nystagmus, which beats in one
direction, is usually peripheral (labyrinthine) or vestibular in origin.[1] Dizziness is one of several terms
used to describe an impending loss of consciousness
and is commonly vascular in origin. However, it is
also associated with a wide spectrum of acute and
chronic disorders, which can range from life-threatening events, such as an acute cerebellar infarction,

to chronic multiple sensory deficits, which commonly afflict elderly patients.[2,3] In a frequently cited university outpatient study of patients presenting with dizziness, the three most common causes of dizziness were peripheral vestibular disorders, hyperventilation, and multiple sensory deficits.[4]

Peripheral Vestibular Disorders

Benign positional vertigo: most frequent cause of dizziness in the adult; patients have paroxysmal positional dizziness and nystagmus[5-7]

External ear impaction: wax and foreign bodies are common causes of mild vertigo.

Otitis media: acute and chronic[8]

Meniere's disease: triad of dizziness, fluctuating low-frequency hearing loss, and tinnitus[9]

Vestibular neuronitis: sudden onset of intense vertigo that usually improves

Disabling positional vertigo: constant vertigo with disabling nausea, often refractory to conventional therapy[10]

Otosclerosis: can present with a wide spectrum of vestibular symptoms, classically associated with conductive or mixed hearing loss with vestibular symptoms, in the absence of middle ear disease[11-13]

Labyrinthine ossification: may be end-stage ossification following inflammation, trauma, cholesteatoma, or surgery[14]

Positional alcohol nystagmus: at alcohol blood levels of 40 mg/dl, alcohol diffuses into the cupula, transforming semicircular canals into gravity-sensitive receptors.[1]

Post-traumatic: temporal bone fractures, hemorrhages into lymphatic regions, perilymphatic fistulas[15-17]

Vestibulotoxic drugs: streptomycin, gentamicin, salicylates, and cisplatin[18]

Organic solvent toxicity[19,20]

Autoimmune inner ear disease[21]

Central Vestibular Disorders

Vestibular nuclei infarction[22]

Vertebrobasilar ischemia: consider in patients with stroke-risk factors and associated symptoms of diplopia, dysarthria, weakness, or numbness[23-25]

Vestibulocerebellar infarction: can sometimes mimic acute labyrinthitis with acute onset of positional vertigo and truncal ataxia[26,27]

Vestibular nuclei or vestibulocerebellar neoplasms: primary or metastatic[28]

Vestibular nuclei inflammation: infection and non-infectious inflammatory processes, such as sarcoidosis or vasculitis

Wernicke's encephalopathy

Post-traumatic central vestibular dysfunction

Multiple sclerosis[29]

Vestibular seizures (vertiginous epilepsy): secondary to temporal lobe or parietal association cortex discharges[1,30]

Posterior fossa neoplasm: cerebellopontine angle tumor, acoustic neuroma, posterior fossa arachnoid cysts[31,32]

Basilar artery aneurysm[33]

Miscellaneous Associations

Cervicogenic disorders: wide spectrum of common degenerative disorders, post-traumatic syndromes and craniovertebral anomalies associated with dizziness[34,35]

Psychogenic vertigo: panic attacks, depression[36-40]

Hyperventilation syndrome[41,42]

Motion sickness

Multiple sensory deficits: often elderly patients with a combination of visual, vestibular, and orthopaedic problems and peripheral neuropathy[1]

Migraine variants: episodic vertigo, particularly in young adults and children[43-45]

Orthostatic hypotension: vasoactive drugs are a common reversible cause in the elderly.[46,47]

Drug toxicity: anticonvulsants, benzodiazepines, psychotropic agents

Cardiac arrhythmias[48]

Mitral valve prolapse: symptoms of dizziness cannot always be correlated with arrhythmias[49,50]

Disorders of autonomic insufficiency: autonomic neuropathy, diabetes[51-53]

Dysequilibrium of aging (presbyastasis): a diagnosis of exclusion in the elderly[54-56]

Parkinson's disease

B_{12} deficiency

Spinal cord tumors

Myxedema

Occult carbon monoxide poisoning: headache dizziness can occur in patients with carboxyhemoglobin levels greater than 10%.[57]

References

1. Brandt T, Daroff RB: The multisensory physiological and pathological vertigo syndromes. Ann Neurol 7:195, 1980.
2. Towler HM: Dizziness and vertigo. Br Med J 288:1739, 1984.
3. Bonikowski FP: Differential diagnosis of dizziness in the elderly. Geriatrics 38(2):89, 1983.
4. Drachman DA, Hart CW: An approach to the dizzy patient. Neurology 22:323, 1972.
5. Baloh RW, Honrubia V, Jacobson K: Benign positional vertigo: clinical and oculographic features in 240 cases. Neurology 37:371, 1987.
6. Gyo K: Benign paroxysmal positional vertigo as a complication of postoperative bedrest. Laryngoscope 98:332, 1988.
7. Bourgeois PM, Dehaene I: Benign paroxysmal positional vertigo (BPPV). Clinical features in 34 cases and review of literature. Acta Neurol Belg 88:65, 1988.
8. Paparella MM, Goycoolea MV, Schachern PA, Sajjadi H: Current clinical and pathological features of round window diseases. Laryngoscope 97:1151, 1987.
9. Wright A: Meniere's syndrome. Br J Hosp Med 34:366, 1985.
10. Jannetta PJ, Moller MB, Moller AR: Disabling positional vertigo. N Engl J Med 310:1700, 1984.
11. Thomas JE, Cody DTR: Neurologic perspectives of otosclerosis. Mayo Clin Proc 56:17, 1981.
12. Forquer BD, Sheehy JL: Cochlear otosclerosis: a review of audiometric findings in 150 cases. Am J Otol 8:1, 1987.
13. Davis GL: Pathology of otosclerosis: a review. Am J Otolaryngol 8:273, 1987.
14. Swartz JD, Mandell DM, Faerber EN, et al: Labyrinthine ossification: etiologies and CT findings. Radiology 157:395, 1985.
15. Lund S: Dizziness and vertigo in the posttraumatic syndrome. A physiological background. Acta Neurochir 36(Suppl):118, 1986.
16. Lehrer JF, Rubin RC, Poole DC, et al: Perilymphatic fistula—a definitive and curable cause of vertigo following head trauma. West J Med 141:57, 1984.
17. Parnes LS, McCabe BF: Perilymph fistula: an important cause of deafness and dizziness in children. Pediatrics 80:524, 1987.
18. Kobayashi H, Ohashi N, Watanabe Y, Mizukoshi K: Clinical features of cisplatin vestibulotoxicity and hearing loss. ORL J Otorhinolaryngol Relat Spec 49:67, 1987.
19. Gyntelberg F, Vesterhauge S, Fog P, et al: Acquired intolerance to organic solvents and results of vestibular testing. Am J Ind Med 9:363, 1986.
20. Fidler AT, Baker EL, Letz RE: Neurobehavioural effects of occupational exposure to organic solvents among construction painters. Br J Ind Med 44:292, 1987.
21. Hughes GB, Barna BP, Kinney SE, et al: Clinical diagnosis of immune inner-ear disease. Laryngoscope 98:251, 1988.

22. Pellegrino TR: Vascular syndromes. Emerg Med Clin North Am 5:751, 1987.
23. Turney TM, Garraway WM, Whisnant JP: The natural history of hemispheric and brainstem infarction in Rochester, Minnesota. Stroke 15:790, 1984.
24. Pessin MS, Gorelick PB, Kwan ES, Caplan LR: Basilar artery stenosis: middle and distal segments. Neurology 37:1742, 1987.
25. Ban M, Ueta H, Nakagawa Y, Matsumoto K: A case of basilar artery occlusion associated with unilateral low origin of the posterior inferior cerebellar artery. Surg Neurol 26:501, 1986.
26. Guiang RL Jr, Ellington OB: Acute pure vertiginous dysequilibrium in cerebellar infarction. Eur Neurol 16:11, 1977.
27. Kattah JC, Kolsky MP, Luessenhop AJ: Positional vertigo and the cerebellar vermis. Neurology 34:527, 1984.
28. Fadul C, Misulis KE, Wiley RG: Cerebellar metastases: diagnostic and management considerations. J Clin Oncol 5:1107, 1987.
29. Daugherty WT, Lederman RJ, Nodar RH, et al: Hearing loss in multiple sclerosis. Arch Neurol 40:33, 1983.
30. Behrman S, Wyke BD: Vestibulogenic seizures. A consideration of vertiginous seizures, with particular reference to convulsions produced by stimulation of labyrinthine receptors. Brain 81:529, 1958.
31. van Swieten JC, Thomeer RT, Vielvoye GJ, Bots GT: Choroid plexus papilloma in the posterior fossa. Surg Neurol 28:129, 1987.
32. Hadley MN, Grahm TW, Daspit CP, Spetzler RF: Otolaryngologic manifestations of posterior fossa arachnoid cysts. Laryngoscope 95:678, 1985.
33. Musiek FE, Geurkink NA, Spiegel P: Audiologic and other clinical findings in a case of basilar artery aneurysm. Arch Otolaryngol Head Neck Surg 113:772, 1987.
34. Fredriksen TA, Hovdal H, Sjaastad O: "Cervicogenic headache": clinical manifestation. Cephalalgia 7:147, 1987.
35. Kumar A, Jafar J, Mafee M, et al: Diagnosis and management of anomalies of the craniovertebral junction. Ann Otol Rhinol Laryngol 95:487, 1986.
36. Tiwari S, Bakris GL: Psychogenic vertigo: a review. Postgrad Med 70(5):69, 1981.
37. Katerndahl DA: The sequence of panic symptoms. J Fam Pract 26:49, 1988.
38. Jacob RG, Mller MB, Turner SM, Wall C III: Otoneurological examination in panic disorder and agoraphobia with panic attacks: a pilot study. Am J Psychiatry 142:715, 1985.
39. Katon W: Panic disorder: epidemiology, diagnosis, and treatment in primary care. J Clin Psychiatry 47(Suppl):21, 1986.
40. Ierodiakonou CS, Iacovides A: Somatic manifestations of depressive patients in different psychiatric settings. Psychopathology 20:136, 1987.
41. Theunissen EJ, Huygen PL, Folgering HT: Vestibular hyperreactivity and hyperventilation. Clin Otolaryngol 11:161, 1986.
42. Perkin GD, Joseph R: Neurological manifestations of

the hyperventilation syndrome. J R Soc Med 79:448, 1986.

43. Kayan A, Hood JD: Neuro-otological manifestations of migraine. Brain 107:1123, 1984.
44. Guidetti G, Bergamini G, Pini LA, et al: Dizziness and headache. Acta Otorhinolaryngol Belg 38:140, 1984.
45. Harker LA, Rassekh C: Migraine equivalent as a cause of episodic vertigo. Laryngoscope 98:160, 1988.
46. Schatz IJ: Orthostatic hypotension. I. Functional and neurogenic causes. Arch Intern Med 144:773, 1984.
47. Venna N: Dizziness, falling, and fainting: differential diagnosis in the aged. Parts I and II. Geriatrics 41(6):30, 1986; 41(7):31, 1986.
48. Rebello R, Brownlee WC: Intermittent ventricular standstill during chronic atrial fibrillation in patients with dizziness or syncope. PACE 10:1271, 1987.
49. Pratt CM, Young JB, Wierman AM, et al: Complex ventricular arrhythmias associated with the mitral valve prolapse syndrome. Effectiveness of moricizine (Ethmozine) in patients resistant to conventional antiarrhythmics. Am J Med 80:626, 1986.
50. Schatz IJ: Mitral valve prolapse. The unresolved questions. Hosp Pract 22(3A):39, 1987.
51. Ewing DJ, Clarke BF: Autonomic neuropathy: its diagnosis and prognosis. Clin Endocrinol Metab 15:855, 1986.
52. Pappas DG, Crawford W: Dizziness due to dysautonomia: response to specific therapy. South Med J 81:531, 1988.
53. Pappas DG, Crawford W, Coghlan HC: Dizziness and the autonomic dysfunction syndrome. Otolaryngol Head Neck Surg 94:186, 1986.
54. Sixt E, Landahl S: Postural disturbances in a 75-year-old population: I. Prevalence and functional consequences. Age Ageing 16:393, 1987.
55. McClure JA: Vertigo and imbalance in the elderly. J Otolaryngol 15:248, 1986.
56. Belal A Jr, Glorig A: The ageing ear. A clinico-pathological classification. J Laryngol Otol 101:1131, 1987.
57. Heckerling PS, Leikin JB, Maturen A, Perkins JT: Predictors of occult carbon monoxide poisoning in patients with headache and dizziness. Ann Intern Med 107:174, 1987.

Selected Readings

Davis EA: Emergency department approach to vertigo. Emerg Med Clin North Am 5:211, 1987.
The approach to dizziness in the emergency room in this clinical review organizes basic and current concepts necessary to make the difficult emergency room distinction between the rare, but potentially life-threatening, central disorders from more benign peripheral and chronic causes of complaints of dizziness, vertigo, and imbalance. Useful clinical pointers and well referenced.

Formby C, Hixson-Robles C, Singleton GT: Correlations between hearing thresholds and caloric responses among a heterogeneous sample of dizzy patients. J Speech Hear Disord 53:65, 1988.
Auditory and vestibular function were compared in a heteroge-

neous group of patients who complained of dizziness. Hearing thresholds for the frequency range of 10 to 14 Hz, but not for conventional audiometric frequencies, correlated with slow-phase eye velocities. Authors conclude that this finding indicates a trend for eye velocity to increase as a function of increasing hearing threshold.

Goldman LB, Izzo KL: Magnetic resonance imaging for vertebral-basilar system infarction. Arch Phys Med Rehabil 69:5, 1988.
MRI offers a noninvasive means of monitoring vascular lesions in the posterior fossa. This study evaluated the usefulness of MRI in patients with suspected vertebral-basilar vascular lesions. Studies were compared with CT. MRI was felt to yield adjunctive information that aided diagnosis, prognosis, and rehabilitation of patients in this study.

Harner SG: Peripheral labyrinthine causes of dizziness. Postgrad Med 81(4):251, 1987.
Useful clinical discussion of the evaluation of dizziness. The article reviews a general otolaryngologic approach to the dizzy patient and reviews five representative labyrinthine diseases.

Kumar A, Valvassori G: An algorithm for neurotologic disorders. Neurol Clin 2:779, 1984.
Still currently useful algorithm for evaluating neurotologic disorders.

Luxon LM: "A bit dizzy." Br J Hosp Med 32:315, 1984.
A discussion of dizziness approached from personal, clinical experience that outlines an outpatient evaluation.

Madlon-Kay DJ: Evaluation and outcome of the dizzy patient. J Fam Pract 21:109, 1985.
Evaluation of 121 patients in an emergency room with the complaint of dizziness. Peripheral vestibular disease was the most common cause of dizziness.

Mller MB, Mller AR, Jannetta PJ, Sekhar L: Diagnosis and surgical treatment of disabling positional vertigo. J Neurosurg 64:21, 1986.
A review of characteristic symptoms of disabling positional vertigo and current tests useful in the differential diagnosis of this disorder.

Norre ME, Forrez G, Beckers A: Vestibulospinal function in two syndromes with spontaneous attacks of vertigo: evaluation by posturography. Clin Otolaryngol 12:215, 1987.
A clinical study of the usefulness of posturography in vestibular syndromes. Authors conclude that this test is a necessary part of the evaluation of certain vestibular syndromes and disturbances of vestibulospinal reflexes.

Thalmann I, Thallinger G, Thalmann R: Otosclerosis: a local manifestation of a generalized connective tissue disorder? Am J Otolaryngol 8:308, 1987.
This study tests the hypothesis that otosclerosis is a local manifestation of a clinically and genetically heterogeneous group of generalized connective tissue disorders by quantitative biochemical techniques. In contrast to previous studies, no significant differences were found in individual glycosaminoglycans excreted in urine of control subjects and patients with otosclerosis.

Wells MD, Yande RD: Vertigo in a district NHS hospital. J Laryngol Otol 101:1235, 1987.
A clincal study that collated experience of three general ENT

clinics in managing the complaint of dizziness over a period of 10 years. The most common cause of vertigo was postural vertigo in the elderly. Meniere's disease was the second most common cause of dizziness in this population. A small percentage (2.4%) of patients had posterior fossa lesions.

44

Drop Attacks: Common and Uncommon Associated Disorders

A drop attack is a sudden fall while standing or walking; there is complete recovery within minutes and no marked loss of consciousness. These attacks overlap with syncopal attacks, both in phenomenology and etiology. Underlying medical conditions, such as hypertension, diabetes mellitus, cardiac disease, and age-related sensory deficits, may be significant risk factors. Drop attacks can be the first manifestation of certain disorders, many of them treatable, such as cervical cord compression, labyrinthitis, and Parkinson's disease. A drop attack can be an epileptic manifestation. The pathophysiology of drop attacks is varied and in some conditions, uncertain. The prognosis of drop attack depends on the coexistent medical condition.

Cardiovascular

Cardiogenic syncope: arrhythmias, atrial myxoma, mitral valve prolapse, aortic stenosis[1,2]

Basilar artery insufficiency and other transient ischemic attacks (TIAs)[3,4]

Orthostatic cerebral ischemia: primary and secondary[5,6]

Vertebral artery compression: often associated with

osteoarthritis; drop attacks can be precipitated by head turning.

Bilateral carotid occlusive disease

Subclavian steal phenomenon

Posterior fossa aneurysms: brain stem, vertebral artery[7]

Transient ischemic attacks (TIAs): causing transient ischemia of corticospinal tracts[3]

Bilateral basis pontis infarction

Basal ganglia infarctions or hemorrhages: loss of postural balance arises contralaterally to unilateral pallidal-putamenal lesions.[8]

Spinal cord ischemia

Impaired Central or Peripheral Postural Reflexes

Old age: decline of postural control and multiple sensory deficits afflicting the elderly[9]

Multiple sensory deficits: particularly neuropathies

Parkinson's disease: loss of postural reflexes can be an initial or chronic manifestation of parkinsonism[10]

Progressive supranuclear palsy

Spinal cord lesions: stenosis, neoplasia, myelopathies

Multiple sclerosis

Movement-induced dystonias

Compressive or Mass Effects

Cervical cord compression: cervical spondylosis, trauma, myelopathies[11,12]

Craniocervical junction anomalies: basilar impression syndromes, such as Chiari malformations, Morquio syndrome[13]

Unstable subluxations of the atlanto-axial joints: rheumatoid arthritis, Down syndrome

Syringomyelia

Odontoid process abnormalities: trauma, rheumatoid arthritis, congenital

Parasagittal tumors: meningiomas

Foramen magnum compression

Fourth ventricle tumors: ependymomas

Third ventricle tumors: colloid cysts, meningiomas[14,15]

Vestibulocerebellar: neoplasia, trauma, congenital, and idiopathic

Cerebellar vermis tumors

Hydrocephalus: gait disturbances are usually prominent; rarely, drop attacks can lead to the diagnosis of unsuspected hydrocephalus.[16–19]

Possible Epileptic Manifestations

Akinetic-myoclonic attacks[20]
Complex-partial seizures[21-23]
Stimulus-sensitive reflex epilepsy
Other unusual seizure types[24]

Miscellaneous Associations

Acute vestibular and labyrinthine disturbances[25]
Chronic vestibular and labyrinthine disturbances: drop attacks of chronic vestibular dysfunction most commonly seen with Meniere's disease[26]
Drug-induced loss of motor control disturbances
Cataplexy: with or without narcolepsy[27]
Diabetes mellitus: may be associated with autonomic neuropathy
B_{12} deficiency: subacute combined dysfunction of the spinal cord is often the first and sometimes exclusive neurologic abnormality with pernicious anemia.
Myxedema
Adrenal insufficiency[28]
Psychogenic: hyperventilation
Idiopathic: cryptogenic drop attacks in women[29]
Syncope: cough, micturition, and hypeventilation-induced syncope with brief lapses of consciousness can mimic drop attacks.

References

1. Dohrmann ML, Cheitlin MD: Cardiogenic syncope. Neurol Clin 4:549, 1986.
2. DiCarlo LA Jr, Morady F: Evaluation of the patient with syncope. Cardiol Clin 3:499, 1985.
3. Brust JCM, Plank CR, Healton EB, et al: The pathology of drop attacks: a case report. Neurology 29:786, 1979.
4. Edwards WH, Mulherin JL Jr: The management of brachiocephalic occlusive disease. Am Surg 49:465, 1983.
5. Stark RJ, Wodak J: Primary orthostatic cerebral ischaemia. J Neurol Neurosurg Psychiatry 46:883, 1983.
6. Thomas JE, Schirger A, Fealey RD, et al: Orthostatic hypotension. Mayo Clin Proc 56:117, 1981.
7. Gautier JC, Morelot D, Gray F, et al: Giant aneurysm of both vertebral arteries. Drop-attacks. Rev Neurol (Paris) 138:63, 1982.
8. Labadie EL, Awerbuch GI, Hamilton RH, Rapcsak SZ: Falling and postural deficits due to acute unilateral basal ganglia lesions. Arch Neurol 46:492, 1989.
9. Lipsitz LA: The drop attack: a common geriatric symptom. J Am Geriatr Soc 31:617, 1983.
10. Klawans HL, Topel JL: Parkinsonism as a falling sickness. JAMA 230:1555, 1974.
11. Maurice-Williams RS: Drop attacks from cervical cord compression. Br J Clin Pract 28:215, 1974.

12. Manabe S, Tateishi A: Epidural migration of extruded cervical disc and its surgical treatment. Spine 11:873, 1986.
13. Bewermeyer H, Dreesbach HA, Hunermann B, Heiss WD: MR imaging of familial basilar impression. J Comput Assist Tomogr 8:953, 1984.
14. Nitta M, Symon L: Colloid cysts of the third ventricle. A review of 36 cases. Acta Neurochir 76:99, 1985.
15. Criscuolo GR, Symon L: Intraventricular meningioma. A review of 10 cases of the National Hospital, Queen Square (1974–1985) with reference to the literature. Acta Neurochir 83:83, 1986.
16. Botez MI: Drop attacks, chalastic fits, and occult hydrocephalus (letter). Neurology 29:1555, 1979.
17. Knutsson E, Lying-Tunell U: Gait apraxia in normal-pressure hydrocephalus: patterns of movement and muscle activation. Neurology 35:155, 1985.
18. Fisher CM: Hydrocephalus as a cause of disturbances of gait in the elderly. Neurology 32:1358, 1982.
19. Sørensen PS, Jansen EC, Gjerris F: Motor disturbances in normal-pressure hydrocephalus. Special reference to stance and gait. Arch Neurol 43:34, 1986.
20. Wang PJ, Omori K, Utsumi H, et al: Partial inhibitory seizures: a report on two cases. Brain Dev 6:553, 1984.
21. Pazzaglia P, D'Alessandro R, Ambrosetto G, et al: Drop attacks: an ominous change in the evolution of partial epilepsy. Neurology 35:1725, 1985.
22. Escueta AVD, Bacsal FE, Treiman DM: Complex partial seizures on closed-circuit television and EEG: a study of 691 attacks in 79 patients. Ann Neurol 11:292, 1982.
23. Holmes GL: Partial seizures in children. Pediatrics 77:725, 1986.
24. Ikeno T, Shigematsu H, Miyakoshi M, et al: An analytic study of epileptic falls. Epilepsia 26:612, 1985.
25. Baloh RW, Honrubia V, Yee RD, et al: Changes in the human vestibulo-ocular reflex after loss of peripheral sensitivity. Ann Neurol 16:222, 1984.
26. Black FO, Effron MZ, Burns DS: Diagnosis and management of drop attacks of vestibular origin: Tumarkin's otolithic crisis. Otolaryngol Head Neck Surg 90:256, 1982.
27. Kales A, Cadieux RJ, Soldatos CR, et al: Narcolepsy-cataplexy. I. Clinical and electrophysiologic characteristics. Arch Neurol 39:164, 1982.
28. Omoigui NA, Cave WT Jr, Chang AY: Adrenal insufficiency. A rare initial sign of metastatic colon carcinoma. J Clin Gastroenterol 9:470, 1987.
29. Stevens DL, Matthews WB: Cryptogenic drop attacks: an affliction of women. Br Med J 1:439, 1973.

Selected Readings

Meissner I, Wiebers DO, Swanson JW, O'Fallon WM: The natural history of drop attacks. Neurology 36:1029, 1986.

A clinical study that grouped 108 patients with drop attacks according to potential mechanisms based on associated medical conditions in decreasing frequency: unknown, 69 (64%); cardiac, 13 (12%); cerebrovascular insufficiency, 9 (8%); combined cardiac and cerebrovascular disease, 8 (7%); seizures, 5 (5%); vestibular,

3 (3%); and, psychogenic, 1 (1%). Authors discuss evaluation and management.

Rapoport S: The management of drop attacks. DM 32:121, 1986.

A review that summarizes current concepts of the physiology of posture and the clinical approach to the evaluation and management of drop attacks. Since brief lapses of consciousness can easily go undetected, major categories of syncope are included in this useful, well-referenced, clinical summary.

Ross RT: Syncope. WB Saunders, London, 1988, pp 131–135.

Comprehensive, scholarly, clinical monograph on syncope full of useful, interesting information for the clinician who evaluates patients with syncope. Chapter 12 is devoted to drop attacks; however, the entire monograph is recommended to those who evaluate patients with symptoms of loss of consciousness.

45
Dementia: Reversible and Irreversible Causes

Dementia is a clinical syndrome manifested by cognitive and intellectual decline sufficient to interfere with social or occupational performance in an alert patient.[1] Personality disturbances are frequently a prominent part of dementia syndromes; therefore, psychiatric syndromes, particularly depression, need to be ruled out. A multitude of irreversible, arrestable, and reversible neurologic, medical, and psychiatric disorders can manifest as dementia. The social and economic cost of dementia justifies a comprehensive evaluation to find such disorders that may underlie a reversible or treatable dementia.[2] Drug toxicity, depression, and coexistent medical disorders are common causes of treatable and reversible dementia. Patients with reversible dementia tend to have a shorter duration dementia and take prescription drugs.[3] Infections limited to the central nervous system can be indolent and mimic chronic, progressive, noninfectious causes of dementia.[4]

A clinical classification of dementia into cortical and subcortical dementias may help in the differential diagnosis, even though both cortical and subcortical dementias have mixed features and, though clinically useful, they cannot be rigidly applied.[5] Examples of cortical deficits include amnesia, aphasia, agnosia, and apraxia. Examples of subcortical deficits include forgetfulness, slowed mentation, apathy, and depression.[6-9] Unfortunately, the major primary neurodegenerative cause of dementia, Alzheimer's disease, still cannot be definitely diagnosed without histologic confirmation and, therefore, remains a diagnosis of exclusion.

Primary Neurodegenerative, Sporadic, and Genetic Disorders

Alzheimer's disease: Alzheimer's disease is the major cause of admission to nursing homes; risk factors include age, occurrence in parent or sibling, serious head trauma, and the presence of trisomy 21.[10,11] Heterogeneous clinical subtypes have suggested a spectrum of severity with severer forms associated with myoclonus and noniatrogenic extrapyramidal disorders.[12-16]

Pick's disease: prominent frontotemporal atrophy on neurodiagnostic imaging[17-20]

Huntington's disease: an autosomal dominant disorder, usually beginning in midlife, characterized by dementia and choreiform movements; aberrant gene localization recently has made presymptomatic testing possible[21-23]

Wilson's disease: an autosomal recessive disorder of copper accumulation with early manifestations that can mimic schizophrenia, particularly in the young adult with a tremor[24-28]

Parkinson's disease with dementia: estimates of the incidence of dementia with Parkinson's disease vary greatly, and the neuropathologic relationship of Parkinson's disease to loss of cognitive function is incompletely understood.[29-36]

Progressive supranuclear palsy: consider this diagnosis in parkinsonian patients who do not respond to conventional antiparkinsonian therapy.[37-43]

Hallervorden-Spatz disease: adult onset with neurofibrillary pathology and dementia[44]

Lewy body dementia: Lewy bodies are found in cortex as well as the brain stem in these patients; a progressive dementia syndrome, often with prominent psychiatric symptoms, occasionally appears parkinsonian[45-47]

Frontal lobe degeneration of non-Alzheimer type[48-51]

Other genetic disorders: though usually diagnosed in children, many of these disorders have reports of late onset of symptoms, including a prominent dementia, Pelizaeus-Merzbacher disease,[52] Lafora's disease,[53] Sanfilippo B-disease,[54] giant axonal neuropathy,[55] metachromatic leukodystrophy,[56] X-linked ataxia,[57] adrenoleukodystrophy,[58] hereditary dentatorubral-pallidoluysian atrophy,[59] adult polyglucosan body disease,[60] Kufs' disease,[61] familial multisystem atrophy,[62] idiopathic familial brain calcifications,[63-65] mitochondrial encephalomyopathy,[66] adult-onset neuronal intranuclear hyaline inclusion disease[67]

Conditions Associated with Vascular Causes of Dementias

Arteriosclerotic and thrombotic large and small vessel disease: multi-infarct dementia, Binswanger chronic progressive subcortical encephalopathy[68-76]

Amyloid angiopathy: amyloid deposition occurs in cortical arteries; multiple intracerebral hematomas, particularly in the frontoparietal and parieto-occipital areas, in the absence of significant hypertension are characteristic clinical findings.[77-80]

Anticardiolipin antibody associated multiple cerebral infarctions: antibody found in patients with and without systemic lupus erythematosus[81,82]

Collagen vascular associated cerebrovascular disease: systemic lupus erythematosus, Cogan's syndrome, Behçet's syndrome[81,83]

Giant cell arteritis

Hemoglobinopathies: sickle cell disease[84]

MELAS syndrome: Mitochondrial myopathy, encephalopathy, lactic acidosis, and strokelike syndrome[85,86]

Angular gyrus syndrome: posterior aphasia, alexia, agraphia, and Gerstmann's syndrome can simulate Alzheimer's disease.[87]

Bilateral thalamic infarction[88-90]

Cardiac arrhythmias and systemic hypotension[91]

Psychiatric Disorders Associated with Dementia

Depression: although depression is the most common cause of pseudodementia, patients can be both depressed and demented.[92-95]

Schizophrenia-like psychoses: organic cerebral disorders occur in a substantial minority of patients diagnosed as schizophrenic.[96-98]

Mania[99]

Drugs Commonly Associated with Reversible Dementia[100]

Multiple drugs in combination may have more than an additive effect.[101]

Alcohol[102–105]

Bromides: found in nonprescription drugs likely to be used by the elderly

Antihistamines: scopolamine and atropine derivatives particularly

Anticonvulsants: phenytoin, phenobarbital, clonazepam, mephenytoin, valproic acid[106,107]

Phenothiazines: chlorpromazine, haloperidol, and fluphenazine

L-dopa: L-dopa toxicity in Parkinson's disease patients is sometimes missed because of presumed associated dementia with Parkinson's disease.

Lithium carbonate[108]

Propanolol hydrochloride

Disulfiram

Anticholinergics

Analgesics: opiates

Digitalis

Sedatives

Antidepressants

Infectious Causes of Dementia

Acquired immune deficiency syndrome (AIDS) dementia complex (AIDS encephalopathy): current evidence suggests direct retrovirus infection, prominent subcortical involvement, and increased risk for secondary central nervous system infections.[109–118]

Creutzfeldt-Jakob disease: rapidly progressive dementia with ataxia and myoclonus[119]

Progressive multifocal leukoencephalopathy (PML): papovavirus infection, usually associated with immunosuppression, recently increasingly diagnosed in the human immunodeficiency virus (HIV)-infected population. PML in the elderly can mimic a primary degenerative disorder causing dementia.[120–123]

Lyme disease: occasionally manifests with neurologic symptoms only, i.e., neuropathy, myelopathy, and encephalitis, without characteristic arthritis or erythema chronicum migrans[124]

Encephalitis: acute and chronic viral encephalitis, postinfectious encephalomyelitis[125]

Chronic meningitis: viral, fungal, mycobacterial, chemical, bacterial (see Section VII, Infectious Disease; Ch. 72)

Cerebral abscess
Neurosyphilis: seen more frequently in association
with HIV infection and sometimes resistant to
conventional therapy[126]
Parasitic: toxoplasmosis, particularly in HIV infections; diffuse cerebral cysticercosis[127-130]
Whipple's disease[131,132]

**Miscellaneous Causes
of Treatable and
Arrestable Dementia**

Primary cerebral tumors: primary central nervous
system lymphomas increasingly seen in younger
patients with HIV infection; meningiomas can be
a treatable cause of dementia in the elderly;
oligodendrogliomas[133-137]
Metastatic carcinoma[138]
Carcinomatosis: gliomatosis[139,140]
Paraneoplastic: limbic encephalitis[141]
Iatrogenic   leukoencephalopathy: antineoplastic
agents, radiation therapy[142,143]
Cardiopulmonary insufficiency[144]
Chronic renal failure and dialysis dementia[145,146]
Portal-systemic or hepatic encephalopathy[147]
Hematologic disorders: severe anemia, polycythemia
vera, multiple myeloma, pernicious anemia (B_{12}
deficiency)[148]
Head trauma: severe postconcussion syndrome, brain
injury of boxers[149,150]
Chronic subdural hematomas: trauma, spontaneous,
anticoagulant therapy
Wernicke's encephalopathy: although usually associated with alcoholism, consider this diagnosis in
patients with gastrointestinal disorders, such as
hyperemesis, status postgastroplasty, in poorly vitamin supplemented parenteral alimentation, and
dialysis.[151-153]
Other vitamin deficiencies: pernicious anemia (B_{12}
deficiency), folate deficiency, pellagra or nicotinic
acid deficiency[154-157]
Endocrinopathies: hyperthyroidism hypothyroidism,
adrenal and pituitary dysfunction, hyperparathyroidism, hypoparathyroidism, Cushing's syndrome,
Addison's disease[158-161]
Dehydration
Pheochromocytoma[162]
Chronic electrolyte abnormalities: hyponatremia, re-
current hypoglycemia, hypophosphatemia[163]
Porphyria
Hydrocephalus: important diagnostic possibility in

patients who develop a significant gait disorder in association with dementia; patients with Paget's disease and rheumatoid arthritis are at risk for developing normal pressure hydrocephalus, a rare secondary manifestation of spinal cord tumors[164–168]

Heavy metal intoxication: mercury, arsenic, lead, thallium, aluminum[169,170]

Industrial toxins: trichloroethylene, toluene, carbon disulfide, carbon monoxide, other organic solvents, and insecticides such as organophosphates[171,172]

Sarcoidosis[173]

Multiple sclerosis[174–177]

Hyperviscosity syndromes: multiple myeloma, macroglobulinemia, polycythemia, leukemia, and others[148,178]

Seizures disorders: nonconvulsive seizures can present as a clinical dementia; intellectual deterioration may occur with recurrent seizures[179,180]

References

1. American Psychiatric Association: Diagnostic and Statistical Manual of Mental Disorders. American Psychiatric Association, Washington DC, 1980.
2. Katzman R: Differential diagnosis of dementing illnesses. Neurol Clin 4:329, 1986.
3. Larson EB, Reifler BV, Featherstone HJ, et al: Dementia in elderly outpatients: a prospective study. Ann Intern Med 100:417, 1984.
4. Beck JC, Benson DF, Scheibel AB, et al: Dementia in the elderly: the silent epidemic (clinical conference). Ann Intern Med 97:231, 1982.
5. Whitehouse PJ: The concept of subcortical and cortical dementia: another look. Ann Neurol 19:1, 1986.
6. Huber SJ, Paulson GW: The concept of subcortical dementia. Am J Psychiatry 142:1312, 1985.
7. Cummings JL, Benson DF: Psychological dysfunction accompanying subcortical dementias. Annu Rev Med 39:53, 1988.
8. Cummings JL: Subcortical dementia. Neuropsychology, neuropsychiatry, and pathophysiology. Br J Psychiatry 149:682, 1986.
9. Cummings JL, Benson F: Subcortical dementia. Review of an emerging concept. Arch Neurol 41:874, 1984.
10. Katzman R: Alzheimer's disease. N Engl J Med 314:964, 1986.
11. Rocca WA: The etiology of Alzheimer's disease: epidemiologic contributions with emphasis on the genetic hypothesis. J Neural Transm 24(Suppl):3, 1987.
12. Chui HC, Teng EL, Henderson VW, et al: Clinical subtypes of dementia of the Alzheimer type. Neurology 35:1544, 1985.
13. Mayeux R, Stern Y, Spanton S: Heterogeneity in dementia of the Alzheimer type: evidence of subgroups. Neurology 35:453, 1985.

14. Black KS, Hughes PL: Alzheimer's disease: making the diagnosis. Am Fam Physician 36:196, 1987.
15. Cummings JL, Benson DF: Dementia of the Alzheimer type. An inventory of diagnostic clinical features. J Am Geriatr Soc 34:12, 1986.
16. Weiler PG: Risk factors associated with senile dementia of the Alzheimer's type. Am J Prev Med 2:297, 1986.
17. Wechsler AF, Verity A, Rosenschein S, et al: Pick's disease. A clinical, computed tomographic, and histologic study with Golgi impregnation observations. Arch Neurol 39:287, 1982.
18. Hansen LA, Deteresa R, Tobias H, et al: Neocortical morphometry and cholinergic neurochemistry in Pick's disease. Am J Pathol 131:507, 1988.
19. Kamo H, McGeer PL, Harrop R, et al: Positron emission tomography and histopathology in Pick's disease. Neurology 37:439, 1987.
20. Heston LL, White JA, Mastri AR: Pick's disease. Clinical genetics and natural history. Arch Gen Psychiatry 44:409, 1987.
21. Martin JB: Huntington's disease: new approaches to an old problem. Neurology 34:1059, 1984.
22. Martin JB, Gusella JF: Huntington's disease. Pathogenesis and management. N Engl J Med 315:1267, 1986.
23. Stewart JT: Huntington's disease. Am Fam Physician 37:105, 1988.
24. Larcher V: Chronic active hepatitis and related disorders. Clin Gastroenterol 15:173, 1986.
25. Prohaska JR: Genetic diseases of copper metabolism. Clin Physiol Biochem 4:87, 1986.
26. Starosta-Rubinstein S, Young AB, Kluin K, et al: Clinical assessment of 31 patients with Wilson's disease. Correlations with structural changes on magnetic resonance imaging. Arch Neurol 44:365, 1987.
27. Rosselli M, Lorenzana P, Rosselli A, Vergara I: Wilson's disease, a reversible dementia: case report. J Clin Exp Neuropsychol 9:399, 1987.
28. Medalia A, Isaacs-Glaberman K, Scheinberg IH: Neuropsychological impairment in Wilson's disease. Arch Neurol 45:502, 1988.
29. Taylor AE, Saint-Cyr JA, Lang AE: Idiopathic Parkinson's disease: revised concepts of cognitive and affective status. Can J Neurol Sci 15:106, 1988.
30. Chui HC, Mortimer JA, Slager U, et al: Pathologic correlates of dementia in Parkinson's disease. Arch Neurol 43:991, 1986.
31. Huber SJ, Shuttleworth EC, Paulson GW: Dementia in Parkinson's disease. Arch Neurol 43:987, 1986.
32. Forno LS: Lewy bodies (letter). N Engl J Med 314:122, 1986.
33. Cummings JL: The dementias of Parkinson's disease: prevalence, characteristics, neurobiology, and comparison with dementia of the Alzheimer type. Eur Neurol 28(Suppl):15, 1988.
34. Mayeux A, Stern Y, Rosenstein R, et al: An estimate of the prevalence of dementia in idiopathic Parkinson's disease. Arch Neurol 45:260, 1988.
35. Yoshimura M: Pathological basis for dementia in el-

derly patients with idiopathic Parkinson's disease. Eur Neurol 28(Suppl):29, 1988.

36. Girotti F, Soliveri P, Carella F, et al: Dementia and cognitive impairment in Parkinson's disease. J Neurol Neurosurg Psychiatry 51:1498, 1988.

37. Maher ER, Lees AJ: The clinical features and natural history of the Steele-Richardson-Olszewski syndrome (progressive supranuclear palsy). Neurology 36:1005, 1986.

38. Ambrosetto P: CT in progressive supranuclear palsy. AJNR 8:849, 1987.

39. Takahashi H, Takeda S, Ikuta F, Homma Y: Progressive supranuclear palsy with limbic system involvement: report of a case with ultrastructural investigation of neurofibrillary tangles in various locations. Clin Neuropathol 6:271, 1987.

40. Duvoisin RC, Golbe LI, Lepore FE: Progressive supranuclear palsy. Can J Neurol Sci 14(Suppl):547, 1987.

41. Sieradzan K, Kwiecinski H, Sawicka E: Progressive supranuclear palsy with lower motor neuron involvement. A case report. J Neurol 234:247, 1987.

42. Daroff RB: Progressive supranuclear palsy: a brief personalized history. Yale J Biol Med 60:119, 1987.

43. Schneider LS, Chui HC: Progressive supranuclear palsy manifesting with depressive features. J Am Geriatr Soc 34:663, 1986.

44. Eidelberg D, Sotrel A, Joachim C, et al: Adult onset Hallervorden-Spatz disease with neurofibrillary pathology. A discrete clinicopathological entity. Brain 110:993, 1987.

45. Popovitch ER, Wisniewski HM, Kaufman MA, et al: Young adult form of dementia with neurofibrillary changes and Lewy bodies. Acta Neuropathol 74:97, 1987.

46. Dickson DW, Davies P, Mayeux R, et al: Diffuse Lewy body disease. Neuropathological and biochemical studies of six patients. Acta Neuropathol 75:8, 1987.

47. Kosaka K, Yoshimura M, Ikeda K, Budka H: Diffuse type of Lewy body disease: progressive dementia with abundant cortical Lewy bodies and senile changes of varying degree—a new disease? Clin Neuropathol 3:185, 1984.

48. Brun A: Frontal lobe degeneration of non-Alzheimer type. I. Neuropathology. Arch Gerontol Geriat 6:193, 1987.

49. Gustafson L: Frontal lobe degeneration of non-Alzheimer type. II. Clinical picture and differential diagnosis. Arch Gerontol Geriatr 6:209, 1987.

50. Risberg J: Frontal lobe degeneration of non-Alzheimer type. III. Regional cerebral blood flow. Arch Gerontol Geriatr 6:225, 1987.

51. Englund E, Brun A: Frontal lobe degeneration of non-Alzheimer type. IV. White matter changes. Arch Gerontol Geriatr 6:235, 1987.

52. Pamphlett R, Silberstein P: Pelizaeus-Merzbacher disease in a brother and sister. Acta Neuropathol 69:343, 1986.

53. Yerby MS, Shaw CM, Watson JM: Progressive demen-

tia and epilepsy in a young adult: unusual intraneuronal inclusions. Neurology 36:68, 1986.

54. van Schrojenstein de Valk HM, van de Kamp JJ: Follow-up on seven adult patients with mild Sanfilippo B-disease. Am J Med Genet 28:125, 1987.

55. Kretzschmar HA, Berg BO, Davis RL: Giant axonal neuropathy. A neuropathological study. Acta Neuropathol 73:138, 1987.

56. Fisher NR, Cope SJ, Lishman WA: Metachromatic leukodystrophy: conduct disorder progressing to dementia. J Neurol Neurosurg Psychiatry 50:488, 1987.

57. Farlow MR, DeMyer W, Dlouhy SR, Hodes ME: X-linked recessive inheritance of ataxia and adult-onset dementia: clinical features and preliminary linkage analysis. Neurology 37:602, 1987.

58. Powers JM, Moser HW, Moser AB, et al: Pathologic findings in adrenoleukodystrophy heterozygotes. Arch Pathol Lab Med 111:151, 1987.

59. Takahashi H, Ohama E, Naito H, et al: Hereditary dentatorubral-pallidoluysian atrophy: clinical and pathologic variants in a family. Neurology 38:1065, 1988.

60. Gray F, Gherardi R, Marshall A, et al: Adult polyglucosan body disease (APBD). J Neuropathol Exp Neurol 47:459, 1988.

61. Berkovic SF, Carpenter S, Andermann F, et al: Kufs' disease: a critical reappraisal. Brain 111:27, 1988.

62. Katz DA, Naseem A, Horoupian DS, et al: Familial multisystem atrophy with possible thalamic dementia. Neurology 34:1213, 1984.

63. Harati Y, Jackson JA, Benjamin E: Adult onset idiopathic familial brain calcifications. Arch Intern Med 144:2425, 1984.

64. Reske-Nielsen E, Jensen PK, Hein-Srensen O, Abelskov K: Calcification of the central nervous system in a new hereditary neurological syndrome. Acta Neuropathol 75:590, 1988.

65. Trautner RJ, Cummings JL, Read SL, Benson DF: Idiopathic basal ganglia calcification and organic mood disorder. Am J Psychiatry 145:350, 1988.

66. Vilming ST, Dietrichson P, Isachsen MM, et al: Late-onset hereditary myopathy with abnormal mitochondria and progressive dementia. Acta Neurol Scand 73:502, 1986.

67. Munoz-Garcia D, Ludwin SK: Adult-onset neuronal intranuclear hyaline inclusion disease. Neurology 36:785, 1986.

68. Cummings JL: Multi-infarct dementia: diagnosis and management. Infarctions produce 20% to 35% of severe dementia cases. Psychosomatics 28:117, 1987.

69. Derix MM, Hijdra A, Verbeeten BW Jr: Mental changes in subcortical arteriosclerotic encephalopathy. Clin Neurol Neurosurg 89:71, 1987.

70. Loeb C: Clinical criteria for the diagnosis of vascular dementia. Eur Neurol 28:87, 1988.

71. Bogousslavsky J, Regli F, Uske A: Leukoencephalopathy in patients with ischemic stroke. Stroke 18:896, 1987.

72. Loeb C, Gandolfo C, Bino G: Intellectual impairment

and cerebral lesions in multiple cerebral infarcts. A clinical-computed tomography study. Stroke 19:560, 1988.

73. De Reuck J, Crevits L, De Coster W, et al: Pathogenesis of Binswanger chronic progressive subcortical encephalopathy. Neurology 30:920, 1980.

74. McQuinn BA, O'Leary DH: White matter lucencies on computed tomography, subacute arteriosclerotic encephalopathy (Binswanger's disease), and blood pressure. Stroke 18:900, 1987.

75. Garcia-Albea E, Cabello A, Franch O: Subcortical arteriosclerotic encephalopathy (Binswanger's disease): a report of five patients. Acta Neurol Scand 75:295, 1987.

76. Roman GC: Senile dementia of the Binswanger type. A vascular form of dementia in the elderly. JAMA 258:1782, 1987.

77. Cosgrove GR, Leblanc R, Meagher-Villemure K, et al: Cerebral amyloid angiopathy. Neurology 35:625, 1985.

78. Yamada M, Tsukagoshi H, Otomo E, Hayakawa M: Cerebral amyloid angiopathy in the aged. J Neurol 234:371, 1987.

79. Esiri MM, Wilcock GK: Cerebral amyloid angiopathy in dementia and old age. J Neurol Neurosurg Psychiatry 49:1221, 1986.

80. Mandybur TI: Cerebral amyloid angiopathy: the vascular pathology and complications. J Neuropathol Exp Neurol 45:79, 1986.

81. Asherson RA, Mercey D, Phillips G, et al: Recurrent stroke and multi-infarct dementia in systemic lupus erythematosus: association with antiphospholipid antibodies. Ann Rheum Dis 46:605, 1987.

82. Coull BM, Bourdette DN, Goodnight SH Jr, et al: Multiple cerebral infarctions and dementia associated with anticardiolipin antibodies. Stroke 18:1107, 1987.

83. Weisberg LA: The cranial computed tomographic findings in patients with neurologic manifestations of systemic lupus erythematosus. Comput Radiol 10:63, 1986.

84. Rothman SM, Fulling KH, Nelson JS: Sickle cell anemia and central nervous system infarction: a neuropathological study. Ann Neurol 20:684, 1986.

85. Mukoyama M, Kazui H, Sunohara N, et al: Mitochondrial myopathy, encephalopathy, lactic acidosis, and stroke-like episodes with acanthocytosis: a clinicopathological study of a unique case. J Neurol 233:228, 1986.

86. Sonninen V, Savontaus ML: Hereditary multi-infarct dementia. Eur Neurol 27:209, 1987.

87. Benson DF, Cummings JL, Tsai SY: Angular gyrus syndrome simulating Alzheimer's disease. Arch Neurol 39:616, 1982.

88. Bewermeyer H, Dreesbach HA, Rackl A, et al: Presentation of bilateral thalamic infarction on CT, MRI, and PET. Neuroradiology 27:414, 1985.

89. Katz DI, Alexander MP, Mandell AM: Dementia following strokes in the mesencephalon and diencephalon. Arch Neurol 44:1127, 1987.

90. Bogousslavsky J, Regli F, Uske A: Thalamic infarcts: clinical syndromes, etiology, and prognosis. Neurology 38:837, 1988.
91. Sulkava R, Erkinjuntti T: Vascular dementia due to cardiac arrhythmias and systemic hypotension. Acta Neurol Scand 76:123, 1987.
92. Reding M, Haycox J, Blass J: Depression in patients referred to a dementia clinic. Arch Neurol 42:894, 1985.
93. Addonizio B, Shamoian CA: Depression, dementia, and pseudodementia. Compr Ther 13:8, 1987.
94. Berrios GE: "Depressive pseudodementia" or "melancholic dementia": a 19th century view. J Neurol Neurosurg Psychiatry 48:393, 1985.
95. Alexopoulos GS, Young RC, Meyers BS, et al: Late-onset depression. Psychiatr Clin North Am 11:101, 1988.
96. Davison K: Schizophrenia-like psychoses associated with organic cerebral disorders: a review. Psychiatr Dev 1:1, 1983.
97. Goldberg TE, Weinberger DR, Berman KF, et al: Further evidence for dementia of the prefrontal type in schizophrenia? A controlled study of teaching the Wisconsin Card Sorting Test. Arch Gen Psychiatry 44:1008, 1987.
98. Lawson WB, Waldman IN, Weinberger DR: Schizophrenic dementia. Clinical and computed axial tomography correlates. J Nerv Ment Dis 176:207, 1988.
99. Casey DA, Fitzgerald BA: Mania and pseudodementia. J Clin Psychiatry 49:73, 1988.
100. Cummings J, Benson DF, LoVerme S Jr: Reversible dementia. Illustrative cases, definition, and review. JAMA 243:2434, 1980.
101. Consensus Conference. Differential diagnosis of dementing diseases. JAMA 258:3411, 1987.
102. Nakada T, Knight RT: Alcohol and the central nervous system. Med Clin North Am 68:121, 1984.
103. Lishman WA: Alcoholic dementia: a hypothesis. Lancet 1:1184, 1986.
104. Martin PR, Adinoff B, Weingartner H, et al: Alcoholic organic brain disease: nosology and pathophysiologic mechanisms. Prog Neuropsychopharmacol Biol Psychiatry 10:147, 1986.
105. Curtis JL, Millman EJ, Joseph M, et al: Prevalence rates for alcoholism, associated depression, and dementia on the Harlem Hospital Medicine and Surgery Services. Adv Alcohol Subst Abuse 6:45, 1986.
106. Thompson PJ, Trimble MR: Anticonvulsant drugs and cognitive functions. Epilepsia 23:531, 1982.
107. Zaret BS, Cohen RA: Reversible valproic acid-induced dementia: a case report. Epilepsia 27:234, 1986.
108. Smith SJ, Kocen RS: A Creutzfeldt-Jakob like syndrome due to lithium toxicity. J Neurol Neurosurg Psychiatry 51:120, 1988.
109. Price RW, Navia BA, Cho ES: AIDS encephalopathy. Neurol Clin 4:285, 1986.
110. Navia BA, Jordan BD, Price RW: The AIDS dementia complex: I. Clinical features. Ann Neurol 19:517, 1986.

111. Navia BA, Cho ES, Petito CK, et al: The AIDS dementia complex: II. Neuropathology. Ann Neurol 19:525, 1986.
112. Elder GA, Sever JL: Neurologic disorders associated with AIDS retroviral infection. Rev Infect Dis 10:286, 1988.
113. Gendelman HE, Leonard JM, Dutko F, et al: Immunopathogenesis of human immunodeficiency virus infection in the central nervous system. Ann Neurol 23(Suppl):S78, 1988.
114. Price RW, Brew B, Sidtis J, et al: The brain in AIDS: central nervous system HIV-1 infection and AIDS dementia complex. Science 239:586, 1988.
115. Beckett A, Summergrad P, Manschreck T, et al: Symptomatic HIV infection of the CNS in a patient without clinical evidence of immune deficiency. Am J Psychiatry 144:1342, 1987.
116. Gabuzda DH, Hirsch MS: Neurologic manifestations of infection with human immunodeficiency virus. Clinical features and pathogenesis. Ann Intern Med 107:383, 1987.
117. Price RW, Sidtis J, Rosenblum M: The AIDS dementia complex: some current questions. Ann Neurol 23(Suppl):S27, 1988.
118. McArthur JC: Neurologic manifestations of AIDS. Medicine 66:407, 1987.
119. Alter M, Sobel E: Creutzfeldt-Jakob disease. Neurol Clin 4:415, 1986.
120. Blum LW, Chambers RA, Schwartzman RJ, et al: Progressive multifocal leukoencephalopathy in acquired immune deficiency syndrome. Arch Neurol 42:137, 1985.
121. Krupp LB, Lipton RB, Swerdlow ML, et al: Progressive multifocal leukoencephalopathy: clinical and radiographic features. Ann Neurol 17:344, 1985.
122. Zochodne DW, Kaufmann JC: Prolonged progressive multifocal leukoencephalopathy without immunosuppression. Can J Neurol Sci 14:603, 1987.
123. Schlitt M, Morawetz RB, Bonnin J, et al: Progressive multifocal leukoencephalopathy: three patients diagnosed by brain biopsy, with prolonged survival in two. Neurosurgery 18:407, 1986.
124. Reik L Jr, Burgdorfer W, Donaldson JO: Neurologic abnormalities in Lyme disease without erythema chronicum migrans. Am J Med 81:73, 1986.
125. Peatfield RC: Basal ganglia damage and subcortical dementia after possible insidious Coxsackie virus encephalitis. Acta Neurol Scand 76:340, 1987.
126. Simon RP: Neurosyphilis. Arch Neurol 42:606, 1985.
127. Sandyk R, Bamford C, Iacono RP, Gillman MA: Cerebral cysticercosis presenting as progressive dementia. Int J Neurosci 35:251, 1987.
128. Torrealba G, Del Villar S, Tagle P, et al: Cysticercosis of the central nervous system: clinical and therapeutic considerations. J Neurol Neurosurg Psychiatry 47:784, 1984.
129. Wadia N, Desai S, Bhatt M: Disseminated cysticercosis. New observations, including CT scan findings and experience with treatment by praziquantel. Brain 111:597, 1988.

130. McCormick GF: Cysticercosis—review of 230 patients. Bull Clin Neurosci 50:76, 1985.
131. Halperin JJ, Landis DMD, Kleinman GM: Whipple disease of the nervous system. Neurology 32:612, 1982.
132. Ryser RJ, Locksley RM, Eng SC, et al: Reversal of dementia associated with Whipple's disease by tri-methoprim-sulfamethoxazole, drugs that penetrate the blood-brain barrier. Gastroenterology 86:745, 1984.
133. Bradshaw JR, Thomson JLG, Campbell MJ: Computed tomography in the investigation of dementia. Br Med J 286:277, 1983.
134. Vakili ST, Muller J, Shidnia H, Campbell RL: Primary lymphoma of the central nervous system: a clinico-pathologic analysis of 26 cases. J Surg Oncol 33:95, 1986.
135. Knight RS, Anslow P, Theaker JM: Neoplastic an-gioendotheliosis: a case of subacute dementia with unusual cerebral CT appearances and a review of the literature. J Neurol Neurosurg Psychiatry 50:1022, 1987.
136. Riisen H, Fossan GO: How shall we investigate de-mentia to exclude intracranial meningiomas as cause? An analysis of 34 patients with meningiomas. Age Ageing 15:29, 1986.
137. Ludwig CL, Smith MT, Godfrey AD, Armbrustmacher VW: A clinicopathological study of 323 patients with oligodendrogliomas. Ann Neurol 19:15, 1986.
138. Madow L, Alpers BJ: Encephalitic form of metastatic carcinoma. Arch Neurol Psychiatry 65:161, 1951.
139. Fischer-Williams M, Bosanquet FD, Daniel PM: Car-cinomatosis of the meninges: a report of 3 cases. Brain 78:42, 1955.
140. Dickson DW, Horoupian DS, Thal LJ, Lantos G: Gliomatosis cerebri presenting with hydrocephalus and dementia. AJNR 9:200, 1988.
141. Torack RM, Morris JC: Mesolimbocortical dementia. A clinicopathologic case study of a putative disorder. Arch Neurol 43:1074, 1986.
142. Hohwieler ML, Lo TC, Silverman ML, Freidberg SR: Brain necrosis after radiotherapy for primary intra-cerebral tumor. Neurosurgery 18:67, 1986.
143. Kuzuhara S, Ohkoshi N, Kanemaru K, et al: Subacute leucoencephalopathy induced by carmofur, a 5-fluo-rouracil derivative. J Neurol 234:365, 1987.
144. Grant I, Heaton RK, McSweeny AJ, et al: Neuropsy-chologic findings in hypoxemic chronic obstructive pulmonary disease. Arch Intern Med 142:1470, 1982.
145. English A, Savage RD, Britton PG, et al: Intellectual impairment in chronic renal failure. Br Med J 1:888, 1978.
146. Fraser CL, Arieff AI: Nervous system complications in uremia. Ann Intern Med 109:143, 1988.
147. Read AE, Sherlock S, Laidlaw J, et al: The neuro-psychiatric syndromes associated with chronic liver disease and an extensive portal-systemic collateral cir-culation. Q J Med 36:135, 1967.
148. Mueller J, Hotson JR, Langston JW: Hyperviscosity-induced dementia. Neurology 33:101, 1983.

149. Battalia JE, Aschenbrener CA, Bennett DR, et al: Brain injury in boxing. Council on Scientific Affairs. JAMA 249:254, 1983.
150. Violon A, De Mol J: Psychological sequelae after head traumas in adults. Acta Neurochir 85:96, 1987.
151. Oczkowski WJ, Kertesz A: Wernicke's encephalopathy after gastroplasty for morbid obesity. Neurology 35:99, 1985.
152. Reuler JB, Girard DE, Cooney TG: Wernicke's encephalopathy. N Engl J Med 312:1035, 1985.
153. Jagadha V, Deck JH, Halliday WC, Smyth HS: Wernicke's encephalopathy in patients on peritoneal dialysis or hemodialysis. Ann Neurol 21:78, 1987.
154. Hart RJ Jr, McCurdy PR: Psychosis in vitamin B_{12} deficiency. Arch Intern Med 128:596, 1971.
155. Strachan RW, Henderson JG: Dementia and folate deficiency. Q J Med 36:189, 1967.
156. Spivak JL, Jackson DL: Pellagra: an analysis of 18 patients and a review of the literature. Johns Hopkins Med J 140:295, 1977.
157. Aikawa H, Suzuki K: Lesions in the skin, intestine, and central nervous system induced by an antimetabolite of niacin. Am J Pathol 122:335, 1986.
158. Bulens C: Neurologic complications of hyperthyroidism. Remission of spastic paraplegia, dementia, and optic neuropathy. Arch Neurol 38:669, 1981.
159. de Fine Olivarius F, Roder E: Reversible psychosis and dementia in myxedema. Acta Psychiatr Scand 46:1, 1970.
160. Joborn C, Hetta J, Frisk P, et al: Primary hyperparathyroidism in patients with organic brain syndrome. Acta Med Scand 219:91, 1986.
161. Friedman JH, Chiucchini I, Tucci JR: Idiopathic hypoparathyroidism with extensive brain calcification and persistent neurologic dysfunction. Neurology 37:307, 1987.
162. White PD, Lishman WA, Wyke MA: Pheochromocytoma as a cause of reversible dementia. J Neurol Neurosurg Psychiatry 49:1449, 1986.
163. Vanneste J, Hage J: Acute severe hypophosphataemia mimicking Wernicke's encephalopathy (letter). Lancet 1:44, 1986.
164. Graff-Radford NR, Godersky JC: Normal-pressure hydrocephalus. Onset of gait abnormality before dementia predicts good surgical outcome. Arch Neurol 43:940, 1986.
165. Martin BJ, Roberts MA, Turner JW: Normal pressure hydrocephalus and Paget's disease of bone. Gerontology 31:397, 1985.
166. Rasker JJ, Jansen ENH, Haan J, et al: Normal-pressure hydrocephalus in rheumatic patients. A diagnostic pitfall. N Engl J Med 312:1239, 1985.
167. Kudo H, Tamaki N, Kim S, et al: Intraspinal tumors associated with hydrocephalus. Neurosurgery 21:726, 1987.
168. Feldmann E, Bromfield E, Navia B, et al: Hydrocephalic dementia and spinal cord tumor. Report of a case and review of the literature. Arch Neurol 43:714, 1986.
169. Reyes PF, Gonzalez CF, Zalewska MK, Besarab A:

Intracranial calcification in adults with chronic lead exposure. AJR 146:267, 1986.

170. Mayor GH, Burnatowska-Hledin M: The metabolism of aluminum and aluminum-related encephalopathy. Semin Nephrol 6(Suppl):1, 1986.
171. O'Flynn RR, Monkman SM, Waldron HA: Organic solvents and presenile dementia: a case referent study using death certificates. Br J Ind Med 44:259, 1987.
172. Gade A, Mortensen EL, Bruhn P: "Chronic painter's syndrome." A reanalysis of psychological test data in a group of diagnosed cases, based on comparisons with matched controls. Acta Neurol Scand 77:293, 1988.
173. Cordingley G, Navarro C, Brust JCM, et al: Sarcoidosis presenting as senile dementia. Neurology 31:1148, 1981.
174. Koenig H: Dementia associated with the benign form of multiple sclerosis. Trans Am Neurol Assoc 93:227, 1968.
175. Beatty WW, Goodkin DE, Monson N, et al: Anterograde and retrograde amnesia in patients with chronic progressive multiple sclerosis. Arch Neurol 45:611, 1988.
176. Huber SJ, Paulson GW, Shuttleworth EC, et al: Magnetic resonance imaging correlates of dementia in multiple sclerosis. Arch Neurol 44:732, 1987.
177. Rao SM: Neuropsychology of multiple sclerosis: a critical review. J Clin Exp Neuropsychol 8:503, 1986.
178. Lechner H, Ott E, Schmidt R: Present state of hemorrheology. Gerontology 33:259, 1987.
179. Dunne JW, Summers QA, Stewart-Wynne EG: Nonconvulsive status epilepticus: a prospective study in an adult general hospital. Q J Med 62:117, 1987.
180. Trimble MR: Cognitive hazards of seizure disorders. Epilepsia 29(Suppl):S19, 1988.

Selected Readings

Aharon-Peretz J, Cummings JL, Hill MA: Vascular dementia and dementia of the Alzheimer type. Cognition, ventricular size, and leuko-araiosis. Arch Neurol 45:719, 1988.

Ventricular size and amount of leuko-araiosis (LA) were compared in groups of patients with multi-infarct dementia (MID) and dementia of the Alzheimer type (DAT). Severity of LA was greater in patients with MID. Correlations with ventricular enlargement and severity of cognitive impairment appeared in patients with MID, but did not appear in patients with DAT.

Alafuzoff I, Iqbal K, Friden H, et al: Histopathological criteria for progressive dementia disorders: clinical-pathological correlation and classification by multivariate data analysis. Acta Neuropathol 74:209, 1987.

A histopathologic study of 55 autopsied brains from patients between 59 and 95 years of age was performed to establish histopathologic criteria for normal aging, Alzheimer's disease (AD), and multi-infarct dementia (MID). Senile/neuritic plaques, neurofibrillary tangles, microscopic infarcts, and perivascular serum protein deposits were quantified in the frontal lobe and hippocampus. Clinical dementias were classified according to DSM-III criteria. Au-

thors present evidence indicating that the pathogenesis of tangles and plaques in nondemented patients differs from the pathogenesis of tangles and plaques in patients with Alzheimer's disease.

Alexopoulos GS, Abrams RC, Young RC, Shamoian CA: Cornell Scale for Depression in Dementia. Biol Psychiatry 23:271, 1988.
The Cornell Scale for Depression in Dementia, a 19-item clinician-administered evaluation that uses interview-derived information from patients and nursing staff members, a test suitable for use in demented patients.

Barclay LL, Weiss EM, Mattis S, et al: Unrecognized cognitive impairment in cardiac rehabilitation patients. J Am Geriatr Soc 36:22, 1988.
Twenty clinically stable patients who were consecutively admitted to a cardiac rehabilitation service were evaluated to determine the prevalence of unrecognized brain dysfunction accompanying chronic severe cardiac disease. Multiple cognitive deficits were present in eight patients (40%), seven of whom were unable to reliably administer their own medications. Authors suggest patients with cardiac disease should undergo early cognitive evaluations.

Becker JT, Huff FJ, Nebes RD, et al: Neuropsychological function in Alzheimer's disease. Pattern of impairment and rates of progression. Arch Neurol 45:263, 1988.
Neuropsychological deficits in Alzheimer's disease include a wide clinical spectrum. From a clinical study of 86 patients with probable Alzheimer's disease and 92 elderly control subjects, certain patterns of neuropsychological impairment in the group of patients with Alzheimer's disease emerged.

Becker PM, Feussner JR, Mulrow CD, et al: The role of lumbar puncture in the evaluation of dementia: the Durham Veterans Admministration/Duke University study. J Am Geriatr Soc 33:392, 1985.
Indications for the use of lumbar puncture (LP) and cerebrospinal fluid (CSF) analysis in the routine, initial evaluation of patients with dementia are examined.

Benson DF, Davis RJ, Snyder BD: Posterior cortical atrophy. Arch Neurol 45:789, 1988.
Five patients with progressive dementia associated at onset with disorders of higher visual function are described. Predominant parieto-occipital atrophy was demonstrated on both CT and MRI in two patients. No pathologic specimens are available for study; however, authors speculate on underlying pathologic conditions, including atypical clinical variants of Alzheimer's disease, a lobar atrophy analogous to Pick's disease, or a previously unrecognized entity.

Chozick B: The nucleus basalis of Meynert in neurological dementing disease: a review. Int J Neurosci 37:31, 1987.
An overview of research and observations of pathologic alterations observed in the nucleus basalis of Meynert, which supplies the major cholinergic innervation of the cerebral cortex. Possible connections between these observations and several dementing neurologic disorders are discussed.

Consensus conference: Differential diagnosis of dementing diseases. JAMA 258:3411, 1987.
Important consensus review of definition, differential diagnosis, and indications for current diagnostic tests available. Priorities for future research on diagnosing dementia are summarized.

Creasey H, Schwartz M, Frederickson H, et al: Quantitative computed tomography in dementia of the Alzheimer type. Neurology 36:1563, 1986.
This study suggests that brain atrophy and ventricular dilatation are related to the severity of dementia.

Davison AN: Pathophysiology of ageing brain. Geronotology 33:129, 1987.
Current concepts of the pathophysiology of aging, which include neurochemical, neuropathologic, and genetic studies related to major neurodegenerative disorders.

Drayer BP: Imaging of the aging brain. Part II. Pathologic conditions. Radiology 166:797, 1988.
MRI of the elderly with a focus on findings in demented elderly are reviewed in this article. MRI findings that correlate clinically with Alzheimer's disease, parkinsonian disorders, and vascular dementias are described, as well as the role of imaging in excluding mass lesions, such as hematomas and neoplasms.

Erkinjuntti T: Differential diagnosis between Alzheimer's disease and vascular dementia: evaluation of common clinical methods. Acta Neurol Scand 76:433, 1987.
A prospective study evaluated consecutively admitted demented patients to evaluate conventional clinical methods in the differential diagnosis between Alzheimer's disease (AD) and vascular dementia. Radiographic evidence of infarction and ischemic scores appeared most useful in determining vascular dementia. Usefulness and limitations of neuropsychology, EEG, cerebral spinal fluid (CSF), and other laboratory investigations were discussed.

Erkinjuntti T, Sulkava R, Kovanen J, Palo J: Suspected dementia: evaluation of 323 consecutive referrals. Acta Neurol Scand 76:359, 1987.
An outpatient study of 323 consecutive referrals for suspected dementia found 135 (41.8%) not demented. Within the nondemented group, 44.1% had a potentially treatable cause for their cognitive symptoms (in 27.4%, it was depression). Of the total 188 patients considered demented (58.2%), 38.8% had primary degenerative and vascular dementias. Potentially treatable causes were found in 10.7% of all demented patients. Treatable causes included metabolic disorders, meningiomas, hydrocephalus, subdural hematomas, and depressive pseudodementia.

Folks DG, Freeman AM III, Sokol RS, et al: Cognitive dysfunction after coronary artery bypass surgery: a case-controlled study. South Med J 81:202, 1988.
Twenty-two patients screened from a sample of 391 patients undergoing coronary artery bypass grafting showed significant decline on the Mini-Mental State Examination, which was administered preoperatively and 4 days postoperatively. Twenty-two matched controls were compared. Among the multiple factors compared, outstanding predictors of increased risk for immediate postoperative cognitive dysfunction include preoperative depression and lower socioeconomic status.

Friedland RP, Koss E, Haxby JV, et al: NIH conference. Alzheimer disease: clinical and biological heterogeneity. Ann Intern Med 109:298, 1988.
An important review of emerging concepts of clinical and biologic characteristics of Alzheimer's disease. The heterogeneity of clinical, anatomic, and physiologic aspects of the disease has resulted in new definitions for several clinical subtypes of Alzheimer's disease based

on behavioral features, time course of progression, age of onset, and the presence or absence of motor deficits.

Gupta SR, Naheedy MH, Young JC, et al: Periventricular white matter changes and dementia. Clinical, neuropsychological, radiological, and pathological correlation. Arch Neurol 45:637, 1988.

Forty-three patients with CT findings of decreased attenuation in the periventricular white matter were studied. MRI correlations in seven patients and pathologic correlations in four patients were made. There was clinical evidence for hypertension in 36 (84%), cerebrovascular risk factors in 41 (95%), and neurologic deficits in 40 patients (93%). Neuropsychological evaluation of 27 patients suggested evidence of subcortical dementia. Pathologic features of these lesions were characterized as areas of infarction, demyelination, and diffuse arteriosclerosis.

Hadley DM, Teasdale GM: Magnetic resonance imaging of the brain and spine. J Neurol 235:193, 1988.

Current concepts and recommendations for clinicians able to choose between computed CT and MRI of the brain when evaluating common neurologic problems, including dementia. Measurement of cerebrospinal fluid volumes and dynamics by MRI is discussed. MRI has an advantage in diseases in which x-ray attenuation of suspected pathology differs slightly from normal parenchyma, such as early edema associated with infarction, infection, low-grade infiltrating neoplasms, and subacute and chronic hemorrhagic lesions of the spinal subarachnoid space and cord.

Hagberg B: Behaviour correlates to frontal lobe dysfunction. Arch Gerontol Geriatr 6:311, 1987.

A review of neuropsychological testing of frontal lobe dysfunction with an emphasis on evaluating cognitive abilities, such as sequences, abstractions, and estimations. Behavior manifestations attributed to the frontal lobe function are reviewed.

Harper CG, Giles M, Finlay-Jones R: Clinical signs in the Wernicke-Korsakoff complex: a retrospective analysis of 131 cases diagnosed at necropsy. J Neurol Neurosurg Psychiatry 49:341, 1986.

A recent necropsy study has shown that 80% of patients with the Wernicke-Korsakoff syndrome were not diagnosed as such during life; only 16% had the classic clinical triad and 19% had no documented clinical signs.

Harrell LE, Callaway R, Sekar BC: Magnetic resonance imaging and the diagnosis of dementia. Neurology 37:540, 1987.

Clinical study suggesting that MRI may be a sensitive way to differentiate multi-infarct dementia and primary degenerative dementia.

Horowitz GR: What is a complete work-up for dementia? Clin Geriatr Med 4:163, 1988.

A clinical discussion, from the perspective of a major geriatric center, about how to evaluate dementia.

Hyman RA, Gorey MT: Imaging strategies for MR of the brain. Radiol Clin North Am 26:471, 1988.

A useful clinical overview of emerging concepts of current indications for choosing MRI and CT when evaluating neurologic disorders. Authors suggest that MRI is the test of choice when evaluating dementia and certain other common neurologic disorders,

such as new-onset seizures, chronic headaches, progressive neurologic deficits, ataxia, vertigo, hearing loss, visual loss, and suspected
multiple sclerosis. CT, however, is the test of choice in emergency
situations and in patients with acute neurologic deficits, such as
stroke, acute onset of severe headaches, and when fine bone detail
is required.

Johnson KA, Davis KR, Buonanno FS, et al: Comparison
of magnetic resonance and roentgen ray computed tomography in dementia. Arch Neurol 44:1075, 1987.
*Merits of MRI and CT in assessing patients with dementia were
compared in 26 patients with Alzheimer's disease (AD), 8 patients
with vascular or mixed dementia, and 2 patients with Parkinson's
disease plus dementia. Subcortical white matter abnormalities, hip-
pocampal abnormalities, enlargement of basal and sylvian cisterns,
and ventriculomegaly were more evident on MRI than CT scans.
Periventricular white matter abnormalities identified on both MRI
and CT images correlated with severity of dementia.*

Jones EG: Neurotransmitters in the cerebral cortex. J
Neurosurg 65:135, 1986.
*A survey of neurotransmitters and modulatory neuropeptides
found in the cerebral cortex.*

Katzman R: Differential diagnosis of dementing illnesses.
Neurol Clin 4:329, 1986.
Useful clinical review.

Kiernan RJ, Mueller J, Langston JW, Van Dyke C: The
Neurobehavioral Cognitive Status Examination: a brief but
quantitative approach to cognitive assessment. Ann Intern
Med 107:481, 1987.
*Authors present a Neurobehavioral Cognitive Status Examina-
tion, a screening examination that assesses cognition in a brief, but
quantitative fashion. The test addresses levels of consciousness, ori-
entation, and attention by using independent tests to evaluate functioning within five major cognitive abilty areas: language, construction, memory, calculations, and reasoning. Cognitive profiles for
several neuropsychiatric disorders illustrate the clinical usefulness.*

Larson EB, Reifler BV, Sumi SM, et al: Diagnostic evaluation of 200 elderly outpatients with suspected dementia.
J Gerontol 40:536, 1985.
*A standardized diagnostic evaluation was performed on 200 con-
secutive patients over age 60 with suspected dementia; over 70%
had Alzheimer's-type dementia. The most common so-called treatable
illnesses were drug toxicity, hypothyroidism, and other metabolic diseases.*

LeMay M: CT changes in dementing diseases: a review.
AJR 147:963, 1986.
*Clinical summary of useful CT findings in dementing disorders.
CT is useful for identifying space-occupying lesions and for aiding
in the recognition of numerous neurodegenerative disorders.*

Lindenbaum J, Healton EB, Savage DG, et al: Neuropsychiatric disorders caused by cobalamin deficiency in the
absence of anemia or macrocytosis. N Engl J Med 318:1720,
1988.
*A study of 141 consecutive patients with neuropsychiatric ab-
normalities due to cobalamin deficiency found that 40 (28%) of
these patients were without anemia or macrocytosis. Most of these
patients benefited from cobalamin therapy, including improvement
in neuropsychiatric abnormalities. Authors conclude that neuro-*

psychiatric disorders due to cobalamin deficiency occur commonly in the absence of anemia or elevated mean cell volume and that measurements of serum methylmalonic acid and total homocysteine before and after treatment are useful in these patients.

Mahler ME, Cummings JL, Benson DF: Treatable dementias. West J Med 146:705, 1987.
Authors present dementia as a syndrome that may be produced by both irreversible and reversible conditions. Evaluation, causes, and management of treatment of reversible conditions are summarized in this useful review.

McGeer PL, Kamo H, Harrop R, et al: Comparison of PET, MRI, and CT with pathology in a proven case of Alzheimer's disease. Neurology 36:1569, 1986.
This study found positron emission tomography (PET) with fluorodeoxyglucose (FDG) a better measure of the severity of Alzheimer's disease than MRI or CT.

Morita K, Kaiya H, Ikeda T, Namba M: Presenile dementia combined with amyotrophy: a review of 34 Japanese cases. Arch Gerontol Geriatr 6:263, 1987.
Thirty-four cases of presenile dementia associated with amyotrophy from Japan are reported. Clinical, radiographic, neurophysiologic, and pathologic findings raise the possibility of a previously undescribed clinical entity that combines progressive dementia and an atypical spinal progressive muscular atrophy.

Neary D, Snowden JS, Northen B, Goulding P: Dementia of frontal lobe type. J Neurol Neurosurg Psychiatry 51:353, 1988.
Seven patients with dementia and a frontal lobe syndrome are described. Comparisons of this clinical picture and Alzheimer's patients found qualitative differences in clinical presentation, neurologic signs, psychological profile, electroencephalography, and PET studies. Authors suggest that dementia of frontal lobe type may represent forms of Pick's disease and may be more common than recognized.

O'Brien MD: Vascular dementia is underdiagnosed. Arch Neurol 45:797, 1988.

Brust JC: Vascular dementia is overdiagnosed. Arch Neurol 45:799, 1988.

Joynt RJ: Vascular dementia: too much, or too little? Arch Neurol 45:801, 1988.
Three-part, well-referenced, pithy series that addresses current concepts and controversies of vascular dementia.

Perl DP, Pendlebury WW: Neuropathology of dementia. Neurol Clin 4:355, 1986.
An overview of pathologic changes in several common disorders that cause dementia. Although the majority of the discussion is devoted to Alzheimer's disease and vascular or multi-infarct dementia, other less common disorders are summarized.

Petito CK: Review of central nervous system pathology in human immunodeficiency virus infection. Ann Neurol 23(Suppl):S54, 1988.
Review of major diseases of the central nervous system associated directly with HIV infection: aseptic meningitis, subacute encephalitis, and vacuolar myelopathy, with an emphasis on neuropathologic findings and clinical correlations.

Sulkava R, Viinikka L, Erkinjuntti T, Roine R: Cerebrospinal fluid neuron-specific enolase is decreased in multi-infarct dementia, but unchanged in Alzheimer's disease. J Neurol Neurosurg Psychiatry 51:549, 1988.

This clinical study supports the opinion that vascular dementia is caused by multiple infarcts and not continuous neuronal ischemia. Cerebrospinal fluid (CSF) neuron-specific enolase (NSE) levels were compared in 22 patients with probable Alzheimer's disease, 35 patients with multi-infarct dementia, and 15 controls. Levels of CSF NSE were lower in patients with multi-infarct dementia without recent vascular events when compared with controls and patients with Alzheimer's disease.

Thal LJ: Dementia update: diagnosis and neuropsychiatric aspects. J Clin Psychiatry 49(Suppl):5, 1988.

Current concepts of neuropsychiatric aspects of dementia. Authors stress that delusions are common in the early phase of Alzheimer's disease.

Thal LJ, Grundman M, Klauber MR: Dementia: characteristics of a referral population and factors associated with progression. Neurology 38:1083, 1988.

Three hundred seventy-five patients who presented with memory loss were evaluated. Diagnoses included senile dementia of Alzheimer's type (SDAT) in 70%, vascular dementia in 5%, mixed (SDAT and vascular) in 9%, and other etiologies in 16%. Clinical features more prominent in vascular dementia than SDAT included incontinence, transient symptoms, gait disturbances, bradykinesia, and pyramidal tract findings. In patients with SDAT, rate of progression of dementia (15 to 55 months) varied inversely with the duration of symptoms at presentation, which may suggest that in this groups of patients, more time may elapse before family or patient recognizes need for medical attention.

Thomsen AM, Brgesen SE, Bruhn P, Gjerris F: Prognosis of dementia in normal-presure hydrocephalus after a shunt operation. Ann Neurol 20:304, 1986.

Forty patients with normal-pressure hydrocephalus (NPH) were examined before and 12 months after ventriculoatrial shunt placement for treatment of NPH. Clinical outcome depended on patient selection. Improvement of cognitive function was seen when three or more of the following preoperative signs were present: known cause, short history, low cerebrospinal fluid outflow, small sulci, and/ or periventricular CT-identified hypodensity.

Torres F, Hutton JT: Clinical neurophysiology of dementia. Neurol Clin 4:369, 1986.

An overview of indications, usefulness, and limitations of clinical neurophysiology in the evaluation of dementia. EEG is useful for differentiation of Alzheimer's type from other treatable dementias and from multi-infarct dementia. Tests of ocular smooth pursuit correlate with severity of dementia in Alzheimer's patients, which may help distinguish them from normal elderly subjects and patients with depression manifesting as pseudodementia. Indications for event-related and sensory evoked potentials are discussed.

Vinters HV, Miller BL, Pardridge WM: Brain amyloid and Alzheimer disease (clinical conference). Ann Intern Med 109:41, 1988.

A review of clinicopathologic features of Alzheimer's disease with a particular focus on lesions with staining properties of amyloid, senile plaque cores, and amyloid angiopathy. Current ideas relating these findings to possible causes and potential treatments are discussed.

46
Excessive Somnolence: Common and Less Common Causes

Disorders of excessive somnolence include a variety of conditions in which the chief complaint is excessive or inappropriate sleepiness that must be initially distinguished from the normal physiologic response to physical fatigue or sleep deprivation. Symptoms of disorders of excessive somnolence (DOES) include excessive napping, difficulty in achieving full arousal on awakening, headache, decreased cognitive and motor performance, and often, complaints of falling asleep quickly in the waking state, particularly when sedentary.[1,2] Sometimes patients will describe episodic, sudden, irresistible sleepiness or "sleep attacks," which may even sound like fainting, blackout spells, or seizure variants[3]. "Sleep attacks" can be objectively measured by the multiple sleep latency test (MLST), which quantifies daytime sleep tendencies.[4] Polysomnography, however, is usually necessary to diagnose two of the most common disorders of excessive somnolence: sleep apnea and narcolepsy.[5–8] Sleep apnea disorders can manifest with a wide variety of symptoms, ranging from annoying snoring to significant cardiorespiratory insufficiency. Occasionally, recent or subacute onset excessive sleepiness can be the first manifestation of an underlying infection, drug effect, or toxic-metabolic-induced encephalopathy.

Obstructive sleep apnea: typical patient is an obese, middle-aged male with a long history of snoring and systemic hypertension; in younger patients, craniofacial anomalies and tonsillar and adenoid hypertrophy may be the cause of obstruction.[9–13]

Obesity: hypoventilation syndrome[14]

Central sleep apnea: characterized by apneic episodes during sleep that are without respiratory effort[15]

Mixed or complex sleep apnea: combination central and obstructive sleep apnea

Narcolepsy: characteristic symptoms include excessive daytime sleepiness, cataplexy, sleep paralysis, and hypnogogic hallucinations. There is a high correlation with HLA-DR2-antigen and narcolepsy. The diagnosis usually requires all-night polysomnography and a daytime multiple sleep latency test.[16-19]

Idiopathic hypersomnolence: can clinically mimic sleep apnea and/or narcolepsy, but is without rapid eye movement (REM) sleep-related symptoms associated with narcolepsy and can be distinguished from sleep apnea by polysomnography[20,21]

Sleep-related myoclonus (nocturnal myoclonus): patients are often unaware of the nocturnal leg jerks causing nocturnal awakenings; symptoms are often first reported by sleeping partner.[22]

Drug-induced: drug-alcohol dependency, excessive sedative usage

Psychiatric conditions leading to transient hypersomnia: reactive depression, acute stress[23-26]

Bipolar disorders

Menstruation-linked periodic hypersomnia: may be linked to ovulatory menstruation[27]

Postconcussive syndrome: often associated with headaches and symptoms that resemble cataplexy[28]

Kleine-Levin syndrome: characterized by hyperphagia, agressive behavior, and hypersomnolence[29-33]

Encephalopathies: infectious, metabolic-toxic, drug-induced, endocrinopathies (hypothyroidism), and multiple possible underlying medical conditions, particularly if associated with cardiac, renal, or hepatic insufficiency

Third ventricle tumors: somnolence can be intermittent with third ventricular colloid cysts, or symptoms can be progressive with slow-growing tumors.[34]

Ventricular shunt malformation[35]

Thalamic and hypothalamic lesions: infarctions, tumors, genetically determined degeneration, infections, sarcoidosis[36-40]

Paramedian diencephalic syndrome: clinical triad of hypersomnolent apathy, amnesic syndrome, and impaired vertical gaze in patients with bilateral diencephalic infarctions[41,42]

Nocturnal epilepsy-related sleep disorder: nocturnal epileptic seizures arouse patients causing daytime hypersomnolence.[43]

References

1. Sleep Disorders Classification Committee: DOES: disorders of excessive somnolence. Sleep 2:58, 1979.
2. Sleep Disorders Classification Committee: DIMS: disorders of initiating and maintaining sleep (insomnias). Sleep 2:21, 1979.
3. Baker TL: Introduction to sleep and sleep disorders. Med Clin North Am 69:1123, 1985.
4. Richardson GS, Carskadon MA, Flagg W, et al: Excessive daytime sleepiness in man: multiple sleep latency measurement in narcoleptic and control subjects. Electroencephalogr Clin Neuropysiol 45:621, 1978.
5. Baker TL, Guilleminault C, Nino-Murcia G, Dement WC: Comparative polysomnographic study of narcolepsy and idiopathic central nervous system hypersomnia. Sleep 9:232, 1986.
6. Coleman RM, Roffwarg HP, Kennedy SJ, et al: Sleep-wake disorders based on a polysomnographic diagnosis. JAMA 247:997, 1982.
7. Guilleminault C: Disorders of excessive sleepiness. Ann Clin Res 17:209, 1985.
8. Orr WC: Utilization of polysomnography in the assessment of sleep disorders. Med Clin North Am 69:1153, 1985.
9. Bradley TD, Phillipson EA: Pathogenesis and pathophysiology of the obstructive sleep apnea syndrome. Med Clin North Am 69:1169, 1985.
10. Guilleminault C: Obstructive sleep apnea. Med Clin North Am 69:1187, 1985.
11. Pollak PT, Vincken W, Munro IR, Cosio MG: Obstructive sleep apnea caused by hemarthrosis-induced micrognathia. Eur J Respir Dis 70:117, 1987.
12. Seggev J, Shapiro MS, Levin S, Schey G: Alveolar hypoventilation and daytime hypersomnia in acromegaly. Eur J Respir Dis 68:381, 1986.
13. Hess CW, Sauter K, Bonfils P: Severe adult hypersomnia—sleep apnea syndrome in craniofacial dysostosis. Respiration 50:147, 1986.
14. Wittels EH: Obesity and hormonal factors in sleep and sleep apnea. Med Clin North Am 69:1265, 1985.
15. White DP: Central sleep apnea. Med Clin North Am 69:1205, 1985.
16. Guilleminault C: Narcolepsy 1985. Sleep 9:99, 1986.
17. Kramer RE, Dinner DS, Braun WE, et al: HLA-DR2 and narcolepsy. Arch Neurol 44:853, 1987.
18. Honda Y, Juji T, Matsuki K, et al: HLA-DR2 and Dw2 in narcolepsy and in other disorders of excessive somnolence without cataplexy. Sleep 9:133, 1986.
19. Poirier G, Montplaisir J, Decary F, et al: HLA antigens in narcolepsy and idiopathic central nervous system hypersomnolence. Sleep 9:153, 1986.
20. Guilleminault C, Faull KF: Sleepiness in nonnarcoleptic, non-sleep apneic EDS patients: the idiopathic CNS hypersomnolence. Sleep 5 (Suppl):S175, 1982.
21. Matsunaga H: Clinical study on idiopathic CNS hypersomnolence. Jpn J Psychiatry Neurol 41:637, 1987.
22. Ohanna N, Peled R, Rubin AHE, et al: Periodic leg movements in sleep: effect of clonazepam treatment. Neurology 35:408, 1985.

23. Hawkins DR, Taub JM, Van de Castle RL: Extended sleep (hypersomnia) in young depressed patients. Am J Psychiatry 142:905, 1985.
24. Greenberg GD, Watson RK, Deptula D: Neuropsychological dysfunction in sleep apnea. Sleep 10:254, 1987.
25. Silberman EK, Sullivan JL: Atypical depression. Psychiatr Clin North Am 7:535, 1984.
26. Ryan ND, Puig-Antich J, Ambrosini P, et al: The clinical picture of major depression in children and adolescents. Arch Gen Psychiatry 44:854, 1987.
27. Sachs C, Persson HE, Hagenfeldt K: Menstruation-related periodic hypersomnia: a case study with successful treatment. Neurology 32:1376, 1982.
28. Guilleminault C, Faull KF, Miles L, et al: Posttraumatic excessive daytime sleepiness: a review of 20 patients. Neurology 33:1584, 1983.
29. Carpenter S, Yassa R, Ochs R: A pathologic basis for Kleine-Levin syndrome. Arch Neurol 39:25, 1982.
30. Striano S, Bilo L, Meo R: An unusual case of Kleine-Levin syndrome associated with sleep terrors. Electroencephalogr Clin Neurophysiol 64:517, 1986.
31. Drake ME Jr: Kleine-Levin syndrome after multiple cerebral infarctions. Psychosomatics 28:329, 1987.
32. Gillberg C: Kleine-Levin syndrome: unrecognized diagnosis in adolescent psychiatry. J Am Acad Child Adolesc Psychiatry 26:793, 1987.
33. Gadoth N, Dickerman Z, Bechar M, et al: Episodic hormone secretion during sleep in Kleine-Levin syndrome: evidence for hypothalamic dysfunction. Brain Dev 9:309, 1987.
34. Beal MF, Kleinman GM, Ojemann RG, et al: Gangliocytoma of third ventricle: hyperphagia, somnolence, and dementia. Neurology 31:1224, 1981.
35. Korfali E, Aksoy K, Safi I: Slit ventricle syndrome presenting with paroxysmal hypersomnia in an adult: case report. Neurosurgery 22:594, 1988.
36. Rubinstein I, Gray TA, Moldofsky H, Hoffstein V: Neurosarcoidosis associated with hypersomnolence treated with corticosteroids and brain irradiation. Chest 94:205, 1988.
37. Gentilini M, De Renzi E, Crisi G: Bilateral paramedian thalamic artery infarcts: report of eight cases. J Neurol Neurosurg Psychiatry 50:900, 1987.
38. Guberman A, Stuss D: The syndrome of bilateral paramedian thalamic infarction. Neurology 33:540, 1983.
39. Kotagal S, Archer CR, Walsh JK, et al: Hypersomnia, bithalamic lesions, and altered sleep architecture in Kearns-Sayre syndrome. Neurology 35:574, 1985.
40. Lugaresi E, Medori R, Montagna P, et al: Fatal familial insomnia and dysautonomia with selective degeneration of thalamic nuclei. N Engl J Med 315:997, 1986.
41. Meissner I, Sapir S, Kokmen E, Stein SD: The paramedian diencephalic syndrome: a dynamic phenomenon. Stroke 18:380, 1987.
42. Biller J, Sand JJ, Corbett JJ, et al: Syndrome of the paramedian thalamic arteries: clinical and neuroimaging correlation. J Clin Neuro Ophthalmol 5:217, 1985.
43. Peled R, Lavie P: Paroxysmal awakenings from sleep associated with excessive daytime somnolence: a form of nocturnal epilepsy. Neurology 36:95, 1986.

Selected Readings

Bannerman C: Sleep disorders in the later years. Postgrad Med 84(1):265, 1988.
Practical, clinical review of sleep disorders presenting in the elderly. A review of age-related sleep changes, as well as current concepts of management and evaluation of complaints of insomnia and hypersomnia in the elderly.

Garvey MJ, Wesner R, Godes M: Comparison of seasonal and nonseasonal affective disorders. Am J Psychiatry 145:100, 1988.
Eighteen patients with seasonal affective disorders were compared to 13 patients with recurrent nonseasonal depressions in this clinical study. Hypersomnia and carbohydrate craving were associated with seasonal depressions.

Guilleminault C, Dement WC: Sleep apnea syndromes. In Guilleminault C, Dement W (eds): Conference on Sleep Apnea Syndromes. Alan R Liss, New York, 1978.
Clinical symposium covering sleep apnea syndromes.

Guilleminault C, Lugaresi E (eds): Sleep/Wake Disorders: Natural History, Epidemiology, and Long-Term Evolution. Raven Press, New York, 1983.
Text includes previously unpublished studies of various clinical aspects of sleep disorders.

Guilleminault C, Mondini S: Mononucleosis and chronic daytime sleepiness. A long-term follow-up study. Arch Intern Med 146:1333, 1986.
Twelve patients between ages 14 and 26 years of age, 10 with infectious mononucleosis and 2 with Guillain-Barré syndrome, developed daytime hypersomnolence. All were suspected of having Epstein-Barr viral infection. Patients have been followed for 3 to 12 years and all have disabling daytime sleepiness.

Orr WC: Utilization of polysomnography in the assessment of sleep disorders. Med Clin North Am 69:1153, 1985.
Useful clinical discussion of the utility of polysomnography in sleep disorders.

Roth B, Nevsimalova S, Sonka K, Docekal P: An alternative to the multiple sleep latency test for determining sleepiness in narcolepsy and hypersomnia: polygraphic score of sleepiness. Sleep 9:243, 1986.
Authors present an alternative technique for quantitative assessment of pathologic diurnal sleepiness. Using this technique, three groups of patients with excessive daytime somnolence are studied: narcoleptic patients, idiopathic hypersomniacs, and sleep apnea ptients.

Sink J, Bliwise DL, Dement WC: Self-reported excessive daytime somnolence and impaired respiration in sleep. Chest 90:177, 1986.
A clinical study to determine which measures of impaired respiration in sleep relate to self-reported excessive daytime somnolence. Authors evaluated 37 elderly clinic patients with symptoms of snoring, a clinical diagnosis of sleep apnea, and varying degrees of self-reported somnolence. When obesity was controlled, results of this study showed a subgroup of somnolent patients who were characterized by more severe oxygen desaturations.

47

Seizures: Major Causes of New Onset Seizures and Epilepsy Presenting at Different Ages*

A new onset seizure can be the initial manifestation of a wide range of obvious or unsuspected conditions, such as genetic influences, trauma, stroke, infection, metabolic disorders, drug abuse, or neoplasia. Seizures are considered epileptic seizures if they are recurrent. Seizure types and epilepsies are classified by clinical characteristics and EEG patterns. Current classification of seizures and epilepsies have significant diagnostic, prognostic, and management implications.[2-5] The major classification distinction is between seizures that generalize (generalized seizures) and seizures that are focal in onset (focal seizures). Both generalized and focal seizures occur with or without loss or disturbance of consciousness. Generalized seizures imply bihemispheric involvement and are manifested by bilateral EEG and clinical signs. A new onset tonic-clonic seizure (grand mal seizure) secondary to alcohol withdrawal is an example of a generalized seizure that is not epileptic.[6] Focal seizures imply onset in one hemisphere and can secondarily generalize. A new onset focal seizure may be a first manifestation of an underlying focal cerebral disorder; therefore, a new onset focal seizure in an adult is an indication for immediate evaluation for cerebral disorders such as meningitis, encephalitis, tumors, or hemorrhage. The underlying focal pathology will determine whether the focal seizure will become recurrent or epileptic. When a first generalized or focal seizure occurs in a clinical setting that does not provide obvious clues, mimics of seizures, such as syncope, pseudoseizures, and transient is-

---

* (Text from Marsden,[1] with permission.)

chemic attacks, need to be ruled out.[7-11] Knowledge of the causes of seizures presenting at different ages can help narrow the wide spectrum of possible underlying causes of a new onset seizure.

Neonate: First Month[12,13]

Birth injury
  Anoxia[14]
  Hemorrhage: focal motor seizures may herald a stroke.[15,16]
Congenital abnormalities: tuberous sclerosis, neurofibromatosis[17,18]
Metabolic disorders: hypoglycemia, hypocalcemia, pyridoxine deficiency, amino acid abnormalities, kernicterus, hypomagnesemia[19]
Intrauterine infection: cytomegalic virus, toxoplasmosis
Meningitis (see Section VII, Infectious Disease, Ch. 71)
  Bacterial: *Escherichia coli* and group B streptococci most common bacterial causes of meningitis in the neonate
Encephalitis: viral, herpes simplex
Drug withdrawal: neonates born to drug-abusing or alcoholic mothers
Occult neonatal seizures[20]

Infancy: 1 to 6 Months

Causes as in neonate
Infantile spasm[21,22]
Brain tumors[23]

Early Childhood: 6 Months to 3 Years

Febrile seizures: usually occurs between 3 months and 5 years of age without evidence of intracranial infection or determined cause[24-28]
Birth injury
Meningitis (see Section VII, Infectious Disease, Ch. 71): *Haemophilus influenzae*, Neisseria meningitis,[29] viral infections, herpes simplex
Miscellaneous infections: acquired immune deficiency syndrome (AIDS)[30]
Trauma
Poisons: lead
Metabolic-endocrine disorders: diabetes, adrenal insufficiency
Cerebral degeneration

Childhood and Adolescence

Idiopathic or primary epilepsy
  Absence (petit mal)[31-36]
  Rolandic epilepsy[37,38]
  Benign myoclonic epilepsy of childhood and adolescence[39,40]
  Benign focal epilepsy of childhood[41,42]
  Periodic spasms[43]
Birth injury
Trauma
Infection (see Section VII, Infectious Disease, Ch. 71): *Haemophilus influenzae,* pneumococcus, meningococcus, viral infections, herpes simplex
Cerebral degenerations
Cardiovascular abnormalities: prolonged QT syndrome[44]
Drug and alcohol-induced
Toxins: lead poisoning, insecticides, herbicides[45]
Occult intracranial vascular malformations[46]

Early Adult Life

Trauma: risk factors that increase the risk of post-traumatic epilepsy include dura penetration, prolonged amnesia, focal neurologic signs, and depressed skull fracture.[47]
Tumor: tumors that most often cause epilepsy include oligodendrogliomas, astrocytomas, meningiomas, and metastatic carcinoma.[48]
Idiopathic or primary epilepsy
Birth injury
Infection (see Section VII, Infectious Disease, Ch. 71)
  Viral: herpes simplex encephalitis
  Bacterial: *Streptococcus pneumoniae*
  Opportunistic infections: consider in human immunodeficiency virus (HIV) high-risk patients
Intracranial vascular malformations: new onset seizures with headache may herald a subarachnoid hemorrhage.[49]
Cerebral degeneration
Drug and alcohol-induced: cocaine, alcohol (see below Later Adult Life: Drug-induced)[50,51]
Metabolic-endocrine disorders: diabetes; pregnancy; hypoglycemia, hyponatremia, hypomagnesemia and hypophosphatemia (often in alcoholics)[52-54]
Systemic disorders: collagen vascular disorders, cardiopulmonary, renal, hepatic insufficiency, porphyria[55]
Arrhythmogenic seizures[56]
Multiple sclerosis

Later Adult Life: After Age 60[57]

Vascular disease: cerebrovascular disease is the most common cause of epilepsy that first develops after age 50; acute and chronic cortical infarctions are a risk for seizures.[48,58–60]

Cerebral degenerations

Fluid and electrolyte disorders: hyponatremia (often drug-induced in the elderly), hypernatremia, hypomagnesemia, hypophosphatemia, hypoglycemia, hypercalcemia, hypocalcemia[55]

Trauma: chronic and acute subdural hematomas

Tumors: primary and metastatic tumors; carcinomatous meningitis[61]

Drug-induced: drugs which commonly cause drug-induced seizures include isoniazid, insulin, lidocaine, psychotropic medications, theophylline, antibiotics, general and local anesthetics, antineoplastic agents, anticonvulsants.[62–69]

Drug withdrawal: tonic-clonic or focal seizures in the elderly may reflect drug withdrawal[70]

Endocrine disorders: a partial seizure (epilepsia partialis) can be the initial manifestation of adult-onset diabetes with elevated serum glucose.

Systemic disorders: cardiopulmonary, hepatic, and renal insufficiency[55]

Infection (see Section VII, Infectious Disease, Ch. 71): bacterial meningitis often secondary to sepsis and/or urinary tract infections; consider mycobacterial meningitis in nursing home patients and elderly patients with a history of previous tuberculosis infection[71]

References

1. Marsden CD, Reynolds EH: Neurology. p. 116. In Laidlaw J, Richens A (eds): A Textbook of Epilepsy, 2nd Ed. Churchill Livingstone, Edinburgh, 1982.
2. Bancaud J, Henriksen O, Rubio-Donnadieu F, et al: Proposal for revised clinical and electroencephalographic classification of epileptic seizures. Epilepsia 22:489, 1981.
3. Wilder BJ, Schmidt RP: Current classification of epilepsies. Postgrad Med 77(4):188, 1985.
4. Porter RJ: Recognizing and classifying epileptic seizures and epileptic syndromes. Neurol Clin 4:495, 1986.
5. Gumnit RJ: Diagnostic difficulties and treatment implications. Epilepsia 28(Suppl):S9, 1987.
6. Morris JC, Victor M: Alcohol withdrawal seizures. Emerg Med Clin North Am 5:827, 1987.
7. Dohrmann ML, Cheitlin MD: Cardiogenic syncope. Seizure versus syncope. Neurol Clin 4:549, 1986.
8. Trimble MR: Pseudoseizures. Neurol Clin 4:531, 1986.

9. Gumnit RJ, Gates JR: Psychogenic seizures. Epilepsia 27(Suppl):S124, 1986.
10. Keranen T, Sillanpaa M, Riekkinen PJ: Distribution of seizure types in an epileptic population. Epilepsia 29:1, 1988.
11. Vining EP, Freeman JM: Seizures which are not epilepsy. Pediatr Ann 14:711, 1985.
12. Painter MJ, Bergman I, Crumrine P: Neonatal seizures. Pediatr Clin North Am 33:91, 1986.
13. Mizrahi EM, Kellaway P: Characterization and classification of neonatal seizures. Neurology 37:1837, 1987.
14. Bergamasco B, Benna P, Ferrero P, et al: Neonatal hypoxia and epileptic risk: a clinical prospective study. Epilepsia 25:131, 1984.
15. Ment LR, Freedman RM, Enrenkranz RA: Neonates with seizures attributable to perinatal complications: computed tomographic evaluation. Am J Dis Child 136:548, 1982.
16. Clancy R, Malin S, Laraque D, et al: Focal motor seizures heralding stroke in full-term neonates. Am J Dis Child 139:601, 1985.
17. Yamamoto N, Watanabe K, Negoro T, et al: Long-term prognosis of tuberous sclerosis with epilepsy in children. Brain Dev 9:292, 1987.
18. Riccardi VM: Neurofibromatosis. Neurol Clin 5:337, 1987.
19. LaFranchi S: Hypoglycemia of infancy and childhood. Pediatr Clin North Am 34:961, 1987.
20. Clancy RR, Legido A, Lewis D: Occult neonatal seizures. Epilepsia 29:256, 1988.
21. Cruse RP: Infantile spasms. Cleve Clin Q 51:273, 1984.
22. Spink DC, Snead OC III, Swann JW, Martin DL: Free amino acids in cerebrospinal fluid from patients with infantile spasms. Epilepsia 29:300, 1988.
23. Rutledge SL, Snead OC III, Morawetz R, Chandra-Sekar B: Brain tumors presenting as a seizure disorder in infants. J Child Neurol 2:214, 1987.
24. Erenberg G: Febrile convulsions: a new look at an old problem. Cleve Clin Q 51:279, 1984.
25. Summary of an NIH consensus statement. Febrile seizures: long-term management of children with fever-associated seizures. Br Med J 281:277, 1980.
26. Kaplan RE: Febrile seizures. When is treatment justified? Postgrad Med 82(5):63, 1987.
27. Rosman NP: Febrile seizures. Emerg Med Clin North Am 5:719, 1987.
28. Wright SW: The child with febrile seizures. Am Fam Physician 36(5):163, 1987.
29. Kaplan SL, Fishman MA: Update on bacterial meningitis. J Child Neurol 3:82, 1988.
30. Biggemann B, Voit T, Neuen E, et al: Neurological manifestations in three German children with AIDS. Neuropediatrics 18:99, 1987.
31. Penry JK: Diagnosis and treatment of absence seizures. Cleve Clin Q 51:283, 1984.
32. Rocca WA, Sharbrough FW, Hauser WA, et al: Risk factors for absence seizures: a population-based case-control study in Rochester, Minnesota. Neurology 37:1309, 1987.

33. Mirsky AF, Duncan CC, Myslobodsky MS: Petit mal epilepsy: a review and integration of recent information. J Clin Neurophysiol 3:179, 1986.
34. Holmes GL, McKeever M, Adamson M: Absence seizures in children: clinical and electroencephalographic features. Ann Neurol 21:268, 1987.
35. Dieterich E, Baier WK, Doose H, et al: Longterm follow-up of childhood epilepsy with absences. I. Epilepsy with absences at onset. Neuropediatrics 16:149, 1985.
36. Dieterich E, Doose H, Baier WK, Fichsel H: Longterm follow-up of childhood epilepsy with absences. II. Absence-epilepsy with initial grand mal. Neuropediatrics 16:155, 1985.
37. Loiseau P, Pestre M, Dartigues JF, et al: Long-term prognosis in two forms of childhood epilepsy: typical absence seizures and epilepsy with rolandic (centrotemporal) EEG foci. Ann Neurol 13:642, 1983.
38. Loiseau P, Duche B, Cordova S, et al: Prognosis of benign childhood epilepsy with centrotemporal spikes: a follow-up study of 168 patients. Epilepsia 29:229, 1988.
39. Aicardi J: Myoclonic epilepsies of infancy and childhood. Adv Neurol 43:11, 1986.
40. Dean C, Hauswald M: Benign juvenile myoclonic epilepsy. Am J Emerg Med 5:496, 1987.
41. Amit R: Benign focal epilepsy of childhood: individual and intrafamilial multifocality of spikes. Clin Electroencephalogr 18:169, 1987.
42. Freeman JM, Tibbles J, Camfield C, Camfield P: Benign epilepsy of childhood: a speculation and its ramifications. Pediatrics 79:864, 1987.
43. Gobbi G, Bruno L, Pini A, et al: Periodic spasms: an unclassified type of epileptic seizure in childhood. Dev Med Child Neurol 29:766, 1987.
44. Horn CA, Beekman RH, Dick M II, Lacina SJ: The congenital long QT syndrome. An unusual cause of childhood seizures. Am J Dis Child 140:659, 1986.
45. Mortensen ML: Management of acute childhood poisonings caused by selected insecticides and herbicides. Pediatr Clin North Am 33:421, 1986.
46. Lobato RD, Perez C, Rivas JJ, Cordobes F: Clinical, radiological, and pathological spectrum of angiographically occult intracranial vascular malformations. Analysis of 21 cases and review of the literature. J Neurosurg 68:518, 1988.
47. Weiss GH, Feeney DM, Caveness WF, et al: Prognostic factors for the occurrence of posttraumatic epilepsy. Arch Neurol 40:7, 1983.
48. Treiman DM: Seizure types and causes of epilepsy. Semin Neurol 1:65, 1981.
49. Steiger JH, Tew JM Jr: Hemorrhage and epilepsy in cryptic cerebrovascular malformations. Arch Neurol 41:722, 1984.
50. Lowenstein DH, Massa SM, Rowbotham MC, et al: Acute neurologic and psychiatric complications associated with cocaine abuse. Am J Med 83:841, 1987.
51. Brennan FN, Lyttle JA: Alcohol and seizures: a review. J R Soc Med 80:571, 1987.
52. Fisher BM, Frier BM: Nocturnal convulsions and in-

sulin-induced hypoglycemia in diabetic patients. Post-grad Med J 63:673, 1987.
53. Dalessio DJ: Seizure disorders and pregnancy. N Engl J Med 312:559, 1985.
54. Knight AH, Rhind EG: Epilepsy and pregnancy: a study of 153 pregnancies in 59 patients. Epilepsia 16:99, 1975.
55. Messing RO, Simon RP: Seizures as a manifestation of systemic disease. Neurol Clin 4:563, 1986.
56. Gilchrist JM: Arrhythmogenic seizures: diagnosis by simultaneous EEG/ECG recording. Neurology 35:1503, 1985.
57. Schold C, Yarnell PR, Earnest MP: Origin of seizures in elderly patients. JAMA 238:1177, 1977.
58. Cocito L, Favale E, Reni L: Epileptic seizure in cerebral arterial occlusive disease. Stroke 13:189, 1982.
59. Luhdorf K, Jensen LK, Plesner AM: Etiology of seizures in the elderly. Epilepsia 27:458, 1986.
60. Cocito L, Loeb C: May focal epileptic seizures be considered a marker of TIAs? Funct Neurol 1:461, 1986.
61. Spencer DD, Spencer SS, Mattson RH, et al: Intracer-ebral masses in patients with intractable partial epilepsy. Neurology 34:432, 1984.
62. Messing RO, Closson RG, Simon RP: Drug-induced seizures: a 10-year experience. Neurology 34:1582, 1984.
63. Hess GP, Walson PD: Seizures secondary to oral viscous lidocaine. Ann Emerg Med 17:725, 1988.
64. Sellers EM: Alcohol, barbiturate and benzodiazepine withdrawal syndromes: clinical management. Can Med Assoc J 139:113, 1988.
65. Fialip J, Aumaitre O, Eschalier A, et al: Benzodiazepine withdrawal seizures: analysis of 48 case reports. Clin Neuropharmacol 10:538, 1987.
66. Theodore WH, Porter RJ, Raubertas RF: Seizures dur-ing barbiturate withdrawal: relation to blood level. Ann Neurol 22:644, 1987.
67. Mahr GC, Berchou R, Balon R: A grand mal seizure associated with desipramine and haloperidol. Can J Psychiatry 32:463, 1987.
68. Paloucek FP, Rodvold KA: Evaluation of theophylline overdoses and toxicities. Ann Emerg Med 17:135, 1988.
69. Lerman P: Seizures induced or aggravated by anticon-vulsants. Epilepsia 27:706, 1986.
70. van Sweden B, Hoste S: Are complex partial seizures an uncommon withdrawal sign in the elderly? Eur Neurol 27:239, 1987.
71. Yaqub BA, Panayiotopoulos CP, Al-Nozha M, et al: Causes of late onset epilepsy in Saudi Arabia: the role of cerebral granuloma. J Neurol Neurosurg Psychiatry 50:90, 1987.

Selected Readings

Anderson VE, Hauser WA, Rich SS; Genetic heteroge-neity in the epilepsies. Adv Neurol 44:59, 1986.
A review of recent research and current concepts of genetic and other heterogeneity in mechanisms leading to epilepsy.

Annegers JF, Hauser WA, Shirts SB, Kurland LT: Factors prognostic of unprovoked seizures after febrile convulsions. N Engl J Med 316:493, 1987.

The risk of unprovoked seizures after febrile convulsions and prognostic factors were examined in a cohort of 687 children who had an initial febrile seizure while residing in Rochester, Minnesota. Overall, children with febrile convulsions had a fivefold excess of unprovoked seizures, and the risk until age 25 was 7%. Risk variables for generalized and complex partial seizures are distinguished. These data appear consistent with the view that the increased risk of generalized-onset unprovoked seizures reflects a predisposition for both simple febrile convulsions and generalized-onset unprovoked seizures.

Bird TD: Genetic considerations in childhood epilepsy. Epilepsia 28(Suppl):S71, 1987.

A review of selected topics pertaining to genetic influences in epilepsy. Topics covered include single gene and chromosomal aberrations associated with epilepsy, multifactorial and polygenic inheritance, and issues of genetic heterogeneity with special reference to idiopathic generalized epilepsy, febrile seizures, and infantile spasms.

Bleck TP: Epilepsy. DM 33:601, 1987.

Clinical monograph covering various aspects of epilepsy, including current concepts of pathophsyiology, treatment, and clinical utility of recent classification related to diagnosis, therapy, prognostication, and genetic counseling. A discussion of therapeutic options includes a discussion of psychological and life-style issues in management of seizure patients.

Camfield PR, Camfield CS, Dooley JM, et al: Epilepsy after a first unprovoked seizure in childhood. Neurology 35:1657, 1985.

A retrospective study of 168 children with initial afebrile, unprovoked seizures who were evaluated for clinical information and recurrence rate. Of the 51.8% of children who had recurrence, 79% of them had additional seizures. High recurrence rates were associated with abnormal neurologic examinations, focal EEG spikes, and complex partial seizures. Low recurrence rates were associated with normal neurologic examinations, normal EEGs, and generalized tonic-clonic seizures.

Dam AM, Fuglsang-Frederiksen A, Svarre-Olsen U, et al: Late-onset epilepsy: etiologies, types of seizure, and value of clinical investigation, EEG, and computerized tomography scan. Epilepsia 26(3):227, 1985.

A study of 221 patients with late-onset epilepsy comparing the relative usefulness of clinical history, EEG, and CT to determine the cause of late-onset epilepsy.

Daras M, Tuchman AJ, Strobos RJ: Computed tomography in adult-onset epileptic seizures in a city hospital population. Epilepsia 28:519, 1987.

CT was performed on 155 patients from a city hospital population. A focal abnormality was found in 71 patients (45.8%). Occurrence of abnormalities on CT was higher (73%) in patients with complex partial seizures.

de la Sayette V, Cosgrove R, Melanson D, Ethier R: CT findings in late-onset epilepsy. Can J Neurol Sci 14:286, 1987.

CT findings were reviewed in 387 patients with new-onset seizures after age of 50. CT findings revealed cerebral atrophy in 113, ischemic lesions in 75, cerebral neoplasms in 20, and no abnormality in 177 patients.

Delgado-Escueta AV, White R, Greenberg DA, et al: Looking for epilepsy genes: clinical and molecular genetic studies. Adv Neurol 44:77, 1986.
Studies of gene expression controlling the development and organization of the CNS lead to insights into the genetic component of epilepsy.

Devinsky D, Nadi S, Theodore WH, Porter RJ: Cerebrospinal fluid pleocytosis following simple, complex partial, and generalized tonic-clonic seizures. Ann Neurol 23:402, 1988.
Postictal pleocytosis was observed in 7 of 62 cerebrospinal fluid (CSF) specimens obtained from 27 patients with epilepsy. All patients had known seizure disorders without other cause for pleocytosis. The maximum number of leukocytes was $12/mm^3$; the maximal number of erythrocytes was $190/mm^3$. Previous studies have found pleocytosis more common after repetitive generalized tonic-clonic seizures. This study found pleocytosis in CSF after a single complex partial seizure or generalized tonic-clonic seizure.

Diamantopoulos N, Crumrine PK: The effect of puberty on the course of epilepsy. Arch Neurol 43:873, 1986.
This study concludes that, in general, puberty does not influence epilepsy; however, in the postmenarche phase of puberty, female patients might experience better seizure control.

Dunne JW, Summers QA, Stewart-Wynne EG: Nonconvulsive status epilepticus: a prospective study in an adult general hospital. Q J Med 62:117, 1987.
A prospective study of nonconvulsive status epilepticus was undertaken to determine the occurrence and characteristics of this condition in adults. The diagnosis was established in 22 of 113 (19%) patients presenting with status epilepticus over a 23-month period. Common clinical observations were (1) a clouding of consciousness characterized by confusion, disorientation, and partial responsiveness; and (2) myoclonic or clonic movements of the face. Precipitating factors included infection, inadequate anticonvulsant medication, and benzodiazepine withdrawal.

Edwards R, Schmidley JW, Simon RP: How often does a CSF pleocytosis follow generalized convulsions? Ann Neurol 13:460, 1983.
The first study documenting the frequency of postictal pleocytosis.

Ellenberg JH, Hirtz DG, Nelson KB: Age at onset of seizures in young children. Ann Neurol 15:127, 1984.
Age at onset of seizures, relationship to prior neurologic status, and outcome were examined in 50,000 children.

Elwes RDC, Johnson AL, Shorvon SD, et al: The prognosis for seizure control in newly diagnosed epilepsy. N Engl J Med 311:944, 1984.
This study concludes that the long-term pattern of seizure control is largely established during the first 2 years of treatment.

Gastaut H, Zifkin BG: The risk of automobile accidents with seizures occurring while driving: relation to seizure type. Neurology 37:1613, 1987.

Based on a study of automobile accidents with epileptic drivers, authors suggest guidelines for licensing restrictions.

Goulatia RK, Verma A, Mishra NK, Ahuja GK: Disappearing CT lesions in epilepsy. Epilepsia 28:523, 1987.
In a series of 46 epileptic patients, a striking and reversible CT lesion, which corresponded to seizure activity, is reported. Maximal radiographic changes corresponded to the area of maximal epileptic discharge; however, multiple lesions were seen in three cases. Authors suggest that these observations and other experimental findings suggest that seizures may occasionally cause a transient CT focal abnormality that may be explained by cerebral edema, which occurs as a consequence of abnormal vascular permeability.

Grabow JD: Diagnosis of epileptic seizures. Postgrad Med 77(4):207, 1985.
Review of the current role of electroencephalography and CT in the diagnosis of epileptic seizures.

Holmes GL: How to evaluate the patient after a first seizure. Postgrad Med 83:199, 1988.
Written for the primary care physician who is approached by a patient and/or parents of a patient who has had a first seizure. Workup, prognosis, and management recommendations are discussed.

Jabbari B, Gunderson CH, Wippold F, et al: Magnetic resonance imaging in partial complex epilepsy. Arch Neurol 43:869, 1986.
Study suggests that MRI is more informative that CT in partial complex epilepsy.

Janz D: Neurological morbidity of severe epilepsy. Epilepsia 29(Suppl):S1, 1988.
A critical review of factors that have an effect on therapeutic prognosis, causes of epilepsy, underlying structural lesions and incidence of convulsive status epilepticus, various types of attacks, and differential epileptic syndromes. Authors conclude that the severity of epilepsy can only be defined from the medical standpoint on the basis of several factors that have predictive value.

Kent DL, Larson EB: Magnetic resonance imaging of the brain and spine. Is clinical efficacy established after the first decade? Ann Intern Med 108:402, 1988.
An overview of the usefulness, limitations, and indications for MRI of the brain and spine.

Mahler ME: Seizures: common causes and treatment in the elderly. Geriatrics 42(7):73, 1987.
Causes of seizures in the elderly reflect effects of aging and invoke special consideration. Stroke and tumor account for the majority of structural brain diseases in the elderly that cause new seizures over age 65. Clinical recomendations for evaluation and special considerations of management of seizures in the elderly.

Mitchell WG, Crawford TO: Intraparenchymal cerebral cysticercosis in children: diagnosis and treatment. Pediatrics 82:76, 1988.
Cerebral cysticercosis often first manifests as a seizure disorder in children and young adults. Intraparenchymal cerebral cysticercosis is diagnosed with increasing frequency in the United States. Clinical, radiographic, and prognostic features are reviewed.

Nelson KB, Ellenberg JH: Predisposing and causative factors in childhood epilepsy. Epilepsia 28(Suppl):916, 1987.

A review of studies of populations to examine factors, particularly prenatal and perinatal, that contribute to the occurrence of nonfebrile seizure disorders of early childhood. From multiple factors explored as predictors of childhood seizure disorders, the following were considered major predictors: congenital malformations of the fetus, family history of certain neurologic disorders, and neonatal seizures.

Rocca WA, Sharbrough FW, Hauser WA, et al: Risk factors for complex partial seizures: a population-based case-control study. Ann Neurol 21:22, 1987.

A population-based, case-control study of risk factors for complex partial seizures (CPS) included patients with onset of CPS before age 35 who were residents of Rochester, Minnesota at time of diagnosis between 1935 and 1979. Conditions significantly more common in patients when compared with controls included history of epilepsy or febrile seizures in the mother, febrile seizures, neonatal convulsions, cerebral palsy, head trauma, and viral encephalitis.

Rocca WA, Sharbrough FW, Hauser WA, et al: Risk factors for generalized tonic-clonic seizures: a population-based case-control study in Rochester, Minnesota. Neurology 37:1315, 1987.

A population-based, case-control study of risk factors for generalized tonic-clonic seizures in patients with onset of seizures before age 30 who were residents of Rochester, Minnesota at the time of diagnosis between 1935 and 1979. Conditions found significantly more frequently in patients than controls included history of convulsions in the mother, febrile seizures, and head trauma.

Rodin E: An assessment of current views on epilepsy. Epilepsia 28:267, 1987.

Assumptions underlying the proposed classification of epilepsies are reviewed. A proposed definition includes ictal and interictal phenomena. Implications for future research are discussed.

Shorvon SD, Farmer PJ: Epilepsy in developing countries: a review of epidemiological, sociocultural, and treatment aspects. Epilepsia 29(Suppl):S36, 1988.

A report of aspects of epilepsy in developing countries. Social effects and local perceptions of etiologies of epilepsies and treatment are discussed from observations made in Africa, Asia, and South America. Poor understanding of principles of drug therapy and an erratic supply of drugs were cited as major reasons for poor compliance with treatment.

Tharp BR: An overview of pediatric seizure disorders and epileptic syndromes. Epilepsia 28(Suppl):S36, 1987.

Comprehensive and well-referenced overview of various aspects of epilepsy in children.

Trimble MR: Cognitive hazards of seizure disorders. Epilepsia 29(Suppl):S19, 1988.

Two investigations are reported in which subgroups of patients with seizures and intellectual deterioration are compared to those without such deterioration. Factors considered most related to decline of cognitive function included recurrent tonic-clonic seizures, head injury, phenytoin therapy, and low folic acid levels. These data suggest some obvious implications for management.

Wachtel TJ, Steele GH, Day JA: Natural history of fever following seizure. Arch Intern Med 147:1153, 1987.

The course of fever following generalized seizures in 93 hospitalized patients was described to help determine factors that may help with timing of appropriate tests to rule out infection during the postictal period. Forty patients (43%) had body temperatures above 37.8°C. No infection was found in two-thirds of the febrile patients, 89% of whom were afebrile in 48 hours. Of the one-third of febrile patients with an infection, all were still febrile after 48 hours.

48
Stroke: Common Risk Factors and Nonatherosclerotic Risk Factors

The devastation of a stroke demands attention to risk factors in patients of all ages. Transient ischemic attacks (TIAs) are the most specific and powerful warning of impending stroke.[1] Stroke prevention depends primarily on modification of risk factors and recognition of TIAs.[1] Diagnosis of a TIA relies on identification of the focal, stereotypic, transient syndromes associated with anterior and posterior circulation insufficiency or ischemia. Carotid artery ischemia classically produces symptoms of monocular blindness, dysphasia, unilateral sensory loss, paresthesias and weakness; whereas, vertebral-basilar disease results in symptoms of bilateral blurred vision, dizziness, diplopia, vertigo, tinnitus, syncope, and loss of consciousness. Disorders that most commonly mimic TIAs and stroke include focal seizures, cardiogenic syncope, acute labyrinthitis, and migraine headaches.[2-11]

In the absence of major stroke risk factors, such as known atherosclerotic disease, diabetes, or hypertension, consider less common nonatherosclerotic causes of stroke or TIA, particularly in the young adult. Although nonatherosclerotic causes of stroke are less common, many are treatable and can manifest initially as a TIA or stroke in a young adult.[12,13] Some common and uncommon nonatherosclerotic causes of young stroke include familial and congenital syndromes, cardiogenic emboli, central nervous system vasculitis, and systemic metabolic-endocrine and hematologic disorders.[14,15]

Stroke: Common Risk Factors

Transient ischemic attacks: 15 to 25% of patients with untreated TIAs develop cerebral infarction, with highest risk in the first year.[16]

Hypertension[17-20]

Hyperlipidemia[21-24]

Atherosclerotic cerebral vascular disease

Atherosclerotic cardiac disease: coronary artery disease is the cause of death in most patients who have TIAs or stroke.[25]

Diabetes mellitus[26-31]

Age

Erythrocytosis: hematocrits greater than 50% have been associated with increased blood viscosity compromising cerebrovascular blood flow[32]

Cigarette smoking[33-40]

Abdominal obesity[41-43]

Heavy alcohol consumption[44-52]

Maternal history of stroke: risk factor for middle-aged men[53]

Disorders Causing Thromboembolic Phenomenon

Atrial fibrillation: thromboembolism often occurs in patients with atrial fibrillation before detection of atrial fibrillation[54-60]

Myocardial thrombosis: following myocardial infarction

Myocardial aneurysms: following large myocardial infarctions

Prosthetic cardiac valves

Mitral stenosis: rheumatic heart disease

Endocarditis: infectious, nonbacterial thrombotic endocarditis[61-66]

Mitral valve prolapse[67-70]

Tumor emboli: cerebral infarction secondary to tumor emboli can be a rare initial manifestation of cancer; lung cancer is the most common neoplasm associated with tumor emboli.[71,72]

Aortic aneurysm and mural thrombosis

Paradoxical emboli: patent foramen ovale and an atrial septal defect[73-76]

Intracardiac tumors: atrial myxoma, papillary fibroelastoma, metastasis[77-80]

Cervical trauma and manipulation[81]

Vertebral artery injury: can occur with even minimal neck trauma[82]

Spontaneous internal carotid artery dissection[83]

Aortoarteritis[84,85]

Fat emboli: associated with trauma[86]

Cardiomyopathies

Hematologic Conditions Causing Hypercoagulable States of Hemorrhage

Coagulation disorders associated with cancer: septic thrombi, disseminated intravascular thrombosis, cerebral venous thrombosis, hemorrhages[87,88]

Metastatic tumors that hemorrhage: malignant melanoma, germ cell tumors, hypernephroma, choriocarcinoma, and bronchogenic carcinoma[89-92]

Primary cerebral tumors: gliomas and meningiomas are rare underlying causes of cerebral hemorrhage[93-95]

Anticoagulant therapy[96-98]

Paroxysmal nocturnal hemoglobinuria

Myeloproliferative disorders: status postsplenectomy, leukemia, essential thrombocythemia[99]

Antithrombin III deficiency[100,101]

Elevated factor VIII[102]

Treatment of vitamin K deficiency leading to a hypercoagulable state[103]

Thrombocythemia[99]

Elevated fibrinogen: appears to be a greater risk factor in men than in women[104]

Hyperviscosity syndromes: polycythemia, hyperglobulinemia

Lupus anticoagulant: common associations include systemic lupus erythematosus, noncerebral venous thrombosis, hypertension, and false-positive VDRLs[105-110]

Anticardiolipin antibodies: may be associated with a lupus anticoagulant-like tendency[105,111,112]

Birth control pills[113-116]

Hemoglobinopathies: sickle cell and hemoglobin SC disease[117-121]

Hemophilia[122]

Vasculitic Disorders That Affect the Central Nervous System

Systemic lupus erythematosus[123]
Temporal arteritis: giant cell arteritis[124-129]
Wegener's granulomatosis[130]
Drug-induced: amphetamines, cocaine, phenylpropanolamine[131,132]
Sarcoidosis[133]
Polyarteritis nodosa
Takayasu's syndrome[134]
Infectious arteritis: tuberculosis, *Listeria monocytogenes*, mycoses, syphilis, *Cryptococcus*, upper respiratory and ear infections, sphenoid sinusitis, herpes zoster[135-141]
Granulomatous angiitis[142-144]

Congenital and Idiopathic Disorders Associated with Stroke

Migraine stroke[145-151]
Intracranial aneurysms: most common cause of subarachnoid hemorrhage in young adults and fatal strokes in persons younger than 45 years[152-157]
Arteriovenous malformations: seizures and headaches can signal cerebral bleeds from occult arteriovenous malformations[158-161]
Carotid artery dissection
Vertebral artery dissection[162-164]
Carotid artery aneurysm
Vertebrobasilar aneurysms
Fibromuscular dysplasia[165-167]
Moyamoya disease[168-172]
Rendu-Osler-Weber disease
von Hippel-Lindau disease
Homocystinuria[173]
Fabry's disease
Ehlers-Danlos disease
Pseudoxanthoma elasticum
Kohlmeier-Degos disease
Tuberous sclerosis
Neurofibromatosis[174]
Mitochondrial myopathy, encephalopathy, lactic acidosis, and strokelike episodes (MELAS)[175-179]
Congenital odontoid aplasia: unsuspected cervical malformations may initially manifest themselves in children or young adults with symptoms of posterior circulation insufficiency.[180]

Miscellaneous

Pregnancy and puerperium: stroke is a major cause of maternal death, and may be associated with eclampsia, metastatic choriocarcinoma, ruptured arteriovenous malformations, and hypercoagulable states.[181-184]

Head trauma: immediate and delayed traumatic intracerebral hematomas[185-187]

Infection-related hemorrhagic lesions: herpes simplex encephalitis, hemorrhagic leukoencephalitis, bacterial abscesses, bacterial endocarditis, mycotic aneurysms, nonbacterial endocarditis[188]

Cerebral amyloid angiopathy: can cause recurrent intracerebral hemorrhages in the elderly[189-191]

Exogenous drug abuse: sympathomimetics, i.e., amphetamine, ephedrine, phenylpropanolamine, alcohol, cocaine, phencyclidine[192-205]

Spontaneous subarachnoid hemorrhage: with normal angiography after subarachnoid hemorrhage[206-211]

Sneddon's syndrome: rare autoimmune disorder characterized clinically by livedo reticularis, cerebral ischemic lesions, and antiphospholipid antibodies[212]

Neuroangiography[213-215]

Chiropractic cervical manipulation[216]

Hypothyroidism[217]

References

1. Mirsen TR, Hachinski VC: Transient ischemic attacks and stroke. Can Med Assoc J 138:1099, 1988.
2. Peled R, Harnes B, Borovich B, Sharf B: Speech arrest and supplementary motor area seizures. Neurology 34:110, 1984.
3. Longo DL, Witherspoon JM: Focal neurologic symptoms in hypercalcemia. Neurology 30:200, 1980.
4. Venna N, Sabin TD: Tonic focal seizures in nonketotic hyperglycemia of diabetes mellitus. Arch Neurol 38:512, 1981.
5. Cerebral Embolism Task Force: Cardiogenic brain embolism. Arch Neurol 43:71, 1986.
6. Hotson JR: Clinical detection of acute vestibulocerebellar disorders. West J Med 140:910, 1984.
7. Little N: Acute head pain. Emerg Med Clin North Am 5:687, 1987.
8. Fisher CM: Late-life migraine accompaniments—further experience. Stroke 17:1033, 1986.
9. Manusov EG: Late-life migraine accompaniments: a case presentation and literature review. J Fam Pract 24(6):591, 1987.
10. Edmeads J: Headache in cerebrovascular disease. A common symptom of stroke. Postgrad Med 81(8):191, 1987.
11. Pfaffenrath V, Pollmann W, Autenrieth G, Rosmanith U: Mitral valve prolapse and platelet aggregation in patients with hemiplegic and non-hemiplegic migraine. Acta Neurol Scand 75:253, 1987.
12. Adams HP Jr, Butler MJ, Biller J, Toffol GJ: Non-

hemorrhagic cerebral infarction in young adults. Arch Neurol 43:793, 1986.

13. Pellegrino TR: Vascular syndromes. Emerg Med Clin North Am 5:751, 1987.
14. Heiskell CA, Conn J Jr: Aortoarterial emboli. Am J Surg 132:4, 1976.
15. Sherman DG, Dyken ML, Fisher M, et al: Cerebral embolism. Chest 89(Suppl):82S, 1986.
16. Toole JF, Yuson CP, Janeway R, et al: Transient ischemic attacks: a prospective study of 225 patients. Neurology 28:746, 1978.
17. Emeriau JP, Decamps A, Manciet G, et al: Hypertension in the elderly. Am J Med 84:92, 1988.
18. Medical Research Council Working Party: Stroke and coronary heart disease in mild hypertension: risk factors and the value of treatment. Br Med J 296:1565, 1988.
19. Dollery CT: Risk predictors, risk indicators, and benefit factors in hypertension. Am J Med 82:2, 1987.
20. Rutan GH, Kuller LH, Neaton JD, et al: Mortality associated with diastolic hypertension and isolated systolic hypertension among men screened for the Multiple Risk Factor Intervention Trial. Circulation 77:504, 1988.
21. Meyer JS, Rogers RL, Mortel KF, Judd BW: Hyperlipidemia is a risk factor for decreased cerebral perfusion and stroke. Arch Neurol 44:418, 1987.
22. Jurgens G, Koltringer P: Lipoprotein(a) in ischemic cerebrovascular disease: a new approach to the assessment of risk for stroke. Neurology 37:513, 1987.
23. Tell GS, Crouse JR, Furberg CD: Relation between blood lipids, lipoproteins, and cerebrovascular atherosclerosis. A review. Stroke 19:423, 1988.
24. Assmann G, Schulte H: The Prospective Cardiovascular Munster Study: prevalence and prognostic significance of hyperlipidemia in men with systemic hypertension. Am J Cardiol 59:9G, 1987.
25. Rokey R, Rolak LA, Harati Y, et al: Coronary artery disease in patients with cerebrovascular disease: a prospective study. Ann Neurol 16:50, 1984.
26. Colwell JA, Halushka PV, Sarji KE, et al: Vascular disease in diabetes. Pathophysiological mechanisms and therapy. Arch Intern Med 139:225, 1979.
27. Abbott RD, Donahue RP, MacMahon SW, et al: Diabetes and the risk of stroke. The Honolulu Heart Program. JAMA 257:949, 1987.
28. Gray CS, Taylor R, French JM, et al: The prognostic value of stress hyperglycaemia and previously unrecognized diabetes in acute stroke. Diabetic Med 4:237, 1987.
29. Barrett-Connor E, Khaw KT: Diabetes mellitus: an independent risk factor for stroke? Am J Epidemiol 128:116, 1988.
30. Lithner F, Asplund K, Eriksson S, et al: Clinical characteristics in diabetic stroke patients. Diabete Metab 14:15, 1988.
31. Laakso M, Ronnemaa T, Pyorala K, et al: Atherosclerotic vascular disease and its risk factors in non-insulin-dependent diabetic and nondiabetic subjects in Finland. Diabetes Care 11:449, 1988.

32. Harrison MJG, Pollock S, Kendall BE, et al: Effect of hematocrit on carotid stenosis and cerebral infarction. Lancet 2:114, 1981.
33. Wilson PWF, Garrison RJ, Castelli WP: Postmenopausal estrogen use, cigarette smoking, and cardiovascular morbidity in women over 50. N Engl J Med 313:1038, 1985.
34. Bonita R, Scragg R, Stewart A, et al: Cigarette smoking and risk of premature stroke in men and women. Br Med J 293:6, 1986.
35. Abbott RD, Yin Y, Reed DM, et al: Risk of stroke in male cigarette smokers. N Engl J Med 315:717, 1986.
36. Oleckno WA: The risk of stroke in young adults: an analysis of the contribution of cigarette smoking and alcohol consumption. Public Health 102:45, 1988.
37. McGill HC Jr: The cardiovascular pathology of smoking. Am Heart J 115:250, 1988.
38. Dollery C, Brennan PJ: The Medical Research Council Hypertension Trial: the smoking patient. Am Heart J 115:276, 1988.
39. Wolf PA, D'Agostino RB, Kannel WB, et al: Cigarette smoking as a risk factor for stroke. The Framingham Study. JAMA 259:1025, 1988.
40. Colditz GA, Bonita R, Stampfer MJ, et al: Cigarette smoking and risk of stroke in middle-aged women. N Engl J Med 318:937, 1988.
41. Björntorp P: Regional patterns of fat distribution. Ann Intern Med 103:994, 1985.
42. Lapidus L, Bengtsson C: Regional obesity as a health hazard in women—a prospective study. Acta Med Scand 723(Suppl):53, 1988.
43. Larsson B: Regional obesity as a health hazard in men—prospective studies. Acta Med Scand 723(Suppl):45, 1988.
44. Gill JS, Zezulka AV, Shipley MJ, et al: Stroke and alcohol consumption. N Engl J Med 315:1041, 1986.
45. Criqui MH: Alcohol consumption, blood pressure, lipids, and cardiovascular mortality. Alcoholism 10:564, 1986.
46. Eichner ER: Alcohol, stroke, and coronary artery disease. Am Fam Physician 37(3):217, 1988.
47. Stampfer MJ, Colditz GA, Willett WC, et al: A prospective study of moderate alcohol consumption and the risk of coronary disease and stroke in women. N Engl J Med 319:267, 1988.
48. Hillbom ME: What supports the role of alcohol as a risk factor for stroke? Acta Med Scand 717(Suppl):93, 1987.
49. Gorelick PB: Alcohol and stroke. Stroke 18:268, 1987.
50. Hillbom M, Kaste M, Rasi V: Can ethanol intoxication affect hemocoagulation to increase the risk of brain infarction in young adults? Neurology 33:381, 1983.
51. Taylor JR, Combs-Orme T: Alcohol and strokes in young adults. Am J Psychiatry 142:116, 1985.
52. Wilkins MR, Kendall MJ: Stroke affecting young men after alcoholic binges. Br Med J 291:1342, 1985.
53. Welin L, Svardsudd K, Wilhelmsen L, et al: Analysis of risk factors for stroke in a cohort of men born in 1913. N Engl J Med 317:521, 1987.

54. Sherman DG, Goldman L, Whiting RB, et al: Thromboembolism in patients with atrial fibrillation. Arch Neurol 41:708, 1984.
55. Kelley RE, Berger JR, Alter M, et al: Cerebral ischemia and atrial fibrillation: prospective study. Neurology 34:1285, 1984.
56. Halperin JL, Hart RG: Atrial fibrillation and stroke: new ideas, persisting dilemmas. Stroke 19:937, 1988.
57. Petersen P, Madsen EB, Brun B, et al: Silent cerebral infarction in chronic atrial fibrillation. Stroke 18:1098, 1987.
58. Petersen P, Godtfredsen J: Risk factors for stroke in chronic atrial fibrillation. Eur Heart J 9:291, 1988.
59. Kempster PA, Gerraty RP, Gates PC: Asymptomatic cerebral infarction in patients with chronic atrial fibrillation. Stroke 19:955, 1988.
60. Weinberger J, Rothlauf E, Materese E, Halperin J: Noninvasive evaluation of the extracranial carotid arteries in patients with cerebrovascular events and atrial fibrillation. Arch Intern Med 148:1785, 1988.
61. Ray H, Wahal KM: Subarachnoid hemorrhage in subacute bacterial endocarditis. Neurology 7:265, 1957.
62. Salgado AV, Furlan AJ, Keys TF: Mycotic aneurysm, subarachnoid hemorrhage, and indications for cerebral angiography in infective endocarditis. Stroke 18:1057, 1987.
63. Lerner PI: Neurologic complications of infective endocarditis. Med Clin North Am 69:385, 1985.
64. Macdonell RA, Kalnins RM, Donnan GA: Non-bacterial thrombotic endocarditis and stroke. Clin Exp Neurol 22:123, 1986.
65. Anderson D, Bell D, Lodge R, Grant E: Recurrent cerebral ischemia and mitral valve vegetation in a patient with antiphospholipid antibodies. J Rheumatol 14:839, 1987.
66. Rogers LR, Cho ES, Kempin S, Posner JB: Cerebral infarction from non-bacterial thrombotic endocarditis. Clinical and pathological study including the effects of anticoagulation. Am J Med 83:746, 1987.
67. Schnee MA, Bucal AA: Fatal embolism in mitral valve prolapse. Chest 83:285, 1983.
68. Jackson AC, Boughner DR, Barnett HJM: Mitral valve prolapse and cerebral ischemic events in young patients. Neurology 34:784, 1984.
69. Kelley RE, Pina I, Lee SC: Cerebral ischemia and mitral valve prolapse: case-control study of associated factors. Stroke 19:443, 1988.
70. Kouvaras G, Bacoulas G: Association of mitral valve leaflet prolapse with cerebral ischemic events in the young and early middle-aged patient. Q J Med 56:387, 1985.
71. O'Neill BP, Dinapoli RP, Okazaki H: Cerebral infarction as a result of tumor emboli. Cancer 60:90, 1987.
72. Kearsley JH, Tattersall MHN: Cerebral embolism in cancer patients. Q J Med 51:279, 1982.
73. Jones HR Jr, Caplan LR, Come PC, et al: Cerebral emboli of paradoxical origin. Ann Neurol 13:314, 1983.
74. Biller J, Adams HP Jr, Johnson MR, et al: Paradoxical

cerebral embolism: eight cases. Neurology 36:1356, 1986.

75. Biller J, Johnson MR, Adams HP Jr, et al: Further observations on cerebral or retinal ischemia in patients with right-left intracardiac shunts. Arch Neurol 44:740, 1987.

76. Lechat P, Mas JL, Lascault G, et al: Prevalence of patent foramen ovale in patients with stroke. N Engl J Med 318:1148, 1988.

77. Sandok BA, von Estorff I, Giuliani ER: CNS embolism due to atrial myxoma. Clinical features and diagnosis. Arch Neurol 37:485, 1980.

78. Milgalter E, Lotan H, Schuger L, et al: Cardiac myxomas—surgical experience with a multi-faceted tumor. Thorac Cardiovasc Surg 35:115, 1987.

79. McFadden PM, Lacy JR: Intracardiac papillary fibroelastoma: an occult cause of embolic neurologic deficit. Ann Thorac Surg 43:667, 1987.

80. Chalmers N, Campbell IW: Left atrial metastasis presenting as recurrent embolic strokes. Br Heart J 58:170, 1987.

81. Mueller S, Sahs AL: Brain stem dysfunction related to cervical manipulation. Report of three cases. Neurology 26:547, 1976.

82. Katirji MB, Reinmuth OM, Latchaw RE: Stroke due to vertebral artery injury. Arch Neurol 42:242, 1985.

83. Mokri B, Sundt TM Jr, Houser OW: Spontaneous internal carotid dissection, hemicrania, and Horner's syndrome. Arch Neurol 36:677, 1979.

84. Wickremasinghe HR, Peiris JB, Thenabadu PN, et al: Transient emboligenic aortoarteritis. Noteworthy new entity in young stroke patients. Arch Neurol 35:416, 1978.

85. Morooka S, Saito Y, Nonaka Y, et al: Clinical features and course of aortitis syndrome in Japanese women older than 40 years. Am J Cardiol 53:859, 1984.

86. Williams AG Jr, Mettler FA Jr, Christie JH, et al: Fat embolism syndrome. Clin Nucl Med 11:495, 1986.

87. Hickey WF, Garnick MB, Henderson IC, et al: Primary cerebral venous thrombosis in patients with cancer—a rarely diagnosed paraneoplastic syndrome. Report of three cases and review of the literature. Am J Med 73:740, 1982.

88. Graus F, Rogers LR, Posner JB: Cerebrovascular complications in patients with cancer. Medicine 64:16, 1985.

89. Mandybur TI: Intracranial hemorrhage caused by metastatic tumors. Neurology 27:650, 1977.

90. Weisberg LA: Hemorrhagic metastatic intracranial neoplasms: clinical-computed tomographic correlations. Comput Radiol 9:105, 1985.

91. Maiuri F, D'Andrea F, Gallicchio B, et al: Intracranial hemorrhages in metastatic brain tumors. J Neurosurg Sci 29:37, 1985.

92. Ross RT: Transient tumor attacks. Arch Neurol 40:633, 1983.

93. Helle TL, Conley FK: Hemorrhage associated with meningioma: a case report and review of the literature. J Neurol Neurosurg Psychiatry 43:725, 1980.

94. Yokota A, Kajiwara H, Matsuoka S, et al: Subarachnoid hemorrhage from brain tumors in childhood. Childs Nerv Syst 3:65, 1987.
95. Scotti G, Filizzolo F, Scialfa G, et al: Repeated subarachnoid hemorrhages from a cervical meningioma. Case report. J Neurosurg 66:779, 1987.
96. Wintzen AR, de Jonge H, Loeliger EA, et al: The risk of intracerebral hemorrhage during oral anticoagulant treatment: a population study. Ann Neurol 16:553, 1984.
97. Ramirez-Lassepas M, Quinones MR: Heparin therapy for stroke: hemorrhagic complications and risk factors for intracerebral hemorrhage. Neurology 34:114, 1984.
98. Atkinson JL, Sundt TM Jr, Kazmier FJ, et al: Heparin-induced thrombocytopenia and thrombosis in ischemic stroke. Mayo Clin Proc 63:353, 1988.
99. Jabaily J, Iland HJ, Laszlo J, et al: Neurologic manifestations of essential thrombocythemia. Ann Intern Med 99:513, 1983.
100. Cosgriff TM, Bishop DT, Hershgold EJ, et al: Familial antithrombin III deficiency: its natural history, genetics, diagnosis, and treatment. Medicine 62:209, 1983.
101. Vomberg PP, Breederveld C, Fleury P, Arts WF: Cerebral thromboembolism due to antithrombin III deficiency in two children. Neuropediatrics 18:42, 1987.
102. Furlow TW Jr: Factor VIII and thrombotic stroke. Ann Neurol 9:620, 1981.
103. Florholmen J, Waldum H, Nordøy A: Cerebral thrombosis in two patients with malabsorption syndrome treated with vitamin K. Br Med J 281:541, 1980.
104. Kannel WB, Wolf PA, Castelli WP, D'Agostino RB: Fibrinogen and risk of cardiovascular disease. The Framingham Study. JAMA 258:1183, 1987.
105. Levine SR, Welch KM: Cerebrovascular ischemia associated with lupus anticoagulant. Stroke 18:257, 1987.
106. Petri M, Rheinschmidt M, Whiting-O'Keefe Q, et al: The frequency of lupus anticoagulant in systemic lupus erythematosus. A study of sixty consecutive patients by activated partial thromboplastin time, Russell viper venom time, and anticardiolipin antibody level. Ann Intern Med 106:524, 1987.
107. Tabachnik-Schor NF, Lipton SA: Association of lupuslike anticoagulant and nonvasculitic cerebral infarction. Arch Neurol 43:851, 1986.
108. Boey ML, Colaco CB, Gharavi AE, et al: Thrombosis in systemic lupus erythematosus: striking association with the presence of circulating lupus anticoagulant. Br Med J (Clin Res) 287:1021, 1983.
109. Fisher M, McGehee W: Cerebral infarct, TIA, and lupus inhibitor. Neurology 36:1234, 1986.
110. Feit H, Frenkel EP, Dunn BR, et al: Acute subdural hematomas with lupus anticoagulant (procoagulant inhibitor). Neurology 34:519, 1984.
111. Levine SR, Kim S, Deegan MJ, Welch KM: Ischemic stroke associated with anticardiolipin antibodies. Stroke 18:1101, 1987.

112. Coull BM, Bourdette DN, Goodnight SH Jr, et al: Multiple cerebral infarctions and dementia associated with anticardiolipin antibodies. Stroke 18:1107, 1987.
113. Bonnar J: Coagulation effects of oral contraception. Am J Obstet Gynecol 157:1042, 1987.
114. Chilvers E, Rudge P: Cerebral venous thrombosis and subarachnoid hemorrhage in users of oral contraceptives. Br Med J (Clin Res) 292:524, 1986.
115. Longstreth WT Jr, Swanson PD: Oral contraceptives and stroke. Stroke 15:747, 1984.
116. Levine SR, Knake JE, Young AB: Atypical progressive stroke syndrome associated with oral contraceptives and cigarette use. Stroke 18:519, 1987.
117. Rothman SM, Fulling KH, Nelson JS: Sickle cell anemia and central nervous system infarction: a neuropathological study. Ann Neurol 20:684, 1986.
118. el Gammal T, Adams RJ, Nichols FT, et al: MR and CT investigation of cerebrovascular disease in sickle cell patients. AJNR 7:1043, 1986.
119. Feldenzer JA, Bueche MJ, Venes JL, Gebarski SS: Superior sagittal sinus thrombosis with infarction in sickle cell trait. Stroke 18:656, 1987.
120. Pavlakis SG, Bello J, Prohovnik I, et al: Brain infarction in sickle cell anemia: magnetic resonance imaging correlates. Ann Neurol 23:125, 1988.
121. Fabian RH, Peters BH: Neurological complications of hemoglobin SC disease. Arch Neurol 41:289, 1984.
122. Federici A, Mannucci PM, Minetti D, et al: Intracranial bleeding in hemophilia. A study of eleven cases. J Neurosurg Sci 27:31, 1983.
123. Kaell AT, Shetty M, Lee BC, et al: The diversity of neurologic events in systemic lupus erythematosus. Prospective clinical and computed tomographic classification of 82 events in 71 patients. Arch Neurol 43:273, 1986.
124. Howard GF III, Ho SU, Kim KS, et al: Bilateral artery occlusion resulting from giant cell arteritis. Ann Neurol 15:204, 1984.
125. Caselli RJ, Hunder GG, Whisnant JP: Neurologic disease in biopsy-proven giant cell (temporal) arteritis. Neurology 38:352, 1988.
126. Save-Soderbergh J, Malmvall BE, Andersson R, Bengtsson BA: Giant cell arteritis as a cause of death. Report of nine cases. JAMA 255:493, 1986.
127. Lipton RB, Rosenbaum D, Mehler MF: Giant cell arteritis causes recurrent posterior circulation transient ischemic attacks which respond to corticosteroid. Eur Neurol 27:97, 1987.
128. Venna N, Goldman R, Tilak S, Sabin TD: Temporal arteritis-like presentation of carotid atherosclerosis. Stroke 17:325, 1986.
129. Sherard RK, Coleridge ST: Giant-cell arteritis. J Emerg Med 4:293, 1986.
130. Hearne CB, Zawada ET Jr: Survival after intracerebral hemorrhage in Wegener's granulomatosis. West J Med 137:431, 1982.
131. Harrington H, Heller HA, Dawson D, et al: Intracerebral hemorrhage and oral amphetamine. Arch Neurol 40:503, 1983.
132. Golbe LI, Merkin MD: Cerebral infarction in a user of free-base cocaine ("crack"). Neurology 36:1602, 1986.

133. Sethi KD, el Gammal T, Patel BR, Swift TR: Dural sarcoidosis presenting with transient neurologic symptoms. Arch Neurol 43:595, 1986.
134. Hall S, Barr W, Lie JT, et al: Takayasu arteritis. A study of 32 North American patients. Medicine 64:89, 1985.
135. Syrjanen J, Valtonen VV, Iivanainen M, et al: Preceding infection as an important risk factor for ischemic brain infarction in young and middle aged patients. Br Med J (Clin Res) 296:1156, 1988.
136. Leiguarda R, Berthier M, Starkstein S, et al: Ischemic infarction in 25 children with tuberculous meningitis. Stroke 19:200, 1988.
137. Holmes MD, Brant-Zawadzki MM, Simon RP: Clinical features of meningovascular syphilis. Neurology 34:553, 1984.
138. Saul RF, Gallagher JG, Mateer JE: Sudden hemiparesis as the presenting sign in cryptococcal meningoencephalitis. Stroke 17:753, 1986.
139. Bourdette DN, Rosenberg NL, Yatsu FM: Herpes zoster ophthalmicus and delayed ipsilateral cerebral infarction. Neurology 33:1428, 1983.
140. Powers JM: Herpes zoster maxillaris with delayed occipital infarction. J Clin Neuro Ophthalmol 6:113, 1986.
141. Verghese A, Sugar AM: Herpes zoster ophthalmicus and granulomatous angiitis. An ill-appreciated cause of stroke. J Am Geriatr Soc 34:309, 1986.
142. Burger PC, Burch JG Vogel FS: Granulomatous angiitis. An unusual etiology of stroke. Stroke 8:29, 1977.
143. Clifford-Jones RE, Love S, Gurusinghe N: Granulomatous angiitis of the central nervous system: a case with recurrent intracerebral hemorrhage. J Neurol Neurosurg Psychiatry 48:1054, 1985.
144. Fukumoto S, Kinjo M, Hokamura K, Tanaka K: Subarachnoid hemorrhage and granulomatous angiitis of the basilar artery: demonstration of the varicella-zoster-virus in the basilar artery lesions. Stroke 17:1024, 1986.
145. Dorfman LJ, Marshall WH, Enzmann DR: Cerebral infarction and migraine: clinical and radiologic correlations. Neurology 29:317, 1979.
146. Fisher CM: Late-life migraine accompaniments—further experience. Stroke 17:1033, 1986.
147. Henrich JB: The association between migraine and cerebral vascular events: an analytical review. J Chronic Dis 40:329, 1987.
148. Broderick JP, Swanson JW: Migraine-related strokes. Clinical profile and prognosis in 20 patients. Arch Neurol 44:868, 1987.
149. Bogousslavsky J, Regli F, Van Melle G, et al: Migraine stroke. Neurology 38:223, 1988.
150. Moen M, Levine SR, Newman DS, et al: Bilateral posterior cerebral artery strokes in a young migraine sufferer. Stroke 19:525, 1988.
151. Rothrock JF, Walicke P, Swenson MR, et al: Migrainous stroke. Arch Neurol 45:63, 1988.
152. Burst JCM: Subarachnoid hemorrhage: early detection and diagnosis. Hosp Pract 17(2):73, 1982.

153. O'Hare TH: Subarachnoid hemorrhage: a review. J Emerg Med 5:135, 1987.
154. Kondziolka D, Bernstein M, ter Brugge K, Schutz H: Acute subdural hematoma from ruptured posterior communicating artery aneurysm. Neurosurgery 22:151, 1988.
155. Di Pasquale G, Andreoli A, Grazi P, et al: Cardioembolic stroke from atrial septal aneurysm. Stroke 19:640, 1988.
156. Vles JS, Lodder J: A rare cause of transient ischemic attacks: saccular aneurysm of the internal carotid artery. J Neurol 226:125, 1981.
157. Steinberger A, Ganti SR, McMurtry JG III, Hilal SK: Transient neurological deficits secondary to saccular vertebrobasilar aneurysms. Report of two cases. J Neurosurg 60:410, 1984.
158. Steiger JH, Tew JM Jr: Hemorrhage and epilepsy in cryptic cerebrovascular malformations. Arch Neurol 41:722, 1984.
159. Kahl W, Anang KD, Meinig G, Schwarz M: Cerebral angiomas: influence of morphological aspects such as size and site on their clinical behavior with special reference to the mode of bleeding. Neurosurg Rev 10:111, 1987.
160. Jellinger K: Vascular malformations of the central nervous system: a morphological overview. Neurosurg Rev 9:177, 1986.
161. Lasjaunias P, Chiu M, ter Brugge K, et al: Neurological manifestations of intracranial dural arteriovenous malformations. J Neurosurg 64:724, 1986.
162. Caplan LR, Baquis GD, Pessin MS, et al: Dissection of the intracranial vertebral artery. Neurology 38:868, 1988.
163. Mas JL, Bousser MG, Hasboun D, Laplane D: Extracranial vertebral artery dissections: a review of 13 cases. Stroke 18:1037, 1987.
164. Katirji MB, Reinmuth OM, Latchaw RE: Stroke due to vertebral artery injury. Arch Neurol 42:242, 1985.
165. Hegedus K, Nemeth G: Fibromuscular dysplasia of the basilar artery. Case report with autopsy verification. Arch Neurol 41:440, 1984.
166. Luscher TF, Lie JT, Stanson AW, et al: Arterial fibromuscular dysplasia. Mayo Clin Proc 62:931, 1987.
167. Pappada G, Panzarasa G, Sani R, Formaggio G: Intracranial fibromuscular dysplasia. Report of two cases and review of literature. J Neurosurg Sci 31:13, 1987.
168. Murphy MJ: Progressive vascular changes in moyamoya syndrome. Stroke 11:656, 1980.
169. Bruno A, Adams HP Jr, Biller J, et al: Cerebral infarction due to moyamoya disease in young adults. Stroke 19:826, 1988.
170. Tagawa T, Haritomi N, Mimaki T, et al: Regional cerebral blood flow, clinical manifestations, and age in children with moyamoya disease. Stroke 18:906, 1987.
171. Chen ST, Liu YH, Hsu CY, et al: Moyamoya disease in Taiwan. Stroke 19:53, 1988.
172. Gomez CR, Hogan PA: Unilateral Moya Moya disease in an adult—a case history. Angiology 38:342, 1987.
173. Scriver CR: Cystinuria (editorial). N Engl J Med 315:1155, 1986.

174. Pellock JM, Kleinman PK, McDonald BM, et al: Childhood hypertensive stroke with neurofibromatosis. Neurology 30:656, 1980.
175. Pavlakis SG, Phillips PC, DiMauro S, et al: Mitochondrial myopathy, encephalopathy, lactic acidosis, and strokelike episodes: a distinctive clinical syndrome. Ann Neurol 16:481, 1984.
176. Ohama E, Ikuta F: Involvement of choroid plexus in mitochondrial encephalomyopathy (MELAS). Acta Neuropathol 75:1, 1987.
177. Hasuo K, Tamura S, Yasumori K, et al: Computed tomography and angiography in MELAS (mitochondrial myopathy, encephalopathy, lactic acidosis and stroke-like episodes): report of 3 cases. Neuroradiology 29:393, 1987.
178. Danks RA, Dorevitch M, Cummins JT, Byrne E: Mitochondrial myopathy, encephalopathy, lactic acidosis and stroke-like episodes (MELAS): adolescent onset with severe cerebral edema. Aust N Z J Med 18:69, 1988.
179. Montagna P, Gallassi R, Medori R, et al: MELAS syndrome: characteristic migrainous and epileptic features and maternal transmission. Neurology 38:751, 1988.
180. Phillips PC, Lorentsen KJ, Shropshire LC, Ahn HS: Congenital odontoid aplasia and posterior circulation stroke in childhood. Ann Neurol 23:410, 1988.
181. Biller J, Adams HP Jr: Cerebrovascular disorders associated with pregnancy. Am Fam Physician 33(6):125, 1986.
182. Handin RI: Thromboembolic complications of pregnancy and oral contraceptives. Prog Cardiovasc Dis 16:395, 1974.
183. Wiebers DO: Ischemic cerebrovascular complications of pregnancy. Arch Neurol 42:1106, 1985.
184. Trommer BL, Homer D, Mikhael MA: Cerebral vasospasm and eclampsia. Stroke 19:326, 1988.
185. Seelig JM, Becker DP, Miller JD, et al: Traumatic acute subdural hematoma. Major mortality reduction in comatose patients treated within four hours. N Engl J Med 304:1511, 1981.
186. Soloniuk D, Pitts LH, Lovely M, et al: Traumatic intracerebral hematomas: timing of appearance and indications for operative removal. J Trauma 26:787, 1986.
187. Dowling G, Curry B: Traumatic basal subarachnoid hemorrhage. Report of six cases and review of the literature. Am J Forensic Med Pathol 9:23, 1988.
188. Ray H, Wahal KM: Subarachnoid hemorrhage in subacute bacterial endocarditis. Neurology 7:265, 1957.
189. Kalyan-Raman UP, Kalyan-Raman K: Cerebral amyloid angiopathy causing intracranial hemorrhage. Ann Neurol 16:321, 1984.
190. Roosen N, Martin JJ, De La Porte C, et al: Intracerebral hemorrhage due to cerebral amyloid angiopathy. J Neurosurg 63:965, 1985.
191. Briceno CE, Resch L, Bernstein M: Cerebral amyloid angiopathy presenting as a mass lesion. Stroke 18:234, 1987.

192. Caplan LR, Hier DB, Banks G: Current concepts of cerebrovascular disease—stroke: stroke and drug abuse. Stroke 13:869, 1982.
193. Matick H, Anderson D, Brumlik J: Cerebral vasculitis associated with oral amphetamine overdose. Arch Neurol 40:253, 1983.
194. Wooten MR, Khangure MS, Murphy MJ: Intracerebral hemorrhage and vasculitis related to ephedrine abuse. Ann Neurol 13:337, 1983.
195. Fallis RJ, Fisher M: Cerebral vasculitis and hemorrhage associated with phenylpropanolamine. Neurology 35:405, 1985.
196. Stoessl AJ, Young GB, Feasby TE: Intracerebral hemorrhage and angiographic beading following ingestion of catecholaminergics. Stroke 16:734, 1985.
197. Glick R, Hoying J, Cerullo L, Perlman S: Phenylpropanolamine: an over-the-counter drug causing central nervous system vasculitis and intracerebral hemorrhage. Case report and review. Neurosurgery 20:969, 1987.
198. Hillbom M, Kaste M: Alcohol intoxication: a risk factor for primary subarachnoid hemorrhage. Neurology 32:706, 1982.
199. Lichtenfeld PJ, Rubin DB, Feldman RS: Subarachnoid hemorrhage precipitated by cocaine snorting. Arch Neurol 41:223, 1984.
200. Lowenstein DH, Massa SM, Rowbotham MC, et al: Acute neurologic and psychiatric complications associated with cocaine abuse. Am J Med 83:841, 1987.
201. Mangiardi JR, Daras M, Geller ME, et al: Cocaine-related intracranial hemorrhage. Report of nine cases and review. Acta Neurol Scand 77:177, 1988.
202. Wojak JC, Flamm ES: Intracranial hemorrhage and cocaine use. Stroke 18:712, 1987.
203. Mody CK, Miller BL, McIntyre HB, et al: Neurologic complications of cocaine abuse. Neurology 38:1189, 1988.
204. Levine SR, Washington JM, Jefferson MF, et al: "Crack" cocaine-associated stroke. Neurology 37:1849, 1987.
205. Boyko OB, Burger PC, Heinz ER: Pathological and radiological correlation of subarachnoid hemorrhage in phencyclidine abuse. Case report. J Neurosurg 67:446, 1987.
206. Hayward RD: Subarachnoid haemorrhage of unknown etiology. J Neurol Neurosurg Psychiatry 40:926, 1977.
207. Brismar J, Sundbärg G: Subarachnoid hemorrhage of unknown origin: prognosis and prognostic factors. J Neurosurg 63:349, 1985.
208. Juul R, Fredriksen TA, Ringkjob R: Prognosis in subarachnoid hemorrhage of unknown etiology. J Neurosurg 64:359, 1986.
209. Alexander MS, Dias PS, Uttley D: Spontaneous subarachnoid hemorrhage and negative cerebral panangiography. Review of 140 cases. J Neurosurg 64:537, 1986.
210. Biller J, Toffol GJ, Kassell NF, et al: Spontaneous subarachnoid hemorrhage in young adults. Neurosurgery 21:664, 1987.

211. Suzuki S, Kayama T, Sakurai Y, et al: Subarachnoid hemorrhage of unknown cause. Neurosurgery 21:310, 1987.
212. Levine SR, Langer SL, Albers JW, Welch KM: Sneddon's syndrome: an antiphospholipid antibody syndrome? Neurology 38:798, 1988.
213. Leow K, Murie JA: Cerebral angiography for cerebrovascular disease: the risks. Br J Surg 75:428, 1988.
214. Theodotou BC, Whaley R, Mahaley MS: Complications following transfemoral cerebral angiography for cerebral ischemia. Report of 159 angiograms and correlation with surgical risk. Surg Neurol 28:90, 1987.
215. Dion JE, Gates PC, Fox AJ, et al: Clinical events following neuroangiography: a prospective study. Stroke 18:997, 1987.
216. Gittinger JW Jr: Occipital infarction following chiropractic cervical manipulation. J Clin Neuro Ophthalmol 6:11, 1986.
217. Edson JR, Fecher DR, Doe RP: Low platelet adhesiveness and other hemostatic abnormalities in hypothyroidism. Ann Intern Med 82:342, 1975.

Selected Readings

Barkovich AJ, Atlas SW: Magnetic resonance imaging of intracranial hemorrhage. Radiol Clin North Am 26:801, 1988.
An overview of intracranial hemorrhage as detected by MRI. The underlying physiology of the evolution of hemorrhagic masses and MRI correlations is complex. Authors describe MRI appearances of benign and neoplastic intraparenchymal hemorrhages.

Biller J, Adams HP Jr: Diagnosis of stroke in young adults. Postgrad Med 81(5):141, 1987.
Clinical review of major diagnostic possibilities and current recommendations for evaluation of stroke in young adults.

Bogousslavsky J, Despland PA, Regli F: Asymptomatic tight stenosis of the internal carotid artery: long-term prognosis. Neurology 36:861, 1986.
The low risk of unheralded ipsilateral infarct questions the usefulness of prophylactic endarterectomy. Diagnosis and treatment of risk factors and heart disease seem more important.

Bogousslavsky J, Hachinski VC, Boughner DR, et al: Cardiac and arterial lesions in carotid transient ischemic attacks. Arch Neurol 43:223, 1986.
Angiography, echocardiography, electrocardiography, and Holter monitoring findings in 250 consecutive patients with carotid TIAs and no previous stroke were evaluated. Potential sources for cardiogenic emboli were found more frequently in patients with known heart disease. Although the yield of possible cardiogenic emboli findings in patients without a history of heart disease was significantly lower, in this study at least 14 such patients had previously undetected potential cardiac sources of emboli.

Bogousslavsky J, Regli F: Vertebrobasilar transient ischemic attacks in internal carotid artery occlusion or tight stenosis. Arch Neurol 42:64, 1985.
This study suggests that vertebrobasilar insufficiency (VBI) may

be an added risk for delayed stroke in patients with carotid artery disease.

Bogousslavsky J, Regli F: Ischemic stroke in adults younger than 30 years of age. Cause and prognosis. Arch Neurol 44:479, 1987.

A clinical study of 41 stroke patients younger than 30 years of age included angiographic and echocardiographic evaluations. Etiologies of strokes in decreasing frequency were mitral valve prolapse and arterial dissection (51%), uncommon causes (34%), and migrainous stroke (15%).

Caplan LR: Carotid-artery disease (editorial). N Engl J Med 315:886, 1986.

Pithy review of current concepts.

Chambers BR, Norris JW: Clinical significance of asymptomatic neck bruits. Neurology 35:742, 1985.

A study assessing the value of auscultation of neck bruits compared to the results of carotid Doppler examination.

Chambers BR, Norris JW: Outcome in patients with asymptomatic neck bruits. N Engl J Med 315:860, 1986.

Data suggest that patients with asymptomatic cervical bruits have a higher risk of a cardiac ischemic event than of a stroke. Although the risk of cerebral ischemic events is highest in patients with severe carotid-artery stenosis, most of these patients do not have strokes without some warning.

Committee on Health Care Issues, American Neurological Association: Does carotid endarterectomy decrease stroke and death in patients with transient ischemic attacks? Ann Neurol 22:72, 1987.

A critical evaluation of carotid endarterectomy in the United States and the evidence that carotid endarterectomy prevents death and stroke in patients with carotid territory TIAs.

Darby DG, Donnan GA, Saling MA, et al: Primary intraventricular hemorrhage: clinical and neuropsychological findings in a prospective stroke series. Neurology 38:68, 1988.

A prospective study of primary intraventricular hemorrhage constituted 3.1% of intracerebral hemorrhages in a series of 2,950 patients. The seven cases reported began with sudden collapse and depressed consciousness. Focal signs were minimal and, if present, were contralateral to the major site of hematoma. Angiography in four patients found three patients with intracranial arteriovenous malformations and one with moyamoya. A persisting amnestic state was a common neurologic deficit in survivors.

Davis PH, Dambrosia JM, Schoenberg BS, et al: Risk factors for ischemic stroke: a prospective study in Rochester, Minnesota. Ann Neurol 22:319, 1987.

A 13-year study of a cohort of 1,804 residents of Rochester, Minnesota who were at least 50 years old and free of stroke when they entered the study were evaluated for major stroke and TIA risk factors. Major risk factors in this study were age, male sex, hypertensive heart disease, coronary heart disease, congestive heart failure, and diabetes mellitus.

Diaz JF, Hachinski VC, Pederson LL, Donald A: Aggregation of multiple risk factors for stroke in siblings of patients with brain infarction and transient ischemic attacks. Stroke 17:1239, 1986.

A study showing that major risk factors tend to cluster in families. Authors suggest that siblings of patients with cerebral infarction and TIAs may have an increased risk of stroke and cardiovascular disease as a result of multiple risk factors operating simultaneously.

Ernst E, Matrai A, Marshall M: Blood rheology in patients with transient ischemic attacks. Stroke 19:634, 1988.
Hematologic parameters in 26 patients with TIAs were evaluated and compared with controls. A hematologic disturbance associated with decreased blood flow was found in those with TIAs. Findings included impairment of blood fluidity such as increased plasma viscosity, changes in blood cell filterability, and erythrocyte aggregation.

Evans WE, Hayes JP: Life history of patients with transient ischemic attacks and essentially normal angiograms. J Vasc Surg 6:548, 1987.
A study of 83 patients with hemispheric TIAs and normal angiograms followed patients from 2 to 132 months. Six patients experienced a cerebrovascular accident, and five had further hemispheric TIAs. These results suggest that the prognosis of patients with hemispheric TIAs and normal angiograms may not be as benign as previously reported.

Ford CS, Frye JL, Toole JF, et al: Asymptomatic carotid bruit and stenosis. Arch Neurol 43:219, 1986.
In patients with asymptomatic carotid bruit and stenosis, myocardial infarctions occur more frequently and are more often the cause of death than are cerebral infarctions.

Foster JW, Hart RG: Hypoglycemic hemiplegia: two cases and a clinical review. Stroke 18:944, 1987.
Two cases of hypoglycemic hemiplegia, which were initially diagnosed as transient ischemic attacks, are described. Angiography was normal in both patients. Attacks resolved with a change in insulin dose.

Foulkes MA, Wolf PA, Price TR, et al: The Stroke Data Bank: design, methods, and baseline characteristics. Stroke 19:547, 1988.
A Stroke Data Bank, a multicenter project to prospectively collect data on the clinical course and sequelae of stroke, has been initiated by the National Institute of Neurological and Communicative Disorders and Stroke.

Gorelick PB, Caplan LR, Langenberg P, et al: Clinical and angiographic comparison of asymptomatic occlusive cerebrovascular disease. Neurology 38:852, 1988.
Clinical and arteriographic characteristics in 106 patients with symptomatic unilateral carotid territory occlusive disease were evaluated to determine the frequency and distribution of occlusive arterial lesions in asymptomatic vessels. Among predominantly young, black, female patients, more asymptomatic lesions were found in the supraclinoid internal carotid artery, anterior cerebral artery stem, and middle cerebral artery stem. Among predominantly elderly, white, male patients, severe occlusive asymptomatic disease was found more frequently at extracranial carotid and vertebral artery sites.

Gorelick PB, Rodin MB, Langenberg P, et al: Is acute alcohol ingestion a risk factor for ischemic stroke? Results of a controlled study in middle-aged and elderly stroke patients at three urban medical centers. Stroke 18:359, 1987.
The risk of acute alcohol ingestion as a stroke risk factor was

assessed in 205 middle-aged and elderly acute ischemic stroke patients and 410 outpatient matched controls. Matched multiple logistic analysis found hypertension and smoking independently associated with stroke, but no correlation with alcohol consumption. Authors conclude that acute alcohol ingestion is not an independent risk factor in middle-aged and elderly patients, and that the apparent association of alcohol and ischemic stroke is the result of confounding effects related to smoking.

Grolimund P, Seiler RW, Aaslid R, et al: Evaluation of cerebrovascular disease by combined extracranial and transcranial Doppler sonography. Experience in 1,039 patients. Stroke 18:1018, 1987.

Usefulness, limitations, and indications for Doppler evaluations are suggested by this study of 1,039 combined cervical and transcranial Doppler examinations. This may offer a promising technique for monitoring cerebral blood flow, vasospasm, and characterizing flow rates of arteriovenous malformations.

Howard G, Toole JF, Frye-Pierson J, Hinshelwood LC: Factors influencing the survival of 451 transient ischemic attack patients. Stroke 18:552, 1987.

Prognostic risk factors were evaluated in 451 patients with TIAs. Proportional hazard analysis revealed decreased survival correlated with increasing age, carotid artery TIAS, cigarette smoking, previous contralateral stroke, ischemic heart disease, and diabetes mellitus.

Jansen PA, Schulte BP, Poels EF, Gribnau FW: Course of blood pressure after cerebral infarction and transient ischemic attack. Clin Neurol Neurosurg 89:243, 1987.

Blood pressure trends in 63 patients admitted for stroke or TIA were studied. This study shows that blood pressure is elevated in the acute phase of cerebral infarction and TIA, but spontaneously becomes normotensive in the first days after the cerebrovascular event. Authors point out that blood pressure may rise within the first few months after discharge.

Johnson JM, Kennelly MM, Decesare D, et al: Natural history of asymptomatic carotid plaque. Arch Surg 120:1010, 1985.

This study suggests that soft plaques have a greater tendency toward subintimal hemorrhage, ulceration, or primary embolization than more well-organized plaques.

Kertesz A, Black SE, Nicholson L, Carr T: The sensitivity and specificity of MRI in stroke. Neurology 37:1580, 1987.

MRI and CT findings in stroke patients were compared in a study of 175 patients. From these data, authors conclude that MRI is more sensitive than CT in the early detection of cerebral infarcts. CT is the method of choice to rule out intracerebral bleeding. However, in later stages, MRI is more specific. MRI was found useful for following the evolution of strokes and distinguishing acute and chronic infarcts without contrast agents.

Landi G, D'Angelo A, Boccardi E, et al: Hypercoagulability in acute stroke: prognostic significance. Neurology 37:1667, 1987.

Coagulation and platelet function were evaluated in 70 patients with recent cerebral infarction or hemorrhage and in 45 age-matched controls. Higher levels of one-stage factor VIII coagulant activity, fibrinopeptide A, and beta-thromboglobulin were associated with stroke.

Landi G, Guidotti M, Valsecchi F: Influence of age on carotid atheroma in patients with reversible ischemic attacks. Stroke 18:43, 1987.
The influence of age on carotid atheroma was reviewed in angiographic findings of 120 patients with reversible ischemic attacks. The prevalence and severity of atherosclerotic lesions increased significantly with age in this study, even after adjusting for hypertension.

Laureno R, Shields RW Jr, Narayan T: The diagnosis and management of cerebral embolism and hemorrhagic infarction with sequential computerized cranial tomography. Brain 110:93, 1987.
Since hemorrhagic infarction is usually not present immediately after a cerebral embolism and spontaneous hemorrhagic transformation can evlove over several days, delayed CT scans are essential to exclude hemorrhagic infarction before initiating anticoagulant therapy.

Lechner H, Schmidt R, Bertha G, et al: Nuclear magnetic resonance image white matter lesions and risk factors for stroke in normal individuals. Stroke 19:263, 1988.
White matter lesions detected by the T2-weighted MRI among 42 volunteers without known cerebrovascular symptoms were correlated with stroke risk factors. Only 11 of the 155 MRI detected abnormalities could be detected by CT. MRI-detected white matter abnormalities appeared to occur with greater frequency in those volunteers with more stroke factors. Authors suggest that white matter lesions in T2-weighted images may represent an early stage of cerebrovascular disease.

Leow K, Murie JA: Cerebral angiography for cerebrovascular disease: the risks. Br J Surg 75:428, 1988.
Cerebral angiography is considered a necessary evaluation before carotid endarterectomy. Analysis of prospective studies of cerebral complications show that over the last decade, major stroke rate after conventional cerebral angiography for patients with TIAs is about 2.4%.

Levy DE: How transient are transient ischemic attacks? Neurology 38:674, 1988.
Duration criteria of ischemic events occurring in 1,343 hospitalized patients were correlated with outcome. Ischemic events were categorized as a TIA if symptoms resolved within 24 hours, a reversible ischemic neurologic deficit (RIND) if symptoms resolved within 1 to 7 days, and ischemic stroke if deficits did not resolve. Data suggest that patients with a deficit persisting at least 60 minutes have less than a 2% chance of resolving spontaneously during any subsequent 1-hour period; therefore, rapid resolution after instituting a new treatment may suggest a therapeutic effect.

Levy DE: Transient CNS deficits: a common, benign syndrome in young adults. Neurology 38:831, 1988.
A study from Cornell University's Department of Neurology of the incidence of transient neurologic loss, i.e., resolution of symptoms in less than 24 hours, in young adults with a median follow-up of 5 years. Authors found transient CNS deficits in the young that were often unexplained, relatively common, and benign. The importance of distinguishing these episodes from true ischemic episodes will become increasingly important as newer, hyperacute stroke therapies emerge.

Loes DJ, Smoker WR, Biller J, Cornell SH: Nontraumatic

lobar intracerebral hemorrhage: CT/angiographic correlation. AJNR 8:1027, 1987.

CT and cerebral angiographic findings of 67 consecutive patients with nontraumatic lobar intracerebral hemorrhages were reviewed. Angiography was more frequently diagnostic in frontal or temporal hematomas than with parietal or occipital lobar hematomas. Authors recommend that all patients with otherwise unexplained nontraumatic lobar intracerebral hemorrhage be evaluated with cerebral angiography.

Maiuri F, Gallicchio B, Donati P, Carandente M: The blood leukocyte count and its prognostic significance in subarachnoid hemorrhage. J Neurosurg Sci 31:45, 1987.

The white blood cell counts in 75 patients with subarachnoid hemorrhages are correlated with the clinical grade of hemorrhage on admission, presence of angiographic spasm, and blood clots in the cisternal space. Low white cell counts were correlated with patients with subarachnoid hemorrhages who had normal angiograms. Higher white cell counts were correlated with ruptured aneurysms. Authors suggest that the white blood cell count appears to have a high prognostic value in predicting neurologic deterioration secondary to arterial spasm.

Meissner I, Wiebers DO, Whisnant JP, O'Fallon WM: The natural history of asymptomatic carotid artery occlusive lesions. JAMA 258:2704, 1987

A retrospective study was conducted to determine the long-term prognosis of patients with asymptomatic hemodynamically significant internal carotid system lesions. Results suggest that patients with asymptomatic pressure-significant carotid system occlusive lesions are at twofold greater risk for stroke than are patients with normal ocular pneumoplethysmography studies and at sevenfold greater risk for stroke than is the general population.

Meyer FB, Sundt TM Jr, Yanagihara T, Anderson RE: Focal cerebral ischemia: pathophysiologic mechanisms and rationale for future avenues of treatment. Mayo Clin Proc 62:35, 1987.

An overview of current and future avenues of newer pharmacologic agents and methods to restore blood flow to areas of focal ischemia suggests that a more aggressive therapeutic approach may soon be offered to selected acute stroke patients.

Mustacchi P: Risk factors in stroke. West J Med 143:186, 1985.

Well-referenced overview.

Natowicz M, Kelley RI: Mendelian etiologies of stroke. Ann Neurol 22:175, 1987.

An important review of genetic disorders associated with increased stroke. Disorders are characterized clinically and biochemically, with proposed pathogenetic mechanisms of stroke. Authors outline appropriate testing for screening and diagnosis.

O'Holleran LW, Kennelly MM, McClurken M, Johnson JM: Natural history of asymptomatic carotid plaque. Five year follow-up study. Am J Surg 154:659, 1987.

A prospective study of 296 carotid arteries in 293 patients quantified carotid stenosis, characterized carotid plaque disease, and correlated these findings with clinical outcome. Patients with hemodynamically significant stenosis and morphologically soft plaque were at greatest risk for TIA or stroke. Patients with calcified plaque and less than 75% stenosis were at lower risk for TIA or stroke.

Passero S, Rossi G, Nardini M, et al: Italian multicenter study of reversible cerebral ischemic attacks. Part 5. Risk factors and cerebral atherosclerosis. Atherosclerosis 63:211, 1987.
A propsective study of 462 patients with reversible cerebral ischemic attacks who underwent angiography studied premorbid and environmental risk factors of atherosclerotic cerebral vessel disease. Authors found age, smoking, and history of hypertension the best predictors of extent and severity of cerebral vessel atherosclerosis.

Quiñones-Baldrich WJ, Moore WS: Asymptomatic carotid stenosis. Rationale for management. Arch Neurol 42:378, 1985.
A review and guidelines for the approach to asymptomatic carotid stenosis.

Ramirez-Lassepas M, Cipolle RJ: Medical treatment of transient ischemic attacks: does it influence mortality? Stroke 19:397, 1988.
Randomized studies published on medical treatment of TIAs in which controls received no treatment or placebo and in which mortality was reported. Data were analyzed using the odds ratio method, and neither treatment modality (chronic anticoagulation or platelet inhibitors) significantly reduced mortality.

Rothrock JF: Clinical evaluation and management of transient ischemic atacks. West J Med 146:452, 1987.
Well-referenced, comprehensive clinical review.

Rothrock JF, Lyden PD, Yee J, Wiederholt WC: "Crescendo" transient ischemic attacks: clinical and angiographic correlations. Neurology 38:198, 1988.
Angiographic or intraoperative correlations of anterior circulation disease were obtained in 47 consecutive patients presenting with repetitive symptoms in the anterior circulation consistent with crescendo TIAs. In 26 patients (55%), anatomically significant disease was found. Positive angiographic findings were more frequently found in patients with amaurosis fugax and signs suggesting cortical ischemia.

Sacco RL, Wolf PA, Bharucha NE, et al: Subarachnoid and intracerebral hemorrhage: natural history, prognosis, and precursive factors in the Framingham Study. Neurology 34:847, 1984.
A prospective study reports that hypertension and heavy smoking are more common among patients with subarachnoid hemorrhages.

Sheng FC, Busuttil RW: Carotid surgery in stroke prevention. Am Fam Physician 33:109, 1986.
Useful clinical review for physicians and for patient information.

Sloan MA: Thrombolysis and stroke. Past and future. Arch Neurol 44:748, 1987.
Thrombolytic (fibrinolytic) therapy of stroke is a recent and hopeful adjunctive therapy that potentially may limit the size of ischemic cerebral infarcts by pharmacologic means. Recent advances reviewed.

Todnem K, Vik-Mo H: Cerebral ischemic attacks as a complication of heart disease: the value of echocardiography. Acta Neurol Scand 74:323, 1986.
The usefulness of echocardiography in detecting cardiac sources of thromboembolic strokes is reviewed in a study of 194 patients with transient ischemic attacks. Ninety-five patients were found to have

heart disease, 63 of whom had positive findings on echocardiogram. Thirty-five patients were found to have a cardiogenic source that caused an embolism. Aortic and mitral valve disease were the two most frequently identified cardiac disorders.

Unger E, Littlefield J, Gado M: Water content and water structure in CT and MR signal changes: possible influence in detection of early stroke. AJNR 9:687, 1988.

MRI has been shown to be more sensitive than CT in early stroke detection. Authors describe experiments with model systems designed to separate the effects of water content and water structure on MRI signal intensity. Data from these experimental designs and subsequent MR images suggest that water structure, and not merely water content, is a significant mechanism underlying relaxation time changes and signal intensity changes produced in acute stroke.

Wang AM, Lin JC, Rumbaugh CL: What is expected of CT in the evaluation of stroke? Neuroradiology 30:54, 1988.

A study of 5,042 CT examinations performed over 2 years, 19.8% of which were obtained to confirm or evaluate a clinically suspected stroke. Eighty-seven percent of clinically suspected strokes were confirmed by CT findings. Intracranial hemorrhages and brain tumors mimicking stroke made up a small but important percentage of findings.

Weir BK: The management of intracranial aneurysms—prospects for improvement. Clin Neurosurg 34:154, 1988.

An overview of current concepts of intracranial aneurysms.

Werdelin L, Juhler M: The course of transient ischemic attacks. Neurology 38:677, 1988.

Seventy-eight patients hospitalized with first episodes of cerebrovascular events of presumed ischemic origin were evaluated to determine if the diagnosis of stroke versus TIAs could be made earlier than 24 hours. Within 1 hour, 50% of the TIAs were resolved; within 4 hours, 90% were resolved. Authors suggest that the persistence of symptoms beyond a few hours and the initial severity of symptoms may provide reliable indicators for predicting which events will be TIAs and which events will be strokes.

Wessler S: Anticoagulants in the prevention of embolic stroke. Part I. Geriatrics 42(2):29, 1987.

A review of the evaluation and indications for anticoagulation therapy in patients with cardiac lesions considered high risk for cardiogenic emboli, including atrial fibrillation, rheumatic mitral valve disease, acute myocardial infarction, prosthetic heart valves, and idiopathic dilated cardiomyopathy. Usefulness of CT in the decision process is stressed.

Winslow CM, Solomon DH, Chassin MR, et al: The appropriateness of carotid endarterectomy. N Engl J Med 318:721, 1988.

Current controversies of usefulness and possible inappropriate use of carotid endarterectomy. Authors suggest that carotid endarterectomy was overused in three geographic areas studied. Appropriate indications and inappropriate reasons for suggesting carotid endarterectomy are discussed.

Yatsu FM, Fields WS: Asymptomatic carotid bruit. Stenosis or ulceration, a conservative approach. Arch Neurol 42:383, 1985.

A concise discussion of the rationale for a conservative approach to the asymptomatic carotid bruit.

Zenker G, Erbel R, Kramer G, et al: Transesophageal

two-dimensional echocardiography in young patients with cerebral ischemic events. Stroke 19:345, 1988.

Authors found transesophageal echocardiography to be a sensitive method for detecting mitral valve prolapse and detecting other valve and cardiac abnormalities that may be the source of cerebrovascular symptoms, particularly in young stroke patients.

49
Restless Legs and Burning Feet: Common and Uncommon Associations

Tingling, burning, prickling, itching, and restless legs are described by patients who usually fall within three major diagnostic categories: (1) sensorimotor and sensory neuropathies, (2) restless leg syndromes, and (3) miscellaneous conditions without objective signs of neuropathy. The clinical history, electrodiagnostic studies, and, in certain cases, sural nerve biopsy are the diagnostic cornerstones. The clinical picture of sensory or sensorimotor neuropathy with primarily sensory symptoms includes numbness, burning, temperature hypersensitivity, and sharp pains, usually felt first in the toes and often limited to distal extremities.[1] Sometimes clinical symptoms at the onset of a polyneuropathy cannot be confirmed with conventional electrodiagnostic studies; occasionally serial studies are helpful. There are a variety of disorders associated with unexplained, yet often persistent, complaints of tingling, numbness, or burning. When these symptoms remain undiagnosed, they plague patients with constant discomfort and plague the patient's physician with concern that these symptoms are manifestations of an undiagnosed disorder. The clinical history can usually quickly narrow a wide range of diagnostic possibilities such as metabolic-endocrine disorders, autoimmune disorders, suspected neoplasms, drug-induced symptoms, infection, vitamin deficiencies, toxic causes, genetic possibilities, restless leg syndromes, and idiopathic neuropathies.[2] If there is clinical evidence for a neuropathy, and certain diseases are suspected, a sural nerve biopsy can be helpful.

Metabolic-Endocrine Disorders

Diabetes: acute forms of diabetic sensory neuropathy usually have minimal signs and better prognosis than the chronic sensorimotor neuropathy often associated with small muscle wasting and patchy stocking and glove sensory loss.[3-7]

Alcoholism: alcoholic polyneuropathy is characterized by a generalized, sensorimotor, distal axonopathy.[8,9]

B_{12} deficiency[10]

Other vitamin deficiencies: thiamine, pantothenic acid, pyridoxine, niacin, and vitamin E[11,12]

Renal failure: particularly with uremia[13-17]

Hypothyroidism[18]

Protein calorie malnutrition[19]

Infection

Syphilis

Herpes zoster

Tick bite (*Ixodes*): Lyme disease[20-22]

Leprosy[23]

Hepatitis B[24]

Human immunodeficiency virus (HIV) infection: six subtypes of polyneuropathy have been described, two are primarily sensory: a predominantly painful polyneuropathy and a sensory ataxic neuropathy secondary to ganglioneuronitis[25-29]

Neoplastic Disorders

Carcinomatous neuropathy: the most commonly identified subtype of carcinomatous neuropathy is the subacute sensory neuropathy, which can precede identification of neoplasm by months and is most often associated with small cell carcinoma of the lung.[30-33]

Paraneoplastic neuropathy[34]

Plasma cell dyscrasias: Waldenström's macroglobulinemia, multiple myeloma, osteosclerotic myeloma, cryoglobulinemia, lymphoma[35-43]

Other cancer associations: subclinical sensory neuropathy occurs in a significant number of patients with cancer and appears directly related to the underlying neoplasm rather than known neuropathy risk factors[44]

Vasculitic, Autoimmune, and Collagen Vascular Disorders

Necrotizing arteritis: associated with rheumatoid arthritis, hepatitis B infections, and HIV infection[45]

Polyarteritis nodosa

Allergic angiitis

Granulomatosis

Systemic necrotizing vasculitis[46]

Wegener's granulomatosis[47]

Hypersensitivity vasculitis: cutaneous hypersensitivity, serum sickness, Henoch-Schönlein purpura, drug- or infection-associated vasculitis[46]

Giant cell arteritis[48]

IgM-associated dysimmune neuropathy: cryoglobulinemia, gamma-heavy chain disease, plasma dyscrasias, paraproteinemias[49-52]

Systemic lupus erythematosus[53]

Behçet's disease[54]

Sjögren's syndrome (sicca syndrome)[55-57]

Nonsystemic vasculitic neuropathy: ischemic neuropathy without systemic vasculitis[58]

Toxic

Drug-induced
  Pyridoxine[59-62]
  Antibiotics: penicillins
  Cisplatin[63-66]
  Adriamycin[67]
  Vincristine[68]
  Almitrine[69]
  Thalidomide[70]
  Chloroquine[71]
  Phenytoin[72]
  Disulfiram
  Isoniazid
  Hydralazine

Toxic metal exposure: lead, arsenic, mercury, gold, thallium, bismuth, antimony[73]

Toxic organic compound exposure: organophosphates, trichlorethylene, carbon disulfide, acrylamide hexacarbons

Idiopathic Neuropathy Syndromes

Acquired inflammatory acute and chronic demyelinating neuropathies: recognition of chronic and dysproteinemic forms are important because they are potentially treatable; dysproteinemic forms may be associated with occult systemic disorders.[74]

Fisher variant Guillain-Barré syndrome: a variation of acquired inflammatory demyelinating polyneuropathy characterized by ophthalmoplegia, ataxia, and areflexia[75,76]

Migrant sensory neuritis of Wartenberg[77]

Acute sensory neuronopathy syndrome[78]

Miscellaneous Associations

Amyloidosis[79]

Biliary cirrhosis[80,81]

Crohn's disease: neuropathies can occur with and without associated vitamin deficiencies or oral metronidazole therapy[82]

Sarcoidosis[83]

Thrombocythemic myeloproliferative disease[84]

Peripheral vascular insufficiency

Trauma: traumatic fascicular neuromas, peripheral nerve trauma[85,86]

Long distance running: can cause multiple small injuries to toes and feet, resulting in transient sensory symptoms[87]

Multiple sclerosis

Restless Legs Syndromes

Ekbom syndrome: tingling, burning, prickly sensations in the legs, relieved by movement[88]

Painful legs and moving toes: characteristic features include pain in the feet or legs and spontaneous involuntary movement of the toes; may be seen following peripheral nerve lesions or minor leg trauma[89–92]

Nocturnal myoclonus and restless legs syndrome: patients characteristically complain of excessive daytime hypersomnolence; bed partners complain of the restless legs.[93]

Muscular pain-fasciculation syndrome: characterized by pain, fasciculations, cramps, occasional paresthesias; with electrophysiologic findings consistent with a benign polyneuropathy[94]

Familial restless legs with periodic movements in sleep[95]

Restless red legs: association of restless leg syndrome with arborizing telangiectasia of the legs[96]

Genetic

Hereditary sensory neuropathy[2,97–105]
Spinocerebellar degeneration[106]
Fabry's disease: alpha-galactosidase deficiency[107–109]
Congenital sensory neuropathy with selective loss of small myelinated fibers[110]
Hereditary motor-sensory neuropathy[111]
Abetalipoproteinemia[112]
Congenital sensory neuropathy with anhidrosis[113]
Hereditary sensory neuropathy with neurotrophic keratitis[114]
Friedreich's ataxia: slowing of distal sensory conduction can be part of the full syndrome or a single clinical finding in relatives[115,116]
Familial amyloid polyneuropathy[117,118]
Group A xeroderma pigmentosum neuropathy[119]

Diseases in Which Sural Biopsy Can Be Diagnostic*

Vasculitic neuropathies: neuropathy seen most frequently in the polyarteritis nodosa group of systemic necrotizing vasculitides, hypersensitivity vasculitides, and Wegener's granulomatosis[58,121,122]
Diabetes mellitus[123–127]
Demyelinating neuropathies[128]
Amyloidosis[129]
Leprosy[23,130]
Hypertrophic form of Charcot-Marie-Tooth disease
Sensory perineuritis
Ataxia telangiectasia
Giant axonal neuropathy[131]
Leukodystrophies
Some neuronal storage disorders[132]
Sarcoidosis[133]
Vitamin E deficiency[134]

References

1. Nakano KK (ed): Peripheral neuropathies. p. 155. In Neurology of Musculoskeletal and Rheumatic Disorders. Houghton Mifflin, Boston, 1979.
2. Dyck PJ, Low PA, Stevens JC: "Burning feet" as the only manifestation of dominantly inherited sensory neuropathy. Mayo Clin Proc 58:426, 1983.
3. Archer AG, Watkins PJ, Thomas PK, et al: The natural history of acute painful neuropathy in diabetes mellitus. J Neurol Neurosurg Psychiatry 46:491, 1983.
4. Heimans JJ, Bertelsmann FW, Van Rooy JCGM: Large and small nerve fiber function in painful diabetic neuropathy. J Neurol Sci 74:1, 1986.

* (From Johnson PC,[120] with permission.)

5. Troni W, Carta Q, Cantello R, et al: Peripheral nerve function and metabolic control in diabetes mellitus. Ann Neurol 16:178, 1984.

6. Report and recommendations of the San Antonio conference on diabetic neuropathy. Consensus statement. Diabetes 37:1000, 1988.

7. Boulton AJ, Ward JD: Diabetic neuropathies and pain. Clin Endocrinol Metab 15:917, 1986.

8. Shields RW Jr: Alcoholic polyneuropathy. Muscle Nerve 8:183, 1985.

9. Melgaard B, Saelan H, Hedegaard L: Symptoms and signs of polyneuropathy and their relation to alcohol intake in a normal male population. Acta Neurol Scand 73:458, 1986.

10. Steiner I, Kidron D, Soffer D, et al: Sensory peripheral neuropathy of vitamin B12 deficiency: a primary demyelinating disease? J Neurol 235:163, 1988.

11. Traber MG, Sokol RJ, Ringel SP, et al: Lack of tocopherol in peripheral nerves of vitamin E-deficient patients with peripheral neuropathy. N Engl J Med 317:262, 1987.

12. Werlin SL, Harb JM, Swick H, Blank E: Neuromuscular dysfunction and ultrastructural pathology in children with chronic cholestasis and vitamin E deficiency. Ann Neurol 13:291, 1983.

13. Asbury AK, Victor M, Adams RD: Uremic polyneuropathy. Arch Neurol 8:413, 1963.

14. D'Amour ML, Dufresne LR, Morin C, Slaughter D: Sensory nerve conduction in chronic uremic patients during the first six months of hemodialysis. Can J Neurol Sci 11:269, 1984.

15. Solders G, Persson A, Wilczek H: Autonomic system dysfunction and polyneuropathy in nondiabetic uremia. A one-year follow-up study after renal transplantation. Transplantation 41:616, 1986.

16. Said G, Boudier L, Selva J, et al: Different patterns of uremic polyneuropathy: clinicopathologic study. Neurology 33:567, 1983.

17. Tegner R, Lindholm B: Uremic polyneuropathy: different effects of hemodialysis and continuous ambulatory peritoneal dialysis. Acta Med Scand 218:409, 1985.

18. Nemni R, Bottacchi E, Fazio R, et al: Polyneuropathy in hypothyroidism: clinical, electrophysiological and morphological findings in four cases. J Neurol Neurosurg Psychiatry 50:1454, 1987.

19. Chopra JS, Dhand UK, Mehta S, et al: Effect of protein calorie malnutrition on peripheral nerves. A clinical, electrophysiological and histopathological study. Brain 109:307, 1986.

20. Vallat JM, Hugon J, Lubeau M, et al: Tick-bite meningoradiculoneuritis: clinical, electrophysiologic, and histologic findings in 10 cases. Neurology 37:749, 1987.

21. Camponovo F, Meier C: Neuropathy of vasculitic origin in a case of Garin-Boujadoux-Bannwarth syndrome with positive *Borrelia* antibody response. J Neurol 233:69, 1986.

22. Dupois MJ: Multiple neurologic manifestations of *Bor-*

relia burgdorferi infection. Rev Neurol (Paris) 144:765, 1988.

23. Gibbels E, Henke U, Klingmuller G, Haupt WF: Myelinated and unmyelinated fibers in sural nerve biopsy of a case with lepromatous leprosy—a quantitative approach. Int J Lepr Other Mycobact Dis 55:333, 1987.

24. Inoue A, Tsukada N, Koh CS, Yanagisawa N: Chronic relapsing demyelinating polyneuropathy associated with hepatitis B infection. Neurology 37:1663, 1987.

25. Lipkin WI, Parry G, Kiprov D, et al: Inflammatory neuropathy in homosexual men with lymphadenopathy. Neurology 35:1479, 1985.

26. Bailey RO, Baltch AL, Venkatesh R, et al: Sensory motor neuropathy associated with AIDS. Neurology 38:886, 1988.

27. Dalakas MC, Pezeshkpour GH: Neuromuscular diseases associated with human immunodeficiency virus infection. Ann Neurol 23(Suppl):S38, 1988.

28. Cornblath DR, McArthur JC: Predominantly sensory neuropathy in patients with AIDS and AIDS-related complex. Neurology 38:794, 1988.

29. Parry GJ: Peripheral neuropathies associated with human immunodeficiency virus infection. Ann Neurol 23(Suppl):S49, 1988.

30. Horwich MS, Cho L, Porro RS, et al: Subacute sensory neuropathy: a remote effect of carcinoma. Ann Neurol 2:7, 1977.

31. Ohnishi A, Ogawa M: Preferential loss of large lumbar primary sensory neurons in carcinomatous sensory neuropathy. Ann Neurol 20:102, 1986.

32. Lamarche J, Vital C: Carcinomatous neuropathy. An ultrastructural study of ten cases. Ann Pathol 7:98, 1987.

33. Donofrio PD, Alessi AG, Albers JW, et al: Electrodiagnostic evolution of carcinomatous sensory neuronopathy. Muscle Nerve 12:508, 1989.

34. Vallat JM, Leboutet MJ, Hugon J, et al: Acute pure sensory paraneoplastic neuropathy with perivascular endoneurial inflammation: ultrastructural study of capillary walls. Neurology 36:1395, 1986.

35. Smith T, Sherman W, Olarte MR, Lovelace RE: Peripheral neuropathy associated with plasma cell dyscrasia: a clinical and electrophysiological follow-up study. Acta Neurol Scand 75:244, 1987.

36. Julien J, Vital C, Vallat JM, et al: Polyneuropathy in Waldenström's macroglobulinemia. Arch Neurol 35:423, 1978.

37. Harbs H, Arfmann M, Frick E, et al: Reactivity of sera and isolated monoclonal IgM from patients with Waldenström's macroglobulinemia with peripheral nerve myelin. J Neurol 232:43, 1985.

38. Lamarca J, Casquero P, Pou A: Mononeuritis multiplex in Waldenström's macroglobulinemia. Ann Neurol 22:268, 1987.

39. Hoppe U, Drager HS, Patzold U, et al: Polyneuropathy in Waldenström's macroglobulinemia. Passive transfer from man to mouse. Acta Neurol Scand 75:112, 1987.

40. Barbieri F, Sinisi L, Santangelo R, et al: Cryoglobuli-

nemic neuropathy. A light and electron microscopic study. Acta Neurol 9:241, 1987.

41. Nemni R, Corbo M, Fazio R, et al: Cryoglobulinemic neuropathy. A clinical, morphological and immunocytochemical study of 8 cases. Brain 111:541, 1988.

42. Lippa CF, Chad DA, Smith TW, et al: Neuropathy associated with cryoglobulinemia. Muscle Nerve 9:626, 1986.

43. Ince PG, Shaw PJ, Fawcett PR, Bates D: Demyelinating neuropathy due to primary IgM kappa B cell lymphoma of peripheral nerve. Neurology 37:1231, 1987.

44. Lipton RB, Galer BS, Dutcher JP, et al: Quantitative sensory testing demonstrates that subclinical sensory neuropathy is prevalent in patients with cancer. Arch Neurol 44:944, 1987.

45. Said G, Lacroix-Ciaudo C, Fujimura H, et al: The peripheral neuropathy of necrotizing arteritis: a clinicopathological study. Ann Neurol 23:461, 1988.

46. Moore PM, Cupps TR: Neurological complications of vasculitis. Ann Neurol 14:155, 1983.

47. Cavaletti G, Marmiroli P, Petruccioli-Pizzini MG, Tredici G: Histological features of nerve fibers and endoneural vessels in a case of Wegener's granulomatosis. Eur Neurol 28:77, 1988.

48. Golbus J, McCune WJ: Giant cell arteritis and peripheral neuropathy: a report of 2 cases and review of the literature. J Rheumatol 14:129, 1987.

49. Galassi G, Nemni R: Sensory action potentials and biopsy of the sural nerve in the neuropathy of nonmalignant IgMk plasma cell dyscrasia. Eur Neurol 25:1, 1986.

50. Jonsson V, Schroder HD, Staehelin-Jensen T, et al: Autoimmunity related to IgM monoclonal gammopathy of undetermined significance. Peripheral neuropathy and connective tissue sensitization caused by IgM M-proteins. Acta Med Scand 223:255, 1988.

51. Sobue G, Yanagi T, Hashizume Y: Chronic progressive sensory ataxic neuropathy with polyclonal gammopathy and disseminated focal perivascular cellular infiltrations. Neurology 38:463, 1988.

52. Meier C: Polyneuropathy in paraproteinemia. J Neurol 232:204, 1985.

53. McCombe PA, McLeod JG, Pollard JD, et al: Peripheral sensorimotor and autonomic neuropathy associated with systemic lupus erythematosus. Clinical, pathological and immunological features. Brain 110:533, 1987.

54. Namer IJ, Karabudak R, Zileli T, et al: Peripheral nervous system involvement in Behçet's disease. Case report and review of the literature. Eur Neurol 26:235, 1987.

55. Malinow K, Yannakakis GD, Glusman SM, et al: Subacute sensory neuronopathy secondary to dorsal root ganglionitis in primary Sjögren's syndrome. Ann Neurol 20:535, 1986.

56. Oddis CV, Eisenbeis CH Jr, Reidbord HE, et al: Vasculitis in systemic sclerosis: association with Sjögren's syndrome and the CREST syndrome variant. J Rheumatol 14:942, 1987.

57. Kennett RP, Harding AE: Peripheral neuropathy as-

sociated with the sicca syndrome. J Neurol Neurosurg Psychiatry 49:90, 1986.

58. Dyck PJ, Benstead TJ, Conn DL, et al: Nonsystemic vasculitic neuropathy. Brain 110:843, 1987.

59. Schaumburg H, Kaplan J, Windebank A, et al: Sensory neuropathy from pyridoxine abuse. N Engl J Med 309:445, 1983.

60. Albin RL, Albers JW, Greenberg HS, et al: Acute sensory neuropathy-neuronopathy from pyridoxine overdose. Neurology 37:1729, 1987.

61. Waterston JA, Gilligan BS: Pyridoxine neuropathy. Med J Aust 146:640, 1987.

62. Friedman MA, Resnick JS, Baer RL: Subepidermal vesicular dermatosis and sensory peripheral neuropathy caused by pyridoxine abuse. J Am Acad Dermatol 14:915, 1986.

63. Roelofs RI, Hrushesky W, Rogin J, et al: Peripheral sensory neuropathy and cisplatin chemotherapy. Neurology 34:934, 1984.

64. Riggs JE, Ashraf M, Snyder RD, Gutmann L: Prospective nerve conduction studies in cisplatin therapy. Ann Neurol 23:92, 1988.

65. Daugaard GK, Petrera J, Trojaborg W: Electrophysiological study of the peripheral and central neurotoxic effect of cis-platin. Acta Neurol Scand 76:86, 1987.

66. Carenza L, Villani C, Framarino-dei-Malatesta ML, et al: Peripheral neuropathy and ototoxicity of dichlorodiamineplatinum: instrumental evaluation. Preliminary results. Gynecol Oncol 25:244, 1986.

67. Cho ES: Toxic effects of adriamycin on the ganglia of the peripheral nervous system: a neuropathological study. J Neuropathol Exp Neurol 36:907, 1977.

68. Legha SS: Vincristine neurotoxicity. Pathophysiology and management. Med Toxicol 1:421, 1986.

69. Gherardi R, Baudrimont M, Gray F, Louarn F: Almitrine neuropathy. A nerve biopsy study of 8 cases. Acta Neuropathol 73:202, 1987.

70. Lagueny A, Rommel A, Vignolly B, et al: Thalidomide neuropathy: an electrophysiologic study. Muscle Nerve 9:837, 1986.

71. Estes ML, Ewing-Wilson D, Chou SM, et al: Chloroquine neuromyotoxicity. Clinical and pathologic perspective. Am J Med 82:447, 1987.

72. Ramirez JA, Mendell JR, Warmolts JR, Griggs RC: Phenytoin neuropathy: structural changes in the sural nerve. Ann Neurol 19:162, 1986.

73. Ehle AL: Lead neuropathy and electrophysiological studies in low level lead exposure: a critical review. Neurotoxicology 7:203, 1986.

74. Albers JW, Kelly JJ Jr: Acquired inflammatory demyelinating polyneuropathies: clinical and electrodiagnostic features. Muscle Nerve 12:435, 1989.

75. de Pablos C, Calleja J, Fernandez F, Berciano J: Miller Fisher syndrome: an electrophysiologic case study. Electromyogr Clin Neurophysiol 28:21, 1988.

76. Jamal GA, Ballantyne JP: The localization of the lesion in patients with acute ophthalmoplegia, ataxia and areflexia (Miller Fisher syndrome). A serial multimodal neurophysiological study. Brain 111:95, 1988.

77. Matthews WB, Esiri M: The migrant sensory neuritis of Wartenberg. J Neurol Neurosurg Psychiatry 46:1, 1983.
78. Sterman AB, Schaumburg HH, Asbury AK: The acute sensory neuronopathy syndrome: a distinct clinical entity. Ann Neurol 7:354, 1980.
79. Dyck PJ, Karnes J, O'Brien PC, Swanson CJ: Neuropathy Symptom Profile in health, motor neuron disease, diabetic neuropathy, and amyloidosis. Neurology 36:1300, 1986.
80. Charron L, Peyronnard JM, Marchand L: Sensory neuropathy associated with primary biliary cirrhosis. Histologic and morphometric studies. Arch Neurol 37:84, 1980.
81. Zeitlhofer J, Mamoli B, Dragosics B, Knoflach P: Electrophysiological studies in primary biliary cirrhosis. Eur Neurol 23:247, 1984.
82. Nemni R, Fazio R, Corbo M, et al: Peripheral neuropathy associated with Crohn's disease. Neurology 37:1414, 1987.
83. Galassi G, Gibertoni M, Mancini A, et al: Sarcoidosis of the peripheral nerve: clinical, electrophysiological, and histological study of two cases. Eur Neurol 23:459, 1984.
84. Salem HH, Van Der Weyden MB, Koutts J, et al: Leg pain and platelet aggregates in thrombocythemic myeloproliferative disease. JAMA 244:1122, 1980.
85. Goebel HH, Besser R: Traumatic fascicular neuroma. Acta Neuropathol (Berl) 75:321, 1988.
86. Asbury AK, Fields HL: Pain due to peripheral nerve damage: an hypothesis. Neurology 34:1587, 1984.
87. Dyck PJ, Classen SM, Stevens JC, O'Brien PC: Assessment of nerve damage in the feet of long-distance runners. Mayo Clin Proc 62:568, 1987.
88. Harriman DGF, Taverner D, Woolf AL: Ekbom's syndrome and burning paraesthesiae. A biopsy study by vital staining and electron microscopy of the intramuscular innervation with a note on age changes in motor nerve endings in distal muscles. Brain 93:393, 1970.
89. Wulff CH: Painful legs and moving toes. A report of 3 cases with neurophysiological studies. Acta Neurol Scand 66:283, 1982.
90. Schoenen J, Gonce M, Delwaide PJ: Painful legs and moving toes: a syndrome with different physiopathologic mechanisms. Neurology 34:1108, 1984.
91. Schott GD: "Painful legs and moving toes": the role of trauma. J Neurol Neurosurg Psychiatry 44:344, 1981.
92. Spillane JD, Nathan PW, Kelly RE, et al: Painful legs and moving toes. Brain 94:541, 1971.
93. Lugaresi E, Cirignotta F, Coccagna G, Montagna P: Nocturnal myoclonus and restless legs syndrome. Adv Neurol 43:295, 1986.
94. Hudson AJ, Brown WF, Gilbert JJ: The muscular pain–fasciculation syndrome. Neurology 28:1105, 1978.
95. Montplaisir J, Godbout R, Boghen D, et al: Familial restless legs with periodic movements in sleep: electro-

physiologic, biochemical, and pharmacologic study. Neurology 35:130, 1985.

96. Metcalfe RA, MacDermott N, Chalmers RJ: Restless red legs: an association of the restless leg syndrome with arborizing telangiectasia of the lower limbs. J Neurol Neurosurg Psychiatry 49:820, 1986.

97. Danon MJ, Carpenter S: Hereditary sensory neuropathy: biopsy study of an autosomal dominant variety. Neurology 35:1226, 1985.

98. Thomas PK: Hereditary motor and sensory neuropathy: evolution of the concept and present status. Electroencephalogr Clin Neurophysiol 39(Suppl):115, 1987.

99. Ouvrier RA, McLeod JG, Conchin TE: The hypertrophic forms of hereditary motor and sensory neuropathy. A study of hypertrophic Charcot-Marie-Tooth disease (HMSN type I) and Dejerine-Sottas disease (HMSN type III) in childhood. Brain 110:121, 1987.

100. Berciano J, Combarros O, Figols J, et al: Hereditary motor and sensory neuropathy type II. Clinicopathological study of a family. Brain 109:897, 1986.

101. Narazaki O, Hanai T, Sakamoto K, Ohnishi A: A case of hereditary motor and sensory neuropathy type III with a decrease in unmyelinated fibers. Brain Dev 8:295, 1986.

102. Ronen GM, Lowry N, Wedge JH, et al: Hereditary motor sensory neuropathy type I presenting as scapuloperoneal atrophy (Davidenkow syndrome) electrophysiological and pathological studies. Can J Neurol Sci 13:264, 1986.

103. Bird TD, Ott J, Giblett ER, et al: Genetic linkage evidence for heterogeneity in Charcot-Marie-Tooth neuropathy (HMSN type I). Ann Neurol 14:679, 1983.

104. Vasilescu C, Alexianu M, Dan A: Neuronal type of Charcot-Marie-Tooth disease with a syndrome of continuous motor unit activity. J Neurol Sci 63:11, 1984.

105. Rozear MP, Pericak-Vance MA, Fischbeck K, et al: Hereditary motor and sensory neuropathy, X-linked: a half century follow-up. Neurology 37:1460, 1987.

106. Bennett RH, Ludvigson P, DeLeon G, et al: Large-fiber sensory neuronopathy in autosomal dominant spinocerebellar degeneration. Arch Neurol 41:175, 1984.

107. Sima AAF, Robertson DM: Involvement of peripheral nerve and muscle in Fabry's disease. Histologic, ultrastructural, and morphometric studies. Arch Neurol 35:291, 1978.

108. Gadoth N, Sandbank U: Involvement of dorsal root ganglia in Fabry's disease. J Med Genet 20:309, 1983.

109. Gemignani F, Marbini A, Bragaglia MM, Govoni E: Pathological study of the sural nerve in Fabry's disease. Eur Neurol 23:173, 1984.

110. Low PA, Burke WJ, McLeod JG: Congenital sensory neuropathy with selective loss of small myelinated fibers. Ann Neurol 3:179, 1978.

111. Phillips LH II, Kelly TE, Schnatterly P, et al: Hereditary motor-sensory neuropathy (HMSN): possible X-linked dominant inheritance. Neurology 35:498, 1985.

112. Wichman A, Buchthal F, Pezeshkpour GH, et al: Peripheral neuropathy in abetalipoproteinemia. Neurology 35:1279, 1985.
113. Ishii N, Kawaguchi H, Miyakawa K, Nakajima H: Congenital sensory neuropathy with anhidrosis. Arch Dermatol 124:564, 1988.
114. Donaghy M, Hakin RN, Bamford JM, et al: Hereditary sensory neuropathy with neurotrophic keratitis. Description of an autosomal recessive disorder with a selective reduction of small myelinated nerve fibers and a discussion of the classification of the hereditary sensory neuropathies. Brain 110:563, 1987.
115. Said G, Marion MH, Selva J, Jamet C: Hypotrophic and dying-back nerve fibers in Friedreich's ataxia. Neurology 36:1292, 1986.
116. Caruso G, Santoro L, Perretti A, et al: Friedreich's ataxia: electrophysiologic and histologic findings in patients and relatives. Muscle Nerve 10:503, 1987.
117. O'Connor CR, Rubinow A, Brandwein S, et al: Familial amyloid polyneuropathy: a new kinship of German ancestry. Neurology 34:1096, 1984.
118. Nakazato M, Kurihara T, Matsukura S, et al: Diagnostic radioimmunoassay for familial amyloidotic polyneuropathy before clinical onset. J Clin Invest 77:1699, 1986.
119. Tachi N, Sasaki K, Kusano T, et al: Peripheral neuropathy in four cases of group A xeroderma pigmentosum. J Child Neurol 3:114, 1988.
120. Johnson PC: Diagnostic peripheral nerve biopsy. BNI Quart 1:2, 1985.
121. Moore PM, Cupps TR: Neurological complications of vasculitis. Ann Neurol 14:155, 1983.
122. Wees SJ, Sunwoo IN, Oh SJ: Sural nerve biopsy in systemic necrotizing vasculitis. Am J Med 71:525, 1981.
123. Sugimura K, Dyck PJ: Sural nerve myelin thickness and axis cylinder caliber in human diabetes. Neurology 31:1087, 1981.
124. Johnson PC: Diabetic neuropathy. p. 406. In Adachi M, Hirano A, Aronson SM (eds): The Pathology of the Myelinated Axon. Igaku-Shoin, New York, 1985.
125. Johnson PC, Doll SC: Dermal nerves in human diabetic subjects. Diabetes 33:244, 1984.
126. Llewelyn JG, Thomas PK, Gilbey SG, et al: Pattern of myelinated fibre loss in the sural nerve in neuropathy related to type 1 (insulin-dependent) diabetes. Diabetologia 31:162, 1988.
127. Johnson PC, Doll SC, Cromey DW: Pathogenesis of diabetic neuropathy. Ann Neurol 19:450, 1986.
128. McCombe PA, Pollard JD, McLeod JG: Chronic inflammatory demyelinating polyradiculoneuropathy. A clinical and electrophysiological study of 92 cases. Brain 110:1617, 1987.
129. Kyle RA, Greipp PR: Amyloidosis (AL). Clinical and laboratory features in 229 cases. Mayo Clin Proc 58:665, 1983.
130. Hamanot RT, Mshana RN, McDougall AC, et al: Sural nerve biopsy in leprosy patients after varying periods of treatment: histopathological and bacteriological findings on light microscopy. Int J Lepr 52:163, 1984.

131. Thomas C, Love S, Powell HC, et al: Giant axonal neuropathy: correlation of clinical findings with postmortem neuropathology. Ann Neurol 22:79, 1987.
132. Ugawa Y, Inoue K, Takemura T, et al: Accumulation of glycogen in sural nerve axons in adult-onset type III glycogenosis. Ann Neurol 19:294, 1986.
133. Nemni R, Galassi G, Cohen M, et al: Symmetric sarcoid polyneuropathy: analysis of a sural nerve biopsy. Neurology 31:1217, 1981.
134. Weder B, Meienberg O, Wildi E, et al: Neurologic disorder of vitamin E deficiency in acquired intestinal malabsorption. Neurology 34:1561, 1984.

Selected Readings

Aminoff MJ: Use of somatosensory evoked potentials to evaluate the peripheral nervous system. J Clin Neurophysiol 4:135, 1987.

An overview of indications and limitations of somatosensory evoked potentials (SEPs) in the evaluation of peripheral neuropathy. SEPs may be useful in distinguishing neurogenic from nonneurogenic thoracic outlet syndromes and may help evaluate other proximal lesions difficult to evaluate with conventional modalities.

Asbury AK, Fields HL: Pain due to peripheral nerve damage: an hypothesis. Neurology 34:1587, 1984.

A hypothesis proposing two distinct pathophysiologies to explain nerve trunk and dysesthetic pain described by patients with peripheral neuropathy.

Chaunu MP, Ratinahirana H, Raphael M, et al: The spectrum of changes on 20 nerve biopsies in patients with HIV infection. Muscle Nerve 12:452, 1989.

Findings from nerve and muscle biopsies performed on 20 patients with HIV infection and peripheral neuropathy. Authors speculate and review current concepts of pathogenesis of HIV-related neuropathies.

Dyck PJ: Detection, characterization, and staging of polyneuropathy: assessed in diabetics. Muscle Nerve 11:21, 1988.

State of the art, limitations, and suggested future directions for the detection and classification of diabetic polyneuropathy. Authors point out the wide variation in reported prevalence of diabetic polyneuropathy and propose a staging approach using neurologic history, examination, and nerve conduction testing, as well as other objective methods of testing neuropathic symptoms and deficits in patients at risk for diabetic neuropathy.

Eichacker PQ, Spiro A, Sherman M, et al: Respiratory muscle dysfunction in hereditary motor sensory neuropathy, type I. Arch Intern Med 148:1739, 1988.

Inspiratory and expiratory muscle testing abnormalities are reported in patients with hereditary motor sensory neuropathy, type I. These findings contrasted with spirometry, static lung volumes, and diffusion capacity, which were all greater than 80% of predicted normal values.

Fox GN: Restless legs syndrome. Am Fam Physician 33(1):147, 1986.

Restless legs syndrome is a common diagnosis in patients evaluated for insomnia in sleep laboratories; symptomatic restless legs syndrome may be more prevalent than believed.

Gjerstad L, Nyberg-Hansen R, Ganes T: Visual evoked responses in hereditary motor and sensory neuropathies. Acta Neurol Scand 77:215, 1988.

A clinical study that supports recent reports of abnormal visual evoked responses in patients with hereditary motor and sensory neuropathies. The study suggests that subclinical involvement of the optic nerve may occur in this disorder and that visual evoked potentials may contribute to its differentiation in patients with similar clinical findings.

Harati Y, Niakan E: Clinical significance of selective nerve fascicular degeneration on sural nerve biopsy specimen. Arch Pathol Lab Med 110:195, 1986.

This study concludes that the presence of selective fascicular degeneration on sural nerve biopsy specimen may represent indirect evidence of angiopathy.

Jamal GA, Hansen S, Weir AI, Ballantyne JP: The neurophysiologic investigation of small fiber neuropathies. Muscle Nerve 10:537, 1987.

A technique for measurement of thermal thresholds as applied to 25 patients referred with symptoms and signs of small fiber peripheral neuropathy is described and compared with conventional electrophysiologic indices. Authors suggest their results indicate that this technique provides an accurate and easily performed index of function in small A delta and C groups of nerve fibers.

LeQuesne PM, Fowler CJ: Quantitative evaluation of toxic neuropathies in man. Electroencephalogr Clin Neurophysiol 39(Suppl):347, 1987.

A review that describes newer techniques used to detect and monitor specific sensory deficits. Major sensory modalities discussed include vibration, pain, and temperature.

Lindenbaum J, Healton EB, Savage DG, et al: Neuropsychiatric disorders caused by cobalamin deficiency in the absence of anemia or macrocytosis. N Engl J Med 318:1720, 1988.

Findings of a cobalamin deficiency in patients with neuropsychiatric abnormalities without anemia or macrocytosis are reported in this clinical study. Symptoms included paresthesias, sensory loss, ataxia, dementia, and psychiatric disorders. Authors suggest that patients benefited from cobalamin therapy and recommend measuring serum methylmalonic acid and total homocysteine before and after treatment.

Mancardi GL, Cadoni A, Zicca A, et al: HLA-DR Schwann cell reactivity in peripheral neuropathies of different origins. Neurology 38:848,1988.

HLA-DR antigens found on Schwann cells in peripheral neuropathies of different origins are reported. From described data, authors suggest that the expression of HLA-DR antigen on Schwann cells does not appear to be related to the inflammatory autoimmune origin of the disorder.

Navarro X, Kennedy WR, Fries TJ: Small nerve fiber dysfunction in diabetic neuropathy. Muscle Nerve 12:498, 1989.

Results from a study of autonomic and sensory small nerve fiber function in 142 type 1 diabetics and 45 control subjects indicate that diabetic neuropathy has a variable presentation in different types of nerve fibers.

Pollock M, Nukada H, Taylor P, et al: Comparison

between fascicular and whole sural nerve biopsy. Ann Neurol 13:65, 1983.

The study concludes that whole nerve biopsy has greater diagnostic potential.

Rance NE, McArthur JC, Cornblath DR, et al: Gracile tract degeneration in patients with sensory neuropathy and AIDS. Neurology 38:265, 1988.

Autopsy findings in four AIDS patients were remarkable for selective degeneration of the gracile tract. These patients experienced lower extremity paresthesias and ankle jerks were reduced to absent. Postmortem spinal cord examinations were remarkable for a striking axonal and myelin sheath loss within the fasciculus gracilis, most severely affecting the cervical and thoracic cord segments. Findings of combined distal sensory neuropathy and gracile tract degeneration suggest a dying-back process of dorsal root ganglia neurons.

Sabin TD: Classification of peripheral neuropathy: the long and the short of it. Muscle Nerve 9:711, 1986.

Thought-provoking paper that challenges classic concepts of traditional root-plexus-nerve analysis of localization. Sprinkled with clinical pearls for those who evaluate patients with suspected peripheral neuropathies.

Sellman MS, Mayer RF: Conduction block in hereditary neuropathy with susceptibility to pressure palsies. Muscle Nerve 10:621, 1987.

Findings in four patients with a hereditary motor and sensory demyelinating neuropathy that were consistent with focal segmental demyelination or conduction block are reported. Authors suggest that long-lasting conduction block may be a clinical feature in this type of hereditary neuropathy.

Thomas PK: Inherited neuropathies related to disorders of lipid metabolism. Adv Neurol 48:133, 1988.

An overview of recent advances in neuropathies of lipid metabolism. The comprehensively referenced topics include phytanic acid storage diseases, lipoprotein deficiencies, Fabry's disease, leukodystrophies, cholestanolosis, Farber's disease, Niemann-Pick disease, Gaucher's disease, Wolman's disease, and gangliosidosis.

Ziegler D, Mayer P, Wiefels K, Gries FA: Assessment of small and large fiber function in long-term type 1 (insulin-dependent) diabetic patients with and without painful neuropathy. Pain 34:1, 1988.

Findings of 12 neural function tests, including thermal discrimination thresholds, pain perception thresholds to heat and cold stimuli, vibration perception thresholds, and motor and sensory nerve conduction velocities assessed in lower and upper extremities, of 60 long-term type 1 diabetic patients are described. Authors suggest that their findings reflect both generalized and selective small or large fiber involvement in long-term type 1 diabetic patients.

50
Carpal Tunnel Syndrome: Common and Uncommon Associated Focal and Systemic Conditions

Carpal tunnel syndrome (CTS) is the most common cause of burning pain, numbness, and tingling in the thumb, index, and middle fingers.[1] Symptoms are caused by median nerve compression at the wrist where the distal median nerve is vulnerable to injury and entrapment by the flexor retinaculum. Acroparesthesias of the hand, which can mimic carpal tunnel, can be caused by cortical lesions; C-6, C-7, and C-8 cervical radiculopathies; median nerve entrapment proximal to the wrist; and peripheral neuropathy.[2] Since multilevel peripheral nerve lesions are not uncommon, it is important to identify those patients with carpal tunnel syndrome who also have a concomitant cervical radiculopathy (double crush syndrome).[3] CTS can be secondary to an isolated focal median nerve lesion or be one manifestation of a more generalized medical disorder. Associated disorders range in seriousness and frequency from common, benign conditions, such as the repetitive wrist flexion activity of daily living, to underlying medical disorders associated with inflammation, tissue infiltration, and peripheral neuropathies.[4,5]

Idiopathic: a nonspecific flexor tenosynovitis within the carpal tunnel[6]

Recurrent wrist flexion-extension: often associated with a frequently used wrist flexion-extension maneuver during occupational or recreational activity[7-16]

Pregnancy: CTS during pregnancy is most common in primiparas with generalized edema[17,18]

Diabetes mellitus: CTS is often superimposed on an underlying peripheral neuropathy.

Hypothyroidism

Obesity

Rheumatologic disorders: rheumatoid arthritis, gout, systemic lupus erythematosus, scleroderma, giant-cell arteritis, eosinophilic fasciitis, sicca complex, trapeziometacarpal arthritis[4,19-30]

Trauma: Colles' and hamate fractures, tourniquets, handcuffs, occupational vibration[31-37]

Infection: infections can be systemic or, rarely, limited to the carpal tunnel, e.g., sporotrichosis tenosynovitis, *Mycobacterium szulgai*, *Mycobacterium chelonei*, Lyme borreliosis, gonococcal tenosynovitis, rubella[38-43]

Infiltrative disorders: acromegaly, sarcoidosis, amyloidosis, mucopolysaccharidoses[44-46]

Hematologic disorders: macroglobulinemia, leukemia, multiple myeloma[47]

Anticoagulant therapy[48]

Focal lesions of the carpal tunnel: cysts, ganglia, anomalous muscles, hamartoma, lipomas, fibromas[49-52]

Bone disorders: osteopetrosis, osteoarthrosis, tumoral calcinosis, osteoarthritis, osteochondroma[53-57]

Hemodialysis: CTS is often superimposed on an underlying peripheral neuropathy associated with renal insufficiency and often with amyloidosis.[58-67]

Carpopedal spasm: cerebral palsy, hypocalcemia[68]

Primary familial bilateral carpal tunnel syndrome[69-71]

Occupationally acquired vibratory angioedema: consider in patients with a history of transient swelling, pruritus, and paresthesias who have been exposed to vibration[7]

Congenital: Madelung's deformity, mallet finger deformity, lipofibromatous hamartoma, hypoplastic scaphoid[72-75]

Pigmented villonodular synovitis of the wrist[76]

Toxic oil syndrome: chemically-induced scleroderma-like syndrome[77]

References

1. Phalen GS: The carpal-tunnel syndrome: seventeen years' experience in diagnosis and treatment of six hundred fifty-four hands. J Bone Joint Surg (Am) 48-A:211, 1966.
2. Stevens JC: AAEE minimonograph #26: the electro-

diagnosis of carpal tunnel syndrome. Muscle Nerve 10:99, 1987.

3. Osterman AL: The double crush syndrome. Orthop Clin North Am 19:147, 1988.
4. Dorwart BB: Carpal tunnel syndrome: a review. Semin Arthritis Rheum 14:134, 1984.
5. Clayburgh RH, Beckenbaugh RD, Dobyns JH: Carpal tunnel release in patients with diffuse peripheral neuropathy. J Hand Surg (Am) 12:380, 1987.
6. Rosenthal EA: Tenosynovitis: tendon and nerve entrapment. Hand Clin 3:585, 1987.
7. Wener MH, Metzger WJ, Simon RA: Occupationally acquired vibratory angioedema with secondary carpal tunnel syndrome. Ann Intern Med 98:44, 1983.
8. Masear VR, Hayes JM, Hyde AG: An industrial cause of carpal tunnel syndrome. J Hand Surg (Am) 11:222, 1986.
9. Barnhart S, Rosenstock L: Carpal tunnel syndrome in grocery checkers. A cluster of a work-related illness. West J Med 147:37, 1987.
10. Margolis W, Kraus JF: The prevalence of carpal tunnel syndrome symptoms in female supermarket checkers. J Occup Med 29:953, 1987.
11. Gibson CT, Manske PR: Carpal tunnel syndrome in the adolescent. J Hand Surg (Am) 12:279, 1987.
12. Silverstein BA, Fine LJ, Armstrong TJ: Occupational factors and carpal tunnel syndrome. Am J Ind Med 11:343, 1987.
13. Bleecker ML: Medical surveillance for carpal tunnel syndrome in workers. J Hand Surg (Am) 12:845, 1987.
14. Feldman RG, Travers PH, Chirico-Post J, Keyserling WM: Risk assessment in electronic assembly workers: carpal tunnel syndrome. J Hand Surg (Am) 12:849, 1987.
15. Mandel S: Neurologic syndromes from repetitive trauma at work. Postgrad Med 82(6):87, 1987.
16. Senveli ME, Turker A, Arda MN, Altinors MN: Bilateral carpal tunnel syndrome in a young carpet weaver. Clin Neurol Neurosurg 89:281, 1987.
17. Noronha A: Neurologic disorders during pregnancy and the puerperium. Clin Perinatol 12:695, 1985.
18. Ekman-Ordeberg G, Salgeback S, Ordeberg G: Carpal tunnel syndrome in pregnancy. A prospective study. Acta Obstet Gynecol Scand 66:233, 1987.
19. Richards AJ: Carpal tunnel syndrome and subsequent rheumatoid arthritis in the "fibrositis" syndrome. Ann Rheum Dis 43:232, 1984.
20. Walther B, Bauer H, Gröbner W, et al: Carpal tunnel syndrome and gout. Dtsch Med Wochenschr 107:942, 1982.
21. Ogilvie C, Kay NR: Fulminating carpal tunnel syndrome due to gout. J Hand Surg (Br) 13:42, 1988.
22. Janssen T, Rayan GM: Gouty tenosynovitis and compression neuropathy of the median nerve. Clin Orthop 216:203, 1987.
23. Sidiq M, Kirsner AB, Sheon RP: Carpal tunnel syndrome. First manifestation of systemic lupus erythematosus. JAMA 222:1416, 1972.
24. Omdal R, Mellgren SI, Husby G: Clinical neuropsy-

chiatric and neuromuscular manifestations in systemic lupus erythematosus. Scand J Rheumatol 17:113, 1988.

25. Barr WG, Blair SJ: Carpal tunnel syndrome as the initial manifestation of scleroderma. J Hand Surg (Am) 13:366, 1988.

26. Lee P, Bruni J, Sukenik S: Neurological manifestations in systemic sclerosis (scleroderma). J Rheumatol 11:480, 1984.

27. Sherard RK, Coleridge ST: Giant-cell arteritis. J Emerg Med 4:293, 1986.

28. Jones HR Jr, Beetham WP Jr, Silverman ML, Margles SW: Eosinophilic fasciitis and the carpal tunnel syndrome. J Neurol Neurosurg Psychiatry 49:324, 1986.

29. Frayha RA: Papular mucinosis, destructive arthropathy, median neuropathy, and sicca complex. Clin Rheumatol 2:277, 1983.

30. Melone CP Jr, Beavers B, Isani A: The basal joint pain syndrome. Clin Orthop 220:58, 1987.

31. Bolton CF, McFarlane RM: Human pneumatic tourniquet paralysis. Neurology 28:787, 1978.

32. Dorfman LJ, Jayaram AR: Handcuff neuropathy. JAMA 239:957, 1978.

33. Carragee EJ, Hentz VR: Repetitive trauma and nerve compression. Orthop Clin North Am 19:157, 1988.

34. Askins G, Finley R, Parenti J, et al: High-energy roller injuries to the upper extremity. J Trauma 26:1127, 1986.

35. Connor DE, Kolisek FR: Vibration-induced carpal tunnel syndrome. Orthop Rev 15:447, 1986.

36. Kongsholm J, Olerud C: Carpal tunnel pressure in the acute phase after Colles' fracture. Arch Orthop Trauma Surg 105:183, 1986.

37. Ali MA: Fracture of the body of the hamate bone associated with compartment syndrome and dorsal decompression of the carpal tunnel. J Hand Surg (Br) 11:207, 1986.

38. Stratton CW, Lichtenstein KA, Lowenstein SR, et al: Granulomatous tenosynovitis and carpal tunnel syndrome caused by *Sporothrix schenckii*. Am J Med 71:161, 1981.

39. Stratton CW, Phelps DB, Reller LB: Tuberculoid tenosynovitis and carpal tunnel syndrome caused by *Mycobacterium szulgai*. Am J Med 65:349, 1978.

40. Zachary LS, Clark GL Jr, Kleinert JM, O'Donovan C III: *Mycobacterium chelonei* tenosynovitis. Ann Plast Surg 20:360, 1988.

41. Halperin JJ, Volkman DJ, Luft BJ, Dattwyler RJ: Carpal tunnel syndrome in Lyme borreliosis. Muscle Nerve 12:397, 1989.

42. DeHertogh D, Ritland D, Green R: Carpal tunnel syndrome due to gonococcal tenosynovitis. Orthopedics 11:199, 1988.

43. Blennow G, Bekassy AN, Eriksson M, Rosendahl R: Transient carpal tunnel syndrome accompanying rubella infection. Acta Paediatr Scand 71:1025, 1982.

44. Jamal GA, Kerr DJ, McLellan AR, et al: Generalized peripheral nerve dysfunction in acromegaly: a study by conventional and novel neurophysiological techniques. J Neurol Neurosurg Psychiatry 50:886, 1987.

45. Nabarro JD: Acromegaly. Clin Endocrinol 26:481, 1987.
46. Pronicka E, Tylki-Szymanska A, Kwast O, et al: Carpal tunnel syndrome in children with mucopolysaccharidoses: needs for surgical tendons and median nerve release. J Ment Defic Res 32:79, 1988.
47. Oken MM: Multiple myeloma. Med Clin North Am 68:757, 1984.
48. Nkele C: Acute carpal tunnel syndrome resulting from hemorrhage into the carpal tunnel in a patient on warfarin. J Hand Surg (Br) 11:455, 1986.
49. McMinn DJ: Carpal tunnel syndrome caused by a simple ganglion. J R Coll Surg Edinb 30:325, 1985.
50. Desai SS, Pearlman HS, Patel MR: Clicking at the wrist due to fibroma in an anomalous lumbrical muscle: a case report and review of literature. J Hand Surg (Am) 11:512, 1986.
51. Asai M, Wong AC, Matsunaga T, Akahoshi Y: Carpal tunnel syndrome caused by aberrant lumbrical muscles associated with cystic degeneration of the tenosynovium: a case report. J Hand Surg (Am) 11:218, 1986.
52. Amadio PC, Reiman HM, Dobyns JH: Lipofibromatous hamartoma of nerve. J Hand Surg (Am) 13:67, 1988.
53. Rakic M, Elhosseiny A, Ramadan F, et al: Adult-type osteopetrosis presenting as carpal tunnel syndrome. Arthritis Rheum 29:926, 1986.
54. Fisk GR: Osteo-arthrosis of the wrist. Clin Rheum Dis 10:571, 1984.
55. Weiber H, Linell F: Tumoral calcinosis causing acute carpal tunnel syndrome. Case report. Scand J Plast Reconstr Surg Hand Surg 21:229, 1987.
56. Dray GJ, Jablon M: Clinical and radiologic features of primary osteoarthritis of the hand. Hand Clin 3:351, 1987.
57. Nather A, Chong PY: A rare case of carpal tunnel syndrome due to tenosynovial osteochondroma. J Hand Surg (Br) 11:478, 1986.
58. Jain VK, Cestero RVM, Baum J: Carpal tunnel syndrome in patients undergoing maintenance hemodialysis. JAMA 242:2868, 1979.
59. Laurent G, Calemard E, Charra B: Dialysis related amyloidosis. Kidney Int 24(Suppl):S32, 1988.
60. Benz RL, Siegfried JW, Teehan BP: Carpal tunnel syndrome in dialysis patients: comparison between continuous ambulatory peritoneal dialysis and hemodialysis populations. Am J Kidney Dis 11:473, 1988.
61. Bardin T: Dialysis related amyloidosis. J Rheumatol 14:647, 1987.
62. Hardouin P, Flipo RM, Foissac-Gegoux P, et al: Current aspects of osteoarticular pathology in patients undergoing hemodialysis: study of 80 patients. Part 1. Clinical and radiological analysis. J Rheumatol 14:780, 1987.
63. Ogawa H, Saito A, Hirabayashi N, Hara K: Amyloid deposition in systemic organs in long-term hemodialysis patients. Clin Nephrol 28:199, 1987.
64. Minami A, Ogino T: Carpal tunnel syndrome in patients undergoing hemodialysis. J Hand Surg (Am) 12:93, 1987.
65. Bardin T, Kuntz D: The arthropathy of chronic hemodialysis. Clin Exp Rheumatol 5:379, 1987.

66. Campistol JM, Cases A, Torras A, et al: Visceral involvement of dialysis amyloidosis. Am J Nephrol 7:390, 1987.
67. Naito M, Ogata K, Goya T: Carpal tunnel syndrome in chronic renal dialysis patients: clinical evaluation of 62 hands and results of operative treatment. J Hand Surg (Br) 12:366, 1987.
68. Alvarez N, Larkin C, Roxborough J: Carpal tunnel syndrome in athetoid-dystonic cerebral palsy. Arch Neurol 39:311, 1982.
69. Gray RG, Poppo MJ, Gottlieb NL: Primary familial bilateral carpal tunnel syndrome. Ann Intern Med 91:37, 1979.
70. Braddom RL: Familial carpal tunnel syndrome in three generations of a black family. Am J Phys Med 64:227, 1985.
71. McDonnell JM, Makley JT, Horwitz SJ: Familial carpal-tunnel syndrome presenting in childhood. Report of two cases. J Bone Joint Surg (Am) 69:928, 1987.
72. Leslie BM, Ruby LK: Congenital carpal tunnel syndrome. A case report. Orthopedics 8:1165, 1985.
73. Luchetti R, Mingione A, Monteleone M, Cristiani G: Carpal tunnel syndrome in Madelung's deformity. J Hand Surg (Br) 13:19, 1988.
74. Jones NF, Peterson J: Epidemiologic study of the mallet finger deformity. J Hand Surg (Am) 13:334, 1988.
75. Radford PJ, Matthewson MH: Hypoplastic scaphoid—an unusual cause of carpal tunnel syndrome. J Hand Surg (Br) 12:236, 1987.
76. Chidgey LK, Szabo RM, Wiese DA: Acute carpal tunnel syndrome caused by pigmented villonodular synovitis of the wrist. Clin Orthop 228:254, 1988.
77. Alonso-Ruiz A, Zea-Mendoza AC, Salazar-Vallinas JM, et al: Toxic oil syndrome: a syndrome with features overlapping those of various forms of scleroderma. Semin Arthritis Rheum 15:200, 1986.

Selected Readings

Bleecker ML, Bohlman M, Moreland R, et al: Carpal tunnel syndrome: role of carpal canal size. Neurology 35:1599, 1985.
A study of carpal canal size as a risk factor for developing CTS in the workplace measured carpal tunnel size in 14 electricians with CT. Seven of the 14 electricians were symptomatic for CTS. The carpal canal size associated with focal electrophysiologic abnormalities ranged from 1.4 to 2.0 cm².

Chaplin E, Kasdan ML: Carpal tunnel syndrome and routine blood chemistries. Plast Reconstr Surg 75:722, 1985.
Authors suggest that patients who meet electrophysiologic criteria for CTS and also have concomitant peripheral neuropathies warrant a laboratory evaluation for primary and treatable disorders.

Fahr LM, Sauser DD: Imaging of peripheral nerve lesions. Orthop Clin North Am 19:27, 1988.
An overview of newer imaging modalities, including ultrasound, CT, and MRI, which allow delineation of lesions that could not be studied with previous conventional techniques. Authors point out that the radiographic imaging of peripheral nerve lesions is still in its infancy.

Fisher MA, Gorelick PB: Entrapment neuropathies. Differential diagnosis and management. Postgrad Med 77(1):160, 1985.
A practical review of clinical features that help evaluate entrapment neuropathies.

Gelberman RH, Rydevik BL, Pess GM, et al: Carpal tunnel syndrome. A scientific basis for clinical care. Orthop Clin North Am 19:115, 1988.
A review of experimental studies supports a clinical classification of median nerve compression at the wrist into early, intermediate, advanced, and acute nerve compression. Authors offer a patient-specific management approach, including recommendations based on the clinical and electrophysiologic findings that can be correlated with previously demonstrated intraneural pathologic changes.

Gellman H, Gelberman RH, Tan AM, et al: Carpal tunnel syndrome. An evaluation of the provocative diagnostic tests. J Bone Joint Surg (Am) 68A:735, 1986.
A study of provocative tests for carpal tunnel syndrome in 50 electrodiagnostically-studied patients with CTS found that wrist-flexion test were most sensitive and that nerve-percussion and tourniquet tests were less helpful.

Hodgkins ML, Grady D: Carpal tunnel syndrome. West J Med 148:217, 1988.
Clinical overview for primary physicians that focuses on evaluation and recommendations for medical management. Indications for surgical management, such as weakness and thenar atrophy, are discussed.

Howard FM: Controversies in nerve entrapment syndromes in the forearm and wrist. Orthop Clin North Am 17:375, 1986.
A review of current management controversies of upper extremity entrapment neuropathies that focuses on indications for surgical management.

Jessurun W, Hillen B, Zonneveld F, et al: Anatomical relations in the carpal tunnel: a computed tomographic study. J Hand Surg (Br) 12:64, 1987.
CT evaluation of carpal tunnel of the hands of patients with CTS and controls in neutral, flexion, and extension positions were performed. Median nerve compression between long flexors and flexor retinaculum was not found in either flexion or extension of the wrist. Cross-sectional areas of carpal tunnels did not differ when patients and controls were compared.

Koenig H, Lucas D, Meissner R, et al: The wrist: a preliminary report on high-resolution MR imaging. Radiology 160:463, 1986.
A magnetic resonance study of the complex region of the wrist.

Logigian EL, Busis NA, Berger AR, et al: Lumbrical sparing in carpal tunnel syndrome: anatomic, physiologic, and diagnostic implications. Neurology 37:1499, 1987.
The observation that CTS is associated with lumbrical muscle sparing is consistent with anatomic relationships of the carpal tunnel. This neuroanatomic gradient also supports the electrodiagnosis of CTS when distal latency to thenar muscles or palm-to-wrist mixed median nerve conduction velocity is normal.

Louis DS, Greene TL, Noellert RC: Complications of carpal tunnel syndrome. J Neurosurg 62:352, 1985.
Neuroma of the palmar cutaneous branch of the median nerve was found to be the most frequent postsurgical complication.

Morgan RF, Terranova W, Nichter LS, et al: Entrapment neuropathies of the upper extremity. Am Fam Physician 31(1):123, 1985.
A helpful, clinical review of upper extremity entrapment neuropathies.

Nathan PA, Meadows KD, Doyle LS: Occupation as a risk factor for impaired sensory conduction of the median nerve at the carpal tunnel. J Hand Surg (Br) 13:167, 1988.
The role of occupational hand activity as a risk factor for developing CTS was evaluated in 471 industrial workers from 27 occupations in 4 industries. No consistent association was found between type and level of occupational hand activity and prevalence or severity of median nerve slowing.

Neal NC, McManners J, Stirling GA: Pathology of the flexor tendon sheath in the spontaneous carpal tunnel syndrome. J Hand Surg (Br) 12:229, 1987.
A study of histologic features of the flexor tendon sheath in spontaneous CTS found: (1) an absence of inflammation and (2) a diversity of pathologic changes, such as connective tissue alterations, particularly when collagen was examined, fibrosis, amyloid deposits, edema, vascular lesions, and foreign body giant cell reactions. Authors suggest that their findings support the view that pressure and ischemia are significant pathogenic factors.

Pfeffer GB, Gelberman RH, Boyes JH, Rydevik B: The history of carpal tunnel syndrome. J Hand Surg (Br) 13:28, 1988.
History of diagnosis and misdiagnosis of carpal tunnel syndrome. Retrospective look with current insights and appreciation for the diversity of clinical manifestations of CTS.

Sainio K, Merikanto J, Larsen TA: Carpal tunnel syndrome in childhood. Dev Med Child Neurol 29:794, 1987.
CTS is rare in childhood; severe pain of short duration can be a clinical feature of childhood CTS.

Seror P: Tinel's sign in the diagnosis of carpal tunnel syndrome. J Hand Surg (Br) 12:364, 1987.
Tinel's sign was found in 63% of patients with CTS and in 45% of control patients. Authors suggest that Tinel's sign may be less helpful diagnostically than previously believed.

Stevens JC, Sun S, Beard CM, et al: Carpal tunnel syndrome in Rochester, Minnesota, 1961 to 1980. Neurology 38:134, 1988.
The incidence of CTS in a Rochester, Minnesota population from 1961 through 1980 determined from the medical records of Rochester Epidemiology Program project at the Mayo Clinic found an annual incidence rate of 99 cases per 100,000 population. Rates were 52 for men, 149 for women, and 105 for both sexes, age adjusted. Age-specific rates increased with age in men, in contrast to a peak between 45 and 54 years of age in women.

Szabo RM, Gelberman RH: The pathophysiology of nerve entrapment syndromes. J Hand Surg (Am) 12:880, 1987.

An overview of current concepts of pathophysiology of nerve entrapment.

Weiss KL, Beltran J, Shamam OM, et al: High-field MR surface-coil imaging of the hand and wrist. Part I. Normal anatomy. Radiology 160:143, 1986.
A study using MRI of the hands and wrists to determine anatomic definition.

Weiss KL, Beltran J, Lubbers LM: High-field MR surface-coil imaging of the hand and wrist. Part II. Pathologic correlations and clinical relevance. Radiology 160:147, 1986.
A study of MRI of the hands and wrists of patients with a variety of suspected pathologic conditions.

51

Progressive Lower Motor Neuron Weakness: Conditions That Can Mimic Guillain-Barré Syndrome

Guillain-Barré syndrome (GBS) is the most common cause of subacute ascending lower motor neuron weakness. Although the clinical presentation is variable, characteristic features include progressive motor weakness that begins in the legs and can progress within weeks to involve all four extremities, trunk, bulbar, facial, and extraocular muscles. Degrees of weakness vary from minimal weakness to total paralysis of all four limbs and respiratory failure.[1-4] Within the first week, patients are usually hyporeflexic and the cerebrospinal fluid (CSF) is characterized by a significantly elevated protein associated with fewer than 50 mononuclear leukocytes/mm^3.[5] Ataxia and autonomic dysfunction are variable parts of the presentation. Part of the history often includes previous infections, inoculations, or preexisting illnesses, such as lupus erythematosus or lymphoma. A variety of rare, life-threatening, usually treatable infectious, metabolic, toxic, and neoplastic disorders can mimic the variety of clinical manifestations associated with GBS.[6] Multiple disorders can cause potential lower motor neuron failure by disrupting the motor unit at the anterior horn cell in the spinal cord, the nerve axon, neuromuscular junction, or muscle. The initial presentation of these disorders can be subclinical to minimal weakness or manifest as a progressive flaccid weakness, which can rapidly progress to life-threatening respiratory failure.

Idiopathic and Immune Dysfunction

Acute demyelinating polyneuropathy (Guillain-Barré syndrome): an inflammatory demyelinating polyradiculoneuropathy, usually an ascending motor weakness, often associated with sensory symptoms, cranial nerve palsies, and autonomic dysfunction[2-7]

Myasthenia gravis: characterized by postexertional, fluctuating weakness with bulbar and ocular symptoms, which often precede limb girdle weakness[8-10]

Psychogenic weakness: chronic overwork and depression are common concomitants[11]

Myasthenic (Eaton-Lambert) syndrome: weakness and aching in the proximal limbs, particularly hips and thighs, are usually a prominent symptom; frequent association with pulmonary small cell carcinoma[12-17]

Systemic lupus erythematosus: can mimic GBS and rarely a myasthenic (Eaton-Lambert) syndrome[18-20]

Rhabdomyolysis: usually associated with muscle tenderness and myoglobinuria[21,22]

Acute intermittent porphyria: episodes of rapidly progressive polyneuropathy, often with abdominal pain and psychosis, are clinical hallmarks of this inherited syndrome[23,24]

Subacute motor neuropathy: subacute, progressive, painless, often patchy and asymmetric lower motor weakness; usually in the legs more than the arms with a history of Hodgkin's disease or other lymphoma[25]

Critically ill polyneuropathy: consider in patients difficult to wean from a ventilator, particularly if there is a history of recent sepsis[26,27]

Polymyositis: sometimes associated with malignancy

Infections

Borrelia burgdorferi: a tick-borne spirochete that causes Lyme disease; can initially manifest as painful radiculoneuritis, or can mimic a GBS with or without a history of rash or tick bite[28-31]

Botulism: wounds, certain foods, and drug abuse are associated risks.[32-39]

Poliomyelitis and postpolio syndrome[40]

Viruses: cytomegalovirus; Epstein-Barr; herpes viruses; varicella zoster; hepatitis A, B, non-A, and non-B; measles; enteroviruses; mumps[41-55]

Diphtheria

Human immunodeficiency virus (HIV) infection: acute GBS, an inflammatory polyradiculoneuropathy presenting as a cauda equina syndrome, and a polymyositis can coincide with HIV seroconversion or be the only clinical indication of chronic, silent HIV infection.[56-59]

Brucellosis: neurobrucellosis can be either peripheral or central (CNS); peripheral forms manifest as proximal polyradiculoneuropathies; cerebellar signs and cranial nerve palsies may accompany central forms.[60]

Campylobacter jejuni[61,62]

Parasitic myositis: trichinosis, toxoplasmosis, cysticercosis

Metabolic-Endocrine

Hypophosphatemia: poorly nourished, hospitalized alcoholics and patients receiving hyperalimentation are at risk for hypophosphatemia.[63,64]

Hyperkalemia and hypokalemia: muscle weakness with periodic paralysis, often occurs at rest after exercise.[65-71]

Thyrotoxic myopathy: associated with periodic paralysis, particularly in Asians, and subacute thyroiditis.[72-76]

Toxins

Acute arsenic intoxication: high-dose arsenic poisoning can produce a subacute onset, progressive polyradiculoneuropathy that mimics the clinical and electrodiagnostic features of GBS[77]

Lead

Organophosphate toxicity[78,79]

Shellfish poisoning

Alcohol: acute alcoholic myopathy can be associated with binge drinking[80]

Animal bites: black widow spider bite (South African *Latrodectus indistinctus*), African scorpion, rabies[81]

Tick paralysis: rapidly progressive ataxia and flaccid weakness with tick attached that resolves when tick is fully extruded[82]

Drugs and Vaccinations[83,84]

Influenza vaccination: associated with GBS[85]

Antibiotics: aminoglycosides and others, frequently implicated in postoperative respiratory depression[86]

Succinylcholine: in cholinesterase deficiency

Procainamide[87]

Psychotropic drugs: lithium, amitriptyline, haloperidol[88,89]

Anticonvulsants: ethosuximide, paraldehyde, phenytoin[90]

Curare

Cholchicine: large doses

Hepatitis B vaccination[91]

Captopril[92]

Tetanus toxoid[93]

Cisplatin[94]

Vincristine[95]

Neoplasm

Acute leukemia[96,97]

Plasma cell dyscrasias[98]

Thymoma: associated with myasthenia gravis[99–103]

References

1. Ropper AH: Severe acute Guillain-Barré syndrome. Neurology 36:429, 1986.
2. Miller RG, Peterson C, Rosenberg NL: Electrophysiologic evidence of severe distal nerve segment pathology in the Guillain-Barré syndrome. Muscle Nerve 10:524, 1987.
3. Koski CL: Guillain-Barré syndrome. Neurol Clin 2:355, 1984.
4. Shuaib A, Becker WJ: Variants of Guillain-Barré syndrome: Miller Fisher syndrome, facial diplegia and multiple cranial nerve palsies. Can J Neurol Sci 14:611, 1987.
5. Asbury AK, Arnason BGW, Karp HR, et al: Criteria for diagnosis of Guillain-Barré syndrome. Ann Neurol 3:565, 1978.
6. Ropper AH: Unusual clinical variants and signs in Guillain-Barré syndrome. Arch Neurol 43:1150, 1986.

7. Dehaene I, Martin JJ, Geens K, et al: Guillain-Barré syndrome with ophthalmoplegia: clinicopathologic study of the central and peripheral nervous system, including the oculomotor nerves. Neurology 36:851, 1986.
8. Drachman DB: Myasthenia gravis (two parts). N Engl J Med 298:136; 298:186, 1978.
9. Herrmann C Jr, Lindstrom JM, Keesey JC, et al: Myasthenia gravis—current concepts (clinical conference). West J Med 142:797, 1985.
10. Engel AG: Myasthenia gravis and myasthenic syndromes. Ann Neurol 16:519, 1984.
11. McCranie EJ: Neurasthenic neurosis: psychogenic weakness and fatigue. Psychosomatics 21:19, 1980.
12. Elmqvist D, Lambert EH: Detailed analysis of neuromuscular transmission in a patient with the myasthenic syndrome sometimes associated with bronchogenic carcinoma. Mayo Clin Proc 43:689, 1968.
13. Jablecki C: Lambert-Eaton myasthenic syndrome. Muscle Nerve 7:250, 1984.
14. Sculier JP, Feld R, Evans WK, et al: Neurologic disorders in patients with small cell lung cancer. Cancer 60:2275, 1987.
15. Sutton GP, Siemers E, Stehman FB, Ehrlich CE: Eaton-Lambert syndrome as a harbinger of recurrent small-cell carcinoma of the cervix with improvement after combination chemotherapy. Obstet Gynecol 72:516, 1988.
16. O'Neill JH, Murray NM, Newsom-Davis J: The Lambert-Eaton myasthenic syndrome. A review of 50 cases. Brain 111:577, 1988.
17. Ramos-Yeo YL, Reyes CV: Myasthenic syndrome (Eaton-Lambert syndrome) associated with pulmonary adenocarcinoma. J Surg Oncol 34:239, 1987.
18. Hughes RL, Katirji MB: The Eaton-Lambert myasthenic syndrome in association with systemic lupus erythematosus. Arch Neurol 43:1186, 1986.
19. Millette TJ, Subramony SH, Wee AS, Harisdangkul V: Systemic lupus erythematosus presenting with recurrent acute demyelinating polyneuropathy. Eur Neurol 25:397, 1986.
20. Morgan SH, Kennett RP, Dudley C, et al: Acute polyradiculoneuropathy complicating systemic lupus erythematosus. Postgrad Med J 62:291, 1986.
21. Rhabdomyolysis. Medical Staff Conference, University of California, San Francisco. West J Med 125:298, 1976.
22. Frank LI, Admire RC: Rhabdomyolysis. Urol Clin North Am 9:267, 1982.
23. Sergay SM: Management of neurologic exacerbations of hepatic porphyria. Med Clin North Am 63:453, 1979.
24. Sekula SA, Tschen JA, Rosen T: The porphyrias. Am Fam Physician 33:219, 1986.
25. Schold SC, Cho ES, Somasundaram M, et al: Subacute motor neuronopathy: a remote effect of lymphoma. Ann Neurol 5:271, 1979.
26. Bolton CF, Laverty DA, Brown JD, et al: Critically ill polyneuropathy: electrophysiological studies and dif-

ferentiation from Guillain-Barré syndrome. J Neurol Neurosurg Psychiatry 49:563, 1986.

27. Bolton CF: Electrophysiologic studies of critically ill patients. Muscle Nerve 10:129, 1987.

28. Dupuis MJ: Multiple neurologic manifestations of *Borrelia burgdorferi* infection. Rev Neurol (Paris) 144:765, 1988.

29. Szyfelbein WM, Ross JS: Lyme disease meningopolyneuritis simulating malignant lymphoma. Mod Pathol 1:464, 1988.

30. Meier C, Grehl H: Vasculitic neuropathy in the Garin-Bujadoux-Bannwarth syndrome. A contribution to the understanding of the pathology and pathogenesis of the neurological complications in Lyme borreliosis. Dtsch Med Wochenschr 113:135, 1988.

31. Halperin JJ, Luft BJ, Anand AK, et al: Lyme neuroborreliosis: central nervous system manifestations. Neurology 39:753, 1989.

32. MacDonald KL, Cohen ML, Blake PA: The changing epidemiology of adult botulism in the United States. Am J Epidemiol 124:794, 1986.

33. Swedberg J, Wendel TH, Deiss F: Wound botulism. West J Med 147:335, 1987.

34. de Jesus PV Jr, Slater R, Spitz LK, et al: Neuromuscular physiology of wound botulism. Arch Neurol 29:425, 1973.

35. Lecour H, Ramos H, Almeida B, Barbosa R: Foodborne botulism. A review of 13 outbreaks. Arch Intern Med 148:578, 1988.

36. MacDonald KL, Spengler RF, Hatheway CL, et al: Type A botulism from sauteed onions. Clinical and epidemiologic observations. JAMA 253:1275, 1985.

37. Sonnabend WF, Sonnabend OA, Grundler P, Ketz E: Intestinal toxicoinfection by *Clostridium botulinum* type F in an adult. Case associated with Guillain-Barré syndrome. Lancet 1:357, 1987.

38. Chia JK, Clark JB, Ryan CA, et al: Botulism in an adult associated with food-borne intestinal infection with *Clostridium botulinum*. N Engl J Med 315:239, 1986.

39. MacDonald KL, Rutherford GW, Friedman SM, et al: Botulism and botulism-like illness in chronic drug abusers. Ann Intern Med 102:616, 1985.

40. Dalakas MC, Elder G, Hallett M, et al: A long-term follow-up study of patients with post-poliomyelitis neuromuscular symptoms. N Engl J Med 314:959, 1986.

41. Dowling P, Menonna J, Cook S: Cytomegalovirus complement fixation antibody in Guillain-Barré syndrome. Neurology 27:1153, 1977.

42. Behar R, Wiley C, McCutchan JA: Cytomegalovirus polyradiculoneuropathy in acquired immune deficiency syndrome. Neurology 37:557, 1987.

43. Cohen JI, Corey GR: Cytomegalovirus infection in the normal host. Medicine 64:100, 1985.

44. Bishopric G, Bruner J, Butler J: Guillain-Barré syndrome with cytomegalovirus infection of peripheral nerves. Arch Pathol Lab Med 109:1106, 1985.

45. Feinberg WM, Zonis J, Minnich LL: Epstein-Barr virus-associated myelopathy in an adult. Arch Neurol 41:454, 1984.

46. Dowling PC, Cook SD: Role of infection in Guillain-Barré syndrome: laboratory confirmation of herpesviruses in 41 cases. Ann Neurol 9(Suppl):44, 1981.

47. Hart IK, Kennedy PG: Guillain-Barré syndrome associated with herpes zoster. Postgrad Med J 63:1087, 1987.

48. Sanders EA, Peters AC, Gratana JW, Hughes RA: Guillain-Barré syndrome after varicella-zoster infection. Report of two cases. J Neurol 234:437, 1987.

49. Murthy JM: Acute inflammatory demyelinating polyradiculoneuropathy following varicella. Postgrad Med J 63:977, 1987.

50. Tabor E: Guillain-Barré syndrome and other neurologic syndromes in hepatitis A, B, and non-A, non-B. J Med Virol 21:207, 1987.

51. Grover B, Dalessandro L, Sanders JG, et al: Severe viral hepatitis A infection, Landry-Guillain-Barré syndrome, and hereditary elliptocytosis. South Med J 79:251, 1986.

52. Tsukada N, Koh CS, Inoue A, Yanagisawa N: Demyelinating neuropathy associated with hepatitis B virus infection. Detection of immune complexes composed of hepatitis B virus surface antigen. J Neurol Sci 77:203, 1987.

53. Macleod WN: Sporadic non-A, non-B hepatitis and Epstein-Barr hepatitis associated with the Guillain-Barré syndrome. Arch Neurol 44:438, 1987.

54. Kumar N, Behari M, Ahuja GK: Encephalomyeloradiculoneuritis following measles. Acta Neurol (Napoli) 9:44, 1987.

55. Melnick JL: Enterovirus type 71 infections: a varied clinical pattern sometimes mimicking paralytic poliomyelitis. Rev Infect Dis 6(Suppl 2):S387, 1984.

56. Dalakas MC, Pezeshkpour GH: Neuromuscular diseases associated with human immunodeficiency virus infection. Ann Neurol 23(Suppl):S38, 1988.

57. Hagberg L, Malmvall BE, Svennerholm L, et al: Guillain-Barré syndrome as an early manifestation of HIV central nervous system infection. Scand J Infect Dis 18:591, 1986.

58. Parry GJ, Clarke S: Multifocal acquired demyelinating neuropathy masquerading as motor neuron disease. Muscle Nerve 11:103, 1988.

59. Gibbels E, Diederich N: Human immunodeficiency virus (HIV)-related chronic relapsing inflammatory demyelinating polyneuropathy with multifocal unusual onion bulbs in sural nerve biopsy. A clinicomorphological study with qualitative and quantitative light and electron microscopy. Acta Neuropathol 75:529, 1988.

60. Shakir RA, Al-Din AS, Araj GF, et al: Clinical categories of neurobrucellosis. A report on 19 cases. Brain 110:213, 1987.

61. Ropper AH: *Campylobacter* diarrhea and Guillain-Barré syndrome. Arch Neurol 45:655, 1988.

62. Sovilla JY, Regli F, Francioli PB: Guillain-Barré syndrome following *Campylobacter jejuni* enteritis. Report

of three cases and review of the literature. Arch Intern Med 148:739, 1988.

63. Knochel JP: Hypophosphatemia in the alcoholic (editorial). Arch Intern Med 140:613, 1980.
64. Weintraub MI: Hypophosphatemia mimicking acute Guillain-Barré-Strohl syndrome. A complication of parenteral hyperalimentation. JAMA 235:1040, 1976.
65. Riggs JE, Moxley RT III, Griggs RC, et al: Hyperkalemic periodic paralysis: an apparent sporadic case. Neurology 31:1157, 1981.
66. Subramony SH, Wee AS: Exercise and rest in hyperkalemic periodic paralysis. Neurology 36:173, 1986.
67. Buruma OJS, Bots GTAM, Went LN: Familial hypokalemic periodic paralysis. 50 year follow-up of a large family. Arch Neurol 42:28, 1985.
68. Cannon L, Bradford J, Jones J: Hypokalemic periodic paralysis. J Emerg Med 4:287, 1986.
69. Zwarts MJ, van Weerden TW, Links TP, et al: The muscle fiber conduction velocity and power spectra in familial hypokalemic periodic paralysis. Muscle Nerve 11:166, 1988.
70. Minaker KL, Meneilly GS, Flier JS, Rowe JW: Insulin-mediated hypokalemia and paralysis in familial hypokalemic periodic paralysis. Am J Med 84:1001, 1988.
71. Rooney RT, Shanahan EC, Sun T, Nally B: Atracurium and hypokalemic familial periodic paralysis. Anesth Analg 67:782, 1988.
72. Bergeron L, Sternbach GL: Thyrotoxic periodic paralysis. Ann Emerg Med 17:843, 1988.
73. Ma JT, Wang C, Lam KS, et al: Fifty cases of primary hyperaldosteronism in Hong Kong Chinese with a high frequency of periodic paralysis. Evaluation of techniques for tumour localisation. Q J Med 61:1021, 1986.
74. Tamai H, Tanaka K, Komaki G, et al: HLA and thyrotoxic periodic paralysis in Japanese patients. J Clin Endocrinol Metab 64:1075, 1987.
75. Ferreiro JE, Arguelles DJ, Rams H Jr: Thyrotoxic periodic paralysis. Am J Med 80:146, 1986.
76. Behar R, Penny R, Powell HC: Guillain-Barré syndrome associated with Hashimoto's thyroiditis. J Neurol 233:233, 1986.
77. Donofrio PD, Wilbourn AJ, Albers JW, et al: Acute arsenic intoxication presenting as Guillain-Barré-like syndrome. Muscle Nerve 10:114, 1987.
78. Lotti M, Becker CE, Aminoff MJ: Organophosphate polyneuropathy: pathogenesis and prevention. Neurology 34:658, 1984.
79. Senanayake N, Karalliedde L: Neurotoxic effects of organophosphorus insecticides. An intermediate syndrome. N Engl J Med 316:761, 1987.
80. Haller RG, Knochel JP: Skeletal muscle disease in alcoholism. Med Clin North Am 68:91, 1984.
81. Gear JHS: Nonpolio causes of polio-like paralytic syndromes. Rev Infect Dis 6(Suppl 2):S379, 1984.
82. Donat JR, Donat JF: Tick paralysis with persistent weakness and electromyographic abnormalities. Arch Neurol 38:59, 1981.

83. Lane RJ, Routledge PA: Drug-induced neurological disorders. Drugs 26:124, 1983.
84. Kaeser HE: Drug-induced myasthenic syndromes. Acta Neurol Scand 100(Suppl):39, 1984.
85. Schonberger LB, Hurwitz ES, Katona P, et al: Guillain-Barré syndrome: its epidemiology and associations with influenza vaccination. Ann Neurol 9(Suppl):31, 1981.
86. Pittinger CB, Eryasa Y, Adamson R: Antibiotic-induced paralysis. Anesthesia Anal 49:487, 1970.
87. Niakan E, Bertorini TE, Acchiardo SR, et al: Procainamide-induced myasthenia-like weakness in a patient with peripheral neuropathy. Arch Neurol 38:378, 1981.
88. Neil JF, Himmelhoch JM, Licata SM: Emergence of myasthenia gravis during treatment with lithium carbonate. Arch Gen Psychiatry 33:1090, 1976.
89. Leys D, Pasquier F, Lamblin MD, et al: Acute polyradiculoneuropathy after amitriptyline overdose. Br Med J (Clin Res) 294:608, 1987.
90. Argov Z, Mastaglia FL: Disorders of neuromuscular transmission caused by drugs. N Engl J Med 301:409, 1979.
91. Shaw FE Jr, Graham DJ, Guess HA, et al: Postmarketing surveillance for neurologic adverse events reported after hepatitis B vaccination. Experience of the first three years. Am J Epidemiol 127:337, 1988.
92. Chakraborty TK, Ruddell WS: Guillain-Barré neuropathy during treatment with captopril. Postgrad Med J 63:221, 1987.
93. Newton N Jr, Janati A: Guillain-Barré syndrome after vaccination with purified tetanus toxoid. South Med J 80:1053, 1987.
94. Wright DE, Drouin P: Cisplatin-induced myasthenic syndrome. Clin Pharm 1:76, 1982.
95. Norman M, Elinder G, Finkel Y: Vincristine neuropathy and a Guillain-Barré syndrome: a case with acute lymphatic leukemia and quadriparesis. Eur J Haematol 39:75, 1987.
96. Phanthumchinda K, Intragumtornchai T, Kasantikul V: Guillain-Barré syndrome and optic neuropathy in acute leukemia. Neurology 38:1324, 1988.
97. Haberland C, Cipriani M, Kucuk O, et al: Fulminant leukemic polyradiculoneuropathy in a case of B-cell prolymphocytic leukemia. A clinicopathologic report. Cancer 60:1454, 1987.
98. Mactier RA, Khanna R: Guillain-Barré syndrome in kappa light chain myeloma. South Med J 80:1054, 1987.
99. DiMario FJ Jr, Lisak RP, Kornstein MJ, Brooks JJ: Myasthenia gravis and primary squamous cell carcinoma of the thymus: a case report. Neurology 38:580, 1988.
100. Maggi G, Giaccone G, Donadio M, et al: Thymomas. A review of 169 cases, with particular reference to results of surgical treatment. Cancer 58:765, 1986.

101. Denayer MA, Rao KR, Wirz D, McNally D: Hepatic metastatic thymoma and myasthenia gravis twenty-two years after the apparent cure of an invasive thymoma. A case report and review of the literature. J Neurol Sci 76:23, 1986.
102. Lewis JE, Wick MR, Scheithauer BW, et al: Thymoma. A clinicopathologic review. Cancer 60:2727, 1987.
103. Bailey RO, Dunn HG, Rubin AM, Ritaccio AL: Myasthenia gravis with thymoma and pure red blood cell aplasia. Am J Clin Pathol 89:687, 1988.

Selected Readings

Amarenco P, Sauron B, Schuller E, et al: Serum and CSF humoral immunity in Guillain-Barré syndrome: clinical correlations. J Neurol Sci 80:129, 1987.
Paired samples of CSF and serum obtained from 29 patients with GBS were analyzed. Various proteins, such as immunoglobulins, and complement levels were measured at various clinical intervals. Findings suggest that intrathecal IgG synthesis is increased in GBS of greater severity and longer duration.

Benson CA, Harris AA: Acute neurologic infections. Med Clin North Am 70:987, 1986.
An overview of acute bacterial, viral, toxin-mediated and parasitic neurologic infections. The focus is on potentially treatable, life-threatening infections.

Bolton CF: Electrophysiologic studies of critically ill patients. Muscle Nerve 10:129, 1987.
An overview of the usefulness of electrophysiologic studies in the critically ill where clinical evaluation of both central and peripheral nervous systems is difficult. In patients with sepsis and critical illness, both encephalopathy and neuropathy are common. The polyneuropathy of critical illness is predominantly axonal with distal axonal degeneration found in motor and sensory fibers.

Cornblath DR, Mellits ED, Griffin JW, et al: Motor conduction studies in Guillain-Barré syndrome: description and prognostic value. Ann Neurol 23:354, 1988.
Electrophysiologic studies reported from the North American study of plasmapheresis in GBS. Prospectively collected motor conduction studies were analyzed during the first 30 days of illness. Mean distal motor and F wave latencies were commonly abnormal in early studies. Authors emphasize the usefulness of recording distal stimulated compound muscle action potential amplitudes as well as usefulness of plasmapheresis early in the course of GBS.

Feasby TE, Gilbert JJ, Brown WF, et al: An acute axonal form of Guillain-Barré polyneuropathy. Brain 109:1115, 1986.
Five cases of acute GBS with electrically inexcitable motor nerves are described. Three patients survived with poor recovery. Autopsy study of the fourth patient was remarkable for severe axonal degeneration in nerve roots and distal nerves without inflammation or demyelination. Authors suggest that these cases represent a variant of GBS.

Frampton G, Winer JB, Cameron JS, Hughes RA: Severe Guillain-Barré syndrome: an association with IgA anticardiolipin antibody in a series of 92 patients. J Neuroimmunol 19:133, 1988.

Ninety-two patients with GBS were studied to determine whether anticardiolipin antibodies (ACA) were associated with acute GBS. IgA ACA titers, but not IgG ACA and IGM ACA titers, were significantly elevated in GBS patients and were associated with peak disease severity.

Genkins G, Kornfeld P, Papatestas AE, et al: Clinical experience in more than 2000 patients with myasthenia gravis. Ann NY Acad Sci 505:500, 1987.

A clinical experience with myasthenia gravis that focuses on therapeutic strategies, particularly their favorable experience with early thymectomy in cases of generalized myasthenia.

Gordon M: Differential diagnosis of weakness—a common geriatric symptom. Geriatrics 41(4):75, 1986.

Clinical overview addressing the evaluation of weakness in the elderly. Common causes include diuretic-induced azotemia and hypokalemia, psychotropic drugs, and peripheral neuropathy associated with diabetes mellitus and alcoholism.

Grob D, Arsura EL, Brunner NG, Namba T: The course of myasthenia gravis and therapies affecting outcome. Ann NY Acad Sci 505:472, 1987.

Clinical features, clinical course, and therapies affecting outcome in 1,487 patients with myasthenia gravis who were followed for a mean of 18 years are reported. The clinical outcome could usually be predicted within the first 1 to 3 years after onset. Men tended to have a more rapid progression and lower rates of remission and improvement than women.

Harrington MG, Kennedy PG: The clinical use of cerebrospinal fluid studies in demyelinating neurological diseases. Postgrad Med J 63:735, 1987.

A clinical overview of current usefulness and limitations of CSF studies in demyelinating diseases. Guidelines offered are particularly useful for evaluation of patients for possible multiple sclerosis and GBS.

Kaur U, Chopra JS, Prabhakar S, et al: Guillain-Barré syndrome. A clinical electrophysiological and biochemical study. Acta Neurol Scand 73:394, 1986.

The clinical features of 56 consecutive patients diagnosed with GBS were evaluated. All patients developed weakness within 1 day to 3 weeks. Most common clinical features included attenuated deep tendon reflexes, paresthesias, cranial nerve involvement, and antecedent infection. The most common patterns of muscle weakness were proximal weakness in all four limbs and proximal leg weakness with distal upper extremity weakness. Maximal incidence of electrophysiologic abnormalities occurred between 4 and 12 weeks after onset of neurologic symptoms.

Levine SR, Welch KM: The spectrum of neurologic disease associated with antiphospholipid antibodies. Lupus anticoagulants and anticardiolipin antibodies. Arch Neurol 44:876, 1987.

Lupus anticoagulants and anticardiolipin antibodies have been associated with several neurologic conditions, including focal cer-

ebral and ocular ischemia, myelopathy of lupoid sclerosis, Degos' disease, GBS, migraine, chorea, and seizures.

Lindstrom J, Shelton D, Fujii Y: Myasthenia gravis. Adv Immunol 42:233, 1988.
An overview of current concepts of the pathophysiology of myasthenia gravis.

McKhann GM, Griffin JW, Cornblath DR, et al: Plasmapheresis and Guillain-Barré syndrome: analysis of prognostic factors and the effect of plasmapheresis. Ann Neurol 23:347, 1988.
This study used multivariate analysis to identify factors associated with differences in recovery time in patients with GBS. Data suggest that the most powerful predictor of outcome was the recording of an abnormally low mean amplitude of compound muscle action potential when stimulating distally. Plasmapheresis was the only variable physicians could influence that had a beneficial effect.

Mendell JR, Kolkin S, Kissel JT, et al: Evidence for central nervous system demyelination in chronic inflammatory demyelinating polyradiculoneuropathy. Neurology 37:1291, 1987.
MRI studies performed in 16 patients with chronic inflammatory demyelinating polyradiculoneuropathy (CIDP) found central nervous system white matter lesions that were indistinguishable from those seen in multiple sclerosis.

Miller RG, Peterson GW, Daube JR, Albers JW: Prognostic value of electrodiagnosis in Guillain-Barré syndrome. Muscle Nerve 11:769, 1988.
Sixty severely ill patients with GBS were electrodiagnostically studied. The most powerful predictor of poor outcome was reduced mean compound muscle action potential amplitudes of less than 10% of the lower limit of normal.

Nelson KR, Gilmore RL, Massey A: Acoustic nerve conduction abnormalities in Guillain-Barré syndrome. Neurology 38:1263, 1988.
Brain stem auditory evoked potentials (BAEPs) were recorded in two patients with GBS. In one acutely deaf patient BAEP waveforms were absent, consistent with acoustic nerve conduction block. Both hearing and BAEP waveforms returned to normal on recovery from GBS. The second patient had bilaterally prolonged wave I latencies.

Osterman PO, Vedeler CA, Ryberg B, et al: Serum antibodies to peripheral nerve tissue in acute Guillain-Barré syndrome in relation to outcome of plasma exchange. J Neurol 235:285, 1988.
Serum antibody levels were measured in 36 patients with acute GBS. Twenty plasma-exchange treated patients were compared with 16 controls. Hemagglutination testing found a significant antibody titer in 19 patients. Thirty patients had complement-fixing antibodies.

Pollard JD: A critical review of therapies in acute and chronic inflammatory demyelinating polyneuropathies. Muscle Nerve 10:214, 1987.
An overview of therapies with the retrospective view of recent randomized or controlled trials. Recommendations for use of plasma exchange and corticosteroids are made for acute and chronic forms of inflammatory demyelinating neuropathies.

Reich SG: Harvey Cushing's Guillain-Barré syndrome: an historical diagnosis. Neurosurgery 21:135, 1987.

Harvey Cushing developed a GBS during the last months of World War I. Neither Cushing nor his physicians made the correct diagnosis.

Ropper AH: Unusual clinical variants and signs in Guillain-Barré syndrome. Arch Neurol 43:1150, 1986.

Limited regional forms of the GBS and unusual focal signs or symptoms that resemble other illnesses are described, including (1) pharyngeal-cervical-brachial weakness with ptosis, sparing power, and reflexes in the legs; (2) paraparesis with normal power and reflexes in the arms; (3) early severe ptosis without other signs of oculomotor weakness and (4) acute severe midline back pain at the onset.

Steiner I, Wirguin I, Abramsky O: Appearance of Guillain-Barré syndrome in patients during corticosteroid treatment. J Neurol 233:221, 1986.

This paper reports three cases of GBS that developed while patients were on corticosteroid treatment. Underlying disorders treated with corticosteroids were ulcerative colitis, multiple sclerosis, and aqueductal stenosis with a shunt malfunction. Authors speculate that GBS in these patients may have been due to a selective effect of low-dose steroids on a specific lymphocyte subpopulation.

van der Meche FG, Meulstee J, Vermeulen M, Kievit A: Patterns of conduction failure in the Guillain-Barré syndrome. Brain 111:405, 1988.

Longitudinal electrophysiologic studies were performed in 13 patients with GBS. Two patterns were distinguished during the progressive phase of the disease. Pattern 1 was a length-dependent reduction of the compound muscle action potential (CMAP). Patients in this group (with one exception) had spared sensory potentials, a prominent clinical motor deficit, and were without clinical sensory deficit. Pattern 2 was a simple reduction of the CMAP. In this pattern, motor and sensory fibers were similarly involved, and patients showed motor and sensory deficits.

Winer JB, Hughes RA, Anderson MJ, et al: A prospective study of acute idiopathic neuropathy. II. Antecedent events. J Neurol Neurosurg Psychiatry 51:613, 1988.

The incidence of antecedent events and serologic evidence of preceding infection in 100 patients with the diagnosis of acute idiopathic neuropathy was studied and compared with age- and sex-matched controls in a prospective study in southeast England. Respiratory infections occurred within 1 month before onset of neuropathic symptoms in 38% of patients and in 12% of controls. Immunizations, insect bites, and animal contact were equally common in patient and controls. Serologic evidence of recent infection with Campylobacter jejuni (14%) and cytomegalovirus (11%) was demonstrated more frequently in patients than controls.

Winer JB, Hughes RA, Osmond C: A prospective study of acute idiopathic neuropathy. I. Clinical features and their prognostic value. J Neurol Neurosurg Psychiatry 51:605, 1988.

A prospective study of 100 patients admitted with the diagnosis of acute idiopathic neuropathy was conducted during 15 months in 1983 and 1984 in southeast England. Major features identified at onset of symptoms that correlated with persistent disability included time taken to become bedbound, ventilator-dependence, age greater than 40 years, and small or absent compound abductor pollicis brevis muscle action potentials when stimulating the median nerve at the wrist.

VI

RHEUMATOLOGY

52
Neck Pain: Associated Cervical and Systemic Disorders

Neck pain is common and can reflect a wide variety of conditions, which are usually benign and self-limiting, but occasionally can be life-threatening. Cervical spine location, anatomy, and structural characteristics make it particularly vulnerable to injury and pain.[1] The neck contains many pain-sensitive tissues in a small area and is surrounded by multiple possible causes of intrinsic and referred pain.[2] Soft tissues, cervical vasculature, neural structures, shoulder joints, and even gastrointestinal and cardiac dysfunction are potential sources of neck pain. The most common causes of neck pain are acute or repeated neck injury and chronic neck strain. However, in a small important group of patients, neck pain can herald serious intrinsic or referred disease.

Cervical and Systemic Disorders Associated with Neck Pain

Cervical sprain: whiplash is the most common cause of neck pain.[3]

Cervical degenerative arthritis[4]

Cervical radiculopathies: cervical root irritation can cause pain, numbness, or weakness in cervical nerve dermatomal distributions, which often refer the presenting symptom to the shoulder, arm, or hand.

Cervical spondylosis and cervical disc degeneration: spondylotic process often occurs at multiple levels at cervical sites subject to great wear.[5]

Cervical disc herniation: lower cervical discs (C4 through C7) most common sites of disc hernation[5]

Postural disorders

Cervical muscle fibrosis: focal trapezius muscle tenderness common

Occipital neuralgia: has been attributed to developmental and post-traumatic lesions involving C1 and C2 nerve roots at the cervicocranial junction region[6]

Superior nuchal ligament strain

Congenital anomalies of the cervical spine: craniocervical malformations[7,8]

Arthritis: osteoarthritis, rheumatoid arthritis,[9] juvenile rheumatoid arthritis,[10] ankylosing spondylitis, ankylosing hyperostosis,[11] gout[12]

Polymyalgia rheumatica: often associated with temporal arteritis

Cervical spinal cord tumors: leg weakness can be the first neurologic sign of a cervical cord tumor; suspect metastatic lesions in the elderly.[13]

Foramen magnum tumors: foramen magnum and high cervical spinal cord tumors often present with a confusing clinical picture, sometimes ascribed initially to hysteria or fibromyositis.[14]

Primary neoplasms of the cervical spine: spinal pain made worse by recumbency can be a clue to spinal cord tumors.[15,16]

Infection: cervical epidural abscess[17]

Osteomyelitis

Multiple myeloma: back pain common

Paget's disease: back pain common[18]

Torticollis

Thyroid masses and inflammation: usually anterior neck pain, tender to palpation[19,20]

Esophageal disorders: esophagitis

Paracervical lymphadenitis

Tracheal irritation: inflammation or neoplasm

Meningeal irritation: usually an acute process, i.e., in association with meningitis or subarachnoid bleeding

Carotid artery dissection: neck pain associated with facial pain or dysesthesias may herald a carotid artery dissection.[21]

Vertebral artery dissection: neck pain, headache, and ipsilateral brain stem ischemic symptoms are clinical clues.[22]

Carotidynia: recurrent vascular neck pain, often associated with carotid tenderness and vascular headaches[23-25]

Glossopharyngeal neuralgia: attacks not uncommonly associated with syncope[26-28]

Crowned dens syndrome: crystalline deposits surrounding the odontoid process can be a rare cause of upper cervical pain.[29]

Referred Symptoms That Can Mask Cervical Disease

Heachache, arm pain, and dysphagia can be symptoms of primary cervical disease. Since cardiovascular, gastrointestinal, and shoulder girdle musculoskeletal structures share cervical root innervation, referred pain to these areas can mask cervical lesions.

Headache: referred pain from occipital neuritis and the first three cervical vertebrae[30]

Arm pain: a common referral pattern of cervical nerves C6–C8.

Shoulder pain[31]

Scapular pain: referred C5–6 irritation

Thoracic outlet syndrome: compression of brachial plexus by a cervical rib or scalene muscles[32]

Dysphagia: anterior osteophyte compression can cause esophageal pain and spasm.[33]

Eye muscle spasms: stimulated by sympathetic nerves surrounding vertebral and carotid vessels[34]

Vertigo: certain neck disorders can cause vertigo.[35]

Pseudoangina pectoris: a C6–7 lesion can cause tenderness at the precordium.

Dyspnea: C4 and C5 lesions can compromise diaphragm function or accessory respiratory muscles.

Nausea and vomiting: C4–5 lesions

References

1. Jackson R: Cervical trauma: not just another pain in the neck. Geriatrics 37(4):123, 1982.
2. Gilbert R, Warfield CA: Evaluating and treating the patient with neck pain. Hosp Pract 22(8):223;28, 1987.
3. Norris SH, Watt I: The prognosis of neck injuries resulting from rear-end vehicle collisions. J Bone Joint Surg (Br) 65-B:608, 1983.
4. Hirsh LF: Cervical degenerative arthritis. Possible cause of neck and arm pain. Postgrad Med 74(1):123, 1983.
5. Schmidek HH: Cervical spondylosis. Am Fam Physician 33(5):89, 1986.
6. Ehni G, Benner B: Occipital neuraliga and the C1–2 arthrosis syndrome. J Neurosurg 61:961, 1984.
7. Nagashima C, Kubota S: Craniocervical abnormalities. Modern diagnosis and a comprehensive surgical approach. Neurosurg Rev 6:187, 1983.
8. Morizono Y, Sakou T, Maehara T: Congenital defect of posterior elements of the axis. Clin Orthop 216:120, 1987.
9. Lipson SJ: Rheumatoid arthritis of the cervical spine. Clin Orthop 182:143, 1984.
10. Hensinger RN, DeVito PD, Ragsdale CG: Changes in the cervical spine in juvenile rheumatoid arthritis. J Bone Joint Surg (Am) 68-A:189, 1986.
11. Spilberg I, Lieberman DM: Ankylosing hyperostosis of the cervical spine. Arthritis Rheum 15:208, 1972.

12. Alarcon GS, Reveille JD: Gouty arthritis of the axial skeleton including the sacroiliac joints. Arch Intern Med 147:2018, 1987.
13. Langfitt TW, Elliott FA: Pain in the back and legs caused by cervical spinal cord compression. JAMA 200:382, 1967.
14. Rosenbaum LH, Nicholas JJ: Early diagnosis of cervical spinal cord meningioma. JAMA 249:1475, 1983.
15. Bohlman HH, Sachs BL, Carter JR, et al: Primary neoplasms of the cervical spine. J Bone Joint Surg (Am) 68-A:483, 1986.
16. Nicholas JJ, Christy WC: Spinal pain made worse by recumbency: a clue to spinal cord tumors. Arch Phys Med Rehabil 67:598, 1986.
17. Lasker BR, Harter DH: Cervical epidural abscess. Neurology 37:1747, 1987.
18. Zlatkin MB, Lander PH, Hadjipavlou AG, et al: Paget's disease of the spine: CT with clinical correlation. Radiology 160:155, 1986.
19. Hamburger JI: The various presentations of thyroiditis. Ann Intern Med 104:219, 1986.
20. Stoffer SS, Loomus M: The painful thyroid. A three-step diagnostic approach. Postgrad Med 81(1):161, 1987.
21. Francis KR, Williams DP, Troost BT: Facial numbness and dysesthesia. New features of carotid artery dissection. Arch Neurol 44:345, 1987.
22. Mokri B, Houser OW, Sandok BA, Piepgras DG: Spontaneous dissections of the vertebral arteries. Neurology 38:880, 1988.
23. Lim RY: Carotodynia exposed: hyoid bone syndrome. South Med J 80:444, 1987.
24. Raskin NH, Prusiner S: Carotidynia. Neurology 27:43, 1977.
25. Orfei R, Meienberg O: Carotidynia: report of eight cases and prospective evaluation of therapy. J Neurol 230:65, 1983.
26. Bruyn GW: Glossopharyngeal neuralgia. Cephalalgia 3:143, 1983.
27. Wilkins RH: Neurovascular compression syndromes. Neurol Clin 3:359, 1985.
28. Wallin BG, Westerberg CE, Sundlof G: Syncope induced by glossopharyngeal neuralgia: sympathetic outflow to muscle. Neurology 34:522, 1984.
29. Bouvet JP, LeParc JM, Michalski B, et al: Acute neck pain due to calcifications surrounding the odontoid process: the crowned dens syndrome. Arthritis Rheum 28:1417, 1985.
30. Jackson R: Headaches associated with disorders of the cervical spine. Headache 6:175, 1967.
31. Grosshandler SL, Stratas NE, Toomey TC, et al: Chronic neck and shoulder pain. Focusing on myofascial origins. Postgrad Med 77(3):149, 1985.
32. Kelly TR: Thoracic outlet syndrome. Current concepts of treatment. Ann Surg 190:657, 1979.
33. Lambert JR, Tepperman PS, Jimenez J: Cervical spine disease and dysphagia. Four new cases and a review of the literature. Am J Gastroenterol 76:35, 1981.
34. Kline LB, McCluer SM, Bonikowski FP: Oculosympath-

etic spasm with cervical spinal cord injury. Arch Neurol 41:61, 1984.
35. Pfaltz CR: Vertigo in disorders of the neck. p. 179. In Dix MR, Hood JD (eds): Vertigo. John Wiley & Sons, New York, 1984.

Selected Readings

Bachulis BL, Long WB, Hynes GD, Johnson MC: Clinical indications for cervical spine radiographs in the traumatized patient. Am J Surg 153:473, 1987.
This study reviews data from 4,941 trauma patients over a 4.5-year period and analyzes clinical factors helpful in deciding indications for cervical spine radiographs. Complete radiographic examinations of the cervical spine are recommended in all patients at risk for cervical spine injury. A screening algorithm for a radiologic screen of cervical spine injuries in trauma patients is presented.

Badami JP, Baker RA, Scholz FJ, et al: Outpatient metrizamide myelography: prospective evaluation of safety and cost effectiveness. Radiology 158:175, 1986.
Data are presented in favor of outpatient metrizamide myelography.

Daniels DL, Grogan JP, Johansen JG, et al: Cervical radiculopathy: computed tomography and myelography compared. Radiology 151:109, 1984.
Study suggests that CT can demonstrate herniations as effectively as myelography.

Kalovidouris A, Mancuso AA, Dillion W: A CT-clinical approach to patients with symptoms related to the V, VII, IX–XII cranial nerves and cervical sympathetics. Radiology 151:671, 1984.
Importance of extending CT examination beyond the skull base is shown in specific cases. Protocols for clinical settings are given.

Moskovich R: Neck pain in the elderly: common causes and management. Geriatrics 43(4):65, 1988.
A clinical review of diagnosis and management of neck pain in the elderly.

O'Driscoll SL, Tomenson J: The cervical spine. Clin Rheum Dis 8:617, 1982.
Study showing normal range of motion for different ages.

Payne R: Neck pain in the elderly: a management review. Part II. Geriatrics 42(2):71, 1987.
A clinical review of neck pain in the elderly that highlights clinical features of common causes of neck pain in the elderly population, such as rheumatoid arthritis and metastatic cancer.

Pech P, Daniels DL, Williams AL, et al: The cervical neural foramina: correlation of microtomy and CT anatomy. Radiology 155:143, 1985.
CT-cryomicrotomic study giving a detailed description of the CT appearance of the cervical neural foramina.

Walter J, Doris PE, Shaffer MA: Clinical presentation of patients with acute cervical spine injury. Ann Emerg Med 13:512, 1984.
Prospective study of 67 patients in an emergency department presenting with acute cervical spine fracture and/or dislocation.

53

Shoulder Pain: Common and Uncommon Causes of Shoulder Pain and Referred Shoulder Pain

Multiple direct and referred causes of shoulder pain can cause similar shoulder discomfort. It is important to identify the source of shoulder pain because delay in appropriate diagnosis can lead to a frozen shoulder and chronic disability. Mechanical problems of the glenohumeral joint, the acromioclavicular joint, and supporting soft tissues cause most shoulder pain.[1] Less common causes of shoulder pain include a wide spectrum of intrinsic and referred disorders, such as cervical spine disease, arthritis, endocrine disease, and even referred intra-abdominal and intrathoracic disease.[2]

Common Causes

Impingement lesions: spectrum of disorders resulting from impingement on rotator cuff, subacromial bursa, or biceps tendon[3]

Acute inflammatory stage: osseous or ligamentous impingement of the rotator cuff and/or biceps tendon producing acute inflammatory process

Chronic inflammatory stage: tendinitis and fibrosis of the rotator cuff and/or biceps tendon[4]

Rupture of the rotator cuff (supraspinatus tendon) or biceps tendon (long head)

Trauma

Fractures: commonly clavicle, proximal humerus

Fracture dislocation

Acromioclavicular instability

Glenohumeral instability: subluxation, dislocation; trauma may be minimal

Adhesive capsulitis ("frozen shoulder"): often following wrist or humerus fractures; must begin early range of motion[5]

Arthritis: osteoarthritis, rheumatoid arthritis, gout, pseudogout, collagen vascular diseases

Cervical spondylosis and degenerative disc disease: most common cervical spine causes of shoulder pain[6]

Reflex sympathetic dystrophy: shoulder-hand syndrome[7]

Myositis ossificans: post-traumatic

Overuse syndromes: seen in athletes[8] and heavy manual laborers[9]

Less Common Causes

Disorders of the shoulder joint and periarticulum

Less common shoulder fractures: scapula, coracoid process

Less common shoulder dislocations: rule out occult posterior glenohumeral dislocation

Cuff tear arthropathy

Postsurgical shoulder pain

Myofascial pain syndromes

Neuropathic arthropathies: postpolio myopathies,[10] hemiplegic shoulder pain[11]

Primary neoplasms: sarcoma, myeloma, osteosarcoma, chondrosarcoma[12]

Metastatic carcinoma: the shoulder is a common site of long bone metastasis.

Neurologic disorders causing referred shoulder pain

Spinal cord lesions: neoplasm, syrinx, infection

Thoracic outlet syndrome[13]

Brachial plexus neuritis: traumatic or inflammatory[14]

Carpal tunnel syndrome: shoulder pain with carpal tunnel syndrome often more prominent at night[15]

Suprascapular nerve entrapment: often presents with shoulder weakness and atrophy of spinatus musculature[16-18]

Axillary nerve entrapment: rare cause of pain in the quadrilateral space[19]

Cervical vascular disorders causing referred shoulder pain

Large vessel arteritis

Axillary-subclavian vein thrombosis[20]

Posterior humeral circumflex artery occlusion[21]

Systemic and miscellaneous disorders

Polymyalgia rheumatica: most common inflammatory rheumatic disorder of the elderly next to rheumatoid arthritis[22]

Milwaukee shoulder syndrome: bilateral shoulder

pain, effusions, and crepitation in elderly women associated with hydroxyapatite crystals[23]

Paget's disease[24]

Endocrine disorders: hypothyroidism, acromegaly, hyperparathyroidism, diabetes[25,26]

Amyloid arthropathy

Osteonecrosis (ischemic necrosis): idiopathic, steroid induced, hemoglobinopathies, chemotherapy and radiation therapy[27]

Osteochondritis dissecans of the humeral head[28]

Hemodialysis[29]

Visceral lesions causing referred shoulder pain: diaphragmatic irritation often refers pain to the scapular upper border.[30]

Pancoast tumors: although the majority of apical tumors appear obvious on chest radiograph, radiographic findings may be limited to apical pleural thickening.[31]

Pulmonary infarction: associated with a pleural or lung apex infarction

Pleural disease: inflammation or neoplasm

Myocardial ischemia (infarction)

Pancreatic disease: pancreatitis, pancreatic pseudocyst

Subphrenic abscess

Splenic trauma

Cholecystitis

Peritonitis

Pneumoperitoneum[32]

References

1. White RH: Shoulder pain. West J Med 137:340, 1982.
2. Bateman JE: Neurologic painful conditions affecting the shoulder. Clin Orthop 173:44, 1983.
3. Post M, Cohen J: Impingement syndrome. A review of late stage II and early stage III lesions. Clin Orthop 207:126, 1986.
4. Mena HR: The pain of acute bursitis/tendinitis of the shoulder. Am J Med 80(S3A):140, 1986.
5. Bulgen DY, Binder AI, Hazleman BL, et al: Frozen shoulder: prospective clinical study with an evaluation of three treatment regimens. Ann Rheum Dis 43:353, 1984.
6. Campbell SM: Referred shoulder pain. An elusive diagnosis. Postgrad Med 73(5):193, 1983.
7. Kozin F: Painful shoulder and the reflex sympathetic dystrophy syndrome. p. 1091. In McCarty DJ (ed): Arthritis and Allied Conditions. A Textbook of Rheumatology, 9th Ed. Lea & Febiger, Philadelphia, 1979.

8. Jobe FW, Jobe CM: Painful athletic injuries of the shoulder. Clin Orthop 173:117, 1983.
9. Herberts P, Kadefors R, Högfors C, et al: Shoulder pain and heavy manual labor. Clin Orthop 191:166, 1984.
10. Bruckner FE, Howell A: Neuropathic joints. Semin Arthritis Rheum 2:47, 1972.
11. Griffin JW: Hemiplegic shoulder pain. Phys Ther 66:1884, 1986.
12. Craig EV, Thompson RC: Management of tumors of the shoulder girdle. Clin Orthop 223:94, 1987.
13. Hawkes CD: Neurosurgical considerations in thoracic outlet syndrome. Clin Orthop 207:24, 1986.
14. Walsh NE, Dumitru D, Kalantri A, Roman AM Jr: Brachial neuritis involving the bilateral phrenic nerves. Arch Phys Med Rehabil 68:46, 1987.
15. Kummel BM, Zazanis GA: Shoulder pain as the presenting complaint in carpal tunnel syndrome. Clin Orthop 92:227, 1973.
16. Hadley MN, Sonntag VKH, Pittman HW: Suprascapular nerve entrapment. J Neurosurg 64:843, 1986.
17. Shabas D, Scheiber M: Suprascapular neuropathy related to the use of crutches. Am J Phys Med 65:298, 1986.
18. Agre JC, Ash N, Cameron MC, House J: Suprascapular neuropathy after intensive progressive resistive exercise: case report. Arch Phys Med Rehabil 68:236, 1987.
19. McKowen HC, Voorhies RM: Axillary nerve entrapment in the quadrilateral space. Case report. J Neurosurg 66:932, 1987.
20. O'Leary MR, Smith MS, Druy EM: Diagnostic and therapeutic approach to axillary-subclavian vein thrombosis. Ann Emerg Med 16:889, 1987.
21. Cormier PJ, Matalon TA, Wolin PM: Quadrilateral space syndrome: a rare cause of shoulder pain. Radiology 167:797, 1988.
22. Allen NB, Studenski SA: Polymyalgia rheumatica and temporal arteritis. Med Clin North Am 70:369, 1986.
23. McCarty DJ, Halverson PB, Carrera GF, et al: "Milwaukee shoulder"—association of microspheroids containing hydroxyapatite crystals, active collagenase and neutral protease with rotator cuff defects. I. Clinical aspects. Arthritis Rheum 24:464, 1981.
24. Wallach S: Chronic joint pain: arthritis or osteitis? Hosp Pract 20(10A):29, 1985.
25. Morén-Hybbinette I, Moritz U, Scherstén B: The painful diabetic shoulder. Acta Med Scand 219:507, 1986.
26. Shinabarger NI: Limited joint mobility in adults with diabetes mellitus. Phys Ther 67:215, 1987.
27. Rossleigh MA, Smith J, Straus DJ, et al: Osteonecrosis in patients with malignant lymphoma. A review of 31 cases. Cancer 58:1112, 1986.
28. Anderson WJ, Guilford WB: Osteochondritis dissecans of the humeral head. An unusual cause of shoulder pain. Clin Orthop 173:166, 1983.
29. Chattopadhyay C, Ackrill P, Clague RB: The shoulder pain syndrome and soft-tissue abnormalities in patients on long-term hemodialysis. Br J Rheumatol 26:181, 1987.

30. Watts GT: Does peritonitis in the upper abdomen cause pain in the tip of the shoulder? Lancet 1:1488, 1986.
31. Attar S, Miller JE, Satterfield J, et al: Pancoast's tumor: irradiation or surgery? Ann Thorac Surg 28:578, 1979.
32. Schriger DL, Rosenberg G, Wilder RJ: Shoulder pain and pneumoperitoneum following a diving accident. Ann Emerg Med 16:1281, 1987.

Selected Readings

Ahovuo J, Paavolainen P, Slatis P: Diagnostic value of sonography in lesions of the biceps tendon. Clin Orthop 202:184, 1986.

A study of the usefulness of sonography in lesions of the biceps tendon compared 10 controls with 30 patients with chronic shoulder pain. The authors conclude that this technique is useful for showing dislocation of the tendons, particularly when the tendon sheath is not well visualized with arthrography.

Bateman JE: Neurologic painful conditions affecting the shoulder. Clin Orthop 173:44, 1983.

Radiating pain associated with motor or sensory changes, particularly below the elbow, suggests a neurologic etiology.

Bonafede RP, Bennett RM: Shoulder pain. Guidelines to diagnosis and management. Postgrad Med 82(1):185, 1987.

Clinical concepts of evaluation and management are reviewed. Authors site supraspinatus tendinitis as the most common cause of shoulder pain followed by bicipital tendinitis, impingement syndromes, supraspinatus rupture, subacromial bursitis, arthritis, frozen shoulder, and various conditions that refer to the shoulder.

Brown C: Compressive, invasive referred pain to the shoulder. Clin Orthop 173:55, 1983.

Another source of shoulder pain should be sought in patients with persistent shoulder pain and no discernable musculoskeletal abnormalities who do not respond to standard therapeutic measures.

Cofield RH, Simonet WT: The shoulder in sports. Mayo Clin Proc 59:157, 1984.

A review of mechanisms and treatment of common sports injuries of the shoulder joint. Sports most commonly associated with shoulder injuries were swimming, baseball, tennis, football, and gymnastics.

Cone RO, Resnick D: Traumatic disorders of the shoulder. JAMA 252:540, 1984.

A concise review of radiographic findings in acute and chronic shoulder injuries.

Crass JR: Current concepts in the radiographic evaluation of the rotator cuff. CRC Crit Rev Diagn Imaging 28:23, 1988.

This review discusses rotator cuff disease and current concepts of available radiographic evaluation such as arthrogram, CT, ultrasonography (US) and MRI.

Curran JF, Ellman MH, Brown NL: Rheumatologic aspects of painful conditions affecting the shoulder. Clin Orthop 173:27, 1983.

Shoulder arthritis often presents to the orthopaedic surgeon with joint pain and loss of shoulder motion.

Epps CH Jr: Painful hematologic conditions affecting the shoulder. Clin Orthop 173:38, 1983.

Shoulder pain can be the presenting symptom of a generalized hematologic disease or disorder.

Gerhart TN, Dohlman LE, Warfield CA: Clinical diagnosis of shoulder pain. Hosp Pract 20(9):134, 1985.
An organized and systematic approach to the diagnosis of shoulder pain.

Johnson JE, Sim FH, Scott SG: Musculoskeletal injuries in competitive swimmers. Mayo Clin Proc 62:289, 1987.
Shoulder pain in young swimmers was evaluated. The most common shoulder complaint was due to supraspinatus or biceps tendinitis. Authors suggest that glenohumeral instability may be a more common cause of shoulder pain in swimmers than is reported.

Mack LA, Nyberg DA, Matsen FA III: Sonographic evaluation of the rotator cuff. Radiol Clin North Am 26:161, 1988.
Ultrasound examination in the diagnosis of rotator cuff syndrome is reviewed. Authors recommend early evaluation of shoulder injuries with this technique before rotator cuff tears occur. This procedure may prevent future shoulder pain.

Rafii M, Firooznia H, Bonamo JJ, et al: Athlete shoulder injuries: CT arthrographic findings. Radiology 162:559, 1987.
CT arthrographic findings in 43 athletes with shoulder pain were evaluated and correlated with surgical results in 19 patients. Clinically unsuspected lesions and instability, as well as early onset of degenerative changes, were defined with this technique.

Seeger LL, Gold RH, Bassett LW, Ellman H: Shoulder impingement syndrome: MR findings in 53 shoulders. AJR 150:343, 1988.
This study found MRI useful in depicting both bony and soft tissue abnormalities associated with the shoulder impingement syndrome (subacromial bursitis, supraspinatus tendinitis, and rotator cuff tears).

Simms RW, Goldenberg DL, Felson DT, Mason JH: Tenderness in 75 anatomic sites. Distinguishing fibromyalgia patients from controls. Arthritis Rheum 31:182, 1988.
Seventy-five unilateral anatomic points of tenderness in 10 patients with fibromyalgia and 10 control patients were studied to determine which sites best identified patients with fibromyalgia. Authors identified 19 sites that best differentiated patients with fibromyalgia from controls.

Van Ouwenaller C, Laplace PM, Chantraine A: Painful shoulder in hemiplegia. Arch Phys Med Rehabil 67:23, 1986.
Two hundred nineteen hemiplegic stroke patients were followed for 1 year to assess clinical factors involved in the shoulder pain, which frequently complicates the care of hemiplegic patients. Anteroinferior subluxation was found to be a frequent cause of shoulder pain, particularly in the spastic patient. Diagnostic and management recommendations are made.

Weaver JK: Skiing-related injuries to the shoulder. Clin Orthop 216:24, 1987.
An analysis of 135 consecutive shoulder injuries associated with skiing found that the anterior dislocation was the most common diagnosis, followed by rotator cuff tears, acromioclavicular separations, and miscellaneous contusions and fractures. The most frequent

isolated fracture was a minimally displaced fracture of the greater tuberosity.

Withrington RH, Girgis FL, Seifert MH: A comparative study of the etiological factors in shoulder pain. Br J Rheumatol 24:24, 1985.

A significant association of shoulder capsulitis with diabetes mellitus and antecedent trauma when compared with supraspinatus tendinitis was found.

Zuckerman JD, Shapiro I: Geriatric shoulder pain: common causes and their management. Geriatrics 42(9):43, 1987.

This article reviews current clinical concepts pertinent to the evaluation of shoulder pain in the geriatric patient.

54

Low Back Pain: Common and Less Common Causes

Low back pain is pain in the area between the lower rib cage and gluteal folds, which often radiates into the thighs.[1] Sciatica and neurologic claudication are important initial symptoms to help localize pathology. Sciatica is a symptom complex of pain and sensory or motor deficits in a lumbar root distribution and is most commonly caused by a herniation of the nucleus pulposus into the L4–L5 or L5–S1 lumbar disc space in patients 20 to 50 years of age.[2] When neurologic claudication accompanies back pain, symptoms are the result of spinal stenosis and are characterized by weakness and paresthesias brought on while walking and relieved by sitting or other positional maneuvers that flex the spine. Lumbosacral strain and sprain are the most common diagnoses of acute low back pain.[3] However, severe pain at rest in a patient with acute back pain should raise concerns of underlying fracture, infection, or neoplasm, particularly in high-risk populations, such as elderly women with osteoporosis, known cancer patients, diabetics, immunosuppressed patients, and drug addicts.

**Common Causes of
Low Back Pain**

Degenerative changes and overuse syndromes cause most chronic back pain. Acute low back pain is most commonly due to traumatic soft tissue or bony injuries that resolve within weeks.

Lumbosacral strain and sprain
Degenerative disc disease: common cause over 40 years old
Spondylolisthesis: degenerative facet joints that usually cause slippage at L4 or L5[4]
Herniated intervertebral disc: usually occurs between 20 and 40 years of age, with an increased incidence in patients with transitional vertebrae[5]
Spinal stenosis: developmental and degenerative processes narrow the lumbar canal; degenerative causes usually result in segmental narrowing with disc slippage and prominent posterior articular processes; commonly found in the elderly, particularly those with osteoporosis and diabetes[1,6]
Compression fracture[7,8]
Ankylosing spondylitis: milder forms of ankylosing spondylitis go unsuspected, particularly in females; if missed, permanent disability is a risk[9,10]
Osteoporosis: postmenopausal women present a high risk category for senile type osteoporosis and possible fracture.[11,12]
Psychogenic: frequent association with reported back pain[13]
Pregnancy: sacroiliac joint dysfunction common cause during pregnancy[14,15]
Menstrual cramps

**Less Common Causes
of Low Back Pain**

Less common causes of back pain should be a concern in the patient with severe pain at rest, particularly in patients at risk for neoplasms, metabolic bone disease, congenital spine deformities, infection, and referred pain from thoracic, abdominal, and pelvic cavities.

Osteoarthritis of facet joints[16]
Missed vertebral fractures: small fractures—particularly those occurring in the apophyseal, transverse, or spinous processes and around vertebral end plates—may be difficult to detect with conventional radiography, but can cause severe pain.[17-19]
Congenital and developmental abnormalities
Scoliosis: pain not always due to curvature[20,21]

Spondylolisthesis: a slippage of one vertebra over another, often associated with spondylolysis, best seen with oblique radiographs. Athletes are considered high risk for this condition.[22]

Achondroplasia[23]

Cystic fibrosis: postural abnormalities or vertebral wedging common cause of pain[24]

Rheumatoid arthritis[25,26]

Reiter's syndrome: back pain is often the first symptom of Reiter's syndrome in young males.

Spondyloarthropathies: inflammatory bowel disease and psoriatic arthritis

Neoplasms: primary, benign, and malignant tumors

    Metastatic tumors: in young men, suspect testicular germ cell tumors.[27]

    Multiple myeloma: bone pain is a frequent presenting complaint.[28,29]

    Ependymoma[30]

    Spinal chordoma[31]

    Sacral schwannomas[32]

    Non-Hodgkin's lymphoma[33]

    Paraganglioma[34]

Paget's disease[35–37]

Primary hyperparathyroidism: back pain and vertebral compression fractures can be the initial symptom of hyperparathyroidism.[38]

Secondary hyperparathyroidism: brown tumor[39]

DISH (diffuse idiopathic skeletal hyperostosis or Forestier disease): an aching spinal stiffness in the elderly, sometimes associated with elbow and heel pain; characteristic radiographic changes include ligament ossification and para-articular osteophytosis[40]

Spinal vascular malformations

    Arteriovenous malformations[41]

    Hemangiomas[42]

Infectious causes

    Vertebral osteomyelitis: may present as back pain and fever at any age, particularly in high-risk patients, such as after genitourinary procedures and in intravenous drug abusers; radiographic changes may be delayed[43,44]

    Discitis[45]

    Epidural abscess: common preceding events include drug abuse, blunt trauma, skin infection; may be rapidly progressive[46,47]

    Tuberculosis: consider in recent immigrants from underdeveloped areas[48,49]

Herpes zoster: may present as lumbar radi-
culopathy[50]
Pyogenic sacroiliitis: consider in drug abusers[51]
Spinal brucellosis[52]

Extraspinal Disease Causing Low Back Pain

Life-threatening, extraspinal disorders, such as intra-
abdominal processes or vascular conditions, can
present with acute back pain.[53]

Peptic ulcer: penetrating into the pancreas or per-
forating duodenal ulcer[54]
Biliary system disease: cholecystitis, carcinoid tumor
of biliary system[55]
Pancreatic disease: pancreatitis, pancreatic carcinoma[56,57]
Renal disease: perinephric abscess, renal stones, pyelonephritis
Pelvic disease: endometriosis, retroperitoneal tumor[58]
Vascular catastrophies: abdominal aortic dissection
or ruptured abdominal aortic aneurysms may
present as back pain without an early clue.[53,59,60]
Lumbar artery aneurysm[61]

References

1. Frymoyer JW: Back pain and sciatica. N Engl J Med 318:291, 1988.
2. Spangfort EV: The lumbar disk herniation: a computer-aided analysis of 2,504 operations. Acta Orthop Scand (Suppl) 142:1, 1972.
3. Nachemson AL: Advances in low-back pain. Clin Orthop 200:266, 1985.
4. Lewinnek GE, Warfield CA: Facet joint degeneration as a cause of low back pain. Clin Orthop 213:216, 1986.
5. Castellvi AE, Goldstein LA, Chan DPK: Lumbosacral transitional vertebrae and their relationship with lumbar extradural defects. Spine 9:493, 1984.
6. Kirkaldy-Willis WH, Paine KWE, Cauchoix J, et al: Lumbar spinal stenosis. Clin Orthop 99:30, 1974.
7. Aebi M, Mohler J, Zach G, Morscher E: Analysis of 75 operated thoracolumbar fractures and fracture dislocations with and without neurological deficit. Arch Orthop Trauma Surg 105:100, 1986.
8. Gertzbein SD, Court-Brown CM: Flexion-distraction injuries of the lumbar spine. Mechanisms of injury and classification. Clin Orthop 227:52, 1988.
9. Calin A, Fries JF: Striking prevalence of ankylosing spondylitis in "healthy" B27 positive males and females. A controlled study. N Engl J Med 293:835, 1975.
10. Jayson MIV: Difficult diagnoses in back pain. Br Med J 288:740, 1984.
11. Lane JM, Vigorita VJ: Osteoporosis. J Bone Joint Surg (Am) 65-A:274, 1983.

12. McHenry MC, Duchesneau PM, Keys TF, et al: Vertebral osteomyelitis presenting as spinal compression fracture. Six patients with underlying osteoporosis. Arch Intern Med 148:417, 1988.

13. Vallfors B: Acute, subacute, and chronic low back pain: clinical symptoms, absenteeism and working environment. Scand J Rehabil Med 11(Suppl):1, 1985.

14. Berg G, Hammar M, Moller-Nielsen J, et al: Low back pain during pregnancy. Obstet Gynecol 71:71, 1988.

15. Melzack R, Schaffelberg D: Low-back pain during labor. Am J Obstet Gynecol 156:901, 1987.

16. Pathria M, Sartoris DJ, Resnick D: Osteoarthritis of the facet joints: accuracy of oblique radiographic assessment. Radiology 164:227, 1987.

17. Holdsworth Sir F: Fractures, dislocations, and fracture-dislocations of the spine. J Bone Joint Surg (Am) 52-A:1534, 1970.

18. Sims-Williams H, Jayson MIV, Baddeley H: Small spinal fractures in back pain patients. Ann Rheum Dis 37:262, 1978.

19. Nussbaum AR, Treves ST, Micheli L: Bone stress lesions in ballet dancers: scintigraphic assessment. AJR 150:851, 1988.

20. Jackson RP, Simmons EH, Stripinis D: Incidence and severity of back pain in adult idiopathic scoliosis. Spine 8:749, 1983.

21. Winter RB, Lonstein JE, Denis F: Pain patterns in adult scoliosis. Orthop Clin North Am 19:339, 1988.

22. Wiltse LL, Widell EH Jr, Jackson DW: Fatigue fracture: the basic lesion is inthmic spondylolisthesis. J Bone Joint Surg (Am) 57:17, 1975.

23. Siebens AA, Hungerford DS, Kirby NA: Achondroplasia: effectiveness of an orthosis in reducing deformity of the spine. Arch Phys Med Rehabil 68:384, 1987.

24. Ross J, Gamble J, Schultz A, Lewiston N: Back pain and spinal deformity in cystic fibrosis. Am J Dis Child 141:1313, 1987.

25. Jacob JR, Weisman MH, Mink JH, et al: Reversible cause of back pain and sciatica in rheumatoid arthritis: an apophyseal joint cyst. Arthritis Rheum 29:431, 1986.

26. Bergstrom G, Bjelle A, Sundh V, Svanborg A: Joint disorders at ages 70, 75, and 79 years—a cross-sectional comparison. Br J Rheumatol 25:333, 1986.

27. Cantwell BM, Mannix KA, Harris AL: Back pain—a presentation of metastatic testicular germ cell tumours. Lancet 1:262, 1987.

28. Kapadia SB: Multiple myeloma: a clinicopathologic study of 62 consecutively autopsied cases. Medicine 59:380, 1980.

29. Doster DR, Folds J, Gabriel DA: Nonsecretory multiple myeloma. Arch Pathol Lab Med 112:147, 1988.

30. Rawlings CE III, Giangaspero F, Burger PC, Bullard DE: Ependymomas: a clinicopathologic study. Surg Neurol 29:271, 1988.

31. de Bruine FT, Kroon HM: Spinal chordoma: radiologic features in 14 cases. AJR 150:861, 1988.

32. Abernathey CD, Onofrio BM, Scheithauer B, et al: Surgical management of giant sacral schwannomas. J Neurosurg 65:286, 1986.

33. Epelbaum R, Haim N, Ben-Shahar M, et al: Non-Hodgkin's lymphoma presenting with spinal epidural involvement. Cancer 58:2120, 1986.
34. Sonneland PR, Scheithauer BW, LeChago J, et al: Paraganglioma of the cauda equina region. Clinico-pathologic study of 31 cases with special reference to immunocytology and ultrastructure. Cancer 58:1720, 1986.
35. Altman RD, Collins B: Musculoskeletal manifestations of Paget's disease of bone. Arthritis Rheum 23:1121, 1980.
36. Altman RD, Brown M, Gargano F: Low back pain in Paget's disease of bone. Clin Orthop 217:152, 1987.
37. Zlatkin MB, Lander PH, Hadjipavlou AG, Levine JS: Paget disease of the spine: CT with clinical correlation. Radiology 160:155, 1986.
38. Dauphine RT, Riggs BL, Scholz DA: Back pain and vertebral crush fractures: an unemphasized mode of presentation for primary hyperparathyroidism. Ann Intern Med 83:365, 1975.
39. Bohlman ME, Kim YC, Eagan J, Spees EK: Brown tumor in secondary hyperparathyroidism causing acute paraplegia. Am J Med 81:545, 1986.
40. Utsinger PD, Resnick D, Shapiro R: Diffuse skeletal abnormalities in Forestier disease. Arch Intern Med 136:763, 1976.
41. Ueda S, Saito A, Inomori S, Kim I: Cavernous angioma of the cauda equina producing subarachnoid hemorrhage. Case report. J Neurosurg 66:134, 1987.
42. Laredo JD, Reizine D, Bard M, Merland JJ: Vertebral hemangiomas: radiologic evaluation. Radiology 161:183, 1986.
43. Musher DM, Thorsteinsson SB, Minuth JN, et al: Vertebral osteomyelitis. Still a diagnostic pitfall. Arch Intern Med 136:105, 1976.
44. McHenry MC, Duchesneau PM, Keys TF, et al: Vertebral osteomyelitis presenting as spinal compression fracture. Six patients with underlying osteoporosis. Arch Intern Med 148:417, 1988.
45. Gozzi G, Stacul F, Zuiani C, et al: The role of computerized tomography in the diagnosis of postoperative intervertebral diskitis. Radiol Med (Torino) 75:287, 1988.
46. Kaufman DM, Kaplan JG, Litman N: Infectious agents in spinal epidural abscesses. Neurology 30:844, 1980.
47. Mooney RP, Hockberger RS: Spinal epidural abscess: a rapidly progressive disease. Ann Emerg Med 16;1168, 1987.
48. Alvarez S, McCabe WR: Extrapulmonary tuberculosis revisited: a review of experience at Boston City and other hospitals. Medicine 63:25, 1984.
49. Pouchot J, Vinceneux P, Barge J, et al: Tuberculosis of the sacroiliac joint: clinical features, outcome, and evaluation of closed needle biopsy in 11 consecutive cases. Am J Med 84:622, 1988.
50. Burkman KA, Gaines RW Jr, Kashani SR, Smith RD: Herpes zoster: a consideration in the differential diagnosis of radiculopathy. Arch Phys Med Rehabil 69:132, 1988.

51. Guyot DR, Manoli A II, Kling GA: Pyogenic sacroiliitis in i.v. drug abusers. AJR 149:1209, 1987.
52. Rajapakse CN, Al-Aska AK, Al-Orainey I, et al: Spinal brucellosis. Br J Rheumatol 26:28, 1987.
53. Hadler NM: Regional back pain (editorial). N Engl J Med 315:1090, 1986.
54. Pearson FG, Cooper JD, Patterson GA, Prakash D: Peptic ulcer in acquired columnar-lined esophagus: results of surgical treatment. Ann Thorac Surg 43:241, 1987.
55. Jutte DL, Bell RH Jr, Penn I, et al: Carcinoid tumor of the biliary system. Case report and literature review. Dig Dis Sci 32:763, 1987.
56. Noda A, Hamano H, Shibata T, et al: Chronic pancreatitis at early age of onset presenting interesting findings through endoscopic retrograde pancreatography and chemical analysis of nonopaque pancreatic concretion. Dig Dis Sci 32:433, 1987.
57. Barkin JS, Goldberg RI, Sfakianakis GN, Levi J: Pancreatic carcinoma is associated with delayed gastric emptying. Dig Dis Sci 31:265, 1986.
58. Jaeckle KA, Young DF, Foley KM: The natural history of lumbosacral plexopathy in cancer. Neurology 35:8, 1985.
59. Jones CS, Reilly MK, Dalsing MC, Glover JL: Chronic contained rupture of abdominal aortic aneurysms. Arch Surg 121:542, 1986.
60. Savarese RP, Rosenfeld JC, DeLaurentis DA: Inflammatory abdominal aortic aneurysm. Surg Gynecol Obstet 162:405, 1986.
61. Kornberg E: Lumbar artery aneurysm with acute aortic occlusion resulting from chiropractic manipulation: a case report. Surgery 103:122, 1988.

Selected Readings

Bates DW, Reuler JB: Back pain and epidural spinal cord compression. J Gen Intern Med 3:191, 1988.
A discussion of the difficult clinical problem of distinguishing which patients with malignancy and back pain have epidural spinal cord compression. Authors point out that a clinical evaluation is inadequate and that the diagnosis depends on radiographic visualization of the spinal cord. Myelography remains the test of choice.

Bernard TN Jr, Kirkaldy-Willis WH: Recognizing specific characteristics of nonspecific low back pain. Clin Orthop 217:266, 1987.
A retrospective study of 1,293 low back pain patients treated for 12 years concludes that sacroiliac and posterior joint syndromes are the most common referred-pain syndromes, and herniated nucleus pulposus and lateral spinal stenosis were the most common causes of nerve root compression lesions. Useful diagnostic recommendations are offered based on a significant amount of clinical data.

Deyo RA, Diehl AK, Rosenthal M: How many days of bed rest for acute low back pain? N Engl J Med 315:1064, 1986.
This study compared the clinical outcome of 2 days versus 7 days of bed rest in patients with acute low back pain. Their data support early return to work.

Durning RP, Murphy ML: Lumbar disk disease. Clinical presentation, diagnosis, and treatment. Postgrad Med 79(5):54, 1986.
Summary of clinical features of lumbar disc disease with helpful suggestions for clinical, radiographic, and electromyographic evaluation.

Gandy S, Payne R: Back pain in the elderly: updated diagnosis and management. Geriatrics 41(12):59,67, 1986.
Current concepts of diagnosis and management of back pain in the elderly. CT findings helpful in distinguishing compression fractures, osteoporosis, and neoplasm are discussed.

Harris LF, Haws FP, Triplett JN Jr, Maccubbin DA: Subdural empyema and epidural abscess: recent experience in a community hospital. South Med J 80:1254, 1987.
Thirty-one cases of localized central nervous system infection were evaluated with a focus on patients with spinal epidural abscess (SEA) and spinal subdural empyema (SSE). Both SEA and SSE presented with fever, spinal pain, loss of motor function, and responded to laminectomy and antibiotics.

Kelen GD, Noji EK, Doris PE: Guidelines for use of lumbar spine radiography. Ann Emerg Med 15:245, 1986.
Recommendations for emergency radiographic evaluation of back pain suggest that plain radiographs are rarely indicated in otherwise healthy patients 20 to 50 years old with mechanical or root pain on initial presentation. Indications for CT are discussed.

Machab I: The Classic. Disc degeneration and low back pain. Clin Orthop 208:3, 1986.
Classic, lucid discussion of disc degeneration and low back pain, which was originally presented at the proceedings of the Royal College of Physicians and Surgeons of Canada, 1952.

Nicholas JJ, Christy WC: Spinal pain made worse by recumbency: a clue to spinal cord tumors. Arch Phys Med Rehabil 67:598, 1986.
Useful clinical observation reported that back pain made worse by recumbency may be an important diagnostic clue suggesting an underlying spinal cord tumor. Four cases described.

Pathria M, Sartoris DJ, Resnick D: Osteoarthritis of the facet joints: accuracy of oblique radiographic assessment. Radiology 164:227, 1987.
Lumbar spine radiography and CT sensitivity and specificity in the assessment of facet joint osteoarthritis were compared. Authors conclude that although conventional radiography is a useful screen for facet joint osteoarthritis, it is insensitive compared with CT.

Portenoy RK, Lipton RB, Foley KM: Back pain in the cancer patient: an algorithm for evaluation and management. Neurology 37:134, 1987.
Back pain is often the first symptom of epidural spinal cord compression in patients with metastatic cancer. An algorithm is proposed which includes the use of myelography, corticosteroids, radiation, and surgery.

Posner JB: Back pain and epidural spinal cord compression. Med Clin North Am 71:185, 1987.
Useful clinical discussion regarding diagnosis and management of back pain, with an emphasis on a rational approach to distinguish self-limited disorders from malignant disease without excessive workup.

Scherokman B, Vukelja S: Diabetic neuropathy simulating

conus medullaris syndrome. Arch Intern Med 148:459, 1988.
Interesting report of two diabetic patients with fecal incontinence, decreased sphincter tone, sacral hypoesthesia, and absent Achilles reflex, which clinically mimicked a conus medullaris syndrome without a mass lesion to explain these findings.

Schwartz CM, Demos TC, Wehner JM: Osteomyelitis of the sacrum as the initial manifestation of Crohn's disease. Clin Orthop 222:181, 1987.
A case report illustrating that low back pain, particularly in young adults, may be osteomyelitis, and in this case, a first manifestation of gastrointestinal tract disease.

Swezey RL: Low back pain in the elderly: practical management concerns. Geriatrics 43(2):39, 1988.
Authors suggest that young adults with low back pain are predisposed to exacerbations and chronic back pain when they are elderly adults.

Waddell G: Clinical assessment of lumbar impairment. Clin Orthop 221:110, 1987.
Discussion offering helpful methods in tackling a common, often sticky problem; that is, how to assess disability in low back pain patients.

Xin SQ, Zhang QZ, Fan DH: Significance of the straight-leg-raising test in the diagnosis and clinical evaluation of lower lumbar intervertebral-disc protrusion. J Bone Joint Surg (Am) 69:517, 1987.
One hundred thirteen patients with lumbar intervertebral disc protrusion were analyzed to determine the relationship between straight-leg-raising test findings and surgical findings. Central protrusions were associated more with pain in the back; lateral protrusions were associated more with pain in the lower extremities.

Yu SW, Sether LA, Ho PS, et al: Tears of the anulus fibrosus: correlation between MR and pathologic findings in cadavers. AJNR 9:367, 1988.
Tears of the anulus fibrosus have been thought to be a cause of back pain. Authors suggest that MRI provides an accurate means of evaluating anulus tears.

55

Sacroiliitis: Conditions Causing Clinical or Radiographic Abnormalities of the Sacroiliac Joint

The sacroiliac joint is a diarthrodial joint linking the sacrum and ilium. Many conditions can produce pain and inflammation of this joint. The most common entities causing sacroiliitis are the seronegative (rheumatoid factor negative) spondyloarthropathies: ankylosing spondylitis, Reiter's syndrome, psoriatic arthritis, and the arthritis of inflammatory bowel disease. These conditions are associated with HLA-B27, peripheral oligoarthritis, and inflammation of the entheses (the sites of attachment of tendons and ligaments to bones). Several other diseases, including rheumatologic, infectious, metabolic, traumatic, degenerative, and miscellaneous conditions can cause sacroiliac joint abnormalities. Many of these entities cause clinical symptoms. Others may be characterized only by radiographic abnormalities. This chapter lists conditions that may cause or mimic sacroiliitis clinically or radiographically.

Spondyloarthropathies

Ankylosing spondylitis[1]: the prototypical seronegative spondyloarthropathy. Bilateral sacroiliitis is a major feature of this disease.

Reactive arthritis[2-4]: immunologically mediated sacroiliitis, usually asymmetric, can follow genital (*Chlamydia trachomatis, Ureaplasma urealyticum*) and enteric (*Shigella, Salmonella, Yersinia* and *Campylobacter*) infections. Reactive arthritis may well be part of a continuum with Reiter's syndrome.[2]

411

Reiter's syndrome[2]: the classic triad of arthritis, conjunctivitis, and urethritis, occurring either together or sequentially, may follow exposure to certain genital or enteric organisms. The sacroiliitis of Reiter's syndrome is usually asymmetric.

Psoriatic arthritis[5]: sacroiliitis occurs in 20 to 40% of patients with psoriatic arthritis. It may be symmetric or asymmetric and is often asymptomatic.

Inflammatory bowel disease[6]: radiographic sacroiliitis can be seen in about 4% of cases of ulcerative colitis and Crohn's disease. It is usually symmetric, and its course is often independent of the intestinal disease.

Whipple's disease[7,8]: about 4% of patients with this condition may have bilateral sacroiliitis resembling ankylosing spondylitis.

Pustulotic arthro-osteitis[9]: this condition is marked by sterile pustules that occur symmetrically on the palms and/or soles and have some clinical and histologic similarity to pustular psoriasis. Sacroiliitis is usually bilateral and occurs in 13% of cases.

Other Inflammatory Conditions

Rheumatoid arthritis[10,11]: although rheumatoid arthritis does not primarily affect the joints of the axial skeleton, sacroiliac joint abnormalities such as radiographic narrowing, sclerosis, and erosions occur in 20 to 40% of cases.

Juvenile chronic arthritis[12,13]: boys with late childhood onset of juvenile chronic arthritis of the pauci-articular type have a high incidence of early ankylosing spondylitis. Most of these children are HLA-B27 positive. Acute anterior uveitis is a common feature.[14]

Behçet's disease[15]: it is not clear if sacroiliitis is an integral feature of Behçet's disease or just a chance association.[16]

Familial Mediterranean fever[17]: sacroiliitis occurs in up to 17% of patients. It does not appear to be associated with HLA-B27.[18]

Polymyalgia rheumatica[19]: up to 28% of patients may have radiographic evidence of sacroiliac abnormalities at 3 years after onset of symptoms.

Relapsing polychondritis[20]: sacroiliac joints may show erosions without accompanying radiologic features of spondylitis. These findings can occur in patients without evidence of rheumatoid arthritis and systemic lupus erythematosus.[21]

Infections

Pyogenic[22]: pyogenic infections of the sacroiliac joint are rare. Staphylococcal organisms are the most frequent causative bacteria. *Escherichia coli*, enterococci, streptococci, *Pseudomonas, Salmonella, Serratia*, and *Yersinia* have also been reported. Intravenous drug abusers have a predilection for developing pyogenic sacroiliac infections. Pyogenic sacroiliitis is usually unilateral.

Salpingitis[23]: sacroiliitis may follow acute salpingitis in both HLA-B27 positive and negative women. This condition may be a form of reactive arthritis.

Brucellosis[24]: 4 to 16% of cases have sacroiliac joint involvement as the result of hematogenous spread.

Tuberculosis[25]: sacroiliac tuberculosis is diagnosed radiographically by the classic triad of signs of bone and joint tuberculosis elsewhere, para-articular osteoporosis, marginal osseous erosions, and gradual narrowing of the joint space.[26]

Syphilis[27]: unilateral sacroiliitis has been reported in association with secondary syphilis.

Metabolic

Gout[28,29]: the sacroiliac joint is involved in 7 to 17% of patients with chronic tophaceous gout.

Calcium pyrophosphate deposition disease (CPPD, pseudogout)[30]: in CPPD, the sacroiliac joints may demonstrate chondrocalcinosis, subchondral pseudocysts, and coalescent contiguous radiolucencies along the subchondral border—the typical radiographic findings of pseudogout.

Hyperparathyroidism[31]: the sacroiliac joint may be involved in both primary and secondary hyperparathyroidism. The patient may develop progressive subchondral bone resorption (usually more prominent on the ilial side of the joint), trabecular thickening and subperiosteal sclerosis. The changes are commonly symmetric, and radiographs can be confused with ankylosing spondylitis.

Hypophosphatemic osteomalacia (X-linked)[32]: 62% have calcific deposits at the sacroiliac joints. The sacroiliac joints typically appear to be sclerotic or fused, without evidence of erosive changes.

Gaucher's disease[33]: patients may develop subarticular sclerosis and apparent joint space obliteration that can resemble ankylosing spondylitis.

Ochronosis (alkaptonuria): the sacroiliac joint can have articular narrowing, sclerosis, and osteophyte formation.

Traumatic/ Degenerative

Osteoarthritis[34]: radiographic changes of degenerative disease, such as loss of joint space, osteophyte formation, sclerosis, and subchondral cyst formation, are fairly common (about 25%) in people over the age of 50.

Paraplegia[35]: radiologic abnormalities of the sacroiliac joint, sometimes resembling ankylosing spondylitis, occur in 4 to 61% of paraplegic patients.

Miscellaneous Conditions

Leg length discrepancy: can lead to sacroiliac joint pain and/or unilateral sacroiliac joint degenerative changes

Mechanical low back pain[36]: up to one-fourth of patients with mechanical or nonspecific low back pain may have abnormal radioisotope uptake in the sacroiliac joint(s) on bone scan. These abnormal scans to not necessarily imply disease of the sacroiliac joint.

Sickle-cell disease[37]: irregular sclerosis and erosion of the sacroiliac joint has been reported.

Pregnancy: increased range of motion of the sacroiliac joint due to the gestational hormone relaxin can lead to sacroiliac joint pain.

Acro-osteolysis (in polyvinyl chloride workers)[38]: chronic polyvinyl chloride exposure can lead to bone resorption around the sacroiliac joint. Radiographic changes include irregular joint contours, joint erosions, and subchondral sclerosis, which are usually bilateral.

Osteitis condensans ilii: a self-limited condition usually found in young, multiparous women, characterized radiographically by bilateral, asymmetric, triangular condensation of bone in the ilium, adjacent to the lower half of the sacroiliac joint.

Paget's disease of bone[39]: may give the radiographic appearance of ankylosis of the sacroiliac joint

Tuberous sclerosis[40]: classically this disorder is marked by epilepsy, mental retardation, and adenoma sebaceum. Medullary osteoblastic deposits may occur around the sacroiliac joint, producing oval or flame-shaped patchy sclerosis.

References

1. Calin A: Ankylosing spondylitis. Clin Rheum Dis 11:41, 1985.
2. Keat A: Reiter's syndrome and reactive arthritis in perspective. N Engl J Med 309:1606, 1983.
3. Aho K, Leirisalo-Repo M, Repo H: Reactive arthritis. Clin Rheum Dis 11:25, 1985.
4. Firestein GS, Zvaifler NJ: Reactive arthritis. Annu Rev Med 38:351, 1987.
5. Laurent MR: Psoriatic arthritis. Clin Rheum Dis 11:61, 1985.
6. Moll JMH: Inflammatory bowel disease. Clin Rheum Dis 11:87, 1985.
7. Canoso JJ, Saini M, Hermos JA: Whipple's disease and ankylosing spondylitis: simultaneous occurrence in HLA-B27 positive male. J Rheumatol 5:79, 1978.
8. Dobbins WO III: HLA antigens in Whipple's disease. Arthritis Rheum 30:102, 1987.
9. Sonozaki H, Mitsui H, Miyanaga Y, et al: Clinical features of 53 cases of pustulotic arthro-osteitis. Ann Rheum Dis 40:547, 1981.
10. Elhabali M, Scherak O, Seidl G, et al: Tomographic examinations of sacroiliac joints in adult patients with rheumatoid arthritis. J Rheumatol 6:417, 1979.
11. DeCarvalho A, Graudal H: Sacroiliac joint involvement in classical or definite rheumatoid arthritis. Acta Radiol [Diagn] 21:417, 1980.
12. Ladd JR, Cassidy JT, Martel W: Juvenile ankylosing spondylitis. Arthritis Rheum 14:579, 1971.
13. Petty RE, Malleson P: Spondyloarthropathies of childhood. Pediatr Clin North Am 33:1079, 1986.
14. Kanski JJ: Uveitis in juvenile chronic arthritis: incidence, clinical features, and prognosis. Eye 2:641, 1988.
15. Shimizu T, Ehrlich GE, Inaba G, et al: Behçet's disease (Behçet syndrome). Semin Arthritis Rheum 8:223, 1979.
16. Yazici H, Tuzlaci M, Yordakul S: A controlled survey of sacroiliitis in Behçet's disease. Ann Rheum Dis 40:558, 1981.
17. Brodey PA, Wolff SM: Radiographic changes in the sacroiliac joints in familial Mediterranean fever. Radiology 114:331, 1975.
18. Lehman TJA, Hanson V, Kornreich H, et al: HLA-B27-negative sacroiliitis: a manifestation of familial Mediterranean fever in childhood. Pediatrics 61:423, 1978.
19. O'Duffy JD, Hunder GG, Wahner HW: A follow-up study of polymyalgia rheumatica: evidence of chronic axial synovitis. J Rheumatol 7:685, 1980.
20. Braunstein EM, Martel W, Stilwill E, et al: Radiological aspects of the arthropathy of relapsing polychondritis. Clin Radiol 30:441, 1979.
21. Kaye R, Sones DA: Relapsing polychondritis: clinical and pathological features in fourteen cases. Ann Intern Med 60:653, 1964.
22. Gordon G, Kabins SA: Pyogenic sacroiliitis. Am J Med 69:50, 1980.
23. Szanto E, Hagenfeldt K: Sacro-iliitis in women—a sequela to acute salpingitis: a follow-up study. Scand J Rheumatol 12:89, 1983.

24. Gotuzzo E, Alarcón GS, Bocanegra TS, et al: Articular involvement in human brucellosis: a restrospective analysis of 304 cases. Semin Arthritis Rheum 12:245, 1982.
25. Seddon HI, St. Clair Strange FG: Sacroiliac tuberculosis. Br J Surg 28:193, 1940.
26. Binet EF, Markanian B (eds): Correlation conferences in radiology and pathology: Unilateral sacroiliitis. NY State J Med 78:1744, 1978.
27. Reginato AJ, Ferreiro-Seoane JL, Falasca G: Unilateral sacroiliitis in secondary syphilis (letter). J Rheumatol 15:717, 1988.
28. Malawista SE, Seegmiller JE, Hathaway BE, et al: Sacroiliac gout. JAMA 194:106, 1965.
29. Alarcón-Segovia D, Cetina JA, Diaz-Jouanen E: Sacroiliac joints in primary gout. Am J Roentgenol Radium Ther Nucl Med 118:438, 1973.
30. Resnick D, Niwayama G, Georgen TG, et al: Clinical, radiographic, and pathologic abnormalities in calcium pyrophosphate dihydrate deposition disease (CPPD): pseudogout. Radiology 122;1, 1977.
31. Resnick D, Dwosh IL, Niwayama G: Sacroiliac joint in renal osteodystrophy: roentgenographic-pathologic correlation. J Rheumatol 2:287, 1975.
32. Polisson RP, Martinez S, Khoury M, et al: Calcification of entheses associated with X-linked hypophosphatemic osteomalacia. N Engl J Med 313:1, 1985.
33. Greenfield GB: Bone changes in chronic adult Gaucher's disease. Am J Roentgenol Radium Ther Nucl Med 110:800, 1970.
34. Resnick D, Niwayama G, Georgen TG: Degenerative disease of the sacroiliac joint. Invest Radiol 10:608, 1975.
35. Khan MA, Kushner I, Freehafer AA: Sacroiliac joint abnormalities in paraplegics. Ann Rheum Dis 38:317, 1979.
36. Lugon M, Torode AS, Travers RL, et al: Sacro-iliac joint scanning with technetium-99 diphosphonate. Rheumatol Rehabil 18:131, 1979.
37. Schumacher HR, Andrews R, McLaughlin G: Arthropathy in sickle-cell disease. Ann Intern Med 78:203, 1973.
38. Dodson VN, Dinman BD, Whitehouse WM, et al: Occupational acro-osteolysis III. A clinical study. Arch Environ Health 22:83, 1971.
39. Franck WA, Bress NM, Singer FR, et al: Rheumatic manifestations of Paget's disease of bone. Am J Med 56:592, 1974.
40. Komar NN, Gabrielsen TO, Holt JF: Roentgenographic appearance of lumbosacral spine and pelvis in tuberous sclerosis. Radiology 89:701, 1967.

Selected Readings

Bellamy N, Park W, Rooney PJ: What do we know about the sacroiliac joint? Semin Arthritis Rheum 12:282, 1983.
Comprehensive review of the embryology, anatomy, radiology, and pathology of the sacroiliac joint. Covers disease processes affecting the sacroiliac joint.

Calin A: Seronegative spondyloarthritides. Med Clin North Am 70:323, 1986.
Current and brief subject review.

Calin A (ed): Spondylarthropathies. Grune & Stratton, Orlando, FL, 1984.
Multiauthored textbook on spondyloarthropathies.

Jacobs JC: Spondyloarthritis and enthesopathy: current concepts in rheumatology. Arch Intern Med 143:103, 1983.
Explains the concepts of spondyloarthritis and enthesopathy.

Moll JMH, Huslock I, Macrae IF, et al: Associations between ankylosing spondylitis, psoriac arthritis, Reiter's disease, the intestinal arthropathies, and Behçet's syndrome. Medicine 53:343, 1974.
Classic paper proposing the concept of the seronegative spondyloarthropathies.

Panayi GS (ed): Seronegative spondyloarthropathies. Clin Rheum Dis 11(1):1, 1985.
This entire issue is devoted to the clinical, genetic, radiologic, and therapeutic aspects of the seronegative spondyloarthropathies.

56
Raynaud's Phenomenon: Primary Disease and Secondary Causes

Raynaud's phenomenon (RP) is characterized by vasospasm in the digits of the hands or feet, which leads to sequential well-demarcated digital pallor, cyanosis, and then rubor in response to cold exposure or stressful stimuli. An attack may be accompanied by pain and may last minutes to hours. There is a strong female predominence for RP, and it crosses all age groups. RP can be divided into idiopathic primary disease or secondary to another cause.

Primary

Patients who have had RP for at least 2 years with no definable underlying etiology are said to have Raynaud's disease and account for up to 75% of RP cases.[1] These patients typically have bilateral involvement and usually do not progress to digital gangrene. Only a small percentage of patients with primary Raynaud's disease will go on to develop a connective tissue disease. If such a disorder does appear, it is more likely that CREST syndrome (calcinosis, Raynaud's, esophageal dysmotility, sclerodactyly, telangiectasia), a variant of scleroderma, will be the eventual diagnosis.[2]

Secondary Causes

A wide variety of disorders have been associated with RP, including collagen vascular diseases, hematologic diseases, drugs, occupational causes, obstructive arterial disease, as well as other conditions.

Collagen Vascular Diseases

Collagen vascular disease is the most common cause of secondary RP, accounting for 10 to 15% of total RP cases.[1]

Scleroderma: 90 to 95% of patients manifest RP, and in at least one-third of patients, it is the presenting symptom.[3,4]

CREST: syndrome of calcinosis, Raynaud phenomenon, esophageal dysmotility, sclerodactyly, and telangiectasias, which is a variant of scleroderma with generally a better prognosis

Mixed connective tissue disease (MCTD): may encompass signs and symptoms of scleroderma, lupus erythematosus, polymyositis, and rheumatoid arthritis and is associated with high titers of antibodies to ribonuclease sensitive extractable nuclear antigens. Typically RP affects 85% of patients with MCTD.[5]

Polymyositis and dermatomyositis: 25 to 30% of these

patients may display RP, which often is one of the earliest symptoms.[6]

Systemic lupus erythematosus: RP occurs in approximately 30% of these patients.[7]

Sjögren's syndrome: RP occurs in approximately 25% of patients with primary Sjögren's syndrome.[8]

Rheumatoid arthritis: RP is seen in less than 10% of patients with rheumatoid arthritis, which approaches the prevalence of RP in the normal population of 5 to 10%.[1]

Occupational Causes

Vibration syndrome: also known as white finger disease and is a combination of vibration and cold exposure, which provides the stimulus for developing RP in occupations such as lumberjacks, jackhammer operators, riveters, and workers using grinding or polishing wheels[9]

Repetitive motions: such as those experienced by pianists, typists, sewing machine operators, and butchers can cause RP[4]

Hypothenar hammer syndrome: a reversible yet uncommon cause of RP due to irregularities or occlusion of the ulnar artery as a result of repeated use of a hammer[10]

Polyvinyl chloride exposure: may create a multisystem disorder that includes RP, acro-osteolysis, thrombocytopenia, pulmonary and portal fibrosis, arthritis, sclerosis of skin, and angiosarcoma of the liver[11]

Industrial arsenic exposure: generally results in mild RP[12]

Obstructive Arterial Disease

Whenever RP occurs in a male, consider obstructive arterial disease.[4]

Traumatic thrombosis of the brachial artery: most commonly an iatrogenic complication of catheterization[13]

Thromboembolism: brachial emboli from a diseased heart, if recurrent, may lead to RP or gangrene.[13]

Arteriosclerosis obliterans: usually occurs after 60 years of age, especially in those with claudication or coronary or cerebrovascular disease[4]

Thromboangiitis obliterans: also known as Buerger's disease; occurs primarily in young male smokers with associated RP, migratory thrombophlebitis, and intermittent claudication[14]

Thoracic outlet obstruction: usually produced by subclavian artery stenosis from a cervical rib or pressure from scalene muscle. The artery stenosis leads to poststenotic aneurysm formation and then migration of small emboli lodge in distal digits to cause RP.[13]

Carpal tunnel syndrome: RP has been seen in the index and middle fingers of an occasional patient with median nerve compression.[15]

Crutch pressure

Drugs

Several pharmacologic agents have been associated with RP.

Beta-adrenergic blockers: RP occurs in approximately 3% of patients using these agents and may arise with either cardioselective or nonselective beta-blocking agents.[16]

Ergotamines: used to treat migraine headaches; can produce RP or severe arteriospasm leading to symmetric gangrene[4]

Methysergide: a synthetic serotonin antagonist, which can cause peripheral vasospasm even in small doses[17]

Chemotherapy: bleomycin alone, by intravenous or intradermal administration, as well as bleomycin in combination with cisplatinum and vinblastine can lead to RP in a significant number of treated patients.[18,19]

Alpha-interferon[20]

Estrogen-progesterone: may occur in women taking birth control pills[15]

Nicotine: associated with cigarette smoking and even chewing nicotine-containing gum[15]

Cyclosporine: can develop in patients treated for idiopathic uveitis[21]

Hematologic Disease

Abnormalities of blood constituents leading to hyperviscosity or increased red cell aggregation may lead to RP or even prolonged vascular occlusion. These patients may not exhibit the typical triphasic color changes of RP, but may have a biphasic pattern.

Cryoglobulinemia: cryoglobulins are the group of proteins that precipitate from cooled serum and are found in association with monclonal or polyclonal gammopathies. Approximately 50% of patients with cryoglobulinemia will exhibit RP.[22]

Cryofibrinogenemia[4]

Macroglobulinemia: predominantly IgM monoclonal gammopathy

Cold hemagglutinins: may be associated with various infections and lymphoma[23]

Polycythemia: may present with RP or with a single cyanotic digit as the "blue toe" syndrome[24]

Miscellaneous Causes

Hypothyroidism: RP has been described in hypothyroid patients and may disappear with thyroid replacement therapy.[25]

Reflex sympathetic dystrophy: characterized by vasomotor and autonomic disturbances with trophic changes in an extremity, which may develop after injury to the extremity or medical illness[4]

Fibromyalgia: a syndrome characterized by chronic diffuse musculoskeletal pain with a sleep disorder without evidence of myositis or arthritis. In one prospective study, a group of 118 fibromyalgia patients demonstrated a 30% incidence of RP with a mean duration of fibromyalgia symptoms of 5 years; none developed further clinical or laboratory evidence of a connective tissue disorder.[26]

Scleromyxedema (generalized lichen myxedematosus): multisystem disorder sometimes associated with RP[27]

Toxic oil syndrome: a multisystem disease with scleroderma-like changes that appeared in Spain in 1981 linked to consumption of toxic cooking oil[28]

Primary pulmonary hypertension: can present simultaneously with RP[4]

Blood transfusion: RP described in a hand distal to the site of an intravenous canula that was precipitated by administration of a blood transfusion.[29]

Adenocarcinoma: lung[30]; small bowel[31]

Subcutaneous parasite: can infest human digital arteries[32]

References

1. Spencer-Green G: Raynaud phenomenon. Bull Rheum Dis 33(5):1, 1983.
2. Gerbracht DD, Steen VD, Ziegler GL, et al: Evolution

of primary Raynaud's phenomenon (Raynaud's disease) to connective tissue disease. Arthritis Rheum 28:87, 1985.

3. Rocco VK, Hurd ER: Scleroderma and scleroderma-like disorders. Semin Arthritis Rheum 16:22, 1986.

4. Coffman JD, Davies WT: Vasospastic diseases: a review. Prog Cardiovasc Dis 18:123, 1975.

5. Ellman MH, Pachman L, Medof ME: Raynaud's phenomenon and initially seronegative mixed connective tissue disease. J Rheumatol 8:632, 1981.

6. Tymms KE, Webb J: Dermatopolymyositis and other connective tissue diseases: a review of 105 cases. J Rheumatol 12:1140, 1985.

7. Passas CM, Wong RL, Peterson M, et al: A comparison of the specificity of the 1971 and 1982 American Rheumatism Association criteria for the classification of systemic lupus erythematosus. Arthritis Rheum 28:620, 1985.

8. Mann DL, Moutsopoulos HM: HLA DR alloantigens in different subsets of patients with Sjögren's syndrome and in family members. Ann Rheum Dis 42:533, 1983.

9. Cohen SR, Bilinski DL, McNutt S: Vibration syndrome: cutaneous and systemic manifestations in a jackhammer operator. Arch Dermatol 121:1544, 1985.

10. Pineda CJ, Weisman MH, Bookstein JJ, et al: Hypothenar hammer syndrome: form of reversible Raynaud's phenomenon. Am J Med 79:561, 1985.

11. Maricq HR, Johnson MN, Whetstone CL, et al: Capillary abnormalities in polyvinyl chloride production workers: examination by in vivo microscopy. JAMA 236:1368, 1976.

12. Lagerkvist BE, Linderholm H: Cold hands after exposure to arsenic or vibrating tools: effects of ketanserin on finger blood pressure and skin temperature. Acta Pharmacol Toxicol 58:327, 1986.

13. Bouhoutsos J, Morris T, Martin P: Unilateral Raynaud's phenomenon in the hand and its significance. Surgery 82:547, 1977.

14. Eadie DGA, Mann CV, Smith PG: Buerger's disease: a clinical and pathological re-examination. Br J Surg 55:452, 1968.

15. Campbell PM, LeRoy EC: Raynaud phenomenon. Semin Arthritis Rheum 16:92, 1986.

16. Eliasson K, Lins LE, Sundqvist K: Vasospastic phenomena in patients treated with beta-adrenoceptor blocking agents. Acta Med Scand 628 (Suppl):39, 1979.

17. Graham JR: Methysergide for prevention of headache: experience in five hundred patients over three years. N Engl J Med 270:67, 1964.

18. Smith EA, Harper FE, LeRoy EC: Raynaud's phenomenon of a single digit following local intradermal bleomycin sulfate injection. Arthritis Rheum 28:459, 1985.

19. Doll DC, Ringenberg QS, Yarbro JW: Vascular toxicity associated with antineoplastic agents. J Clin Oncol 4:1405, 1986.

20. Roy V, Newland AC: Raynaud's phenomenon and cryoglobulinaemia associated with the use of recombinant human alpha-interferon (letter). Lancet 1:944, 1988.

21. Deray G, LeHoang P, Achour L, et al: Cyclosporin and Raynaud phenomenon (letter). Lancet 2:1092, 1986.
22. Winfield JB: Cryoglobulinemia. Hum Pathol 14:350, 1983.
23. Ritzmann SE, Levin WC: Cryopathies: a review. Rev Intern Med 107:186, 1961.
24. Coffman JD: Evaluation of the patient with Raynaud's phenomenon. Postgrad Med 78(2):175, 1985.
25. Shagan BP, Friedman SA: Raynaud's phenomenon in hypothyroidism. Angiology 27:19, 1976.
26. Dinerman H, Goldenberg DL, Felson DT: A prospective evaluation of 118 patients with the fibromyalgia syndrome: prevalence of Raynaud's phenomenon, sicca symptoms, ANA, low complement, and Ig deposition at the dermal-epidermal junction. J Rheumatol 13:368, 1986.
27. Gabriel SE, Perry HO, Oleson GB, Bowles CA: Scleromyxedema: a scleroderma-like disorder with systemic manifestations. Medicine 67:58, 1988.
28. Alonso-Ruiz A, Zea-Mendosa AC, Salazar-Vallinas JM, et al: Toxic oil syndrome: a syndrome with features overlapping those of various forms of scleroderma. Semin Arthritis Rheum 15:200, 1986.
29. Moore JK, Proctor DW: Raynaud's phenomenon precipitated by blood transfusion. Anaesthesia 41:398, 1986.
30. Wilmalaratna HS, Sachdev D: Adenocarcinoma of the lung presenting with Raynaud's phenomenon, digital gangrene and multiple infarctions in the internal organs (letter). Br J Rheumatol 26:473, 1987.
31. Wytock DH, Bartholomew LG, Sheps SG: Digital ischemia associated with small bowel malignancy. Gastroenterology 84:1025, 1983.
32. Beaver PC, Brenes R, Ardon J: Dirofilaria from the index finger of a man in Costa Rica. Am J Trop Med Hyg 35:988, 1986.

Selected Readings

Bouhoutsos J, Morris T, Martin P: Unilateral Raynaud's phenomenon in the hand and its significance. Surgery 82:547, 1977.
Review of 88 cases of unilateral RP and their outcome after attempted surgical treatment.

Campbell PM, LeRoy EC: Raynaud phenomenon. Semin Arthritis Rheum 16:92, 1986.
A review that includes evaluation of 112 patients with RP, including several interesting and medically reversible cases of RP.

Coffman JD, Davies WT: Vasospastic diseases: a review. Prog Cardiovasc Dis 18:123, 1975.
A comprehensive, well-referenced review of the associated diseases and causes of RP, as well as pathophysiology and treatment options.

Smith CR, Rodeheffer RJ: Treatment of Raynaud's phenomenon with calcium channel blockers. Am J Med 78:39, 1985.

Outlines pharmacologic treatment options of RP, as well as reporting data from placebo-controlled, double-blind trial of nifedipine in treatment of patients with RP.

Spencer-Green G: Raynaud phenomenon. Bull Rheum Dis 33(5):1, 1983.

A concise overview.

57

Elevated Erythrocyte Sedimentation Rate: Common Clinical Correlations

The erythrocyte sedimentation rate (ESR) is a simple, inexpensive, and widely used laboratory test that measures the distance in millimeters that erythrocytes fall during 1 hour. An elevated ESR can be used to (1) aid in the determination of the presence or absence of disease in some settings, (2) monitor progression or improvement of previously recognized disease, or (3) measure the response to therapy.[1] However, in asymptomatic persons, the ESR is seldom the sole clue to disease.[2]

The Westergren method for determining the ESR has been recommended by the International Committee for Standardization in Hematology[3]; however, an elevated ESR has not been consistently defined in the literature.

Both gender and age significantly affect baseline ESR.[4] A simple algorithm for calculating normal ESR is applicable in ages greater than 20 years: in men, age in years divided by 2; in women, age in years plus 10 divided by 2.[5,6]

Infections

Any infection may lead to an elevated ESR, bacterial infections more commonly than viral infections.[1] Fever and leukocytosis are better indicators of acute infection in its early stages than an increased ESR.[2]

Bacterial infections: virtually all significant bacterial infections result in an elevated ESR.[7]

Viral infections: most uncomplicated viral infections, such as the common cold, rubeola, mumps and influenza, demonstrate a normal ESR or one only minimally elevated; however, a significantly elevated ESR may reflect complications, such as in mumps orchitis.[7]

Pelvic inflammatory disease: commonly ESR is increased early in the course of the disease[8]; may reflect acute salpingitis with chlamydial infection.[9]

Meningococcemia: characteristically associated with elevated ESR; low or normal rate may be associated with overwhelming sepsis[10]

Infective endocarditis: greater than 90% of patients have elevated ESR at time of admission.[11]

Brain abscesses: increased ESR seen in approximately 70% of patients[12]

Primary atypical pneumonia: extremely high ESR is frequently seen in first and second weeks of the illness[13]

Osteomyelitis: more than 80% of patients with hematogeneous and post-traumatic osteomyelitis will have elevated ESR, and these levels will be even higher with contiguous septic arthritis.[14]

Septic arthritis: elevated ESR is seen in more than 90% of these patients.[14]

Lumbar disc space infections: ESR is elevated in 85 to 100% of cases and can be the only abnormal laboratory value.[14]

Tuberculosis: increased ESR is to be expected in active pulmonary tuberculosis, but normal rates in the presence of active disease are not uncommon.[7]

Systemic fungal infections[7]

Leptospirosis: ESR may be significantly elevated.[15]

Neoplastic Disease

Malignancy is not uncommon in symptomatic patients with an increased ESR. However, patients with malignancy can have normal ESR, particularly within the early weeks following a histologic diagnosis of cancer.[16] Extreme elevation of the ESR (greater than 100 mm/h) can be a clue to metastatic disease, especially skeletal metastasis, though a normal ESR does not exclude metastases.[2]

Multiple myeloma: commonly associated with elevated ESR[16]

Waldenström's macroglobulinemia: may be associated with elevated ESR[17] or may cause lowering of ESR if associated with hyperviscosity[1]

Hodgkin's disease: ESR may be useful in serial monitoring of this malignancy.[18]

Leukemia: in acute lymphoblastic leukemia, the ESR is usually increased to greater than 40 mm/h.[19]

Carcinoma: elevated ESR is more common in bronchogenic carcinoma than in other types, but frequently can be seen in colonic, lung, prostatic, pancreatic, breast, and gastric carcinomas and especially in patients who develop skeletal metastases.[16]

Collagen Vascular Diseases

The ESR is usually elevated in patients with active rheumatologic or immunologic diseases; it is a nonspecific indicator of inflammation.[20]

Rheumatic fever: patients with untreated acute rheumatic fever almost always demonstrate elevated ESR, especially in those with joint involvement or pancarditis.[21]

Rheumatoid arthritis: the ESR tends to parallel disease activity, but 5 to 10% of patients with active disease will have a normal ESR.[2]

Polymyalgia rheumatica (PMR): syndrome characterized by severe aching and stiffness in the neck, shoulder girdle, or pelvic girdle muscles in which an elevated ESR is the most consistent laboratory abnormality; clinical relapse can occur when the ESR is normal[2]

Temporal arteritis (TA): almost always elevated in these patients and is typically markedly elevated. It is suggested that if normal ESR is obtained initially, then it should be repeated serially, as it may be subsequently elevated; also measurement of C-reactive protein may be elevated in such a case.[22] In both PMR and TA, the ESR usually falls rapidly with corticosteroid treatment.[2] In a small percentage of patients with PMR and TA, the ESR has been normal at presentation.[23]

Takayasu arteritis: in the early inflammatory phase,

the ESR is typically elevated, but may return to normal during the occlusive or pulseless phase.[24]

Inflammatory arthritides: gout, pseudogout, and the spondyloarthropathies (ankylosing spondylitis, Reiter's syndrome, enteritis-associated arthritis, and psoriatic arthritis); all typically are associated with elevated ESR, but a significant percentage of these patients will have a normal ESR.

Systemic lupus erythematosus: elevated ESR typically associated with active phases of disease, though a few patients may maintain markedly elevated ESR even though their disease has been in remission several years, and others will never exhibit an elevated ESR, even during episodes of severe illness.[25]

Systemic vasculitides: polyarteritis nodosa, systemic leukocytoclastic vasculitis (LCV), Henoch-Schönlein purpura (HSP), Churg-Strauss allergic granulomatosis, Wegener's granulomatosis, Kawasaki disease, and lymphomatoid granulomatosis may all be associated with elevated ESR during active disease. Approximately 75% of patients with HSP have increased rates,[26] and rates greater than 100 mm/h are not unusual in systemic LCV.[27]

Dermatomyositis and polymyositis: ESR is elevated in about half the patients and is greater than 50 mm/h in 20% of patients during active disease.[28]

Gastrointestinal Diseases

Several gastrointestinal inflammatory disorders, chronic liver disease, and various causes of acute abdomen have been associated with elevated ESR.

Inflammatory bowel disease: ulcerative colitis and regional enteritis have elevated ESRs, but the rate may be normal with quiescent disease.[7]

Chronic liver disease: can lead to a hypoalbuminemic state that will cause an elevated ESR.[29]

Appendicitis: generally associated with normal ESR, but if perforation or abscess formation has occurred, then an elevated ESR is likely.[8,30]

Amebic hepatitis or liver abscess: common cause of elevated ESR in the tropics[15]

Other causes of acute abdomen: acute pancreatitis, incarcerated hernia, acute cholecystitis, diverticulitis, and peritonitis have associated elevated ESRs[4,30]

Acute gastrointestinal hemorrhage: may result in an increased ESR even in the absence of significant associated disease[31]

Renal Diseases

Various renal diseases from bacterial pyelonephritis to acute and chronic glomerulonephritis or other causes of renal failure can lead to an elevated ESR.

Acute pyelonephritis: typically causes ESR elevation, but the rate may be normal if the urinary tract infection is localized to the lower tract[7]

Nephrotic syndrome: with associated hypoalbuminemia or renal failure leads to an increased ESR[7]

Chronic renal failure: patients both on and off hemodialysis showed elevated ESR in the absence of infectious, rheumatologic, or oncologic complications.[32]

Acute glomerulonephritis (GN): 80% of children with acute GN have an increased ESR.[33]

Hemolytic-uremic syndrome: accelerated ESRs out of proportion to the degree of anemia may be found in these patients.[34]

Miscellaneous

An elevated ESR has been associated with various other conditions from drugs to trauma.

Drugs: benzathine penicillin G injections,[35] oral contraceptives,[36] and intravenous heparin[37] all elevate ESR.

Anemia: although a lowered hematocrit causes elevation of the ESR by the Westergren method,[7] significant elevation of the ESR in otherwise healthy persons without systemic disease does not usually occur until the hematocrit is less than 20%.[38]

Benign monoclonal gammopathy: increase in gamma globulin in the plasma causes increase in red cell aggregation; thus increasing the ESR.[2]

Cryoglobulinemia: cryoglobulins also cause increased red cell aggregation.[2]

Hyperlipidemia: increase in serum lipids has been demonstrated to elevate ESR.[39]

Stress[10]

Pregnancy: a rise in ESR begins in the fourth month

of pregnancy and peaks in the first week of the puerperium.[41]

Menses: reduced during the period of menstrual flow and then rises in the premenstrual phase[4]

Dermatitis: especially in skin conditions with significant inflammation, such as psoriasis.

Myocardial infarction: the increase in ESR occurs about 48 hours after infarction, peaks 5 days later, and generally returns to normal in the 14th to 32nd day[1] or may reflect a postcardiac injury syndrome[42]

Thyroid disease: hypothyroidism[43] and subacute thyroiditis[44] both may exhibit elevated ESR.

Diabetic acidosis[7]

Chronic granulomatous disease: sarcoidosis[7]

Surgery and trauma: the degree of elevation of ESR is proportional to the amount of tissue destruction.[7] Postoperative elevations can occur with major surgery, particularly major orthopaedic surgery.[14]

Extremely Elevated ESR

An ESR of greater than 100 mm/h is highly specific for disease: typically infection, malignancy, or collagen vascular disease. Only 5 to 7% of patients with an extreme ESR elevation remain undiagnosed.[17,45] Approximately 15% of all patients with markedly elevated ESRs will have cancer.[45]

Conditions That Lower ESR

In order to properly evaluate an ESR, the conditions that tend to lower ESR must be recognized.

Drugs: aspirin, nonsteroidal anti-inflammatory drugs, corticosteroids, asparaginase[1]

Congestive heart failure: widely accepted, but poorly documented as cause of low ESR[1]

Hemoglobinopathies: especially in sickle-cell disease, since abnormally shaped cells do not form rouleaux pattern normally; thus lowering ESR[7]

Polycythemia[7]

Hereditary spherocytosis[1]

Hemolytic anemia[1]

Pyruvate kinase deficiency[1]

Chronic lymphocytic leukemia: when associated with extreme elevation of white blood count[46]

Hypofibrinogenemia: can be hereditary or secondary to diseases in which fibrinogen is consumed, such as disseminated intravascular coagulation[1]

Bile salt excess[7]
Trichinosis[1]

Laboratory Sources of Error in the Evaluation of ESR

The accuracy of the ESR depends on several mechanical, environmental, and technical factors in its measurement.

False elevation of ESR
  Large bore tube or relatively tall column[1]
  High room temperature[7]
  Inadequate mixing of blood: may lead to preformed rouleaux formation[7]
  Excessive anticoagulant: lowers concentration of macromolecules[32]
  Use of heparin as anticoagulant[32]
  Vibration or centrifugation: may inhibit settling of red cells[1]
False reduction of ESR
  Refrigerated blood: must be returned to room temperature[7]
  Delay in running ESR greater than 2 hours[7]
  Clotting in collecting tube: leads to consumption of fibrinogen.[7]

References

1. Bedell SE, Bush BT: Erythrocyte sedimentation rate: from folklore to facts. Am J Med 78:1001, 1985.
2. Sox HC Jr, Liang MH: The erythrocyte sedimentation rate: guidelines for rational use. Ann Intern Med 104:515, 1986.
3. International Committee for Standardization in Hematology: Recommendation for measurement of erythrocyte sedimentation rate of human blood. Am J Clin Pathol 68:505, 1977.
4. Lawrence JS: Assessment of the Activity of Disease. Paul B. Hoeber, New York, 1961.
5. Miller A, Green M, Robinson D: Simple rule for calculating normal erythrocyte sedimentation rate. Br Med J 286:266, 1983.
6. Griffiths RA, Good WR, Watson NP, et al: Normal erythrocyte sedimentation rate in the elderly. Br Med J 289:724, 1984.
7. Lascari AD: The erythrocyte sedimentation rate. Pediatr Clin North Am 19:1113, 1972.
8. Bannick EG, Gregg RO, Guernsey CM: The erythrocyte sedimentation rate. JAMA 109:1257, 1937.
9. Wølner-Hanssen P, Mårdh PA, Svensson L, et al: Laparoscopy in women with chlamydial infection and pelvic pain: a comparison of patients with and without salpingitis. Obstet Gynecol 61:299, 1983.
10. Stiehm ER, Damrosch DS: Factors in the prognosis of meningococcal infection. Review of 63 cases with emphasis on recognition and management of the severely ill patient. J Pediatr 68:457, 1966.

11. Von Reyn CF, Levy BS, Arbeit RD, et al: Infective endocarditis: an analysis based on strict case definitions. Ann Intern Med 94:505, 1981.

12. Hass WK, Harter DH: Erythrocyte sedimentation rate in patients with intracranial mass lesions. Neurology 7:480, 1957.

13. Galbraith HJB, Jones KW: Primary atypical pneumonia and high sedimentation rates. Br Med J 1:1144, 1958.

14. Schulak DJ, Rayhack JM, Lippert FG III, et al: The erythrocyte sedimentation rate in orthopaedic patients. Clin Orthop 167:197, 1982.

15. Cheah JS, Ransome GA: Significance of very high erythrocyte sedimentation rates (100 mm or above in one hour) in 360 cases in Singapore. J Trop Med Hyg 74:28, 1971.

16. Peyman MA: The effect of malignant disease on the erythrocyte sedimentation rate. Br J Cancer 16:56, 1962.

17. Zacharski LR, Kyle RA: Significance of extreme elevation of erythrocyte sedimentation rate. JAMA 202:116, 1967.

18. Margerison ACF, Mann JR: Serum copper, serum ceruloplasmin, and erythrocyte sedimentation rate measurements in children with Hodgkin's disease, non-Hodgkin's lymphoma, and non-malignant lymphadenopathy. Cancer 55:1501, 1985.

19. Iversen T: Leukemia in infancy and childhood: a material of 570 Danish cases. Acta Pediatr Scand 167(Suppl):73, 1966.

20. McCarty GA: Update on laboratory studies and relationship to rheumatic and allergic diseases. Ann Allergy 55:421, 1985.

21. Barnert AL, Terry EE, Persellin RH: Acute rheumatic fever in adults. JAMA 232:925, 1975.

22. Jones JG, Hazelman BL: ESR in polymyalgia rheumatica and giant cell arteritis (letter). Ann Rheum Dis 42:702, 1983.

23. Ellis ME, Ralston S: The ESR in the diagnosis and management of the polymyalgia rhematica/giant cell arteritis syndrome. Ann Rheum Dis 42:168, 1983.

24. Conn DL, Hunder GG: Takayasu's arteritis. p. 1159. In Kelley WN, Harris ED Jr, Ruddy S, Sledge CB (eds): Textbook of Rheumatology, 2nd Ed. WB Saunders, Philadelphia, 1985.

25. Rothfield N: Clinical features of systemic lupus erythematosus. p. 1070. In Kelley WN, Harris ED Jr, Ruddy S, Sledge CB (eds): Textbook of Rheumatology, 2nd Ed. WB Saunders, Philadelphia, 1985.

26. Allen DM, Diamond LK, Howell DA: Anaphylactoid purpura in children (Schönlein-Henoch syndrome): review with a follow-up of the renal complications. Am J Dis Child 99:833, 1960.

27. McCombs RP: Systemic "allergic" vasculitis. JAMA 194:1059, 1965.

28. Bradley WG: Inflammatory diseases of muscle. p. 1225. In Kelley WN, Harris ED Jr, Ruddy S, Sledge CB (eds): Textbook of Rheumatology, 2nd Ed. WB Saunders, Philadelphia, 1985.

29. Talkers R: Erythrocyte sedimentation rate/zeta sedimentation rate. Emerg Med Clin North Am 4:87, 1986.

30. Lesser A, Goldberger HA: The blood sedimentation test and its value in the differential diagnosis of acute appendicitis. Surg Gynecol Obstet 60:157, 1935.
31. Chapman RS, Mohamed SD: Pyrexia and elevated erythrocyte sedimentation rate in acute gastro-duodenal hemorrhage. Postgrad Med J 44:238, 1968.
32. Shusterman N, Kimmel PL, Kiechle FL, et al: Factors influencing erythrocyte sedimentation in patients with chronic renal failure. Arch Intern Med 145:1796, 1985.
33. Rubin MI, Rapoport M, Waltz AD: A comparison of routine urinalysis, addis count, and blood sedimentation rate as criteria of activity in acute glomerulonephritis. J Pediatr 20:32, 1942.
34. Lieberman E, Heuser E, Donnell GN, et al: Hemolytic-uremic syndrome: clinical and pathological considerations. N Engl J Med 275:227, 1966.
35. Haas RC, Taranta A, Wood HF: Effect of intramuscular injections of benzathine penicillin G on some acute-phase reactants. N Engl J Med 256:152, 1957.
36. Burton JL: Effect of oral contraceptives on erythrocyte sedimentation rate in healthy young women. Br Med J 3:214, 1967.
37. Penchas S, Stern Z, Bar-Or D: Heparin and the ESR (letter). Arch Intern Med 138:1864, 1978.
38. Poole JCF, Summers GAC: Correction of ESR in anemia: experimental study based on interchange of cells and plasma between normal and anaemic subjects. Br Med J 1:353, 1952.
39. Schimmelpfennig RW Jr, Chusid MJ: Illnesses associated with extreme elevation of the erythrocyte sedimentation rate in children. Clin Pediatr 19:175, 1980.
40. Palmblad J, Karlsson C-G, Levi L, et al: The erythrocyte sedimentation rate and stress. Acta Med Scand 205:517, 1979.
41. Fahraeus R: The suspension-stability of the blood. Acta Med Scand 55:1, 1921.
42. Stelzner TJ, King TE Jr, Antony VB, et al: The pleuropulmonary manifestations of the postcardiac injury syndrome. Chest 84:383, 1983.
43. Larsson SO: On serum proteins and erythrocyte sedimentation rate in hypothyroidism. Acta Med Scand 172:545, 1962.
44. Nikolai TF, Brosseau J, Kettrick MA, et al: Lymphocytic thyroiditis with spontaneously resolving hyperthyroidism (silent thyroiditis). Arch Intern Med 140:478, 1980.
45. Wyler DJ: Diagnostic implications of markedly elevated erythrocyte sedimentation rate: a reevaluation. South Med J 70:1428, 1977.
46. Glass R: Factitiously low ESR with chronic lymphocytic leukemia (letter). N Engl J Med 285:921, 1971.

Selected Readings

Bedell SE, Bush BT: Erythrocyte sedimentation rate: from folklore to facts. Am J Med 78:1001, 1985.
Excellent comprehensive review of the history of the ESR, physical and chemical properties of red cells and methods used to measure ESR, and clinical significance of a low or elevated ESR.

Crawford J, Eye-Boland MK, Cohen HJ: Clinical utility

of erythrocyte sedimentation rate and plasma protein analysis in the elderly. Am J Med 82:239, 1987.
Good discussion of use and interpretation of ESR in the elderly, with evaluation of ESR and other laboratory parameters in a defined population of 111 ambulatory retirement home residents.

Lascari AD: The erythrocyte sedimentation rate. Pediatr Clin North Am 19:1113, 1972.
Good review with emphasis on disease states associated with elevated ESR.

Peyman MA: The effect of malignant disease on the erythrocyte sedimentation rate. Br J Cancer 16:56, 1962.
Extensive evaluation of 300 patients with malignant neoplasms with description of effect of various malignancies, presence or absence of metastases, and secondary infection on the ESR.

Schulak DJ, Rayhack JM, Lippert FG, et al: The erythrocyte sedimentation rate in orthopaedic patients. Clin Orthop 167:197, 1982.
Well-referenced review of the usefulness of the ESR in orthopaedic patients.

Sox HC Jr, Liang MH: The erythrocyte sedimentation rate: guidelines for rational use. Ann Intern Med 104:515, 1986.
Excellent review with special attention given to the interpretation and use of ESR in clinical decision making.

Wong RL, Korn JH: Temporal arteritis without an elevated erythrocyte sedimentation rate: case report and review of the literature. Am J Med 80:959, 1986.
Evaluation of 36 reported patients with biopsy-proven temporal arteritis, but without an elevated ESR.

Wyler DJ: Diagnostic implications of markedly elevated erythrocyte sedimentation rate: a reevaluation. South Med J 70:1428, 1977.
Analysis of 200 hospitalized patients with ESR greater than or equal to 100 mm/h and comparison with other similar studies.

58
Antinuclear Antibodies

Conditions Associated with a Positive Test and Disease Association of Specific Autoantibodies

The fluorescent antinuclear antibody (FANA) test is often performed as a "screening" test for systemic lupus erythematosus or one of the other connective tissue diseases. Although a positive test for antinuclear antibodies (ANA) is a diagnostic criterion for systemic lupus erythematosus, it is not specific for the disease. Many other rheumatologic, hematologic, hepatic, infectious, neoplastic, and pulmonary conditions are associated with circulating ANAs. Furthermore, many drugs, most notably hydralazine and procainamide, can induce the production of ANAs.

The pattern or patterns (homogeneous, nucleolar, peripheral, or rim) seen on a FANA screen can often be a clue to the type of autoantibody being produced. Many of the ANAs have specific disease associations. A few of the autoantibodies (Sm, dsDNA, centromere, and Scl-70) are marker antibodies for certain diseases. Others, such as antibodies to histones, nRNP, SS-A, and PM-1, are highly sensitive for certain conditions; but they are not specific for them. The prevalence of a positive FANA and of a particular pattern for a given autoantibody will depend on the test substrate used in performing the test. Furthermore, many of the ANAs are not found on the routine FANA screen and must be assayed individually. In fact, some "ANAs" are not truly antibodies to nuclear antigens, but are antibodies to other cellular antigens such as cytoplasmic, ribosomal, and nucleolar proteins.

Conditions Associated with a Positive Antinuclear Antibody Test

Rheumatologic	Systemic lupus erythematosus[1,2] Sjögren's syndrome[1-3] Polymyositis[1,2] Dermatomyositis[1,2] Progressive systemic sclerosis (diffuse scleroderma)[1,2,4] CREST syndrome (calcinosis, Raynaud's phenomenon, esophageal dysmotility, sclerodactyly, telangiectasias)[1,2] Linear scleroderma[5] Morphea[6] Mixed connective tissue disease[2] Overlap connective tissue syndromes[1,2] Rheumatoid arthritis[1,2] Juvenile rheumatoid arthritis[7] Raynaud's phenomenon, primary[1] Behçet's syndrome[8] Henoch-Schönlein purpura[9]
Hematologic	Benign monoclonal gammopathy[10] Multiple myeloma[10] Waldenström's macroglobulinemia[10]
Hepatic	Chronic active hepatitis[11] Chronic biliary cirrhosis[11] Primary sclerosing cholangitis[12]
Infectious	Infectious mononucleosis[1] Leprosy (Hansen's disease)[1] Malaria[13]

	Subacute bacterial endocarditis[1]
	Human immunodeficiency virus[14]
Neoplastic	Leukemia, acute and chronic[2]
	Lymphoma[1]
	Melanoma[15]
	Nasopharyngeal carcinoma[2]
Pulmonary	Idiopathic pulmonary fibrosis[1]
	Fibrosing alveolitis[16]
	Primary pulmonary hypertension[17]
Miscellaneous Conditions	Chronic glomerulonephritis[18]
	Myasthenia gravis[18,19]
	Pregnancy[20]
	Silent thyroiditis (thyrotoxic phase)[21]
	Graves' disease[22]
	Cholesterol emboli[23]
Drugs	Antiarrhythmics
	Procainamide[24-26]
	Propafenone[27]
	Quinidine[28]
	Antibiotics
	Isoniazid[29,30]
	Griseofulvin[30]
	Nitrofurantoin[29,30]
	Penicillin[30]
	Streptomycin[30]
	Sulphonamides[30]
	Tetracycline[30]
	Anticonvulsants
	Carbamazepine[31]
	Ethosuximide[29,30]
	Mephenytoin[29,30]
	Phenytoin[29,30]
	Primidone[29,30]
	Trimethadione[29,30]
	Antihypertensives
	Acetabutolol[32]
	Atenolol[32]
	Captopril[33]
	Guanethidine[32]
	Hydralazine[29,30]

Labetolol[32]
Methyldopa[29,30]
Metoprolol[32]
Minoxidil[34]
Oxprenolol[32]
Practolol[32]
Pindolol[30]
Reserpine[30]
Tertatolol[35]
Antithyroid
   Methimazole[36]
   Propylthiouracil[29,30]
Psychotropic
   Chlorpromazine[37]
   Lithium carbonate[38]
   Nomifensine[39]
Rheumatologic
   Allopurinol[30]
   Gold salts[30]
   Penicillamine[40]
   Phenylbutazone[30]
   Sulfasalazine[41]
Miscellaneous drugs
   Aminoglutethimide[30]
   Methysergide[30]
   Oral contraceptives[30]

Specific Antigens and Their Disease Associations (Organized by Fluorescent Antinuclear Antibody Pattern)

This section lists the various antigens to which auto-antibodies have been demonstrated and the diseases that have been associated with them. The antigens have been organized according to the pattern seen on FANA screen, if such a pattern has been identified. It should be noted, however, that some of the auto-antibodies do not always appear in every FANA screen and that a few can give more than one immunofluorescence pattern.

Homogeneous (Diffuse)

Histones: SLE,[42] drugs+,[42] RA[42]
Histone complexes: drug-induced SLE (symptomatic)[26,42]
DNP: SLE,[1] drug-induced SLE,[1] RA[1]

Nucleolar

Nucleolar RNA: PSS,[1] Raynaud's phenomenon[1]
RNA polymerase I: PSS[43]
U3 RNP: PSS[43]

Peripheral (Rim)

Doublestranded (ds) DNA: SLE*,[1,42] MCTD,[44] RA,[44] SS,[44] PSS[44]
Singlestranded (ss) DNA: occasionally causes peripheral pattern[1]
Histones: occasionally causes peripheral pattern[1]
DNP: occasionally causes peripheral pattern[1]

Speckled

Nuclear (n) RNP: MCTD+,[2] SLE,[2] PSS,[2] UCTS[45]
Sm: SLE*[1,2]
SS-A (Ro)[46,47]: SS,[1,2] SLE,[1,2] neonatal SLE+,[48] discoid lupus erythematosus,[49] subacute cutaneous lupus erythematosus,[47] MCTD,[44] RA,[44] paraproteins,[10] primary biliary cirrhosis[1]
SS-B (La, Ha): SS,[1,2] SLE,[1,2] mothers of neonatal SLE,[47] paraproteins[10]
Centromere (kinetochore): CREST*,[1,2] PSS,[50] Raynaud's phenomenon,[50] primary biliary cirrhosis[50]
Jo-1: PM[2,51]
Ki (SL): SLE,[42,52] MCTD,[52] vasculitis[52]
Ku: Overlap of PM-PSS[2,49]
Ma: SLE[1,2]
Me: SLE,[45] MCTD,[45] UCTS[45]
Mi-1: DM,[2,45] SLE[45]
Mi-2: DM[53]
NuMA (nuclear mitotic apparatus antigen): RA,[1] SS,[1] SLE[1]
PCNA (proliferating cell nuclear antigen): SLE[2,49]
Perinuclear factor: Seronegative RA[54]
PM-1: PM,[44,45] DM,[44,51] overlap of PM-PSS[2,55]

RANA (rheumatoid arthritis associated nuclear antigen): RA[+2, 49]
Ribosomal P protein: SLE[56,57]
Ribosomal (r) RNP: SLE,[42] MCTD,[19] SS[19]
Scl-70 (Topoisomerase I): PSS*[2,58]
Scl-86: PSS[4]
Su: SLE,[45] UCTS[45]
U1-RNA: MCTD,[42] SLE[42]

Miscellaneous (Do Not Always Fall in a Recognized Pattern)

Single-stranded (ss) DNA: SLE,[44] PSS,[18] linear scleroderma,[18] morphea,[18] RA,[18] SS,[18,44] MCTD,[18,44] PM,[18,44] DM,[18,44] chronic active hepatitis,[18] chronic glomerulonephritis,[18] infectious mononucleosis,[18] myasthenia gravis,[18] primary biliary cirrhosis[18]
Cytoskeletal: PM,[59] DM,[59] PSS,[59] RA[59]
Golgi: SLE[1]
Granulocyte-specific nuclear antigen: RA[2]
Guanosine: procainamide-induced SLE,[25] SLE[60]
HaT-1: RA[61]
Lamins: produce a ringlike nuclear immunofluorescent staining distinct from the peripheral pattern; associated with hepatitis, blood cytopenias, and vasculitis[62]
LAMP (lupus-associated membrane proteins): SLE[63]
LANA (leukemia-associated nuclear antigen): acute and chronic leukemia[2]
Liver-disease associated antigens: chronic active hepatitis[2]
Lysosomes: SLE[1]
Melanoma-associated antigens: melanoma[2]
Mitochondria: SLE,[1] primary biliary cirrhosis,[1] chronic active hepatitis, PSS[64]
Neurofilament: SLE[65]
Neuronal: SLE[66]
Neutrophil cytoplasm: Wegener's granulomatosis,[67] systemic vasculitis[67]
NPC (nasopharyngeal carcinoma) associated nuclear antigens: nasopharyngeal carcinoma.[2]
Nucleosomes: SLE[1]
Nuclear matrix: SLE[1]
Phospholipids (cardiolipin): SLE,[1,68] lupus anticoagulant,[68] other connective tissue diseases,[68] thromboses,[68] recurrent fetal loss[68]
PL-7: myositis,[1] SLE[1]
SL: overlap of SS and SLE[1,2]
Smooth muscle actin: SLE,[1] chronic active hepatitis[1]
Synthetases: PM[69]
Vimetin intermediate filaments: SLE,[1] RA[1]

VLS (variable large speckles): UCTS[2]
XR: SLE,[1,70] chronic active hepatitis[1,70]

Autoantibodies and Their Prevalence in Selected Conditions

This final part lists selected diseases and the prevalance of various autoantibodies that have been associated with them. Percentages reflect values culled from several sources,[1,2,18,42,44,45,49,51,71] with values strikingly higher or lower than those found in most other sources eliminated.

Systemic Lupus Erythematosus

FANA: (95 to 98% positive[1,44,71]
DNP: 70%[1]
dsDNA*: 50 to 70%[1,51]—associated with nephritis[1]
Guanosine[60]
Histones: 60 to 80%[1,42,51]
Ki: 10%[42,52]
LAMP: 88%[63]
Ma: 10%[1,49,51]—associated with nephritis[1]
Me[1,45]
Neurofilament: associated with CNS disease[65]
Neuronal: associated with CNS disease[66]
nRNP: 30 to 50%[44,51,71]
PCNA: 2 to 10%[1,2,42,49,51]
Ribosomal P protein: 12%[56]—associated with psychosis[56,57]
rRNP: 6 to 10%[1,42]
Sm*: 30%[1,2,42,49]
SS-A: 30 to 40%[1,2,49,51]—associated with lower incidence of nephritis[18]
SS-B: 10–15%[1,2,49,51]—associated with lower incidence of nephritis[18]
ssDNA: 70 to 80%[18,51]
Su: rare[1]—associated with a decreased frequency of malar rash, alopecia, and arthritis, but a higher frequency of Raynaud's phenomenon[1]
U1-RNP: 40%[42]—associated with the absence of nephritis[1]

"ANA-negative" Systemic Lupus Erythematosus

Two to 5% of patients with SLE will have a negative FANA screen. However, most of these patients will have antibodies to other antigens as follows:

Phospholipid[72]
SS-A: 60%[1,47]
SS-B: 32%[47]
ssDNA: 30%[47]

Drug-induced Systemic Lupus Erythematosus (Almost 100% FANA-Positive[71])

dsDNA: 50% with procainamide and hydralazine[18]
Guanosine: 83% of patients on procainamide with symptoms of SLE[25]
Histones[+]: 95 to 100%[2,49,51]

Neonatal Systemic Lupus Erythematosus

SS-A[+]: 83% of mothers of infants with neonatal SLE and congenital heart block[47]
SS-B: 41% of mothers of infants with neonatal SLE and congenital heart block[47]

Sjögren's Syndrome, Primary (75 to 80% FANA-positive[71])

NuMA[1]
RANA: 30%[44]
SS-A: 60–70%[1,42,45,49,51]—associated with extraglandular disease[1,47]
SS-B: 50–60%[1,42,49,51]
ssDNA: 20%[18]

Polymyositis

FANA: 30 to 40% positive[44,71]
Jo-1: 30 to 40%[1,2,44,49,51]—associated with interstitial lung disease[73,74]
PL-7[1]
PM-1: 60%[44,45]
ssDNA: 15%[18]
Synthetases[69]

Dermatomyositis (30 to 40% FANA-positive[71])

dsDNA: 25%[44]
Jo-1: rare[45,74]
Mi-1: 11%[49,51]
Mi-2: 21%[53]
PM-1: 17%[2,49,51]
ssDNA: 15%[18]

Progressive Systemic Sclerosis (50 to 60% FANA-positive[44,49,71])

Centromere: 10 to 15%[1,44,50,51,71]
Mitochondria: 8%[64]
Nucleolar RNA: 60 to 70%[49,51]
RNA polymerase I: 15%[43]
rRNP: 20%[49,51,71]
Scl-70*: 15 to 20%[1,2,44,49,51,58]
Scl-86: 59%[4]
SS-A: 33%[44]
ssDNA: 15%[18,49]
u3 RNP: 48%[43]

CREST Syndrome (90 to 95% FANA-positive[44])

Centromere*: 70%[44,45,49]

Mixed Connective Tissue Disease (About 100% FANA-positive[71])

dsDNA: 25%[44]
Ki: 14%[52]
Me[45]
Mi[45]
nRNP+: 95 to 100%[49,51]
ssDNA: 35%[45]

Polymyositis-scleroderma Overlap

Ku: 55%[2,49,51]
PM-1+: 70 to 90%[2,45,49,51,57]

Undifferentiated Connective Tissue Syndromes

Me[45]
nRNP[45]
Su[45]

Rheumatoid Arthritis (30 to 50% FANA-positive[1,44,71,75])

HaT-1: 24%[61]
Histones: 15 to 20%[2,42,44,49,51]
NuMA[1]
RANA+: 90 to 95%[2,49]
nRNP: 10%[71]
Perinuclear factor: 37% seronegative RA[54]
SS-A: 10%[71]
ssDNA: 50 to 60%[18]

Chronic Active Hepatitis

Mitochondria[1]
Smooth muscle actin[1]
ssDNA: 60%[18]

Primary Biliary Cirrhosis (38% FANA-positive[11])

Centromere: 10%[11,50]
Mitochondria[1]
SS-A[1]
ssDNA: 15%[18]

Abbreviations

CREST: calcinosis, Raynaud's phenomenon, esophageal dysmotility, sclerodactyly, telangectasias
DM: dermatomyositis
MCTD: mixed connective tissue disease
PM: polymyositis
PSS: progressive systemic sclerosis (diffuse scleroderma)
RA: rheumatoid arthritis
SLE: systemic lupus erythematosus
SS: Sjögren's syndrome
UCTS: undifferentiated connective tissue syndrome
*: marker antibody for this condition[2]
+: antibodies that are very sensitive, but not specific for the condition listed

References

1. McCarty GA: Autoantibodies and their relation to rheumatic diseases. Med Clin North Am 70:237, 1986.
2. Tan EM: Autoantibodies to nuclear antigens (ANA): their immunobiology and medicine. Adv Immunol 33:167, 1982.
3. Harley JB, Alexander EL, Bias WB, et al: Anti-Ro (SS-A) and anti-La (SS-B) in patients with Sjögren's syndrome. Arthritis Rheum 29:196, 1986.
4. van Venrooij WJ, Stapel SO, Houben H, et al: Scl-86, a marker antigen for diffuse scleroderma. J Clin Invest 75:1053, 1985.
5. Piette WW, Dorsey JK, Foucar E: Clinical and serologic expression of localized scleroderma: case report and review of the literature. J Am Acad Dermatol 13:342, 1985.
6. Falanga V, Medsger TA Jr, Reichlin M: Antinuclear and anti-single-stranded DNA antibodies in morphea and generalized morphea. Arch Dermatol 123:350, 1987.
7. Leak AM: Autoantibody profile in juvenile chronic arthritis. Ann Rheum Dis 47:178, 1988.
8. Moroi Y, Takeuchi A, Mori M, et al: Antinuclear antibodies in Behçet's disease (letter). J Rheumatol 9:809, 1982.
9. Saulsbury FT: Antinuclear antibody in Henoch-Schönlein purpura. Am J Med Sci 291:180, 1986.
10. Sestak AL, Harley JB, Yoshida S, Reichlin M: Lupus/Sjögren's autoantibody specificities in sera with paraproteins. J Clin Invest 80:138, 1987.
11. Bernstein RM, Neuberger JM, Bunn CC, et al: Diversity of autoantibodies in primary biliary cirrhosis and chronic active hepatitis. Clin Exp Immunol 55:553, 1984.
12. el-Shabrawi M, Wilkinson ML, Portmann B, et al: Primary sclerosing cholangitis in childhood. Gastroenterology 92:1226, 1987.
13. Adu A, Williams DG, Quakyi IA, et al: Anti-ssDNA and

antinuclear antibodies in malaria. Clin Exp Immunol 49:310, 1982.

14. Kopelman RG, Zolla-Pazner S: Association of human immunodeficiency virus infection and autoimmune phenomena. Am J Med 84:82, 1988.
15. Thomas PJ, Kaur JS, Aitcheson CT, et al: Antinuclear, antinucleolar, and anticytoplasmic antibodies in patients with malignant melanoma. Cancer Res 43:1372, 1983.
16. Holgate ST, Haslam P, Turner-Warwick M: The significance of antinuclear and DNA antibodies in cryptogenic fibrosing alveolitis. Thorax 38:67, 1983.
17. Rich S, Kieras K, Hart K, et al: Antinuclear antibodies in primary pulmonary hypertension. J Am Coll Cardiol 8:1307, 1986.
18. Koffler D, Miller TE, Faiferman I: Antipolynucleotide antibodies: the rheumatic connection. Hum Pathol 14:406, 1983.
19. Alarcón-Segovia D: Antibodies to nuclear and other intracellular antigens in the connective tissue diseases. Clin Rheum Dis 9:161, 1983.
20. Farnam J, Lavastida MT, Grant JA, et al: Antinuclear antibodies in the serum of normal pregnant women: a prospective study. J Allergy Clin Immunol 73:596, 1984.
21. Tajiri J, Higashi K, Morita M, et al: Elevation of anti-DNA antibody titer during thyrotoxic phase of silent thyroiditis. Arch Intern Med 146:1623, 1986.
22. Baethge BA, Levine SN, Wolf RE: Antibodies to nuclear antigens in Graves' disease. J Clin Endocrinol Metab 66:485, 1988.
23. Cappiello RA, Espinoza LR, Vasey FB, Germain BF: Cholesterol emboli mimicking systemic vasculitis. Arthritis Rheum 31 (Suppl 1):R39, 1988.
24. Gorsulowsky DC, Bank PW, Goldberg AD, et al: Antinuclear antibodies as indicators for the procainamide-induced systemic lupus erythematosus-like syndrome and its clinical presentations. J Am Acad Dermatol 12:245, 1985.
25. Weisbart RH, Yee WS, Colburn KK, et al: Antiguanosine antibodies: a new marker for procainamide-induced systemic lupus erythematosus. Ann Intern Med 104:310, 1986.
26. Totoritis MC, Tan EM, McNally EM, Rubin RL: Association of antibody to histone complex H2A-H2B with symptomatic procainamide-induced lupus. N Engl J Med 318:1431, 1988.
27. Guindo J, de la Serna AR, Borja J, et al: Propafenone and a syndrome of the lupus erythematosus type (letter). Ann Intern Med 104:589, 1986.
28. Cohen MG, Kevat S, Prowse MV, Ahern MJ: Two distinct quinidine-induced rheumatic syndromes. Ann Intern Med 108:369, 1988.
29. Weinstein A: Drug-induced systemic lupus erythematosus. Prog Clin Immunol 4:1, 1980.
30. Harmon CE, Portanova JP: Drug-induced lupus: clinical and serological studies. Clin Rheum Dis 8:121, 1982.
31. Alballa S, Fritzler M, Davis P: A case of drug induced lupus due to carbamazepine. J Rheumatol 14:599, 1987.
32. Wilson JD: Antinuclear antibodies and cardiovascular drugs. Drugs 19:292, 1980.

33. Reidenberg MM, Case DB, Drayer DE, et al: Development of antinuclear antibody in patients treated with high doses of captopril. Arthritis Rheum 27:579, 1984.
34. Tunkel AR, Shuman M, Popkin M, et al: Minoxidil-induced systemic lupus erythematosus. Arch Intern Med 147:599, 1987.
35. Roudier J, Delmas PD: Tertatolol-induced lupus (letter). Arthritis Rheum 31:145, 1988.
36. Shabtai R, Shapiro MS, Orenstein D, et al: The antithyroid arthritis syndrome reviewed. Arthritis Rheum 27:227, 1984.
37. Canoso RT, de Oliveira RM: Characterization and antigenic specificity of chlorpromazine-induced antinuclear antibodies. J Lab Clin Med 108:213, 1986.
38. Presley AP, Kahn A, Williamson N: Antinuclear antibodies in patients on lithium carbonate. Br Med J 2:280, 1976.
39. Garcia-Morteo O, Maldonado-Cocco JA: Lupus-like syndrome during treatment with nomifensine (letter). Arthritis Rheum 26:936, 1983.
40. Chalmers A, Thompson D, Stein HE, et al: Systemic lupus erythematosus during penicillamine therapy for rheumatoid arthritis. Ann Intern Med 97:659, 1982.
41. Clementz GL, Dolin BJ: Sulfasalazine-induced lupus erythematosus. Am J Med 84:535, 1988.
42. Wilson MR, Tan EM: Antibodies to nonhistone antigens. p. 291. In Lahita RG (ed): Systemic Lupus Erythematosus. Churchill Livingstone, New York, 1987.
43. Reimer G, Steen VD, Penning CA, et al: Correlates between autoantibodies to nucleolar antigens and clinical features in patients with systemic sclerosis (scleroderma). Arthritis Rheum 31:525, 1988.
44. Smeenk R, Westgeest T, Swaak T: Antinuclear antibody determination: the present state of diagnostic and clinical relevance. Scand J Rheumatol 56 (Suppl):78, 1985.
45. Sharp GC, Alspaugh MA: Autoantibodies to nonhistone nuclear antigens: their immunobiology and clinical relevance. p. 197. In Gupta S, Talal N (eds): Immunology of Rheumatic Diseases. Plenum, New York, 1987.
46. Hymes SR, Russell TJ, Jordon RE: The anti-Ro antibody system. Int J Dermatol 25:1, 1986.
47. Tsokos GC, Pillemer SR, Klippel JH: Rheumatic disease syndromes associated with antibodies to the Ro (SS-A) ribonuclear protein. Semin Arthritis Rheum 16:237, 1987.
48. Lee LA, Weston WL: New findings in neonatal lupus syndrome. Am J Dis Child 138:233, 1984.
49. Nakamura RM, Tan EM: Autoantibodies to nonhistone nuclear antigens and their clinical significance. Hum Pathol 14:392, 1983.
50. Powell FC, Winkelmann RK, Venencie-Lemarchand F, et al: The anticentromere antibody: disease specificity and clinical significance. Mayo Clin Proc 59:700, 1984.
51. Fritzler MJ: Antinuclear antibodies in the investigation of rheumatic diseases. Bull Rheum Dis 35 (6):1, 1985.
52. Riboldi P, Asero R, Origgi L, Crespi S: The SL/Ki system in connective tissue diseases: incidence and clinical associations. Clin Exp Rheumatol 5:29, 1987.
53. Targoff IN, Reichlin M: The association between Mi-2

antibodies and dermatomyositis. Arthritis Rheum 28:796, 1985.

54. Westgeest AAA, Boerbooms AMT, Jongmans M, et al: Antiperinuclear factor: indicator of more severe disease in seronegative rheumatoid arthritis. J Rheumatol 14:893, 1987.

55. Treadwell EL, Alspaugh MA, Wolfe JF, Sharp GC: Clinical relevance of PM-1 antibody and physiochemical characterization of PM-1 antigen. J Rheumatol 11:658, 1984.

56. Bonfa E, Elkon KB: Clinical and serologic associations of the antiribosomal P protein antibody. Arthritis Rheum 29:981, 1986.

57. Bonfa E, Golombek SJ, Kaufman LD, et al: Association between lupus psychosis and anti-ribosomal P protein antibodies. N Engl J Med 317:265, 1987.

58. Catoggio LJ, Skinner RP, Maddison PJ: Frequency and clinical significance of anticentromere and anti-Scl-70 antibodies in an English connective tissue disease population. Rheumatol Int 3:19, 1983.

59. Senecal JL, Oliver JM, Rothfield N: Anticytoskeletal autoantibodies in the connective tissue diseases. Arthritis Rheum 28:889, 1985.

60. Wong AL, Colburn KK, Leyba MK, Gusewitch G: Antiguanosine antibodies and SLE activity: a longitudinal analysis. Arthritis Rheum 31 (Suppl 2):S87, 1988.

61. Abe Y, Inada S, Torikai K: A new autoantibody in patients with rheumatoid arthritis: characterization of the anti-HaT-1 antibody system. Arthritis Rheum 31:135, 1988.

62. Lassoued K, Guilly MN, Danon F, et al: Antinuclear autoantibodies specific for lamins: characterization and clinical significance. Ann Intern Med 108:829, 1988.

63. Jacob L, Viard JP, Choquette D, et al: Anti-LAMP (lupus-associated membrane protein) antibodies: a new marker of systemic lupus erythematosus (SLE). Arthritis Rheum 31 (Suppl 2):S29, 1988.

64. Fregeau DR, Leung PSC, Coppel RL, et al: Autoantibodies to mitochondria in systemic sclerosis: frequency and characterization using recombinant cloned autoantigen. Arthritis Rheum 31:386, 1988.

65. Robbins ML, Kornguth SE, Bell CL, et al: Antineurofilament antibody evaluation in neuropsychiatric systemic lupus erythematosus. Combination with anticardiolipin antibody assay and magnetic resonance imaging. Arthritis Rheum 31:623, 1988.

66. How A, Dent PB, Liao SK, Denburg JA: Antineuronal antibodies in neuropsychiatric systemic lupus erythematosus. Arthritis Rheum 28:789, 1985.

67. Parlevliet KJ, Henzen-Logmans SC, Oe PL, et al: Antibodies to components of neutrophil cytoplasm: a new diagnostic tool in patients with Wegener's granulomatosis and systemic vasculitis. Q J Med 66:55, 1988.

68. Harris EN, Gharavi AE, Hughes GRV: Anti-phospholipid antibodies. Clin Rheum Dis 11:591, 1985.

69. Sthoeger Z, Reeves WH: Identification of subpopulations of anti-ku (p70/p80) autoantibodies reactive with distinct epitopes using natural and cloned antigens. Arthritis Rheum 31 (Suppl):S13, 1988.

70. Hughes GR: Autoantibodies in lupus and its variants: experience in 1000 patients. Br Med J 289:339, 1984.
71. White RH, Robbins DL: Clinical significance and interpretation of antinuclear antibodies. West J Med 147:210, 1987.
72. Colaco CB, Elkon KB: The lupus anticoagulant. A disease marker in antinuclear antibody negative lupus that is cross-reactive with autoantibodies to double-stranded DNA. Arthritis Rheum 28:67, 1985.
73. Yoshida S, Akizuki M, Mimori T, et al: The precipitating antibody to an acidic nuclear protein antigen, the Jo-1, in connective tissue diseases. A marker for a subset of polymyositis with interstitial pulmonary fibrosis. Arthritis Rheum 26:604, 1983.
74. Hochberg MC, Feldman D, Stevens MB, et al: Antibody to Jo-1 in polymyositis/dermatomyositis: association with interstitial pulmonary disease. J Rheumatol 11:663, 1984.
75. Garcia-de la Torre I, Miranda-Mendez L: Studies of antinuclear antibodies in rheumatoid arthritis. J Rheumatol 9:603, 1982.

Selected Readings

Feltkamp TEW, Smeenk RJT (eds): Nuclear antigens and antinuclear antibodies. Scand J Rheumatol Suppl 56:1, 1985.
This entire issue is a series of reports of the fourth Bertine Koperberg Conference held at Ousterbeek, The Netherlands in May 1984. There are valuable articles on the clinical relevance, immunotaxonomy, and biology of ANAs.

Fritzler MJ: Antinuclear antibodies in the investigation of rheumatic diseases. Bull Rheum Dis 35:1, 1985.
Excellent introduction to the diagnostic use of ANA.

Harmon CE, Portanova JP: Drug-induced lupus: clinical and serological studies. Clin Rheum Dis 8:121, 1982.
Review of drug-induced lupus.

Harris EN, Gharavi AE, Hughes GRV: Anti-phospholipid antibodies. Clin Rheum Dis 11:591, 1985.
Thorough review of recently characterized antibodies that have been associated with thromboses, recurrent fetal loss, and the lupus anticoagulant.

Hess E: Drug-related lupus (editorial). N Engl J Med 318:1460, 1988.
Current editorial review of diagnosis and pathogenesis of drug-induced lupus.

McCarty GA: Autoantibodies and their relation to rheumatic diseases. Med Clin North Am 70:237, 1986.
Excellent review of ANAs, covering diagnostic tests, specific autoantibodies, and disease association.

Nakamura RM, Tan EM: Autoantibodies to nonhistone nuclear antigens and their clinical significance. Hum Pathol 14:392, 1983.
General subject review.

Richardson B, Epstein WV: Utility of the fluorescent antibody test in a single patient. Ann Intern Med 95:333, 1981.

Application of Bayes' theorum to the FANA with positive predictive values given for various patient populations.

Sharp GC, Alspaugh MA: Autoantibodies to nonhistone nuclear antigens: their immunobiology and clinical relevance. p. 197. In Gupta S, Talal N (eds): Immunology of Rheumatic Diseases. Plenum, New York, 1987.
General subject review.

Tan EM: Autoantibodies to nuclear antigens (ANA): their immunobiology and medicine. Adv Immunol 33:167, 1982.
Comprehensive review of the immunobiology and disease relationship of ANAs by one of the leading experts on ANAs. Extensively referenced.

Tsokos GC, Pillemer SR, Klippel JH: Rheumatic disease syndromes associated with antibodies to the Ro (SS-A) ribonuclear protein. Semin Arthritis Rheum 16:237, 1987.
Review of the association of ANA-negative lupus, subacute cutaneous lupus, neonatal lupus syndrome, and extraglandular Sjögren's syndrome and their relationship to the auto-SS-A antibody.

Weinstein A: Drug-induced systemic lupus erythematosus. Prog Clin Immunol 4:1, 1980.
General subject review.

59

Rheumatoid Factor: Conditions Associated with a Positive Test

Rheumatoid factors are a group of autoantibodies against certain structures in the Fc portion of the IgG molecule. As detected by the common serologic procedures, rheumatoid factors are usually IgM proteins. About three-fourths of patients with rheumatoid arthritis have detectable rheumatoid factor in their serum. Although the presence of rheumatoid factor is a diagnostic criterion for rheumatoid arthritis, a positive test for rheumatoid factor should not be used as the sole criterion for the diagnosis of rheumatoid arthritis because a positive test can be found in a small percentage of healthy young people and in diseases other than rheumatoid arthritis. The incidence of positive rheumatoid factor detection increases with age. The method of detection of rheumatoid factor may influence whether or not rheumatoid factor is found. Furthermore, the titer of rheumatoid factor should be considered in determining whether or not a patient has a significant level of rheumatoid factor. This chapter lists those conditions in which the prevalence of positive rheumatoid factor tests may be greater than that found in the general population.

Rheumatologic Diseases	Rheumatoid arthritis[1] Juvenile rheumatoid arthritis[2,3]: especially in the polyarticular form Systemic lupus erythematosus[4] Sjögren's syndrome[5] Progressive systemic sclerosis (scleroderma)[6] Mixed connective tissue disease[4] Raynaud's phenomenon[7] Polyarteritis nodosa[8] Hypersensitivity vasculitis[8] Wegener's granulomatosis[8] Takayasu's arteritis[9] Behçet's disease[10] Mixed cryoglobulinemia[11]
Acute Viral Infections	Cytomegalovirus[12] Hepatitis B[13] Infectious mononucleosis[14] Influenza[15] Rubella[16]
Bacterial Infections	Subacute bacterial endocarditis[17] Acute bacterial endocarditis[18] Shunt nephritis[19] Periodontal disease[20] Otitis media[21]: in the ear effusions only; not found in the serum Nephropathia epidemica[22] Lyme disease[23] Brucellosis[4] Leprosy (Hansen's disease)[24] *Mycoplasma* pneumonia[25] Salmonellosis[4]

Syphilis[26]
Tuberculosis[27]
Yaws[4]
Yersiniosis[28]

Parsasitis Infections

Filariasis[4]
Kala-azar[29]
Parasitic migrans[30]
Leishmaniasis[31]
Malaria[32]
Schistosomiasis[31]
Trypanosomiasis[32]

Neoplastic Diseases

Bladder cancer[33]
Breast cancer[34]
Colorectal cancer[35]
Gastric cancer[35]
Leukemia[36]
Lung cancer (squamous cell)[34]
Melanoma[37]
Pancreatic cancer[35]
Reticulum cell sarcoma[14]

Metabolic Disease

Graves' disease[38]
Hyperlipidemia, type IV[39]
Cholesterol emboli[40]

Pulmonary Diseases

Asbestosis[41]
Coal workers' pneumoconiosis[42]: these patients have an increased prevalence of rheumatoid factor even if they do not have Caplan's syndrome.
Idiopathic pulmonary fibrosis[43]
Sarcoidosis[44]
Silicosis[45]

Hepatic Diseases

Chronic liver disease[46]
Primary biliary cirrhosis[47]

Other Conditions

Aging[48]
Graft-versus-host disease[48]
Hypergammaglobulinemic purpura[49]

Idiopathic cardiomyopathy[50]
Open heart surgery[51]
Thermal injury[52]

References

1. Koopman WJ, Schrohenloher RE: Rheumatoid factor. p. 217. In Utsinger PD, Zvaifler NJ, Ehrlich GE (eds): Rheumatoid Arthritis: Etiology, Diagnosis, Management. JP Lippincott Philadelphia, 1985.
2. Eichenfield AH, Athreya BH, Doughty RA, et al: Utility of rheumatoid factor in the diagnosis of juvenile rheumatoid arthritis. Pediatrics 78:480, 1986.
3. Leak AM: Autoantibody profile in juvenile chronic arthritis. Ann Rheum Dis 47:178, 1988.
4. Carson DA: Rheumatoid factor. p. 664. In Kelley WN, Harris ED Jr, Ruddy S, Sledge CB (eds): Textbook of Rheumatology, 2nd Ed. WB Saunders, Philadelphia, 1985.
5. Alexander M: Clinical aspects of Sjögren's syndrome. South Med J 79:857, 1986.
6. Seibold JR, Medsger TA Jr, Winkelstein A, et al: Immune complexes in progressive systemic sclerosis (scleroderma). Arthritis Rheum 25:1167, 1982.
7. Kallenberg CG, Wouda AA, The TH: Systemic involvement and immunologic findings in patients presenting with Raynaud's phenomenon. Am J Med 69:675, 1980.
8. Cupps TR, Fauci AS: The vasculitides, Vol. XXI. In Smith LH (ed): Major Problems in Internal Medicine. WB Saunders, Philadelphia, 1981.
9. Kanzaki S, Kanda S: Coombs' antibodies and rheumatoid factors in Takayasu's arteritis (letter). JAMA 254:232, 1985.
10. Shimizu T, Katsuta Y, Oshima Y: Immunological studies on Behçet's syndrome. Ann Rheum Dis 24:494, 1965.
11. Gorevic PD, Kassab HJ, Levo Y, et al: Mixed cryoglobulinemia: clinical aspects and long-term follow-up of 40 patients. Am J Med 69:287, 1980.
12. Langenhuysen MMAC: Antibody against γ-globulin after blood transfusion and cytomegalovirus-infection. Clin Exp Immunol 9:393, 1971.
13. Anderson-Visona K, Villarejos VM: Identity of antibody to hepatitis B e/1 antigen as an atypical rheumatoid factor. J Infect Dis 141:603, 1980.
14. Capra JD, Winchester RJ, Kunkel HG: Cold-reactive rheumatoid factors in infectious mononucleosis and other diseases. Arthritis Rheum 12:67, 1969.
15. Svec KH, Dingle JH: The occurrence of rheumatoid factor in association with antibody response to influenza A2 (Asian) virus. Arthritis Rheum 8:524, 1965.
16. Johnson RE, Hall AP: Rubella arthritis: report of cases studied by latex tests. N Engl J Med 258:743, 1958.
17. Carson DA, Bayer AS, Eisenberg RA, et al: IgG rheumatoid factor in subacute bacterial endocarditis: relationship to IgM rheumatoid factor and circulating immune complexes. Clin Exp Immunol 31:100, 1978.
18. Sheagren JN, Tuazon CU, Griffin C, Padmore N:

Rheumatoid factor in acute bacterial endocarditis. Arthritis Rheum 19:887, 1976.

19. Dobrin RS, Day NK, Quie PG, et al: The role of complement, immunoglobulin, and bacterial antigen in coagulase-negative staphylococcal shunt nephritis. Am J Med 59:660, 1975.

20. Hirsch HZ, Tarkowski A, Koopman WJ, Mestecky J: Rheumatoid factor production in adult periodontitis patients. Arthritis Rheum 31 (Suppl 2):S92, 1988.

21. DeMaria TF, McGhee RB Jr, Lim DJ: Rheumatoid factor in otitis media with effusion. Arch Otolaryngol 110:279, 1984.

22. Penttinen K, Lahdevirta J, Kekomaki R, et al: Circulating immune complexes, immunoconglutinins, and rheumatoid factors in nephropathia epidemica. J Infect Dis 143:15, 1981.

23. Kujala GA, Steere AC, Davis JS IV: IgM rheumatoid factor in Lyme disease: correlation with disease activity, total serum IgM, and IgM antibody to *Borrelia burgdorferi*. J Rheumatol 14:772, 1987.

24. Petchclai B, Chuthanondh R, Rungruong S, Ramasoota T: Autoantibodies in leprosy among Thai patients. Lancet 1:1481, 1973.

25. Mizutani H, Mizutani H: Immunoglobulin M rheumatoid factor in patients with mycoplasmal pneumonia. Am Rev Respir Dis 134:1237, 1986.

26. Peltier A, Christian CL: The presence of the "rheumatoid factor" in sera from patients with syphilis. Arthritis Rheum 2:1, 1959.

27. Singer JM, Plotz CM, Peralta FM, Lyons HC: The presence of anti-gamma globulin factors in sera of patients with active pulmonary tuberculosis. Ann Interm Med 56:545, 1962.

28. Kekomaki R, Granfors K, Leino R, et al: Clinical correlates of circulating immune complexes in patients with recent yersiniosis. J Infect Dis 148:223, 1983.

29. Kunkel HG, Simon HJ, Fudenberg H: Observations concerning positive serologic reactions for rheumatoid factor in certain patients with sarcoidosis and other hyperglobulinemic states. Arthritis Rheum 1:289, 1958.

30. Huntley CC, Costas MG, Williams RC, et al: Anti-γ-globulin factors in visceral larva migrans. JAMA 197:552, 1966.

31. Carvalho EM, Andrews BS, Martinelli R, et al: Circulating immune complexes and rheumatoid factor in schistosomiasis and visceral leishmaniasis. Am J Trop Med Hyg 32:61, 1983.

32. Houba V, Alison AC: M-antiglobulins (rheumatoid-factor-like globulins) and other gammaglobulins in relation to tropical parasitic infections. Lancet 1:848, 1966.

33. Gupta NP, Malaviya AN, Singh SM: Rheumatoid factor in bladder tumors. J Urol 120:296, 1978.

34. Twomey JJ, Rossen RD, Lewis VM, et al: Rheumatoid factor and tumor-host interaction. Proc Natl Acad Sci USA 73:2106, 1976.

35. Schattner A, Shani A, Talpaz M, Bentwich Z: Rheumatoid factors in the sera of patients with gastrointestinal carcinoma. Cancer 52:2156, 1983.

36. Sherry MG: The incidence of positive RA tests in

Hodgkin's disease and leukemia. Am J Clin Pathol 50:398, 1968.

37. Giuliano AE, Irie R, Morton DL: Rheumatoid factor in melanoma patients: alterations of humoral tumor immunity in vitro. Cancer 43:1624, 1979.
38. Silverberg J, Row VV, Volpe R: Rheumatoid factor in Graves' disease. Ann Intern Med 88:216, 1978.
39. Goldman JA, Glueck CJ, Abrams NR, et al: Musculoskeletal disorders associated with type-IV hyperlipoproteinaemia. Lancet 2:449, 1972.
40. Cappiello RA, Espinoza LR, Vasey FB, Germain BF: Cholesterol emboli mimicking systemic vasculitis. Arthritis Rheum 31 (Suppl 1):R39, 1988.
41. Pernis B, Vigliani EC, Selikoff IJ: Rheumatoid factor in serum of individuals exposed to asbestos. Ann NY Acad Sci 132:112, 1965.
42. Pearson DJ, Mentrech MS, Elliot JA, et al: Serologic changes in pneumoconiosis and progressive massive fibrosis of coal workers. Am Rev Resp Dis 124:696, 1981.
43. Tomasi TB Jr, Fudenberg HH, Finby N: Possible relationship of rheumatoid factors and pulmonary disease. Am J Med 33:243, 1962.
44. Mitchell DN, Scadding JG: Sarcoidosis. Am Rev Resp Dis 110:774, 1974.
45. Doll NJ, Stankus RP, Hughes J, et al: Immune complexes and autoantibodies in silicosis. J Allergy Clin Immunol 68:281, 1981.
46. Bonomo L, LoSpalluto J, Ziff M: Anti-gamma globulin factors in liver disease. Arthritis Rheum 6:104, 1963.
47. Culp KS, Fleming CR, Duffy J, et al: Autoimmune associations in primary biliary cirrhosis. Mayo Clin Proc 57:365, 1982.
48. Williams RC Jr: Rheumatoid factors. Hum Pathol 14:386, 1983.
49. Capra JD, Winchester RJ, Kunkel HG: Hypergammaglobulinemic purpura: studies of the unusual anti-γ-globulins characteristic of the sera of these patients. Medicine 50:125, 1971.
50. Kirsner AB, Hess EV, Fowler NO: Immunologic findings in idiopathic cardiomyopathy: a prospective serial study. Am Heart J 86:625, 1973.
51. Pretty HM, Fudenberg HH, Perkins HA, Gerbode F: Anti-γ-globulin antibodies after open heart surgery. Blood 32:205, 1968.
52. Hutchinson R, Patel R, MacArthur J: Rheumatoid, antinuclear, and antileukocyte cytotoxic factors in patients with burns. Am J Surg 122:520, 1971.

Selected Readings

Bartfeld H: Distribution of rheumatoid factor activity in nonrheumatoid states. Ann NY Acad Sci 168:30, 1969.
Thorough compilation of reports of rheumatoid factor in nonrheumatoid states through 1969.

Carson DA: Rheumatoid factor. p. 664. In Kelley WN, Harris ED Jr, Ruddy S, Sledge CB (eds): Textbook of Rheumatology. 2nd Ed. WB Saunders, Philadelphia, 1985.
General subject review.

Dresner E, Trombly P: The latex-fixation reaction in nonrheumatic diseases. N Engl J Med 261:981, 1959.
Classic article on rheumatoid factor in hepatic and viral diseases.

Koopman WJ, Schrohenloher RE: Rheumatoid factor. p. 217. In Utsinger PD, Zvaifler NJ, Ehrlich GE (eds): Rheumatoid Arthritis: Etiology, Diagnosis, Management. JB Lippincott, Philadelphia, 1985.
General subject review.

Mannik M: Rheumatoid factors. p. 660. In McCarty DJ (ed): Arthritis and Allied Conditions: A Textbook of Rheumatology. 10th Ed. Lea & Febiger, Philadelphia, 1985.
General subject review.

Williams RC Jr: Rheumatoid factors. Hum Pathol 14:386, 1983.
General subject review.

60
Acute Arthritis: Common and Less Common Causes

Acute arthritis can be the first sign of chronic arthritis or reflect an underlying systemic disorder. Polyarthritis (more than one joint involved) and monoarthritis (one joint) are useful clinical distinctions because certain conditions almost always present as either polyarthritis or monoarthritis.

Acute Polyarthritis: Common Causes

Most inflammatory arthritides can occur at any age, but are more common between 30 and 50 years of age. Rheumatoid arthritis and systemic lupus erythematosus are much more common in females. Reiter's syndrome, psoriatic arthritis, and reactive arthritis are more frequently recognized in males because their cases are usually more severe.

Rheumatoid arthritis: usually subacute, but the acute presentation is not rare[1]

Psoriatic arthritis: acute arthritis occasionally pre-cedes psoriatic skin changes[2]

Reactive arthritis: Reiter's-like arthritis following enteritis[3]

Reiter's syndrome: triad of urethritis, ocular inflam-mation, and arthritis; triad does not always occur simultaneously[4]

Systemic lupus erythematosus[5]

Infectious arthritis

Viral arthritis: rubella, rubella vaccine,[6] hepatitis, infectious mononucleosis,[7] mumps, chickenpox,[8] coxsackie virus[9]

Lyme arthritis: characteristic rash, erythema marginatum[10]

Erythema nodosum: arthritis may precede skin changes; more common associations include tuber-culosis, streptococcal infection, sarcoidosis, and coccidioidomycosis[11]

Juvenile onset arthritis: Still's disease; may occur in adults[12]

Sarcoidosis[13]

Osteoarthritis: although inflammation is a common finding in acute osteoarthritis, be cautious about attributing inflammation to radiographic changes. Radiographic changes associated with osteoarthritis are far more typical of chronic osteoarthritis.

Acute Monoarthritis: Common Causes

Consider acute monoarthritis infectious until proven otherwise. Aspirated joint fluid should be sent for appropriate smears, cultures, and crystal identifica-tion. Some common infectious agents, such as *Neis-seria gonorrhoeae* and *Haemophilus influenzae,* are dif-ficult to culture. Gout, pseudogout, and osteoarthritis are rare before age 40; gout is uncommon in females.

Infections

Pyogenic arthritis: gonococcus[14] (may be polyartic-ular), streptococcus,[15] staphylococcus,[16] *Pseudo-monas,*[17] meningococcus, salmonella,[18] *Haemophi-lus influenzae,*[19] polymicrobia,[20] *Yersinia*[21,22]

Gouty arthritis: tender, swollen, warm, red joints[23]

Pseudogout: calcium pyrophosphate crystals in syn-ovial fluid[24]

Trauma: loose body, mechanical derangement, os-teochondritis dissecans

Reiter's disease: more frequently polyarthritis[25]

Psoriatic arthritis: more frequently polyarthritis

Osteoarthritis: be wary, osteoarthritis can coexist with infection, gout, or pseudogout.

Eosinophilic synovitis: acute self-limited monoarthritis in patients with synovial fluid eosinophilia and dermatographism[26]

Lipid microspherule-associated acute monoarthritis[27,28]

Acute Polyarthritis: Less Common Causes

Inflammatory bowel disease arthritis[29,30]

Rheumatic fever: often precedes evidence of carditis[31]

Ankylosing spondylitis and new peripheral involvement

Sjögren's syndrome[32]

Bowel bypass: arthritis-dermatitis syndrome[33]

Neoplasia: leukemia,[34] carcinomatosis, melanoma[35]

Serum sickness: history of drug exposure

Whipple's disease[36]

Brucellosis[37]

Relapsing polychondritis[38]

Acute Monoarthritis: Less Common Causes

Infectious: sporotrichosis,[39] tuberculosis, fungal[40]

Hematologic disorders: hemophilia,[41] sickle-cell disease,[42] thalassemia,[43] myeloid metaplasia,[44] acute leukemia in children[45]

Neuropathic arthropathy: often diffuse calcium and bony deposition

Pigmented villonodular synovitis

Congenital dysplasia with joint space collapse

Synovial and soft tissue tumors

Reflex sympathetic dystrophy: hand or foot

Neoplastic: malignant metastatic deposits near joints can cause a nonspecific inflammatory monoarthritis[46]

Carcinomatous arthritis: one report of elbow monoarthritis due to metastatic breast carcinoma[47]

Ewing's sarcoma[48]

References

1. Krane SM, Simon LS: Rheumatoid arthritis: clinical features and pathogenic mechanisms. Med Clin North Am 70:263, 1986.
2. Bachmann E, Clemmensen OJ, Dyrbye M, et al: Joint involvement in psoriasis: scintigraphic, radiologic, and clinical findings. Dermatologica 166:250, 1983.
3. Keat A: Reiter's syndrome and reactive arthritis in perspective. N Engl J Med 309:1606, 1983.
4. Willkens RF, Arnett FC, Bitter T, et al: Reiter's syn-

drome. Evaluation of preliminary criteria for definite disease. Arthritis Rheum 24:844, 1981.

5. Labowitz R, Schumacher HR Jr: Articular manifestations of systemic lupus erythematosus. Ann Intern Med 74:911, 1971.

6. Tingle AJ, Chantler JK, Pot KH, et al: Postpartum rubella immunization: association with development of prolonged arthritis, neurological sequelae, and chronic rubella viremia. J Infect Dis 152:606, 1985.

7. Sigal LH, Steere AC, Niederman JC: Symmetric polyarthritis associated with heterophile-negative infectious mononucleosis. Arthritis Rheum 26:553, 1983.

8. Williams AJ, Freemont AJ, Barnett DB: Pericarditis and arthritis complicating chickenpox. Br J Clin Pract 37:226, 1983.

9. Hurst NP, Martynoga AG, Nuki G, et al: Coxsackie B infection and arthritis. Br Med J 286:605, 1983.

10. Meyerhoff J: Lyme disease. Am J Med 75:663, 1983.

11. Reece RM: Erythema nodosum. Am Fam Physician 13 (3):99, 1976.

12. Corbett AJ, Zizic TM, Stevens MB: Adult-onset Still's disease with an associated severe restrictive pulmonary defect: a case report. Ann Rheum Dis 42:452, 1983.

13. Swaak AJG, Hissink-Muller WH, Van Soesbergen RM: Sarcoidosis presenting with severe thrombocytopenia and arthritis. Clin Rheumatol 1:212, 1982.

14. Goldman JA: Patterns of gonococcal arthritis (editorial). J Rheumatol 8:707, 1981.

15. Vartian C, Lerner PI, Shlaes DM, et al: Infections due to Lancefield group G streptococci. Medicine 64:75, 1985.

16. Lurie DP, Musil G: Staphylococcal septic arthritis presenting as acute flare of pseudogout: clinical, pathological, and arthroscopic findings with a review of the literature. J Rheumatol 10:503, 1983.

17. Dan M, Jedwab M, Shibolet S: Recurrent septic arthritis due to *Pseudomonas* sp. Postgrad Med J 57:257, 1981.

18. Brodie TD, Ehresmann GR: *Salmonella dublin* arthritis: an initial case presentation. J Rheumatol 10:144, 1983.

19. Borenstein DG, Simon GL: *Haemophilus influenzae* septic arthritis in adults. A report of four cases and a review of the literature. Medicine 65:191, 1986.

20. Petty BG, Sowa DT, Charache P: Polymicrobial polyarticular septic arthritis. JAMA 249:2069, 1983.

21. Bernstein RM, Mackworth-Young CG, Saverymutu SH, et al: *Yersinia* arthritis: demonstration of occult enteritis by [111]indium leucocyte scanning. Ann Rheum Dis 43:493, 1984.

22. Leirisalo-Repo M, Suoranta H: Ten-year follow-up study of patients with *Yersinia* arthritis. Arthritis Rheum 31:533, 1988.

23. German DC, Holmes EW: Hyperuricemia and gout. Med Clin North Am 70:419, 1986.

24. McCarty DJ: Arthritis associated with crystals containing calcium. Med Clin North Am 70:437, 1986.

25. Amor B: Reiter's syndrome and reactive arthritis (editorial). Clin Rheumatol 2:315, 1983.

26. Brown JP, Rola-Pleszczynski M, Menard HA: Eosinophilic synovitis: clinical observations on a newly recog-

nized subset of patients with dermatographism. Arthritis Rheum 29:1147, 1986.

27. Reginato AJ, Schumacher HR, Allan DA, et al: Acute monoarthritis associated with lipid liquid crystals. Ann Rheum Dis 44:537, 1985.

28. Trostle DC, Schumacher HR Jr, Medsger TA Jr, et al: Lipid microspherule-associated acute monarticular arthritis. Arthritis Rheum 29:1166, 1986.

29. Jordan JM, Zizic TM, Dorsch CA: Possible pathogenetic role for ulcerative colitis in the arthritis, hepatomegaly, and erythema nodosum of common variable immunodeficiency. Johns Hopkins Med J 151:54, 1982.

30. Al-Hadidi S, Khatib G, Chhatwal P, et al: Granulomatous arthritis in Crohn's disease. Arthritis Rheum 27:1061, 1984.

31. Zagala JG, Feinstein AR: The preceding illness of acute rheumatic fever. JAMA 179:863, 1962.

32. Castro-Poltronieri A, Alarcón-Segovia D: Articular manifestations of primary Sjögren's syndrome. J Rheumatol 10:485, 1983.

33. Leff RD, Towles W, Aldo-Benson MA, et al: A prospective analysis of the arthritis syndrome and immune function in jejunoileal bypass patients. J Rheumatol 10:612, 1983.

34. Luzar MJ, Sharma HM: Leukemia and arthritis: including reports on light, immunofluorescent, and electron microscopy of the synovium. J Rheumatol 10:132, 1983.

35. Speerstra F, Boerbooms AMTh, van de Putte LBA, et al: Arthritis caused by metastatic melanoma. Arthritis Rheum 25:223, 1982.

36. Khan MA: Axial arthropathy in Whipple's disease. J Rheumatol 9:928, 1982.

37. Alarcon GS, Bocanegra TS, Gotuzzo E, et al: Reactive arthritis associated with brucellosis: HLA studies. J Rheumatol 8:621, 1981.

38. McAdam LP, O'Hanlan MA, Bluestone R, et al: Relapsing polychondritis: prospective study of 23 patients and a review of the literature. Medicine 55:193, 1976.

39. Crout JE, Brewer NS, Tompkins RB: Sporotrichosis arthritis. Clinical features in patients. Ann Intern Med 86:294, 1977.

40. Haapasaari J, Essen RV, Kahanpää A, et al: Fungal arthritis simulating juvenile rheumatoid arthritis. Br Med J 285:923, 1982.

41. Wilkins RM, Wiedel JD: Septic arthritis of the knee in a hemophiliac: a case report. J Bone Joint Surg (Am) 65-A:267, 1983.

42. de Ceulaer K, Forbes M, Roper D, et al: Non-gouty arthritis in sickle cell disease: report of 37 consecutive cases. Ann Rheum Dis 43:599, 1984.

43. Gerster JC, Dardel R, Guggi S: Recurrent episodes of arthritis in thalassemia minor. J Rheumatol 11:352, 1984.

44. Heinicke MH, Zarrabi MH, Gorevic PD: Arthritis due to synovial involvement by extramedullary hematopoiesis in myelofibrosis with myeloid metaplasia. Ann Rheum Dis 42:196, 1983.

45. Saulsbury FT, Sabio H: Acute leukemia presenting as arthritis in children. Clin Pediatr 24:625, 1985.

46. Gerster JC, Jaquier E, Ribaux C: Nonspecific inflammatory monoarthritis in the vicinity of bony metastases. J Rheumatol 14:844, 1987.
47. Garcia-Morteo D, Lema B, Maldonado-Cocco JA, Garcia-Morteo O: Carcinomatous arthritis of the elbow caused by metastatic breast carcinoma. Clin Rheumatol 6:273, 1987.
48. Halla JT, Hirsch V: Monoarthritis as the presenting manifestation of localized Ewing's sarcoma in an older patient. J Rheumatol 14:628, 1987.

Selected Readings

Caldwell DS, McCallum RM: Rheumatologic manifestations of cancer. Med Clin North Am 70:385, 1986.
A variety of musculoskeletal syndromes may be the presenting manifestation of an occult neoplastic process.

Decker JL, Malone DG, Haraoui B, et al: NIH conference. Rheumatoid arthritis: evolving concepts of pathogenesis and treatment. Ann Intern Med 101:810, 1984.
NIH conference reviewing rheumatoid arthritis. Well referenced.

Freeman R, Jones MR: Microbiology. Clin Rheum Dis 9:3, 1983.
Review of methods and procedures needed to diagnose common arthropathies.

Goldenberg DL, Reed JI: Bacterial arthritis. N Engl J Med 312:764, 1985.
Current approaches to diagnosis and treatment. Well referenced.

Parker JD, Capell HA: An acute arthritis clinic—one year's experience. Br J Rheumatol 25:293, 1986.
Gout and reactive arthritis were the most common diagnoses in 150 patients seen in an acute arthritis clinic for a period of 12 months.

Raja SN, Meyer RA, Campbell JN: Peripheral mechanisms of somatic pain. Anesthesiology 68:571, 1988.
Interesting review of recent data that correlates subjective estimates of pain in humans with activity of single nerve fibers, activity of certain nociceptors, and chemical mediators. Authors suggest possible mechanisms of pain associated with inflammation-induced changes affecting articular afferents, such as can be seen in acute and chronic arthritis.

Rodnan GP, Schumacher HR, Zvaifler NJ (eds): Primer on the Rheumatic Diseases. 8th Ed. Arthritis Foundation, Atlanta, 1983.
Summary of major diseases and clinical findings.

Sequeira W, Stinar D: Serum angiotensin-converting enzyme levels in sarcoid arthritis. Arch Intern Med 146:125, 1986.
Levels of serum angiotensin-converting enzyme may be helpful in differential diagnosis of patients with "seronegative polyarthritis."

Willkens RF: Rheumatoid arthritis: clinical considerations in diagnosis and management. Am J Med 83:31, 1987.
Review of clinical concepts, with an emphasis on current concepts of the immune response, immunogenetics, and improved identification of infectious agents in patients with acute and chronic symptoms associated with rheumatoid arthritis.

61
Uveitis and Arthritis: Associated Diseases

Inflammation of the uveal tract is associated with a variety of systemic diseases that include joint inflammation. Uveitis may be subdivided by its location: anterior (iris and ciliary body inflammation also called iridocyclitis or iritis) versus posterior (choroid inflammation also called chorioretinitis). Subsets of both uveitis and arthritis can be distinguished on the basis of clinical course, histologic appearance, and immunogenetic association, such as HLA-B27 association.[1]

HLA-B27-Related Diseases

The presence of the histocompatibility antigen HLA-B27 in all patients with acute anterior uveitis is approximately 55 to 60%, and approximately 15% of those patients will have a systemic disease such as ankylosing spondylitis, Reiter's syndrome, or inflammatory bowel disease.[2]

Ankylosing spondylitis (AS): between 15 to 30% of patients with AS will have associated anterior uveitis, which is characterized by acute, recurrent attacks of red, painful eye with photophobia.[3,4] Most patients with uveitis and AS will be HLA-B27-positive.[5] The activity of the spondylitis does not necessarily parallel the uveitis.

Reiter's syndrome: classically presents as a triad of arthritis, nonspecific urethritis and conjunctivitis; but recurrent acute anterior uveitis will occur in approximately 30% of patients and is similar to the uveitis seen in AS patients.[2] Reiter's syndrome with uveitis has been associated with several infectious agents including *Chlamydia*-induced urethritis and enteritis due to *Salmonella, Shigella,* or *Yersinia.*[5]

Inflammatory bowel disease: anterior uveitis occurs with a frequency varying from 5 to 12% in ulcerative colitis and 2 to 13% in Crohn's disease. The activity of the uveitis tends to parallel the activity of the colitis.[6] Patients with uveitis, colitis, and spondylitis are more likely to be HLA-B27 positive.[7]

Psoriatic arthritis: less than 10% of these patients will develop acute recurrent anterior uveitis, which will rarely lead to chronic uveitis.[8] HLA-B27-positivity occurs in about 15% of patients with peripheral psoriatic arthropathy and approximately 50% with psoriatic spondylitis-sacroiliitis.[9]

Non-HLA-B27-Related Diseases

Several diseases with inflammatory joint findings are associated with uveitis, but do not have a relation to HLA-B27 positivity including juvenile rheumatoid arthritis, sarcoidosis, Behçet's syndrome, and other less common diseases.

Juvenile rheumatoid arthritis (JRA): chronic nongranulomatous uveitis occurs almost exclusively in the pediatric population, especially in girls who present with oligoarticular arthritis. Uveitis is rare in JRA patients with polyarticular or systemic onset.[10]

Behçet's syndrome: multisystem disorder with oral, genital, and skin lesions; arthritis; and bilateral anterior uveitis, which may be associated with hypopyon and/or retinal vasculitis and is seen primarily in Turkish or Japanese men aged 20 to 40 years. Uveitis may occur in as many as 60 to 70% of these patients.[8]

Sarcoidosis: systemic diseases of noncaseating granuloma with chronic unilateral or bilateral anterior or posterior granulomatous uveitis, which may produce few symptoms and occurs in 30 to 40% of patients with sarcoidosis.[11]

Relapsing polychondritis (RP): characterized by inflammatory episodes involving auricular, nasal, or laryngotracheal cartilage and an inflammatory arthritis. Uveitis is frequently associated with scleritis or episcleritis.[12]

Kawasaki disease: also known as mucocutaneous lymph node syndrome, which is a form of necrotizing polyarteritis with cardiac involvement and polyarthritis; approximately 80% of patients will develop bilateral acute, nongranulomatous anterior uveitis.[13]

Wegener's granulomatosis: ocular manifestations are common, but uveitis occurs in less than 5% of patients.[14]

Leukocytoclastic vasculitis: episodic symmetric polyarthritis and anterior uveitis[15]

Hypocomplementemic urticarial vasculitis: diagnosis rests on typical urticarial skin lesions, low serum complement levels, plus two of the following: dermal venulitis, arthritis, glomerulonephritis, episcleritis or uveitis, recurrent abdominal pain, and C1q precipitin in plasma.[16]

Gonococcal arthritis: may be associated with unilateral uveitis and its onset; can occur weeks or months after abatement of urethritis[17]

Stevens-Johnson syndrome: characterized by erythema multiforme exudativum, mucocutaneous ulceration, and polyarthralgia and may be associated with uveitis or panophthalmitis[7]

Cogan's syndrome: characterized by interstitial keratitis in association with vertigo, tinnitus, or a hearing loss. Uveitis may occur in 15 to 30% of patients and joint symptoms in up to 50% of patients[18]

References

1. Rosenbaum JT, Cousins SW: Uveitis and arthritis: experimental models and clinical correlates. Semin Arthritis Rheum 11:383, 1982.
2. Scharf Y, Zonis S: Histocompatibility antigens (HLA) and uveitis. Surv Ophthalmol 24:220, 1980.
3. Marks SH, Barnett M, Calin A: Ankylosing spondylitis in women and men: a case-control study. J Rheumatol 10:624, 1983.
4. Coles RS: Ocular manifestations of connective tissue disease. Hosp Pract 20:70, 1985.
5. O'Connor GR: Endogenous uveitis. p. 90. In Kraus-Mackiw E, O'Connor GR (eds): Uveitis: Pathophysiology and Therapy. Thieme-Stratton, New York, 1983.
6. Friedman AH, Luntz MH, Henley WL: Diagnosis and Management of Uveitis: An Atlas Approach. p. 66. Williams & Wilkins, Baltimore, 1982.
7. James DG: Acute anterior uveitis. Clin Rheum Dis 3:299, 1977.
8. Rosenbaum JT, Nozik RA: Uveitis: many diseases, one diagnosis. Am J Med 79:545, 1985.
9. Catsarou-Catsari A, Katsambas A, Theodoropoulos P, et al: Ophthalmological manifestations in patients with psoriasis. Acta Derm Venereol (Stockh) 64:557, 1984.
10. Rosenberg AM: Uveitis associated with juvenile rheumatoid arthritis. Semin Arthritis Rheum 16:158, 1987.
11. Obenauf CD, Shaw HE, Syndor CF, et al: Sarcoidosis and its ophthalmic manifestations. Am J Ophthalmol 86:648, 1978.
12. Isaak BL, Liesegang TJ, Michet CJ Jr: Ocular and systemic findings in relapsing polychondritis. Ophthalmology 93:681, 1986.
13. Ohno S, Miyajima T, Higuchi M, et al: Ocular mani-

festations of Kawasaki's disease (mucocutaneous lymph node syndrome). Am J Ophthalmol 93:713, 1982.

14. Haynes BF, Fishman ML, Fauci AS, et al: The ocular manifestations of Wegener's granulomatosis: fifteen years experience and review of the literature. Am J Med 63:131, 1977.

15. Ryan LM, Kozin F, Eiferman R: Immune complex uveitis: a case. Ann Intern Med 88:62, 1978.

16. Schwartz HR, McDuffie FC, Black LF, et al: Hypocomplementemic urticarial vasculitis: association with chronic obstructive pulmonary disease. Mayo Clin Proc 57:231, 1982.

17. Regan CDJ, Foster CS: Retinal vascular diseases: clinical presentation and diagnosis. Int Ophthalmol Clin 26:25, 1986.

18. Vollertsen RS, McDonald TJ, Younge BR, et al: Cogan's syndrome: 18 cases and a review of the literature. Mayo Clin Proc 61:344, 1986.

Selected Readings

Coles RS: Ocular manifestations of connective tissue disease. Hosp Pract 20:70, 1985.
Good general review of uveitis as well as other eye findings in rheumatic diseases.

Rosenbaum JT, Cousins SW: Uveitis and arthritis: experimental models and clinical correlates. Semin Arthritis Rheum 11:383, 1982.
Proposes experimental models for the study of uveitis and arthritis and lists associated systemic diseases.

Rosenbaum JT, Nozik RA: Uveitis: many diseases, one diagnosis. Am J Med 79:545, 1985.
Concise review of diverse presentations of uveitis in arthritis syndromes.

Rosenberg AM: Uveitis associated with juvenile rheumatoid arthritis. Semin Arthritis Rheum 16:158, 1987.
Thorough review of anatomy, physiology, and immunology of uveal tract, as well as the clinical features and management of uveitis associated with juvenile rheumatoid arthritis.

62
Joint Pain and Abdominal Symptoms: Common and Uncommon Associations

Arthritis, followed by anti-inflammatory medication with subsequent gastritis, is the most common cause of joint pain and abdominal symptoms. Diagnostic possibilities include inflammatory bowel disorders, immune disorders, infections, and a few rare inherited disorders. Anti-inflammatory-induced gastritis is more common in the elderly. Inflammatory bowel diseases and systemic lupus erythematosus are more common in females.

Anti-inflammatory-induced gastritis
Inflammatory bowel disease: Ulcerative colitis,[1] Crohn's disease[2]
Systemic lupus erythematosus
Vasculitis: polyarteritis nodosa,[3] Henoch-Schönlein purpura
Pelvic inflammatory disease: gonorrhea,[4] syphilis
Acute infections: *Salmonella*,[5] meningococcemia, Rocky Mountain spotted fever, infectious mononucleosis,[6] *Yersinia* entercolitis,[7,8] acute rheumatic fever[9]
Haemophilus influenzae[10]
Hepatitis[11]
Hyperparathyroidism[12]
Scleroderma
Pancreatitis[13,14]
Hemoglobinopathies: sickle cell,[15] thalassemia minor[16]
Amebic colitis[17]
Gout: urate nephrolithiasis[18]
Bowel bypass arthritis-dermatitis syndrome
Behçet's syndrome[19]
Relapsing polychondritis[20]
Whipple's disease[21]
Familial Mediterranean fever: periodic peritonitis[22]

Porphyria[23]
Hemochromatosis[24]
Sarcoidosis[25]
Pyogenic sacroiliitis: sacroiliac joint infection can mimic the acute abdomen[26]
Collagenous colitis[27]

References

1. Greenstein AJ, Janowitz HD, Sachar DB: The extra-intestinal complications of Crohn's disease and ulcerative colitis: a study of 700 patients. Medicine 55:401, 1976.
2. Al-Hadidi S, Khatib G, Chhatwal P, et al: Granulomatous arthritis in Crohn's disease. Arthritis Rheum 27:1061, 1984.
3. Cohen RD, Conn DL, Ilstrup DM: Clinical features, prognosis, and response to treatment in polyarteritis. Mayo Clin Proc 55:146, 1980.
4. Goldman JA: Patterns of gonococcal arthritis (editorial). J Rheumatol 8:707, 1981.
5. Brodie TD, Ehresmann GR: *Salmonella dublin* arthritis: an initial case presentation. J Rheumatol 10:144, 1983.
6. Sigal LH, Steere AC, Niederman JC: Symmetric polyarthritis associated with heterophile-negative infectious mononucleosis. Arthritis Rheum 26:553, 1983.
7. Bernstein RM, Mackworth-Young CG, Saverymutu SH, et al: *Yersinia* athritis: demonstration of occult enteritis by [111]indium leucocyte scanning. Ann Rheum Dis 43:493, 1984.
8. Feeney GF, Kerlin P, Sampson JA: Clinical aspects of infection with *Yersinia enterocolitica* in adults. Aust NZ J Med 17:216, 1987.
9. Lahat E, Azizi E, Eshel G, Mundel G: Recurrent abdominal and cervical pains. An unusual clinical presentation of acute rheumtic fever. Helv Paediatr Acta 41:549, 1987.
10. Borenstein DG, Simon GL: *Haemophilus influenzae* septic arthritis in adults. A report of 4 cases and review of the literature. Medicine 65:191, 1986.
11. Bayer AS: Arthritis associated with hepatitis. Clinical and pathogenetic considerations. Postgrad Med 67 (4):175, 1980.
12. Pritchard MH, Jessop JD: Chondrocalcinosis in primary hyperparathyroidism. Influence of age, metabolic bone disease, and parathyroidectomy. Ann Rheum Dis 36:146, 1977.
13. Lucas PF, Owen TK: Subcutaneous fat necrosis, "polyarthritis", and pancreatic disease. Gut 3:146, 1962.
14. Bregeon C, Sentenac P, Queinnec JY, Renier JC: Pancreatic cytosteatonecrosis. Rev Rhum Mal Osteoartic 54:129, 1987.
15. Schumacher HR, Andrews R, McLaughlin G: Arthropathy in sickle-cell disease. Ann Intern Med 78:203, 1973.
16. Gerster JC, Dardel R, Guggi S: Recurrent episodes of

arthritis in thalassemia minor. J Rheumatol 11:352, 1984.

17. Kasliwal RM: Chronic colitis and arthritis with special emphasis on amoebic colitis. Am J Proctol Gastroenterol Colon Rectal Surg 32:12, 1981.
18. Yü T: Nephrolithiasis in patients with gout. Postgrad Med 63 (5):164, 1978.
19. Thach BT, Cummings NA: Behçet syndrome with "aphthous colitis." Arch Intern Med 136:705, 1976.
20. McAdam LP, O'Hanlan MA, Bluestone R, et al: Relapsing polychondritis: prospective study of 23 patients and a review of the literature. Medicine 55:193, 1976.
21. Khan MA: Axial arthropathy in Whipple's disease. J Rheumatol 9:928, 1982.
22. Meyerhoff J: Familial Mediterranean fever: report of a large family, review of the literature, and discussion of the frequency of amyloidosis. Medicine 59:66, 1980.
23. Grossman ME, Bickers DR, Poh-Fitzpatrick MB, et al: Porphyria cutanea tarda. Clinical features and laboratory findings in 40 patients. Am J Med 67:277, 1979.
24. Askari AD, Muir WA, Rosner IA, et al: Arthritis of hemochromatosis. Clinical spectrum, relation to histocompatibility antigens, and effectiveness of early phlebotomy. Am J Med 75:957, 1983.
25. Rosenberg AM, Yee EH, MacKenzie JW: Arthritis in childhood sarcoidosis. J Rheumatol 10:987, 1983.
26. Cohn SM, Schoetz DJ Jr: Pyogenic sacroiliitis: another imitator of the acute abdomen. Surgery 100:95, 1986.
27. Wengrower D, Pollak A, Okon E, Stalnikowicz R: Collagenous colitis and rheumatoid arthritis with response to sulfasalazine. A case report and review of the literature. J Clin Gastroenterol 9:456, 1987.

Selected Readings

Hindmarsh JT: The porphyrias: recent advances. Clin Chem 32:1255, 1986.
Current concepts and recent research.

Inman RD, Hodge M, Johnston MEA, et al: Arthritis, vasculitis, and cryoglobulinemia associated with relapsing hepatitis A virus infection. Ann Intern Med 105:700, 1986.
Two patients with relapsing hepatitis A complicated by arthritis are described.

Moll JM: Inflammatory bowel disease. Clin Rheum Dis 11:87, 1985.
A review of inflammatory bowel disorders with particular emphasis on arthropathies of ulcerative colitis and Crohn's disease.

Pease C, Keat A: Arthritis as the main or only symptom of hepatitis B infection. Postgrad Med J 61:545, 1985.
Three patients with hepatitis B who presented with severe joint pain are discussed.

Senécal JL, Oliver JM, Rothfield N: Anticytoskeletal autoantibodies in the connective tissue diseases. Arthritis Rheum 28:889, 1985.
A report of 103 patients with connective tissue diseases were studied for the presence of anticytoskeletal antibodies.

63

The Swollen Knee: Causes of Acute and Chronic Knee Effusions

The most common cause of an acutely swollen knee is trauma. Even trivial sounding trauma can result in significant knee injury by causing meniscal tears, sprains, or ligamentous instability. A knee joint effusion is not always present in a swollen knee. Less common causes of knee swelling, such as synovial cysts or bursitis, can simulate the presence of a knee effusion. In certain populations, such as the elderly, chronically ill, or immunocompromised patients, a swollen knee may be the first manifestation of a more generalized illness, such as infection or metabolic-degenerative disorder.

Causes of Acute Knee Effusions

Fractures: lipohemarthrosis
Soft tissue injuries: rule out quadriceps-patellar tendon injury
Meniscal tears[1]
Ligamentous instability: cruciate, collaterals, and combinations[2]
Postsurgical: loose prosthesis/infection[3]
Rheumatoid arthritis[4]
Osteoarthritis[5]
Septic arthritis: *Neisseria gonorrhoeae*, a frequent infectious agent[6]
Pseudogout: calcium pyrophosphate dihydrate crystal deposition
Gout
Reiter's syndrome

Psoriatic arthritis: can have significantly elevated white cell counts

Viral arthropathy: mumps, coxsackievirus, adenovirus, hepatitis[7]

Lyme arthritis: a multisystem disease transmitted by ticks[8,9]

Acute monocytic arthritis: syndrome characterized by acute polyarthritis, rash, fever, synovial fluid monocytosis, and biopsy findings similar to a hypersensitivity angiitis[10]

Ankylosing spondylitis: knee effusions more common in females with ankylosing spondylitis

Sporotrichosis arthritis: diagnosis often delayed because of absence of associated skin and lung involvement[11]

Inflammatory bowel disease

Causes of Chronic Knee Effusions

A chronically swollen knee raises a wide spectrum of possibilities. Many degenerative, metabolic, infectious, neoplastic, and neuropathic conditions develop commonly in the knee.

Chronic stages of all causes of acute knee effusions: inflammatory arthritides

Osteochondritis dissecans: more common in children[12]

Osteoarthritis

Patellofemoral pain syndrome: anterior knee pain in young adults is a common presentation.[13,14]

Osteonecrosis: idiopathic, steroid-induced

Osgood-Schlatter's disease: more common in adolescents

Juvenile chronic arthritis[15]

Osteochondral loose bodies

Osteomyelitis: frequently associated with osteoarthritis or previous knee trauma

Chondrocalcinosis (CPPD): diseases other than pseudogout associated with CPPD: hemochromatosis, hyperparathyroidism, severe osteoarthritis, ochronosis, Wilson's disease, acromegaly, gout, and diabetes mellitus

Neoplasms: pigmented villonodular synovitis, sarcomas, giant cell tumors, and fibroma[16]

Sarcoidosis[17]

Hemophilia: hemarthrosis and musculoskeletal bleeding are the most common clinical manifestations of severe hemophilia.[18]

Hypothyroidism

Sickle-cell arthropathy

Hyperlipoproteinemia type IV: clinical findings more severe in homozygous patients than in heterozygous patients[19]

Systemic lupus erythematosus (SLE) and other collagen vascular disease: articular symptoms are most common clinical manifestation of SLE[20]

Reflex sympathetic dystrophy

Inflammatory bowel disease

Wegener's granulomatosis[21]

Chronic infections: particularly mycobacteria and fungi

References

1. Fahmy NRM, Williams EA, Noble J: Meniscal pathology and osteoarthritis of the knee. J Bone Joint Surg (Br) 65-B:24, 1983.
2. Funk FJ Jr: Osteoarthritis of the knee following ligamentous injury. Clin Orthop 172:154, 1983.
3. Pun WK, Chow SP, Chan KC, et al: Effusions in the knee in elderly patients who were operated on for fracture of the hip. J Bone Joint Surg (Am) 70:117, 1988.
4. Goldie I: A synopsis of surgery for rheumatoid arthritis (excluding the hand). Clin Orthop 191:185, 1984.
5. McDermott M, Freyne P: Osteoarthrosis in runners with knee pain. Br J Sports Med 17:84, 1983.
6. Goldenberg DL, Cohen AS: Acute infectious arthritis. A review of patients with nongonococcal joint infections (with emphasis on therapy and prognosis). Am J Med 60:369, 1976.
7. Bayer AS: Arthritis associated with common viral infections: mumps, coxsackievirus, and adenovirus. Postgrad Med 68 (1):55, 1980.
8. Mertz LE, Wobig GH, Duffy J, et al: Ticks, spirochetes, and new diagnostic tests for Lyme disease. Mayo Clin Proc 60:402, 1985.
9. Culp RW, Eichenfield AH, Davidson RS, et al: Lyme arthritis in children. An orthopaedic perspective. J Bone Joint Surg (Am) 69:96, 1987.
10. Brawer AE, Cathcart ES: Acute monocytic arthritis. Arthritis Rheum 22:294, 1979.
11. Crout JE, Brewer NG, Tompkins RB: Sporotrichosis arthritis. Ann Intern Med 86:294, 1977.
12. Hughston JC, Hergenroeder PT, Courtenay BG: Osteochondritis dissecans of the femoral condyles. J Bone Joint Surg (Am) 66-A:1340, 1984.
13. Schutzer SF, Ramsby GR, Fulkerson JP: Computed tomographic classification of patellofemoral pain patients. Orthop Clin North Am 17:235, 1986.
14. Dye SF, Boll DA: Radionuclide imaging of the patellofemoral joint in young adults with anterior knee pain. Orthop Clin North Am 17:249, 1986.

15. Pettersson H, Rydholm U: Radiologic classification of knee joint destruction in juvenile chronic arthritis. Pediatr Radiol 14:419, 1984.
16. Ogata K, Ushijima M: Tenosynovial fibroma arising from the posterior cruciate ligament. Clin Orthop 215:153, 1987.
17. Kaplan H: Sarcoid arthritis. A review. Arch Intern Med 112:924, 1963.
18. Soreff J: Joint debridement in the treatment of advanced hemophilic knee arthropathy. Clin Orthop 191:179, 1984.
19. Buckingham RB, Bole GG, Bassett DR: Polyarthritis associated with type IV hyperlipoproteinemia. Arch Intern Med 135:286, 1975.
20. Labowitz R, Schumacher HR Jr: Articular manifestations of systemic lupus erythematosus. Ann Intern Med 74:911, 1971.
21. Noritake DT, Weiner SR, Bassett LW, et al: Rheumatic manifestations of Wegener's granulomatosis. J Rheumatol 14:949, 1987.

Selected Readings

Burk DL Jr, Kanal E, Brunberg JA, et al: 1.5-T surface-coil MRI of the knee. AJR 147:293, 1986.
MRI studies of normal knees were compared with 20 knees with suspected menisci or articular surface pathology. Authors conclude that although MRI is useful in studying the integrity of articular cartilage and in detecting gross arthritic cartilage lesions, it is still less sensitive than arthroscopy in evaluating moderate changes in hyaline cartilage.

Insall JN (ed): Surgery of the Knee. 1st Ed. Churchill Livingstone, New York, 1984.
A comprehensive work written by authorities in the field, which covers most of the advances in the knowledge of knee joint biomechanics, diagnostic methods, and surgical management.

Li KC, Henkelman RM, Poon PY, et al: MR imaging of the normal knee. J Comput Assist Tomogr 8:1147, 1984.
MRI is particularly helpful in visualizing menisci and cruciate ligaments without the use of contrast agents.

Reicher MA, Hartzman S, Bassett LW, et al: MR imaging of the knee Part 1. Traumatic disorders. Radiology 162:547, 1987.
One hundred thirty patients with knee joint injuries were evaluated with high-resolution MRI. Authors report a high accuracy of identification of suspected meniscal and ligament tears, and patellar tendon injuries.

Sartoris DJ, Guerra J Jr, Mattrey RF, et al: Perfluoroctylbromide as a contrast agent for computed tomographic imaging of septic and aseptic arthritis. Invest Radiol 21:49, 1986.
Perfluoroctylbromide (PFOB) was added to CT imaging of septic and aseptic arthritis animal models. Results suggest PFOB and CT imaging may provide a useful technique for distinguishing sterile from septic arthritis.

Schwimmer M, Edelstein G, Heiken JP, et al: Synovial cysts of the knee: CT evaluation. Radiology 154:175, 1985.

This study found CT useful in evaluating atypical synovial cysts and cysts that were difficult to define with arthroscopy.

Sternbach GL: Evaluation of the knee. J Emerg Med 4:133, 1986.

Author outlines current clinical concepts in acute care of the traumatic knee. The basic physical examination of the knee joint is reviewed, as well as indications for joint aspiration and radiographic studies.

Zarins B, Adams M: Knee injuries in sports. N Engl J Med 318:950, 1988.

A comprehensive, well-referenced review of current concepts of pathophysiology, evaluation, and management of knee injuries.

64

Crystals and Other Refractile Elements in Synovial Fluid: Pathologic Associations and Refractile Artifacts*

Synovial fluid analysis is critical in the evaluation of undiagnosed arthropathy. Crystals and other refractile elements can provide significant diagnostic clues to the cause of acute or chronic arthritis or be only incidental or artifactual findings. It is clinically helpful to understand and categorize some optical characteristics of joint fluid refractile elements, such as positive and negative elongation, less correctly referred to as positive or negative birefringence. As per Gatter,[1] two optic terms are essential, but often

* (Adapted from Gatter,[1] with permission.)

misused in crystal analysis: (1) birefringence is the quality of splitting incident light into two refracted rays, that vibrate at different angles; (2) elongation is the process of determining the optic sign as being positive or negative, depending on the color of the crystal when its long axis is parallel to the orienting line of the compensator, i.e., positive elongation when the crystal is blue in this position or negative elongation when it is yellow in this position.

Crystals and Refractile Elements with Pathologic Associations

Monosodium urate monohydrate crystals: strong negative elongation, usually needle-shaped, and are diagnostic for gout. (Urate may also appear as symmetric spheres.[2])

Calcium pyrophosphate dihydrate (CPPD) crystals: weak positive elongation, rod or rhomboid shape and are diagnostic for pseudogout, also are commonly associated with osteoarthritis[3,4]

Hydroxyapatite crystals: may be missed by light microscopy, may be better identified by scanning electron microscopy or alizarin red S staining[5] and have been associated with osteoarthritis,[3,4] Milwaukee shoulder syndrome with rotator cuff tears,[6] calcific tendonitis,[7] and erosive polyarticular arthropathy[8]

Cholesterol crystals: variable elongation and shape, most commonly associated with rheumatoid arthritis; however, chylous synovial effusions are also associated with rheumatoid arthritis, systemic lupus erythematosus, filariasis, pancreatitis, and trauma.[9]

Lipid: "Maltese cross"-appearing lipid microspherules, or lipid liquid crystals, are associated with acute inflammatory arthritis in a few reports.[10–12] Larger lipid droplets may indicate intra-articular trauma.[9]

Calcium oxalate crystals: positive elongation and variable shape; seen in patients on hemodialysis with clinical manifestations that can mimic gout, pseudogout, or apatite deposition disease[13]

Calcium hydrogen phosphate dihydrate crystals: rod-shaped with strong birefringence and positive elongation and may be involved in acute arthritis[14]

Cryoprotein: can occur with erosive arthritis and tenosynovitis[15]

Amyloid: occurs with primary amyloidosis or chronic hemodialysis patients[16,17]

Thorns: plant thorns embedded in synovial tissue

have varying fragmented shapes with birefringence and may lead to synovitis.[18]

Charcot-Leyden crystals: hexagonal bipyramid crystals with positive elongation have been described in acute monoarticular arthritis with associated eosinophilia of synovial fluid.[19,20]

Refractile Artifacts

Several artifacts seen in synovial fluid are refractile and should be identified as nonpathologic entities.

Calcium oxalate crystals: can form in synovial fluid placed in test tube containing oxalate as an anticoagulant

Lithium heparin crystals: appear as small variable-shaped crystals with positive elongation when lithium heparin is used as anticoagulant in test tubes[21]

Corticosteroid crystals: the morphologic and elongation properties of corticosteroid crystals vary with the specific preparation. Steroid crystals occasionally produce transient clinical synovitis and may be present for weeks or months after intra-articular injection.[22]

Prosthetic debris: fragments of polymethylemethacrylate and polyethylene are birefringent and have been found in synovial biopsies of patients after total joint replacement[23]

Talc: from surgical gloves may appear as bright Maltese crosses[1]

Nail polish: used to seal cover slips; can result in large number of bright rods with positive elongation at the cover-slip margin[1]

Immersion oil: may contain crystals of varying sizes and shapes with positive elongation, but will be eliminated as source of confusion if the microscope is focused on the proper plane of the slide[1]

Dust and fibers: from lens paper; are irregularly shaped with branching structure and are birefringent[1]

References:

1. Gatter R: A Practical Handbook of Joint Fluid Analysis. pp. 31,81. Lea & Febiger, Philadelphia, 1984.
2. Fiechtner JJ, Simkin PA: Urate spherulites in gouty synovia. JAMA 245:1533, 1981.
3. Gibilisco PA, Schumacher HR Jr, Hollander JL, et al: Synovial fluid crystals in osteoarthritis. Arthritis Rheum 28:511, 1985.

4. Halverson PB, McCarty DJ: Patterns of radiographic abnormalities associated with basic calcium phosphate and calcium pyrophosphate dihydrate crystal deposition in the knee. Ann Rheum Dis 45:603, 1986.
5. Paul H, Reginato AJ, Schumacher HR: Alizarin red S staining as a screening test to detect calcium compounds in synovial fluid. Arthritis Rheum 26:191, 1983.
6. McCarty DJ, Halverson PB, Carrera GF, et al: "Milwaukee shoulder"—association of microspheroids containing hydroxyapatite crystals, active collagenase, and neutral protease with rotator cuff defects. I. Clinical aspects. Arthritis Rheum 24:464, 1981.
7. Faure G, Daculsi G: Calcified tendinitis: a review. Ann Rheum Dis 42(Suppl 49):50, 1983.
8. Schumacher HR, Miller JL, Ludivico C, Jessar RA: Erosive arthritis associated with apatite crystal deposition. Arthritis Rheum 24:31, 1981.
9. Wise CM, White RE, Agudelo CA: Synovial fluid lipid abnormalities in various disease states: review and classification. Semin Arthritis Rheum 16:222, 1987.
10. Weinstein J: Synovial fluid leukocytosis associated with intracellular lipid inclusions. Arch Intern Med 140:560, 1980.
11. Schlesinger PA, Stillman MT, Peterson L: Polyarthritis with birefringent lipid within synovial fluid macrophages: case report and ultrastructural study. Arthritis Rheum 25:1365, 1982.
12. Trostle DC, Schumacher HR Jr, Medsger TA Jr, et al: Lipid microspherule-associated acute monarticular arthritis. Arthritis Rheum 29:1166, 1986.
13. Reginato AJ, Ferreio Seoane JL, Barbazan Alvarez C, et al: Arthropathy and cutaneous calcinosis in hemodialysis oxalosis. Arthritis Rheum 29:1387, 1986.
14. Utsinger PD: Dicalcium phosphate deposition disease; a suspected new crystal-induced arthritis. Presented 14th International Congress of Rheumatology, San Francisco, June 1977.
15. Langlands DR, Dawkins RL, Matz LR, et al: Arthritis associated with a crystallizing cryoprecipitable IgG paraprotein. Am J Med 68:461, 1980.
16. Lakhanpal S, Li CY, Gertz MA, et al: Synovial fluid analysis for diagnosis of amyloid arthropathy. Arthritis Rheum 30:419, 1987.
17. Munoz-Gomez J, Bergada-Barado E, Gomez-Perez R, et al: Amyloid arthropathy in patients undergoing periodical haemodialysis for chronic renal failure: a new complication. Ann Rheum Dis 44:729, 1985.
18. Sugarman M, Stobie DG, Quismorio FP, et al: Plant thorn synovitis. Arthritis Rheum 20:1125, 1977.
19. Menard HA, de Medicis R, Lussier A, et al: Charcot-Leyden crystals in synovial fluid (letter). Arthritis Rheum 24:1591, 1981.
20. Dougados M, Benhamou L, Amor B: Charcot-Leyden crystals in synovial fluid (letter). Arthritis Rheum 26:1416, 1983.
21. Tanphaichitr K, Spilberg I, Hahn BH: Lithium heparin crystals simulating CPPD crystals (letter). Arthritis Rheum 19:966, 1976.
22. Kahn CB, Hollander JL, Schumacher HR: Corticosteroid crystals in synovial fluid. JAMA 211:807, 1970.

23. Crugnola A, Schiller A, Radin E: Polymeric debris in synovium after total joint replacement: histological identification. J Bone Joint Surg 59A:860, 1977.

Selected Readings

Gatter RA: A Practical Handbook of Joint Fluid Analysis. Lea & Febiger, Philadelphia, 1984.
Most comprehensive source of information on synovial fluid and its analysis. It includes color plates and photographs, as well as technical notes on optics, techniques of joint aspiration, and the clinical significance of joint fluid findings.

Gatter RA: Use of the compensated polarizing microscope. Clinics Rheum Dis 3:91, 1977.
Concise review of important information needed to analyze joint fluid using polarized light.

Kahn CB, Hollander JL, Schumacher HR: Corticosteroid crystals in synovial fluid. JAMA 211:807, 1970.
Includes descriptions and photographs of crystals of five corticosteroid esters used in joint injections.

Paul H, Reginato AJ, Schumacher HR: Alizarin red S staining as a screening test to detect calcium compounds in synovial fluid. Arthritis Rheum 26:191, 1983.
Describes a simple, rapid screening test to detect microcrystalline calcium salts on wet drop preparations of synovial fluid using alizarin red S stain and light microscopy.

Platt PN: Examination of synovial fluid. Clinics Rheum Dis 9:51, 1983.
Good general review article.

Wise CM, White RE, Agudelo CA: Synovial fluid lipid abnormalities in various disease states: review and classification. Semin Arthritis Rheum 16:222, 1987.
Review and discussion of synovial fluid lipid abnormalities

65

Neuropathic or Charcot Joints: Conditions Associated with Charcot Joints

In 1868, Jean Charcot described anesthetic joints susceptible to repeated injury in patients with tabes dorsalis.[1] Neuropathic or Charcot joints currently refer to joint changes associated with many diseases involving the spinal cord and peripheral nerves and are thought to be secondary to repeated mechanical trauma associated with loss of pain.[2]

Tabes dorsalis[3,4]
Diabetes mellitus[5,6]
Syringomyelia[7,8]
Spina bifida with meningomyelocele[9]
Nerve injury secondary to mass effect or trauma[10]
Spinal cord injury[11,12]
Steroid intra-articular injections[13]
Familial peripheral neuropathy
Dejerine-Sottas disease: familial interstitial hypertrophic polyneuropathy
Hereditary sensory neuropathy[14]
Charcot-Marie-Tooth disease (CMT): peroneal muscular atrophy
Toxic peripheral neuropathies: arsenic, lead, and selenium
Riley-Day syndrome: familial dysautonomia[15]
Pernicious anemia: combined systems degeneration[16]
Congenital insensitivity to pain[17]
Pituitary gigantism[18]
Leprosy[19]
Familial amyloid polyneuropathy[20]
Juvenile rheumatoid arthritis[21]
Calcium pyrophosphate dihydrate deposition disease (CPPD)[22]
Dialysis[23]

References

1. Bruckner FE, Howell A: Neuropathic joints. Semin Arthritis Rheum 2:47, 1972.
2. Brower AC, Allman RM: The neuropathic joint: a neurovascular bone disorder. Radiol Clin North Am 19:571, 1981.
3. Pomeranz MM, Rothberg AS: A review of 58 cases of tabetic arthropathy. Am J Syphilis 25:103, 1941.
4. Fishel B, Dan M, Yedwab M, et al: Multiple neuropathic arthropathy in a patient with syphilis. Clin Rheum 4:348, 1985.
5. Raju UB, Fine G, Partamian JO: Neuropathic neuroarthropathy (Charcot's joint). Arch Pathol Lab Med 106:349, 1982.
6. Reiner M, Scurran BL, Karlin JM, Silvani SH: The neuropathic joint in diabetes mellitus. Clin Podiatr Med Surg 5:421, 1988.
7. Williams B: Orthopaedic features in the presentation of syringomyelia. J Bone Joint Surg (Br) 61-B:314, 1979.
8. Rhoades CE, Neff JR, Rengachary SS, et al: Diagnosis of post-traumatic syringohydromyelia presenting as neuropathic joints. Clin Orthop 180:182, 1983.
9. Carr TL: The orthopaedic aspects of one hundred cases of spina bifida. Postgrad Med J 32:201, 1956.
10. Johnson JTH: Neuropathic fractures and joint injuries. J Bone Joint Surg (Am) 49-A:1, 1967.
11. Crim JR, Bassett LW, Gold RH, et al: Spinal neuroarthropathy after traumatic paraplegia. AJNR 9:359, 1988.
12. Foderaro AE, el-Khoury GY, Hingtgen WL, et al: General case of the day. Neuropathic arthropathy of the thoracic spine (T8–T9). Radiographics 7:395, 1987.
13. Chandler GN, Jones DT, Wright V, et al: Charcot's arthropathy following intra-articular hydrocortisone. Br Med J 1:952, 1959.
14. Dyck PJ, Stevens JC, O'Brien PC, et al: Neurogenic arthropathy and recurring fractures with subclinical inherited neuropathy. Neurology 33:357, 1983.
15. Brunt PW: Unusual cause of Charcot joints in early adolescence (Riley-Day syndrome). Br Med J 4:277, 1967.
16. Halonen PI, Jarvinen KAJ: On the occurrence of neuropathic arthropathies in pernicious anaemia. Ann Rheum Dis 7:152, 1948.
17. Greider TD: Orthopedic aspects of congenital insensitivity to pain. Clin Orthop 172:177, 1983.
18. Daughaday WH: Extreme gigantism. Analysis of growth velocity and occurrence of severe peripheral neuropathy and neuropathic arthropathy (Charcot joints). N Engl J Med 297:1267, 1977.
19. Faget GH, Mayoral A: Bone changes in leprosy: a clinical and roentgenologic study of 505 patients. Radiology 42:1, 1944.
20. Pruzanski W, Baron M, Shupak R: Neuroarthropathy (Charcot joints) in familial amyloid polyneuropathy. J Rheumatol 8:477, 1981.
21. Rothschild BM, Hanissian AS: Severe generalized (Charcot-like) joint destruction in juvenile rheumatoid arthritis. Clin Orthop 155:75, 1981.

22. Helms CA, Chapman GS, Wild JH: Charcot-like joints in calcium pyrophosphate dihydrate deposition disease. Skeletal Radiol 7:55, 1981.
23. Meneghello A, Bertoli M: Neuropathic arthropathy (Charcot's joint) in dialysis patients. ROFO 141:180, 1984.

Selected Readings

Bruckner FE, Howell A: Neuropathic joints. Semin Arthritis Rheum 1:47, 1972.
An extensive review of neuropathic joints.

Fahr LM, Sauser DD: Imaging of peripheral nerve lesions. Orthop Clin North Am 19:27, 1988.
Imaging of peripheral nerve lesions is possible with MRI technology. A discussion of current abilities of CT, ultrasound, and MRI technology in evaluating peripheral nerves in trauma, nerve entrapment syndromes, and tumors.

66
Amyloidosis: Common and Uncommon Presentations

Amyloidosis is a disease complex that results in the extracellular deposition of insoluble fibrillar protein materials that is Congo red-sensitive.[1] Amyloid deposits can occur in various organs and tissues throughout the body as systemic disease or be manifested in a localized area at one specific site. The classification of amyloidosis is based on the structure of various amyloid fibrils and clinical syndromes. One classification scheme includes seven categories of amyloidosis: (1) primary or myeloma-associated form with light chain protein (AL); (2) secondary form, which occurs as response to underlying inflammatory or infectious disease with amyloid A protein (AA); (3) familial form, which has been described in several kinships throughout the world (AF); (4) endocrine tissue-related form, especially associated with medullary carcinoma of the thyroid (AE); (5) senile amyloidosis with cardiac, brain, and other organ involvement (AS); (6) cutaneous form (AD); and (7) hemodialysis-associated form (AH).[2] Amyloidosis can present withspread systemic findings or be limited to one organ system.

Common Presentations

Systemic Features

Weakness and fatigue: initial symptoms in up to 50% of patients with AL amyloidosis[3]

Weight loss: common presenting symptom in AL disease; the amount of weight loss may be striking[3]

Throat Features

Hoarseness or voice change: may be initial symptom in AL amyloidosis[3]

Cardiovascular or Respiratory Features

Amyloid infiltration of the heart is the leading cause of death in AL amyloidosis, but less often the cause of death in the AA form.[4]

Congestive heart failure: occurs in 25 to 35% of cases of AL amyloidosis and is typically a low output state that mimics constrictive pericarditis or restrictive cardiomyopathy[1,3,4]

Electrocardiogram abnormalities: include low voltage QRS complexes in the limb leads or "pseudoinfarct" patterns[4]

Arrhythmias or conduction disorders: patients with cardiac amyloidosis can be especially sensitive to digitalis[5]

Dyspnea: may be secondary to congestive heart failure or diffuse amyloid deposition within the respiratory tract[3]

Gastrointestinal Features

Macroglossia: may be severe enough to interfere with eating or cause sleep apnea[3,6]

Hepatomegaly: usually associated with only mild abnormalities of hepatic function[3]

Diarrhea: may be secondary to autonomic dysfunction rather than amyloid deposition[7]

Renal Features

Proteinuria or nephrotic syndrome: nonselective proteinuria is present at time of diagnosis in approximately 80% of patients with AL amyloidosis; may be severe enough to produce a nephrotic syndrome[3]

Nervous System Features

Autonomic dysfunction
Peripheral neuropathy: present in approximately 15% of cases of AL amyloidosis, but may be most prominent symptom in cases of AF amyloidosis[8]
Carpal tunnel syndrome: often bilateral; the combination of carpal tunnel syndrome and an arthropathy in a patient with multiple myeloma strongly suggests a diagnosis of amyloidosis[3,9]

Features in Skin and Extremities

Purpura and ecchymosis: intracutaneous bleeding is common and frequently involves the neck and face[3]
Edema: common finding[3]

Uncommon Presentations

Amyloidosis has been associated with many presentations that occur less commonly and may be rare or unusual.

Eye, Ear or Mouth Features

Visual loss: results from amyloid-induced vitreous opacities and may occur in AL or AF forms[10,11]
Scalloped pupils: bilateral irregular pupillary margins and fringed edges have rarely been seen in familial amyloidosis.[12]
Proptosis and ophthalmoplegia[13,14]
Glaucoma[15]
External auditory canal occlusion: may occlude bilateral external canals[3]
Sicca syndrome[16]
Ageusia: loss of taste may precede macroglossia[17]

Oral cavity lesions: recurrent hemorrhagic bullae,[3] swelling in the floor of the mouth, or a papular lesion on tongue and buccal mucosa[18]

Jaw claudication: may be associated with other ischemic vascular symptoms[19]

Breast Features

Breast mass: due to predilection of amyloid deposits for adipose tissue, differential diagnosis of multiple nontender, nonmalignant breast masses should include amyloidosis[20]

Cardiovascular Features

Myocardial infarction: amyloid deposition sometimes occurs in the coronary arteries[21]

Myocardial rupture[22]

Pericardial disease: amyloidosis limited to pericardium is rare[6,23]

Hypertension: associated with long-standing renal amyloidosis[3]

Claudication[19]

Respiratory Features

Respiratory amyloidosis occurs in three characteristic forms: tracheobronchial, nodular, and diffuse parenchymal and may be associated with systemic or localized amyloidosis.[24]

Hemoptysis: most frequent complaint in tracheobronchial form of respiratory amyloidosis[24]

Tracheobronchopathia osteoplastica: characterized by nodular or diffuse ossification of tracheobronchial mucosa[24]

Pulmonary nodules: nodular amyloidosis in lung may result in solitary nodule, but more commonly in multiple nodules[24]

Diffuse lung disease: when radiographic changes are evident, usually associated with cough and dyspnea[24]

Gastrointestinal Features

Involvement of the gastrointestinal (GI) tract is common in AL amyloidosis and often is asymptomatic, but widespread dysfunction may occur.[25]

Dysmotility: may occur in any location in GI tract and may be due to autonomic dysfunction or effects of amyloid on smooth muscle.[7]

Dysphagia: amyloid deposition in the esophagus may result in dysphagia[26]

Malabsorption[3]

Achlorhydria or vitamin B_{12} deficiency: rarely occur[27]

Gastrointestinal bleeding: caused by amyloid infiltration of blood vessels and can lead to severe blood loss from any site in the GI tract[28]

Gastric mass: amyloidosis of stomach may mimic carcinoma of stomach as a mass or absence of rugal patterns and decreased motility[3]

Intestinal obstruction: apparent mechanical obstruction in amyloidosis may actually be pseudo-obstruction[29]

Intestinal infarction or perforation[30]

Rectal mass: may resemble rectal carcinoma[31]

Intrahepatic cholestasis: can occur with AL[32]

Ascites[33]

Portal hypertension[34]

Splenomegaly: initial finding in less than 5% of AL cases[3]

Functional hyposplenism: results in Howell-Jolly bodies on peripheral blood smear[35]

Splenic rupture[36]

Urinary Tract Features

Hematuria: usually due to amyloid deposition in lower urinary tract[27]

Ureteral obstruction[23]

Nervous System Features

Intracerebral hematoma: cerebral amyloid angiopathy occurs in hereditary and nonhereditary form, not associated with systemic amyloidosis, but accounts for 5 to 10% of primary nontraumatic brain hemorrhages[37]

Paraplegia: spinal cord compresssion by amyloid tissue[38]

Adie's pupil: sluggish pupillary action[6]

Anal incontinence[6]

Endocrine Features

Panhypopituitarism[39]

Thyroid mass: thyroid enlargement may be rapid and may lead to thyroid dysfunction.[1,3] Focal amyloid deposits are characteristically found in medullary carcinoma.

Addison's disease[40]

Diabetes insipidus: nephrogenic form[27]

Musculoskeletal Features	The three patterns of amyloid involvement in the musculoskeletal system are synovial articular form, diffuse marrow infiltration, and localized amyloidosis of bone.[41]

Arthropathy: AL amyloid arthropathy is relatively noninflammatory with frequent symmetric involvement of shoulders, wrists, knees, and fingers and may be associated with subcutaneous nodules; thus mimicking rheumatoid arthritis.[5,42]

Shoulder arthropathy ("shoulder pad sign"): shoulder joints are often swollen, firm, and nontender with massive amyloid accummulation in the glenohumeral joints, pathognomonic for amyloidosis.[43]

Osteoporosis: may lead to painful compression fractures[41]

Osteolytic lesions: localized amyloidosis of bone is rare.[44]

Pseudohypertrophy of skeletal muscles: amyloid infiltration of muscles may lead to enlargement of skeletal muscles, giving them a firm, "wooden" consistency and be associated with stiffness and weakness.[45]

Myopathy[46]

Lymphatic and Hematologic

Lymphadenopathy: generalized, hilar and mediastinal adenopathy have been described rarely.[3,24]

Acquired deficiency of coagulation factors: factor X deficiency or occasionally factor IX deficiency may result in hemorrhagic complications[47]

Dermal Features

Amyloid deposits occur frequently in the skin in AL amyloidosis, but very rarely in AA forms. There are also several localized types of cutaneous amyloidosis that are virtually never associated with systemic disease.[48]

Cutaneous lesions: most commonly in AL amyloidosis, the lesions are nonpruritic, yellow, waxy papules that typically involve the face, scalp, neck, and especially the eyelids.[48]

Scleroderma-like skin: the skin becomes thick and tightened and can mimic scleroderma.[49]
Postproctoscopic periorbital purpura[50]

References

1. Scott PP, Scott WW Jr, Siegelman SS: Amyloidosis: an overview. Semin Roentgenol 21:103, 1986.
2. Cohen AS, Connors LH: The pathogenesis and biochemistry of amyloidosis. J Pathol 151:1, 1987.
3. Kyle RA, Greipp PR: Amyloidosis (AL): clinical and laboratory features in 229 cases. Mayo Clin Proc 58:665, 1983.
4. Smith TJ, Kyle RA, Lie JT: Clinical significance of histopathologic patterns of cardiac amyloidosis. Mayo Clin Proc 59:547, 1984.
5. Glenner GG: Amyloid deposits and amyloidosis: the beta-fibrilloses (second of two parts). N Engl J Med 302:1333, 1980.
6. Cohen AS: An update of clinical, pathologic, and biochemical aspects of amyloidosis. Int J Dermatol 20:515, 1981.
7. Battle WM, Rubin MR, Cohen S, et al: Gastrointestinal-motility dysfunction in amyloidosis. N Engl J Med 301:24, 1979.
8. Kyle RA: Amyloidosis. Clin Haematol 11:151, 1982.
9. Hickling P, Wilkins M, Newman GR, et al: A study of amyloid arthropathy in multiple myeloma. Q J Med 50:417, 1981.
10. Hitchings RA, Tripathi RC: Vitreous opacities in primary amyloid disease: a clinical, histochemical, and ultrastructural report. Br J Ophthalmol 60:41, 1976.
11. Benson MD, Wallace MR, Tejada E, et al: Hereditary amyloidosis: description of a new American kindred with late onset cardiomyopathy. Appalachian amyloid. Arthritis Rheum 30:195, 1987.
12. Rubinow A, Cohen AS: Scalloped pupils in familial amyloid polyneuropathy. Arthritis Rheum 29:445, 1986.
13. Knowles DM II, Jakobiec FA, Rosen M, et al: Amyloidosis of the orbit and adnexae. Surv Ophthalmol 19:367, 1975.
14. Raflo GT, Farrell TA, Sioussat RS: Complete ophthalmoplegia secondary to amyloidosis associated with multiple myeloma. Am J Opthalmol 92:221, 1981.
15. O'Doherty DP, Neoptolemos JP, Wood KF: Place of surgery in the management of amyloid disease. Br J Surg 74:83, 1987.
16. Simon BG, Moutsopoulos HM: Primary amyloidosis resembling sicca syndrome. Arthritis Rheum 22:932, 1979.
17. Ujike H, Yamamoto M, Hara I: Taste loss as an initial symptom of primary amyloidosis (letter). J Neurol Neurosurg Psychiatry 50:111, 1987.
18. Flick WG, Lawrence FR: Oral amyloidosis as initial symptom of multiple myeloma: a case report. Oral Surg Oral Med Oral Pathol 49:18, 1980.

19. Gertz MA, Kyle RA, Griffing WL: Jaw claudication in primary systemic amyloidosis. Medicine 65:173, 1986.
20. O'Connor CR, Rubinow A, Cohen AS: Primary (AL) amyloidosis as a cause of breast masses. Am J Med 77:981, 1984.
21. Barth RF, Willerson JT, Buja LM, et al: Amyloid coronary artery disease, primary systemic amyloidosis and paraproteinemia. Arch Intern Med 126:627, 1970.
22. Lindberg J: Rupture of the right ventricle of the heart in a case of advanced heart amyloidosis. Acta Pathol Microbiol Scand 79:53, 1971.
23. Weinrauch LA, Desautels RE, Christlieb AR, et al: Amyloid deposition in serosal membranes: its occurrence with cardiac temponade, bilateral ureteral obstruction, and gastrointestinal bleeding. Arch Intern Med 144:630, 1984.
24. Gross BH, Felson B, Birnberg FA: The respiratory tract in amyloidosis and the plasma cell dyscrasias. Semin Roentgenol 21:113, 1986.
25. Gilat T, Spiro HM: Amyloidosis and the gut. Am J Dig Dis 13:619, 1968.
26. Rubinow A, Burakoff R, Cohen AS, et al: Esophageal manometry in systemic amyloidosis: a study of 30 patients. Am J Med 75:951, 1983.
27. Havlir D, Tierney LM Jr: Biochemical and clinical aspects of amyloidosis. West J Med 147:65, 1987.
28. Yood RA, Skinner M, Rubinow A, et al: Bleeding manifestations in 100 patients with amyloidosis. JAMA 249:1322, 1983.
29. Legge DA, Wollaeger EE, Carlson HC: Intestinal pseudo-obstruction in systemic amyloidosis. Gut 11:764, 1970.
30. Akbarian M, Fenton J: Perforation of small bowel in amyloidosis. Arch Intern Med 114:815, 1964.
31. Williamson RCN: Primary amyloidosis of the rectum. Proc R Soc Med 65:74, 1972.
32. Rubinow A, Koff RS, Cohen AS: Severe intrahepatic cholestasis in primary amyloidosis. A report of four cases and a review of the literature. Am J Med 64:937, 1978.
33. Gregg JA, Herskovic T, Bartholomew LG: Ascites in systemic amyloidosis. Arch Intern Med 116:605, 1965.
34. Kapp JP: Hepatic amyloidosis with portal hypertension. JAMA 191:497, 1965.
35. Gertz MA, Kyle RA, Greipp PR: Hyposplenism in primary systemic amyloidosis. Ann Intern Med 98:475, 1983.
36. Polliack A, Hershko C: Spontaneous rupture of the spleen in amyloidosis. Israel J Med Sci 8:57, 1972.
37. Vinters HV: Cerebral amyloid angiopathy: a critical review. Stroke 18:311, 1987.
38. McAnena OJ, Feely MP, Kealy WF: Spinal cord compression by amyloid tissue. J Neurol Neurosurg Psychiatry 45:1067 1982.
39. Feinberg DH, Harlan WK: Amyloidosis of the pituitary gland linked with multiple myeloma. Pa Med 64:761, 1961.
40. Pear BL: Other organs and other amyloids. Semin Roentgenol 21:150, 1986.

41. Goldman AB, Pavlov H, Bullough P: Case report 137: primary amyloidosis involving the skeletal system. Skeletal Radiol 6:69, 1981.
42. Cohen AS, Canoso JJ: Rehumatological aspects of amyloid disease. Clin Rheum Dis 1;149, 1975.
43. Katz GA, Peter JB, Pearson CM, et al: The shoulder-pad sign—a diagnostic feature of amyloid arthropathy. N Engl J Med 288:354, 1973.
44. Lai KN, Chan KW, Siu DLS, et al: Pathologic hip fractures secondary to amyloidoma: case report and review of the literature. Am J Med 77:937, 1984.
45. Ringel SP, Claman HN: Amyloid-associated muscle pseudohypertrophy. Arch Neurol 39:413, 1982.
46. Bruni J, Bilbao JM, Pritzker KPH: Myopathy associated with amyloid angiopathy. Can J Neurol Sci 4:77, 1977.
47. Furie B, Voo L, McAdam KPWJ, et al: Mechanism of factor X deficiency in systemic amyloidosis. N Engl J Med 304:827, 1981.
48. Franklin EC: Amyloid and amyloidosis of the skin. J Invest Dermatol 67:451, 1976.
49. Rubinow A, Cohen AS: Skin involvement in generalized amyloidosis. Ann Intern Med 88:781, 1978.
50. Kyle RA, Bayrd ED: Amyloidosis: review of 236 cases. Medicine 54:271, 1975.

Selected Readings

Cohen AS, Connors LH: The pathogenesis and biochemistry of amyloidosis. J Pathol 151:1, 1987.
Good discussion of pathogenetic and biochemical aspects of amyloidosis with updated classification system, including systemic and localized amyloidosis.

Glenner GG: Amyloid deposits and amyloidosis: the beta-fibrilloses (second of two parts). N Engl J Med 302:1333, 1980.
General overview with classification by chemical categorization of clinicopathologic entities in amyloidosis, including discussion of systemic, organ-limited, and localized amyloidosis.

Havlir D, Tierney LM Jr: Biochemical and clinical aspects of amyloidosis. West J Med 147:65, 1987.
Concise discussion with emphasis on clinical aspects of amyloidosis.

Kyle RA: Amyloidosis. Clin Haematol 11:151, 1982.
Well-referenced discussion of all types of amyloidosis.

Kyle RA, Greipp PR: Amyloidosis (AL): Clinical and laboratory features in 229 cases. Mayo Clin Proc 58:665, 1983.
Review of AL amyloidosis, with emphasis on clinical presentation and laboratory data.

O'Doherty DP, Neoptolemos JP, Wood KF: Place of surgery in the management of amyloid disease. Br J Surg 74:83, 1987.
Review of the presentation and treatment of surgical complications of amyloidosis.

Scott PP, Scott WW Jr, Siegelman SS: Amyloidosis: an overview. Semin Roentgenol 21:103, 1986.
Concise review of the subject.

67
Subcutaneous Nodules: Disorders That Can Mimic Rheumatoid Nodules

Rheumatoid subcutaneous nodules are small (few millimeters to 2 cm), colorless, firm nodules that usually occur at pressure points, such as the extensor surface of the arms. They are found in about 20% of patients with rheumatoid arthritis and are a diagnostic criterion for this condition. Many other conditions, including rheumatologic, immunologic, dermatologic, metabolic, infiltrative, and infectious diseases, are associated with subcutaneous nodules. In many instances, these nodules can only be differentiated from rheumatoid nodules histologically. This chapter lists nodules that might be confused with rheumatoid nodules, either because of appearance, histology, location, or association with arthritis.

Rheumatologic and Immunologic Diseases

Rheumatoid arthritis[1]
Juvenile rheumatoid arthritis[2]: may histologically more closely resemble rheumatic fever nodules[3]
Rheumatoid nodulosis[4]: a syndrome consisting of rheumatoid nodules, musculoskeletal complaints, and minimal or no synovitis.
Benign rheumatoid nodules[5,6]: rheumatoid nodules (histologically) with no musculoskeletal signs or symptoms or evidence of rheumatoid arthritis; much more common in children
Palindromic rheumatism[1]: acute, recurrent attacks of arthritis with symptom-free intervals between attacks. Patients are rheumatoid-factor negative.
Rheumatic fever[7]: nodules can be differentiated histologically from rheumatoid nodules
Jaccoud's arthritis[8]
Systemic lupus erythematosus[9,10]: nodules are histologically identical to rheumatoid nodules.

Osteoarthritis (Heberden's nodes): caused by bony spurs

Tophaceous gout: aspiration or biopsy of a tophus will show negatively birefringent (urate) crystals.

Agammaglobulinemia with polyarthritis[11]: patients have polyarthritis and nodules histologically consistent with rheumatoid nodules.

Polyarteritis nodosum[12,13]: biopsy shows vasculitis. Nodules are rare in the era of immunosuppressive treatment.

Scleroderma[13]: histologically resemble rheumatoid nodules, but have no area of necrosis

Behçet's disease[13]: erythema nodosum and arthritis are common manifestations. Erythema nodosum lesions are red, painful, and only rarely somewhat nodular.

Whipple's disease[14]: biopsy shows specific diagnostic features of Whipple's disease, including macrophages laden with phagosomes.

Weber-Christian disease (nodular panniculitis)[13]: characteristic histologic findings will distinguish this entity.

Dermatologic Diseases

Granuloma annulare[15]: can be difficult to distinguish histologically from rheumatoid nodules

Erythema elevatum diutinum[16]: benign cutaneous small vessel vasculitis characterized by the appearance of red, brown, purple, or orange-yellow nodules over the acral extremities and buttocks; may be associated with arthralgias

Acrodermatitis chronica atrophicans[15]: this condition may include subcutaneous fibrous nodules near the joints along with inflammation of the extensor surfaces near the joints.

Chondrodermatitis nodularis chronica helicis: painful nodule on the upper third of the helix of the ear. Biopsy shows underlying perichondritis with fibrinoid degeneration of the cartilage.

Basal cell carcinoma[17]

Epithelioid sarcoma[18]: can be differentiated by immunohistologic stains for epithelial and hematopoietic antigens[19]

Amelanotic melanoma

Metabolic Diseases

Type II hyperlipoproteinemia (tendonous and tuberous xanthomas)[13]: xanthomas can occur over Achilles, patellar, or extensor tendons of the hands

and feet. Patients with type II hyperlipoproteinemia may have a migratory polyarthritis.[20,21]
Necrobiosis lipoidica diabeticorum[15]: can closely resemble rheumatoid nodules histologically
Tophaceous gout

Infiltrative Diseases

Multicentric reticulohistiocytosis[22,23]: nodules appear
on the dorsum of fingers, face, ears, chest, and
olecranon process. Patients have a symmetric polyarthritis, especially of the hands, which can lead
to arthritis mutilans. Biopsy of nodules or synovium
shows multinucleated giant cells.

Sarcoidosis: biopsy shows noncaseating granuloma.

Amyloidosis[24,25]: nodules can occur juxta-articularly
and are frequently associated with amyloid arthropathy.[24] Diagnosis is made by Congo red staining of
biopsy material.

Infectious Diseases

Synovial tuberculosis[26]: biopsy reveals acid-fast bacilli.

Subacute bacterial endocarditis (Osler's nodes): Osler's nodes are usually red or purple and tender.
Subacute bacterial endocarditis may be associated
with arthritis.[27]

Poststreptococcal state[28]: subcutaneous nodules have
been reported with arthritis in the absence of the
Jones' criteria for rheumatic fever.

Leprosy (Hansen's disease)[13]: erythema nodosum leprosum often results from the treatment of lepromatous leprosy. The nodules are usually red and
tender and occur on the trunk and face. A rheu-
matoid-like arthritis can coexist.[29]

Spirochetal infections[13]: syphilitic juxta-articular
gumma often occur over the extensor surface of
the ulna. Biopsy reveals treponemal organisms.
Yaws and bejel can directly invade the synovial and
perisynovial tissues and may produce subcutaneous
nodules. Pinta has also been associated with nodules.

Coccidioidomycosis[13]: one-third of pulmonary cases
are associated with joint symptoms; many patients
have erythema nodosum lesions.

Sporotrichosis[30]: arthritis and red juxta-articular
nodules about the infected joints; occasionally
occur in patients with disseminated infections

Miscellaneous Conditions

Ganglions of the hand and wrist
Foreign body reactions[26]
Chemical irritations[26]
Corticosteroid injections[31]

References

1. Kaye BR, Kaye RL, Bobrove A: Rheumatoid nodules: review of the spectrum of associated conditions and proposal of a new classification, with a report of four seronegative cases. Am J Med 76:279, 1984.
2. Calabro JJ: Other extra-articular manifestations of juvenile rheumatoid arthritis. Arthritis Rheum 20(Suppl 2):237, 1977.
3. Bywaters EGE, Cardoe N: Multiple nodules in juvenile chronic polyarthritis. Ann Rheum Dis 31:421, 1972.
4. Wisnieski JJ, Askari AD: Rheumatoid nodulosis: a relatively benign rheumatoid variant. Arch Intern Med 141:615, 1981.
5. Simons FE, Schaller JG: Benign rheumatoid nodules. Pediatrics 56:29, 1975.
6. Pye RJ, Greaves MW: Benign rheumatoid nodules of the skin. Br J Dermatol 101 (Suppl):58, 1979.
7. Benedek TG: Subcutaneous nodules and the differentiation of rheumatoid arthritis from rheumatic fever. Semin Arthritis Rheum 13:305, 1984.
8. Ruderman JE, Abruzzo JL: Chronic postrheumatic fever arthritis (Jaccoud's): report of a case with subcutaneous nodules. Arthritis Rheum 9:640, 1966.
9. Hahn BH, Yardley JH, Stevens MB: "Rheumatoid" nodules in systemic lupus erythematosus. Ann Intern Med 72:49, 1970.
10. Dubois EL, Friou GJ, Chandor S: Rheumatoid nodules and rheumatoid granulomas in systemic lupus erythematosus. JAMA 220:515, 1972.
11. Barnett EV, Winkelstein A, Weinberger HJ: Agammaglobulinemia with polyarthritis and subcutaneous nodules. Am J Med 48:40, 1970.
12. Lyell A: The cutaneous manifestations of polyarteritis nodosa. Br J Dermatol 66:335, 1954.
13. Moore CP, Willkens RF: The subcutaneous nodule: its significance in the diagnosis of rheumatic disease. Semin Arthritis Rheum 7:63, 1977.
14. Good AE, Beals TF, Simmons JL, Ibrahim MAH: A subcutaneous nodule with Whipple's disease: key to early diagnosis? Arthritis Rheum 23:856, 1980.
15. Wood MG, Beerman H: Necrobiosis lipoidica, granuloma annulare, and rheumatoid nodule. J Invest Dermatol 34:139, 1960.
16. Watt TL, Baumann RR: Pseudoxanthomatous rheumatoid nodules. Arch Dermatol 95:156, 1967.
17. Healey LA, Wilske KR, Sagebiel RW: Rheumatoid nodules simulating basal-cell carcinoma. N Engl J Med 277:7, 1967.
18. Heenan PJ, Quirk CJ, Papadimitriou JM: Epithelioid sarcoma. A diagnostic problem. Am J Dermatopathol 8:95, 1986.
19. Wick MR, Manivel JC: Epithelioid sarcoma and isolated

necrobiotic granuloma: a comparative immunocyto-chemical study. J Cutan Pathol 13:253, 1986.
20. Glueck CJ, Levy RI, Frederickson DS: Acute tendinitis and arthritis. A presenting symptom of familial type II hyperlipoproteinemia. JAMA 206:2895, 1968.
21. Khachadurian AK: Migratory polyarthritis in familial hypercholesterolemia (type II hyperlipoproteinemia). Arthritis Rheum 11:385, 1968.
22. Barrow MV, Holubar K: Multicentric reticulohistiocytosis. A review of 33 patients. Medicine 48:287, 1969.
23. Ginsburg WW, O'Duffy JD: Multicentric reticulohistiocytosis. p. 1563. In Kelley WN, Harris ED Jr, Ruddy S, Sledge CB (eds): Textbook of Rheumatology. 3rd Ed. WB Saunders, Philadelphia, 1989.
24. Wiernik PH: Amyloid joint disease. Medicine 51:465, 1972.
25. Gordon DA, Pruzanski W, Ogryzlo MA, et al: Amyloid arthritis simulating rheumatoid disease in five patients with multiple myeloma. Am J Med 55:142, 1973.
26. Gardner DL: The Pathology of Rheumatoid Arthritis. p. 122. Williams & Wilkins, Baltimore, 1972.
27. Churchill MA Jr, Geraci JE, Hunder GG: Musculoskeletal manifestations of bacterial endocarditis. Ann Intern Med 87:754, 1977.
28. Dagan B, Herman J, Kaufman B: Pseudorheumatoid subcutaneous nodules and the poststreptococcal state: a case report. Arch Intern Med 143:2316, 1983.
29. Karat AB, Karat S, Job CK, et al: Acute exudative arthritis in leprosy-rheumatoid-arthritis-like syndrome in association with erythema nodosum leprosum. Br Med J 3:770, 1967.
30. Lynch PJ, Voorhees JJ, Harrell ER: Systemic sporotrichosis. Ann Intern Med 73:23, 1970.
31. Balogh K: The histologic appearance of corticosteroid injection sites. Arch Pathol Lab Med 110:1168, 1986.

Selected Readings

Benedek TG: Subcutaneous nodules and the differentiation of rheumatoid arthritis from rheumatic fever. Semin Arthritis Rheum 13:305, 1984.
This article reviews the clinical and pathologic characteristics of rheumatoid nodules and rheumatic fever nodules, as well as their differential diagnosis.

Kaye BR, Kaye RL, Bobrove A: Rheumatoid nodules: review of the spectrum of associated conditions and proposal of a new classification, with a report of four seronegative cases. Am J Med 76:279, 1984.
Review of prevalence, characteristics, differential diagnosis, histologic features, pathogenesis, and complication of rheumatoid nodules. Also classifies rheumatoid nodules into prognostic and clinical groups.

Keil H: The rheumatic subcutaneous nodules and simulating lesions. Medicine (Baltimore) 17:261, 1938.
Classic and exhaustive review of conditions simulating rheumatic nodules.

Moore CP, Willkens RF: The subcutaneous nodule: its significance in the diagnosis of rheumatic disease. Semin Arthritis Rheum 7:63, 1977.

Review of features of almost every type of subcutaneous nodule even remotely related to rheumatology.

VII

INFECTIOUS
DISEASE

68

Fever of Unknown Origin: Common and Less Common Causes

Fever of unknown origin (FUO) is classically defined as recurrent fever of 38.3°C or greater, lasting 3 weeks or longer, and undiagnosed after 1 week of hospital evaluation.[1] Prolonged undiagnosed fever is usually an atypical manifestation of more common diseases rather than a manifestation of an exotic illnesses.[2] The three most common causes of FUO (in patients without known immune compromise) are infection, neoplasia, and diseases of autoimmunity and hypersensitivity or collagen vascular disease.

Infections Causing Fever

The most common infections are tuberculosis and subacute endocarditis, followed by hepatic and subphrenic abscesses, pyelitis, and perinephric abscesses.[3]

Systemic infections
 Tuberculosis: usually miliary,[4] increasing case reports of tuberculosis in pregnant immigrants and in human immunodeficiency virus (HIV)-infected patients[5,6]
 Subacute and chronic endocarditis
Localized infections: the intra-abdominal cavity is a common site for abscess formation, particularly after trauma, surgery, or colonic disease.
Miscellaneous visceral infections: pancreatitis, tubo-ovarian abscesses, gall bladder empyemas, pericholecystic abscesses, cholecystitis[7]
Intraperitoneal abscesses: subhepatic, subphrenic, paracolic, pelvic, appendiceal rupture with abscess
Urinary tract: pyelonephritis, renal carbuncle, perinephric abscess, prostatic abscess
Neurologic abscesses: brain, spinal cord
Dental abscesses
Osteomyelitis

495

Sinusitis
Thrombophlebitis: chronically ill, spinal cord injury[8]

Other Infectious Causes of Fever

Viral: Epstein-Barr, mononucleosis, cytomegalovirus, hepatitis, cat-scratch fever
Fungal: histoplasmosis, blastomycosis, coccidioidomycosis, candidiasis
Mycoplasma: Mycoplasma pneumonia[9]
Parasitic: toxoplasmosis, malaria, trichinosis, leishmaniasis, trypanosomiasis, amebiasis
Spirochetes: leptospira, treponema, *Borrelia* tick-bite and rat-bite fevers, syphilis[10]
Rickettsia
Chlamydia: psittacosis.
Brucellosis[11]

Neoplasms Causing Fever

Lymphoma, particularly Hodgkin's, and leukemia are common neoplastic causes of obscure fever.

Lymphoma
Leukemias: often acute leukemia with superimposed infection
Renal carcinoma: particularly hypernephroma
Osteosarcoma
Hepatic carcinoma: primary or metastatic
Pancreatic carcinoma
Carcinoma of the stomach
Cancer of the colon: may be associated with a paracolonic abscess, necrotic polyps, and unusual infections[12,13]
Leiomyoma[14]
Craniopharyngioma: may simulate chronic neutrophilic meningitis[15]
Adrenal tumors[16]

Collagen, Vascular, Autoimmune, and Hypersensitivity Diseases Causing Fever

Scleroderma
Dermatomyositis
Temporal arteritis: with or without associated polymyalgia rheumatica[17,18]
Rheumatoid arthritis
Inflammatory bowel disease: common cause in young adults
Still's disease
Vasculitis: necrotizing, allergic
Systemic lupus erythematosus

Polyarteritis nodosa
Polymyositis
Gout
Wegener's granulomatosis: often associated with sinusitis and mastoiditis
Serum sickness
Rheumatic fever
Drug fever: any drug can cause drug fever; some common offending drugs are sulfonamides, penicillins, phenytoin, iodides, antihistamines, barbiturates, ibuprofen, isoniazid, nitrofurantoin, quinidine, salicylates[19]
Erythema multiforme

Fever and Recent Travel

Malaria: malaria may be the third most common disease in the world, after the common cold and trachoma.
Typhoid fever
Amebiasis
Brucellosis
Arbovirus
Arenavirus: including the potentially contagious Lassa fever virus
Leptospirosis
See also Chapter 77

Miscellaneous and Less Common Causes of Fever

Granulomatous disease: sarcoidosis, granulomatous hepatitis
Pulmonary emboli[20]
Factitious fever[21]
Atrial myxoma: can mimic endocarditis[22,23]
Hepatitis: cirrhosis
Whipple's disease
Mediterranean fever
Porphyria
Hormonal hyperthermia: thyrotoxicosis, thyroiditis, pituitary-hypothalamic abnormalities, adrenal insufficiency, pheochromocytoma[24]
Radiation therapy
Acquired immune deficiency syndrome (AIDS): patients with AIDS can initially have lymphadenopathy, fever, and no certain source of infection.
Undiagnosed: in the majority of patients discharged without a diagnosis, fever will resolve spontaneously without subsequent serious disease development.[25]

Thyroiditis
Histiocytosis
Dissecting aortic aneurysm[26]
Kikuchi's disease: necrotizing lymphadenitis in young
patients that may mimic malignant disease[27]
Complex partial status epilepticus: fever may occur
with seizures and may rarely be the presenting
manifestation[28]
Dental infection[29,30]

References

1. Petersdorf RG, Beeson PB: Fever of unexplained origin:
report on 100 cases. Medicine 40:1, 1961.
2. Jacoby GA, Swartz MN: Fever of undetermined origin.
N Engl J Med 289:1407, 1973.
3. Demirjian ZN, Harris NL: A 78-year-old woman with
persistent fever of unknown origin. N Engl J Med
308:705, 1983.
4. Cucin RL, Coleman M, Eckardt JJ, et al: The diagnosis
of miliary tuberculosis: utility of peripheral blood abnormalities, bone marrow, and liver needle biopsy. J
Chron Dis 26:355, 1973.
5. Brar HS, Golde SH, Egan JE: Tuberculosis presenting
as puerperal fever. Obstet Gynecol 70:488, 1987.
6. Pedersen C, Nielsen JO: Tuberculosis in homosexual
men with HIV disease. Scand J Infect Dis 19:289, 1987.
7. Johnson LB: The importance of early diagnosis of acute
acalculus cholecystitis. Surg Gynecol Obstet 164:197,
1987.
8. Weingarden DS, Weingarden SI, Belen J: Thromboembolic disease presenting as fever in spinal cord injury.
Arch Phys Med Rehabil 68:176, 1987.
9. Lam K, Bayer AS: *Mycoplasma pneumoniae* as a cause of
the "fever of unknown origin" syndrome. Arch Intern
Med 142:2312, 1982.
10. Chung WM, Pien FD, Grekin JL: Syphilis: a cause of
fever of unknown origin. Cutis 31:537, 1983.
11. Rumley RL, Chapman SW: *Brucella canis:* an infectious
cause of prolonged fever of undetermined origin. South
Med J 79:626, 1986.
12. Panwalker AP: Unusual infections associated with colorectal cancer. Rev Infect Dis 10:347, 1988.
13. Kelleher JP, Sales JE: Pyrexia of unknown origin and
colorectal carcinoma. Br Med J (Clin Res) 293:1475,
1986.
14. Witt JH, Marks MI, Smith EI, et al: Leiomyoma presenting as prolonged fever, anemia, and thrombocytosis.
Cancer 52:2359, 1983.
15. Krueger DW, Larson EB: Recurrent fever of unknown
origin, coma, and meningismus due to a leaking craniopharyngioma. Am J Med 84:543, 1988.
16. Klausner JM, Nakash R, Inbar M, et al: Prolonged fever
as a presenting symptom in adrenal tumors. Oncology
45:15, 1988.
17. Calamia KT, Hunder GG: Giant cell arteritis (temporal

arteritis) presenting as fever of undetermined origin. Arthritis Rheum 24:1414, 1981.

18. Wilke WS, Wysenbeek AJ, Krall PL, et al: Masked presentation of giant-cell arteritis. Cleve Clin Q 52:155, 1985.

19. Lipsky BA, Hirschmann JV: Drug fever. JAMA 245:851, 1981.

20. Watanakunakorn C, Hayek F: High fever (greater than 39 degrees C) as a clinical manifestation of pulmonary embolism. Postgrad Med J 63 (745):951, 1987.

21. Aduan RP, Fauci AS, Dale DC, et al: Factitious fever and self-induced infection. Ann Intern Med 90:230, 1979.

22. Roeltgen DP, Weimer GR, Patterson LF: Delayed neurologic complications of left atrial myxoma. Neurology 31:8, 1981.

23. Milgalter E, Lotan H, Schuger L, et al: Cardiac myxomas—surgical experience with a multi-faceted tumor. Thorac Cardiovasc Surg 35:115, 1987.

24. Simon HB, Daniels GH: Hormonal hyperthermia. Endocrinologic causes of fever. Am J Med 66:257, 1979.

25. Esposito AL, Gleckman RA: A diagnostic approach to the adult with fever of unknown origin. Arch Intern Med 139:575, 1979.

26. Smith MA, Singer C: Fever of unknown origin: unusual presentation of dissecting aortic aneurysm. Am J Med 85:126, 1988.

27. Rudniki C, Kessler E, Zarfati M, et al: Kikuchi's necrotizing lymphadenitis: a cause of fever of unknown origin and splenomegaly. Acta Haematol 79:99, 1988.

28. Semel JD: Complex partial status epilepticus presenting as fever of unknown origin. Arch Intern Med 147:1571, 1987.

29. Samra Y, Barak S, Shaked Y: Dental infection as the cause of pyrexia of unknown origin—two case reports. Postgrad Med J 62 (732):949, 1986.

30. Huebner GR, Groat D: The role of dental disease in fever of unknown origin. Postgrad Med 79 (5):275, 1986.

Selected Readings

Bodey GP: Infection in cancer patients. A continuing association. Am J Med 81:11, 1986.
Useful review of factors predisposing to infection in patients with malignant disease. Neutropenia is the most significant predisposing factor. Gram-negative bacilli cause the majority of infections in this patient population. Fungal infections are often the cause of fevers of unknown origin in this population.

Chang JC: How to differentiate neoplastic fever from infectious fever in patients with cancer: usefulness of the naproxen test. Heart Lung 16:122, 1987.
Authors propose that the naproxen test helps diagnose etiology of fever of unknown origin in patients with cancer. Early and complete lysis of fever during naproxen therapy in this patient population would support the diagnosis of neoplasm as the source of fever.

Gleckman RA, Esposito AL: Fever of unknown origin in the elderly: diagnosis and treatment. Geriatrics 41 (3):45, 1986.

Authors offer a useful perspective for the evaluation of fever of unknown origin in the elderly. They advise against checklist evaluations and emphasize the importance of discontinuing potential fever-causing drugs.

Kauffman CA, Jones PG: Diagnosing fever of unknown origin in older patients. Geriatrics 39 (2):46, 1984.
A useful discussion that outlines common causes and a diagnostic approach to fever of unknown origin in the elderly. Authors point out that hepatic abscesses occur more frequently in the elderly, often without known source of infection, and that giant cell arteritis accounts for 16% of fever of unknown origin in elderly patients.

Keating HJ III, Klimek JJ, Levine DS, et al: Effect of aging on the clinical significance of fever in ambulatory adult patients. J Am Geriatr Soc 32:282, 1984.
A study of the effect of age on the ultimate outcome of febrile illness presenting in the ambulatory setting was prospectively carried out on 1,202 adults presenting with fever; 58.2% of patients aged 17 to 39 years had viral syndromes, otitis media, or pharyngitis. In contrast, only 4.1% of patients 60 years or older had viral syndromes. Advancing age was significantly correlated with more serious disease, higher rate of bacterial pathogen isolation, and life-threatening consequences.

Kochenour NK, Branch DW, Rote NS, Scott JR: A new postpartum syndrome associated with antiphospholipid antibodies. Obstet Gynecol 69:460, 1987.
A postpartum syndrome of pleuropulmonary disease, fever, cardiac manifestations, and antiphospholipid antibodies is described in three patients. Authors suggest that such patients with antiphospholipid antibodies are at risk for a previously unreported and serious autoimmune postpartum syndrome.

Larson EB, Featherstone HJ, Petersdorf RG: Fever of undetermined origin: diagnosis and follow-up of 105 cases, 1970–1980. Medicine 61:269, 1982.
Important review.

Marantz PR, Linzer M, Feiner CJ, et al: Inability to predict diagnosis in febrile intravenous drug abusers. Ann Intern Med 106:823, 1987.
A study to determine the predictive value of available initial clinical information in febrile intravenous drug abusers was prospectively carried out on 87 consecutive admissions involving 75 febrile intravenous drug abusers. No correlation with emergency room diagnostic predictions or clinical data was found with final diagnosis. Diagnoses made in decreasing frequency included pneumonia, trivial illness (such as viral syndrome, pharyngitis, or pyrogen reaction), endocarditis, and other conditions.

McCartney AC, Robertson MR, Piotrowicz BI, Lucie NP: Endotoxemia, fever and clinical status in immunosuppressed patients: a preliminary study. J Infect 15:201, 1987.
A prospective study to evaluate the usefulness of endotoxemic assays in neutropenic patients was carried out in a group of 10 immunocompromised patients. Endotoxemia was associated with gram-negative bacteremia, but gram-negative bacteria did not always produce endotoxemia. Raised endotoxin values were also seen with gram-positive bacteria and administration of blood products. Authors conclude that, although endotoxemic assays may clarify mechanisms of fever, they are probably of little help in routine clinical management in fever in the immunocompromised patient.

Mellors JW, Horwitz RI, Harvey MR, Horwitz SM: A

simple index to identify occult bacterial infection in adults with acute unexplained fever. Arch Intern Med 147:666, 1987.

In an attempt to develop a management strategy for patients with unexplained fever, authors studied 880 adults who presented with acute fever in an emergency room. One hundred thirty-five (15%) had unexplained fever, bacterial infection was found in 48 (35%), and bacteremia was found in 21 (44%) of 48 infected patients. The index of features predictive of occult bacterial infection includes age 50 years or older, diabetes mellitus, white blood cell count greater than or equal to 15,000/mm³, and Wintrobe erythrocyte sedimentation rate greater than or equal to 30 mm/h.

Montanaro A: Vasculitis in older patients: presentations and significance. Geriatrics 43 (3):75, 1988.

A classification system based on clinical features of vasculitic syndromes as they present in the elderly. Common, as well as unique, presentations of vasculitis in the elderly are discussed.

Nolan SM, Fitzgerald FT: Fever of unknown origin. The general internist's approach. Postgrad Med 81 (5):190, 1987.

Useful two-part clinical review of current concepts of differential diagnosis and evaluation of patients with fever of unknown origin.

Petersdorf RG: FUO. How it has changed in 20 years. Hosp Pract 20 (4):841, 1985.

Outstanding clinical review of the subject. Author points out that malignant diseases have replaced infection as a leading cause of fever of undetermined origin.

Petersdorf RG, Beeson PB: Fever of unexplained origin: report on 100 cases. Medicine 40:1, 1961.

A classic monograph.

Rodbard D: The role of regional body temperature in the pathogenesis of disease. N Engl J Med 305:808, 1981.

Still current concepts of the pathophysiology of fever.

Schmidt KG, Rasmussen JW, Srensen PG, Wedebye IM: Indium-111-granulocyte scintigraphy in the evaluation of patients with fever of undetermined origin. Scand J Infect Dis 19:339, 1987.

Authors suggest this method may prove useful in the detection of occult infections.

Smith JW: Fever of undetermined origin: not what it used to be. Am J Med Sci 292:56, 1986.

Eighty cases of fever of undetermined origin in Dallas from 1979 to 1985 were analyzed. Infectious etiologies were found in 50%. Compared to older series, viral infections were more common; however, tuberculosis and malaria were less common. Solid tumors were the most common noninfectious cause of fever in this series.

Weinstein L: Clinically benign fever of unknown origin: a personal retrospective. Rev Infect Dis 7:692, 1985.

Author defines a clinically distinct group of patients with fever of unknown origin that he considers clinically benign. An important perspective.

69
Postsurgical Fever: Causes of Postoperative Infection

Postoperative infections are usually relatively uncomplicated wound infections limited to skin or subcutaneous infection; however, postoperative infection can also result in unexpected sepsis, leading to life-threatening systemic toxicity. Despite chemoprophylaxis and improved surgical and antiseptic techniques, postoperative wound infections are a major cause of infection in hospitals. Awareness of major risk factors, commonly identified bacteria causing wound infections, and noninfectious causes of postoperative fever can help prevent, diagnose, and manage the postoperative infection.[1]

Factors Predisposing Surgical Patients to Postoperative Infections

Most postoperative infection is found in the surgical incision or postoperative body cavity. Other common sites include lungs, urinary tract, and veins used for intravenous therapy. Life-threatening sepsis can develop, particularly if postoperative conditions include certain high-risk associations with infection, such as incisional pain, visceral stasis, and colonization by potential pathogens of otherwise sterile tissue or new species supplanting otherwise normal flora.[2] Advanced age and medical disorders, which create a relatively immunocompromised state, obviously increase the risk for infection.

Dead space
Necrotic tissue
Foreign bodies: grafts,[3] prostheses,[4] shrapnel, surgical instruments
Hematoma
Preoperative trauma and contamination
Immunocompromised host: malignancy, immunodeficiency, chemotherapy, postorgan transplantation[5–8]

Diabetes mellitus and obesity[9,10]
Systemic illness
Malnutrition
Shock
Presurgical treatment with broad spectrum antibiotics
Decreased vascular perfusion: local or systemic
Prolonged preoperative hospitalization
Osteomyelitis[11]
Splenectomized patients[12,13]
Radiation-induced injury[14]

Bacteria Most Commonly Found in Postoperative Infections

The patient and operative room personnel are the primary source of wound contamination. Most surgical infections are due to multiple bacterial pathogens, most commonly a combination of aerobic and anaerobic species.[2] Gram-negative bacteria are the most common organisms following gastrointestinal tract surgery.[1]

Staphylococcus aureus and other staphylococcal species
Escherichia coli
Proteus species
Pseudomonas species

Common Noninfectious Causes of Postoperative Fever

Atelectasis: can progress to pneumonia
Phlebitis: intravascular catheter sites
Deep vein thrombosis: particularly in the lower extremities
Drug fever
Transfusion reactions
Pyoderma gangrenosum: a rare noninfectious cause of postoperative wound necrosis
Graves' disease

References

1. Nichols RL: Postoperative infections and antimicrobial prophylaxis. p. 1637. In Mandell GL, Douglas RG Jr, Bennett JE (eds): Principles and Practice of Infectious Diseases. 2nd Ed. Churchill Livingstone, New York, 1985.
2. Stone HH: Infection in postoperative patients. Am J Med 81 (S1A):39, 1986.
3. Doscher W, Krishnasastry KV, Deckoff SL: Fungal graft infections: case report and review of the literature. J Vasc Surg 6:398, 1987.
4. Koch AE: *Candida albicans* infection of a prosthetic knee replacement: a report and review of the literature. J Rheumatol 15:362, 1988.

5. Dindzans VJ, Schade RR, Van Thiel DH: Medical problems before and after transplantation. Gastroenterol Clin North Am 17:19, 1988.
6. Peterson PK, Anderson RC: Infection in renal transplant recipients. Current approaches to diagnosis, therapy, and prevention. Am J Med 81:2, 1986.
7. Charpentier B: Viral infections in renal transplant recipients: an evolutionary problem. Adv Nephrol 15:353, 1986.
8. Kusne S, Dummer JS, Singh N, et al: Infections after liver transplantation. An analysis of 101 consecutive cases. Medicine 67:132, 1988.
9. Lilienfeld DE, Vlahov D, Tenney JH, McLaughlin JS: Obesity and diabetes as risk factors for postoperative wound infections after cardiac surgery. Am J Infect Control 16:3, 1988.
10. Diamond MP, Entman SS, Salyer SL, et al: Increased risk of endometritis and wound infection after cesarean section in insulin-dependent diabetic women. Am J Obstet Gynecol 155:297, 1986.
11. Wald ER: Risk factors for osteomyelitis. Am J Med 78 (S6B):206, 1985.
12. Abdi EA, Ding JC, Cooper IA: *Nocardia* infection in splenectomized patients: case reports and a review of the literature. Postgrad Med J 63:455, 1987.
13. Mower WR, Hawkins JA, Nelson EW: Postsplenectomy infection in patients with chronic leukemia. Am J Surg 152:583, 1986.
14. Himmel PD, Hassett JM: Radiation-induced chronic arterial injury. Semin Surg Oncol 2:225, 1986.

Selected Readings

Abraham E: Immunologic mechanisms underlying sepsis in the critically ill surgical patient. Surg Clin North Am 65:991, 1985.
Article describing the range of immunologic abnormalities that follows accidental and operative trauma.

Becker GD: Identification and management of the patient at high risk for wound infection. Head Neck Surg 8:205, 1986.
Authors review experimental, clinical data and their personal experience of wound infection associated with head and neck cancer surgery. Guidelines for controlling wound infection are offered.

Brown BM, Johnson JT, Wagner RL: Etiologic factors in head and neck wound infections. Laryngoscope 97:587, 1987.
Records of 245 major head and neck surgery patients were reviewed to determine causes of wound infection that occurred in 17 patients. Factors considered major associations with infection risk included stage IV tumors, myocutaneous flap reconstructions, and probable errors in surgical technique. Authors offer a strategy to minimize postoperative infection.

Burchard KW, Barrall DT, Reed M, Slotman GJ: *Enterobacter* bacteremia in surgical patients. Surgery 100:857, 1986.
Sixty-three surgical patients with positive blood cultures for Enterobacter *were reviewed to determine clinical, epidemiologic, and*

mortality risk factors. Enterobacter *bacteremia occurred more frequently in male patients, after antibiotic therapy, with placement of central venous catheters, after gastrointestinal tract surgery, and with respiratory failure. Sputum, open skin wounds, and central venous lines were the most common portals of entry.*

Claesson BE, Holmlund DE: Predictors of intraoperative bacterial contamination and postoperative infection in elective colorectal surgery. J Hosp Infect 11:127, 1988.
A prospective study of 238 patients undergoing colorectal operations that investigated risk factors for intraoperative bacterial contamination and postoperative infection. Intraoperative infection was strongly associated with intraoperative contamination. Abdominal drains correlated with contamination, but not with infection.

Fernand R, Lee CK: Postlaminectomy disc space infection. A review of the literature and a report of three cases. Clin Orthop 209:215, 1986.
Three cases of iatrogenic postlaminectomy disc space infection are reported with a review of the literature. Most common clinical signs included recurrent pain, muscle spasm, fever, and positive straight leg raising test. Sedimentation rate is usually increased. Radioisotope and CT scans are helpful earlier because roentgenographic findings may appear weeks after initial symptoms.

Flint LM: Early postoperative acute abdominal complications. Surg Clin North Am 68:445, 1988.
Clinical discussion that highlights clinical features allowing rapid diagnosis and problems associated with decisions to reoperate for diagnosis and therapy.

Galicier C, Richet H: A prospective study of postoperative fever in a general surgery department. Infect Control 6:487, 1985.
A prospective study of 693 surgical patients was carried out to investigate the cause of postoperative fever. Only 50% of postoperative infections were associated with fever.

Garibaldi RA: Postoperative pneumonia and urinary tract infection: epidemiology and prevention. J Hosp Infect 11 (Suppl A):265, 1988.
A review of current concepts and management suggestions involving hospital-acquired pneumonias and urinary tract infections. New nonantibiotic approaches to infection control are discussed.

Garibaldi RA, Brodine S, Matsumiya S, Coleman M: Evidence for the non-infectious etiology of early postoperative fever. Infect Control 6:273, 1985.
A prospective study of infections in 871 general surgery patients identified 81 patients with unexplained postoperative fevers. Patients with unexplained early fevers tended to be younger, had less severe underlying disease, and underwent less extensive operations. Authors suggest that most of these cases were noninfectious.

Holt GR, Garner ET, McLarey D: Postoperative sequelae and complications of rhinoplasty. Otolaryngol Clin North Am 20:853, 1987.
An overview of complications of rhinoplasty. The discussion includes postoperative infection syndromes, such as localized Staphylococcus aureus *or* Pseudomonas *abscess, cavernous sinus thrombosis, basilar meningitis, postoperative toxic shock syndrome, and bacteremia.*

Hoogewoud HM, Rubli E, Terrier F, et al: The role of computerized tomography in fever, septicemia and multiple

system organ failure after laparotomy. Surg Gynecol Obstet 162:539, 1986.
Study proposing that as soon as sepsis is suspected in postlaparotomy patients, an abdominal and pelvic CT study should be performed.

Levin S, Goodman LJ: Selected overview of nongynecologic surgical intra-abdominal infections. Am J Med 79 (S5B):146, 1985.
A focused overview of nongynecologic surgical intra-abdominal infections.

Mollman HD, Haines SJ: Risk factors for postoperative neurosurgical wound infection. A case-control study. J Neurosurg 64:902, 1986.
Postoperative infection in neurosurgical patients was studied at the University of Minnesota for a 14-year period. Three major risk factors emerged: cerebrospinal fluid leak, concurrent noncentral nervous system infection, and perioperative antibiotic therapy.

Nagachinta T, Stephens M, Reitz B, Polk BF: Risk factors for surgical-wound infection following cardiac surgery. J Infect Dis 156:967, 1987.
A prospective study of 1,009 elective cardiac surgery evaluated preoperative and operative factors to determine the risk of postoperative sternal-mediastinal wound infection. Determined risk factors included reduced serum albumin, obesity, diabetes mellitus, preoperative length of hospital stay, and concurrent smoking habits.

Nelson CL: Prevention of sepsis. Clin Orthop 222:66, 1987.
Overview of current concepts of surgical technique and prophylactic management, with a focus on orthopaedic surgical problems and techniques.

Nichols RL, Smith JW, Klein DB, et al: Risk of infection after penetrating abdominal trauma. N Engl J Med 311:1065, 1984.
Discussion of risk factors for development of infection after penetrating abdominal trauma.

Nishi M, Hiramatsu Y, Hioki K, et al: Risk factors in relation to postoperative complications in patients undergoing esophagectomy or gastrectomy for cancer. Ann Surg 207:148, 1988.
Three hundred sixty-four elderly patients with cancer undergoing esophagectomy and/or gastrectomy were evaluated for risk factors contributing to postoperative complications. Significant correlations included vital organ disorders, reduction in maximum response of stress hormones to surgical procedures, and functional variability of target organs; all were more closely related to postoperative course than age.

Ortona L, Federico G, Fantoni M, et al: A study on the incidence of postoperative infections and surgical sepsis in a university hospital. Infect Control 8:320, 1987.
From 1,505 patients on 10 wards of a university hospital in Rome, data was gathered to determine the overall incidence and factors related to surgical infections. Infection rate was most influenced by age, immunosuppressive diseases, and immunosuppressive therapy. Most frequent etiologic agents were Pseudomonas aeruginosa, S. aureus, and E. coli.

Ottino G, DePaulis R, Pansini S, et al: Major sternal wound infection after open-heart surgery: a multivariate analysis of risk factors in 2,579 consecutive operative procedures. Ann Thorac Surg 44:173, 1987.

Major sternal wound infections developed in 48 of 2,579 consecutive patients on a university cardiac surgical service. Out of multiple possible risk factors evaluated, six significant factors emerged: hospital environment, interval between admission and surgery, reoperation, blood transfusions, early chest reexploration, and sternal rewiring.

Roberts J, Barnes W, Pennock M, Browne G: Diagnostic accuracy of fever as a measure of postoperative pulmonary complications. Heart Lung 17:166, 1988.

This study evaluated the diagnostic accuracy of fever as a measure of postoperative pulmonary complications. Fever was an accurate indicator of radiograph evidence of atelectasis in only 56% of subjects.

Rogers PN, Wright IH: Postoperative intra-abdominal sepsis. Br J Surg 74:973, 1987.

The clinical spectrum of postoperative intraabdominal sepsis is reviewed, including clinical examination and useful current imaging techniques. Diagnostic laparotomy and surgical intervention are stressed.

Shapiro M, Munoz A, Tager IB, et al: Risk factors for infection at the operative site after abdominal or vaginal hysterectomy. N Engl J Med 307:1661, 1982.

Prospective study of 323 patients and the factors associated with higher risk of infection.

Simpson LC, Peters GE: Poststernotomy infections presenting as deep neck abscess. Arch Otolaryngol Head Neck Surg 114:909, 1988.

Two cases of poststernotomy mediastinitis presenting as deep neck infections are described.

Smith EB: Anaerobic infections in surgery. J Natl Med Assoc 76:206, 1984.

Presentation of principles and practical concepts of anaerobic surgical infections.

Wheeland RG: The newer surgical dressings and wound healing. Dermatol Clin 5:393, 1987.

Interesting update on new synthetic surgical dressing materials available, with an emphasis on cutaneous wound care.

Wilson RF: Special problems in the diagnosis and treatment of surgical sepsis. Surg Clin North Am 65:965, 1985.

Sepsis is the most frequent single cause of death after surgery or trauma. A clinical review of current concepts and diagnostic approaches, with a special focus on patients with impaired host defenses, such as the elderly and patients with severe trauma.

70

Hypothermia: Causes and Associated Disorders

A diagnosis of hypothermia can be made when the core temperature is below 35°C.[1] Even though the patient may appear dead, decreased oxygen requirements may sustain life for long periods, even after cardiac arrest.[2] Hypothermia occurs most frequently in alcoholics, elderly patients, and the debilitated who are also at high risk for serious associated infections, such as pneumonia, cellulitis, and bacteremia, which hypothermia can dangerously mask.[3]

Endocrine Dysfunction Causing Hypothermia

The most frequent endocrine disorders causing hypothermia are myxedema and diabetic ketoacidosis.[4]

Myxedema: hypothermic myxedema coma can mimic an acute myocardial infarction with elevated creatine phosphokinase (CPK).[5,6]
Diabetes mellitus: autonomic dysfunction and diabetic ketoacidosis[7-9]
Hypopituitarism
Adrenal insufficiency: Addison's disease

Toxic-Metabolic Disorders Causing Hypothermia

Starvation
Alcoholism[10,11]
Uremia: renal failure
Drug toxicity: barbiturates, opiates, anesthesia, phenothiazines, ethylene glycol, chemotherapy[12]
Magnesium sulfate therapy[13]
Antipsychotic drugs[14]

Neurologic Dysfunction Causing Hypothermia

Hypothalamic disorders: tumors, cerebral vascular infarctions[15]
Autonomic dysfunction
Spinal cord lesions[16]
Wernicke's encephalopathy[17,18]
Head trauma[19]
Subarachnoid hemorrhage[20]

Craniovertebral and upper cervical spine disorders: associated autonomic dysfunction[21,22]
Multiple sclerosis[23]
Parkinsonism

Miscellaneous Causes and Associations with Hypothermia

Accidental hypothermia: environmental exposure, cold water immersion, near drowning[24–30]
Bacterial sepsis
Iatrogenic: hypothermic therapy during surgery, cold blood, gastric lavage, hypothermic blankets, peritoneal dialysis, antipyretics
Dermatologic disorders: exfoliative dermatitis,[31] erythroderma,[32] psoriasis[33]
Severe burns[34]
Pancreatitis[35]
Shapiro's syndrome: periodic attacks of hypothermia associated with agenesis of the corpus callosum[36]
Spontaneous periodic hypothermia[37]
Anorexia nervosa[38,39]
Acute myocardial infarction[40]
Tetanus[41]

References

1. Milner JE: Hypothermia (editorial). Ann Intern Med 89:565, 1978.
2. Fell RH, Gunning AJ, Bardhan KD, et al: Severe hypothermia as a result of barbiturate overdose complicated by cardiac arrest. Lancet 1:392, 1968.
3. Lewin S, Brettman LR, Holzman RS: Infections in hypothermic patients. Arch Intern Med 141:920, 1981.
4. Exton-Smith AN: Hypothermia (editorial). West J Med 133:431, 1980.
5. Angel JH, Sash L: Hypothermic coma in myxoedema. Br Med J 1:1855, 1960.
6. Nee PA, Scane AC, Lavelle PH, et al: Hypothermic myxedema coma erroneously diagnosed as myocardial infarction because of increased creatine kinase MB. Clin Chem 33:1083, 1987.
7. Scott AR, Bennett T, MacDonald IA: Diabetes mellitus and thermoregulation. Can J Physiol Pharmacol 65:1365, 1987.
8. Guerin JM, Meyer P, Segrestaa JM: Hypothermia in diabetic ketoacidosis. Diabetes Care 10:801, 1987.
9. Scott AR, MacDonald IA, Bennett T, Tattersall RB: Abnormal thermoregulation in diabetic autonomic neuropathy. Diabetes 37:961, 1988.
10. Weyman AE, Greenbaum DM, Grace WJ: Accidental hypothermia in an alcoholic population. Am J Med 56:13, 1974.
11. Smith GS, Kraus JF: Alcohol and residential, recreational, and occupational injuries: a review of the epi-

demiologic evidence. Annu Rev Public Health 9:99, 1988.
12. Jackson MJ, Proctor SJ, Leonard RCF: Hypothermia during chemotherapy for Hodgkin's disease. Br Med J 286:1183, 1983.
13. Rodis JF, Vintzileos AM, Campbell WA, et al: Maternal hypothermia: an unusual complication of magnesium sulfate therapy. Am J Obstet Gynecol 156:435, 1987.
14. Noto T, Hashimoto H, Sugae S, et al: Hypothermia caused by antipsychotic drugs in a schizophrenic patient. J Clin Psychiatry 48:77, 1987.
15. Fox RH, Davies TW, Marsh FP, et al: Hypothermia in a young man with an anterior hypothalamic lesion. Lancet 2:185, 1970.
16. Altus P, Hickman JW, Nord HJ: Accidential hypothermia in a healthy quadriplegic patient. Neurology 35:427, 1985.
17. Lipton JM, Payne H, Garza HR, et al: Thermolability in Wernicke's encephalopathy. Arch Neurol 35:750, 1978.
18. Reuler JB, Girard DE, Cooney TG: Wernicke's encephalopathy. N Engl J Med 312:1035, 1985.
19. Ratcliffe PJ, Bell JI, Collins KJ, et al: Late onset post-traumatic hypothalamic hypothermia. J Neurol Neurosurg Psychiatry 46:72, 1983.
20. Nussey SS, Ang VT, Jenkins JS: Chronic hypernatremia and hypothermia following subarachnoid hemorrhage. Postgrad Med J 62:467, 1986.
21. Rosomoff HL: Occult respiratory and autonomic dysfunction in craniovertebral anomalies and upper cervical spinal disease. Spine 11:345, 1986.
22. Gray HH, Smith LD, Moore RH: Idiopathic periodic hypothermia and bizarre behaviour in the presence of occult syringomyelia. Postgrad Med J 62:289, 1986.
23. Sullivan F, Hutchinson M, Bahandeka S, Moore RE: Chronic hypothermia in multiple sclerosis. J Neurol Neurosurg Psychiatry 50:813, 1987.
24. Davidson M, Grant E: Accidental hypothermia. Postgrad Med 70 (5):42, 1981.
25. Moss J: Accidental severe hypothermia. Surg Gynecol Obstet 162:501, 1986.
26. Lnning PE, Skulberg A, Abyholm F: Accidental hypothermia. Review of the literature. Acta Anaesthesiol Scand 30:601, 1986.
27. Purdue GF, Hunt JL: Cold injury: a collective review. J Burn Care Rehabil 7:331, 1986.
28. Sinks T: Hazards of working in cold weather include frostbite, hypothermia. Occup Health Saf 57:20, 1988.
29. Ornato JP: Special resuscitation situations: near drowning, traumatic injury, electric shock, and hypothermia. Circulation 74:IV23, 1986.
30. Orlowski JP: Drowning, near-drowning, and ice-water submersions. Pediatr Clin North Am 34:75, 1987.
31. Krook G: Hypothermia in patients with exfoliative dermatitis. Acta Derm Venereol 40:142, 1960.
32. Reuler JB, Jones SR, Girard DE: Hypothermia in the erythroderma syndrome. West J Med 127:243, 1977.
33. Grice KA, Bettley FR: Skin water loss and accidental hypothermia in psoriasis, ichthyosis, and erythroderma. Br Med J 4:195, 1967.

34. Roe CF, Kinney JM, Blair C: Water and heat exchange in third degree burns. Surgery 56:212, 1964.
35. Read AE, Emslie-Smith D, Gough KR, et al: Pancreatitis and accidental hypothermia. Lancet 2:1219, 1961.
36. Shapiro WR, Williams GH, Plum F: Spontaneous recurrent hypothermia accompanying agenesis of the corpus callosum. Brain 92:423, 1969.
37. Mooradian AD, Morley GK, McGeachie R, et al: Spontaneous periodic hypothermia. Neurology 34:79, 1984.
38. Smith DK, Ovesen L, Chu R, et al: Hypothermia in a patient with anorexia nervosa. Metabolism 32:1151, 1983.
39. Palla B, Litt IF: Medical complications of eating disorders in adolescents. Pediatrics 81:613, 1988.
40. Doherty NE, Ades A, Shah PK, et al: Hypothermia with acute myocardial infarction. Ann Intern Med 101:797, 1984.
41. MacWalter RS, McFadden JP, Griffiths RA: Tetanus presenting as hypothermia. J R Soc Med 79:616, 1986.

Selected Readings

Celestino FS, Van Noord GR, Miraglia CP: Accidental hypothermia in the elderly (clinical conference). J Fam Pract 26 (3):259, 1988.

Case report and clinical conference. Useful clinical diagnostic definitions and review of predisposing conditions and altered physiology predisposing elderly patients to hypothermia.

Collins KJ: Effects of cold on old people. Br J Hosp Med 38:506, 1987.

Factors related to the increased morbidity and mortality from cardiovascular and respiratory disease in the elderly are reviewed in light of recent physiologic investigations on the effects of cold in the elderly.

Danzl DF, Pozos RS, Auerbach PS, et al: Multicenter hypothermia survey. Ann Emerg Med 16:1042, 1987.

A multicenter survey of clinical presentations, treatment, and outcome of accidental hypothermia presents a plethora of data relating clinical outcome to presentation and treatment. Authors propose a refinement of current American Heart Association cardiopulmonary resuscitation standards in hypothermia.

Dean NC: Hypothermia. Lifesaving procedures. Postgrad Med 82 (8):48, 1987.

A clinical review of current concepts of management of severe hypothermia, including techniques of active core rewarming when necessary.

Fischbeck KH, Simon RP: Neurological manifestations of accidental hypothermia. Ann Neurol 10:384, 1981.

Neurologic findings in 97 patients presenting with hypothermia are reported. Alcohol and Wernicke's encephalopathy were frequent causes in this study. Even at temperatures of 20 to 27°C, 6 of 18 patients remained verbally responsive, and 10 had intact reflexes. No correlation with eye movement abnormalities or extensor plantar responses with the degree of hypothermia could be made.

Hart LE, Sutton JR: Environmental considerations for exercise. Cardiol Clin 5:245, 1987.

An interesting review of current concepts of the human physiologic response to environmental temperature and exercise, with a focus on cardiorespiratory function and adaptation.

Hauty MG, Esrig BC, Hill JG, Long WB: Prognostic factors in severe accidental hypothermia: experience from the Mt. Hood tragedy. J Trauma 27:1107, 1987.
Prognostic indicators that may help predict survival in patients with accidental hypothermia include underlying medical illnesses, duration of cold exposure, initial core temperature, mental status, presence of spontaneous respirations, cardiac rate and rhythm, and arterial oxygen tension. Important initial laboratory markers included hyperkalemia and elevated serum ammonia, indicating cell lysis, and hypofibrinogenemia, suggesting intravascular thrombosis.

Kafetz K: Hypothermia and elderly people. Practitioner 231:864, 1987.
Concise clinical review of hypothermia in the elderly written for the general practitioner.

Kortelainen ML: Drugs and alcohol in hypothermia and hyperthermia related deaths: a retrospective study. J Forensic Sci 32:1704, 1987.
An interesting review from a forensic medicine department examining factors related to the death of patients who presented with drug- or alcohol-related hyperthermia or hypothermia. The poikilothermic effect of alcohol is discussed. Drugs most commonly associated with hypothermia included antidepressants, neuroleptics, and barbiturates.

Lloyd EL: Hypothermia in the elderly. Med Sci Law 28:107, 1988.
Well-referenced, excellent review with a focus on environmental factors endangering the elderly. Author notes that many symptoms of hypothermia mimic senility in the elderly; for example, a change in personality may be one of the earliest signs of hypothermia in the elderly.

Matz R: Hypothermia: mechanisms and countermeasures. Hosp Pract 21 (1A):45, 1986.
A thoughtful, useful review of clinical concepts and the physiology of the hypothermic patient that stresses the slowness of body processes during hypothermia from which practical diagnostic and therapeutic concepts are drawn.

Morris DL, Chambers HF, Morris MG, Sande MA: Hemodynamic characteristics of patients with hypothermia due to occult infection and other causes. Ann Intern Med 102:153, 1985.
From a prospective study of 85 consecutive patients with hypothermia, authors suggest that hemodynamic characteristics can distinguish infection-related hypothermia. Infection-related hypothermic patients in this study had lower calculated systemic vascular resistances and higher cardiac indices compared with hypothermic patients without severe infections.

Moss J: Accidental severe hypothermia. Surg Gynecol Obstet 162:501, 1986.
A well-referenced clinical review.

National Center for Health Statistics: Leads from the MMWR: Hypothermia-associated deaths—United States, 1968–1980. JAMA 255:307, 1986.
Mortality data from the National Center for Health Statistics during 1968 to 1980 attribute 6,460 deaths to effects of cold. Elderly are at highest risk; men are at higher risk than women.

Reuler JB: Hypothermia: pathophysiology, clinical settings, and management. Ann Intern Med 89:519, 1978.

Still current review. Well referenced.

Slater DN: Death from hypothermia: are current views on causative factors well founded? Br Med J (Clin Res) 296:1643, 1988.
Causes of mortality were studied in 43 elderly patients in a Yorkshire East District who were reportedly hypothermic before death. Most frequent causes were inadequate heating and mentally ill patients wandering away from supervised care.

Swain JA: Hypothermia and blood pH. A review. Arch Intern Med 148:1643, 1988.
A useful review summarizing laboratory, theoretical, and clinical evidence that the management of blood pH during hypothermia may be significant in altering the clinical outcome.

Vuori I: The heart and the cold. Ann Clin Res 19:156, 1987.
This review presents evidence that cold environments contribute to increased cardiovascular disease, particularly coronary heart disease-related morbidity and mortality.

Wong KC: Physiology and pharmacology of hypothermia. West J Med 138:227, 1983.
Current concepts of the physiologic changes that correlate with the severity of hypothermia with implications for rational management.

71

Acute Meningitis: Common Infectious Etiologies

Acute meningitis is a life-threatening disorder. Appropriate treatment depends on prompt recognition of the bacterial, fungal, mycobacterial, or viral infectious agent. The most common clinical presentation includes fever, meningism, headache, and mental status changes. Important factors in determining the most probable pathogen include age, presence of concomitant infection, history of exposure, and the presence of immunosuppression. Physical findings of infection, particularly possible parameningeal foci from trauma or shunts, or infected sinuses, ears, throat, neck, lungs, and urinary tract can lead to early recognition of the infectious agent. Obtaining a history of possible exposure to tuberculosis, viral disease, rodents, ticks, dairy products, and farm animals is important. The presence of immuno-suppression is increasingly important to establish and should include determining human immunodeficiency virus (HIV)-infection and HIV-risk factors, history of leukemia, lymphoma, or drug-induced immunosuppression such as chemotherapy or corticosteroid use.[1] Many infectious and noninfectious causes of chronic meningitis can mimic acute bacterial meningitis. Spinal fluid culture is essential to the etiologic diagnosis of meningitis. Gram stain cultures of other potentially infectious body fluids such as urine may be helpful.[2]

Common Causes of Acute Bacterial Meningitis

Although most cases of bacterial meningitis occur in children under 5 years of age, it is seen increasingly in the elderly and patients infected with HIV.[3,4] Common bacterial etiologies of acute meningitis include Group B streptococci and *Escherichia coli* in neonates; *Haemophilus influenzae* and *Neisseria meningitidis* in children; *Streptococcus pneumoniae* and *N. meningitidis* in adults.

H. influenzae B: occurs most often in children 3 months to 2 years of age, often following otitis media, sinusitis, or respiratory tract infections; sterile effusions are common.[5-8]

S. pneumoniae: the most common cause of adult bacterial meningitis, often associated with pneumonia, otitis media, and endocarditis; alcoholics and the elderly are at risk[9]

N. meningitidis: skin manifestations include macular rashes, petechiae, purpura, and ecchymoses.[10,11]

E. coli: adult risk factors include sepsis associated with urinary tract infections, trauma, and neurosurgery.[2,12]

Other gram-negative bacteria: *Salmonellae, Klebsiella, Proteus,* and *Pseudomonas;* less commonly involved than *E. coli,* these gram-negative organisms are also found in newborns, after neurosurgery, trauma, in the elderly, and in the immunocompromised.[13]

Staphylococcus aureus: can follow furunculosis and postoperative wound infections and is often associated with a parameningeal infection[14,15]

Listeria monocytogenes: neonates, pregnant women, compromised hosts (particularly lymphoma and leukemia), and the elderly are at risk.[16,17]

Streptococci, group B: occurs in the neonate[18]

Enterobacteriaceae: occurs in the neonate

Mixed bacterial meningitis: affects a largely adult population, with risk factors including infection at contiguous foci such as tumors or fistulous communications with the CNS[19]

Viruses and Nonbacterial Agents

Enteroviruses: coxsackievirus,[20] echoviruses, poliomyelitis[21]

Mumps virus: associated parotitis[22,23]

Arboviruses

Herpes simplex virus: types 1 and 2 infect the CNS. Type 1 usually is associated with a meningoencephalitis. Type 2 more often presents as aseptic meningitis[24-27]

Treponema pallidum: secondary syphilis can present as acute meningitis[28,29]

HIV: a self-limited aseptic meningitis during which HIV can be sometimes isolated from blood and cerebrospinal fluid or associated with HIV-seroconversion; cranial nerves are often affected[30-32]

Mycobacterium tuberculosis: patients with pulmonary and disseminated tuberculosis are at particular risk for this meningitis, which is usually of insidious onset.

Mycobacterium avium-intracellulare: an opportunistic infection in humans, an increasingly seen organism in HIV-infected patients[33]

Cryptococcus neoformans: most common fungal infection of the brain, usually insidious; can present abruptly with acute confusional state, particularly in immunocompromised patients[34]

Other fungi: *Coccidioides immitis, Histoplasma capsulatum,* and *Candida albicans*

Lyme disease: meningitis, cranial neuritis, and radiculoneuritis caused by a spirochete transmitted by *Ixodes dammini* and related ticks[35]

References

1. Francke E: The many causes of meningitis. Postgrad Med 82 (2):175, 1987.
2. LeFrock JL, Smith BR, Molavi A: Gram-negative bacillary meningitis. Med Clin North Am 69:243, 1985.
3. Gold R: Bacterial meningitis—1982. Proceedings of a

symposium: body fluids and infectious diseases. Clinical and microbiologic advances. Am J Med 75(Suppl 1B):98, 1983.

4. Witt DJ, Craven DE, McCabe WR: Bacterial infections in adult patients with the acquired immune deficiency syndrome (AIDS) and AIDS-related complex. Am J Med 82:900, 1987.

5. Frazier JP, Cleary TG, Pickering LK: Meningitis due to *Haemophilus parainfluenzae.* Pediatr Infect Dis 1 (2):117, 1982.

6. Spagnuolo PJ, Ellner JJ, Lerner PI, et al: *Haemophilus influenzae* meningitis: the spectrum of disease in adults. Medicine 61:74, 1982.

7. Bol P, Spanjaard L, van Alphen L, Zanen HC: Epidemiology of *Haemophilus influenzae* meningitis in patients more than 6 years of age. J Infect 15:81, 1987.

8. van Alphen L, van Dam A, Bol P, et al: Types and subtypes of 73 strains of *Haemophilus influenzae* isolated from patients more than 6 years of age with meningitis in the Netherlands. J Infect 15:95, 1987.

9. Bohr V, Paulson OB, Rasmussen N: Pneumococcal meningitis. Late neurologic sequelae and features of prognostic impact. Arch Neurol 41:1045, 1984.

10. Cann KJ, Rogers TR, Jones DM, et al: *Neisseria meningitidis* in a primary school. Arch Dis Child 62:1113, 1987.

11. Achtman M, Crowe BA, Olyhoek A, et al: Recent results on epidemic meningococcal meningitis. J Med Microbiol 26:172, 1988.

12. Rahal JJ, Simberkoff MS: Host defense and antimicrobial therapy in adult gram-negative bacillary meningitis. Ann Intern Med 96:468, 1982.

13. Gower DJ, Barrows AA III, Kelly DL Jr, Pegram S Jr: Gram-negative bacillary meningitis in the adult: review of 39 cases. South Med J 79:1499, 1986.

14. Phair JP: Meningitis due to *Staphylococcus aureus.* Am J Med 78:965, 1985.

15. Schlesinger LS, Ross SC, Schaberg DR: *Staphylococcus aureus* meningitis: a broad-based epidemiologic study. Medicine 66:148, 1987.

16. Bouvet E, Suter F, Gibert C, et al: Severe meningitis due to *Listeria monocytogenes.* Scand J Infect Dis 14:267, 1982.

17. Berk SL, Alvarez S: Bacterial infections in the elderly. Postgrad Med 77 (3):168, 1985.

18. Mulder CJJ, Zanen HC: Neonatal group B streptococcal meningitis. Arch Dis Child 59:439, 1984.

19. Downs NJ, Hodges GR, Taylor SA: Mixed bacterial meningitis. Rev Infect Dis 9:693, 1987.

20. Reyes MP, Zalenski D, Smith F, et al: Coxsackievirus—positive cervices in women with febrile illnesses during the third trimester in pregnancy. Am J Obstet Gynecol 155:159, 1986.

21. Wilfert CM, Lehrman SN, Katz SL: Enteroviruses and meningitis. Pediatr Infect Dis 2:333, 1983.

22. Nagai H, Morishima T, Morishima Y, et al: Local T cell subsets in mumps meningitis. Arch Dis Child 58:927, 1983.

23. Jubelt B: Enterovirus and mumps virus infections of the nervous system. Neurol Clin 2:187, 1984.

24. White WB, Hanna M, Stewart JA: Systemic herpes simplex virus type 2 infection. Arch Intern Med 144:826, 1984.
25. Ratzan KR: Viral meningitis. Med Clin North Am 69:399, 1985.
26. Stuart-Harris C: The epidemiology and clinical presentation of herpes virus infections. J Antimicrob Chemother 12 (SB):1, 1983.
27. Barnes DW, Whitley RJ: CNS diseases associated with varicella zoster virus and herpes simplex virus infection. Pathogenesis and current therapy. Neurol Clin 4:265, 1986.
28. Bayne LL, Schmidley JW, Goodin DS: Acute syphilitic meningitis. Arch Neurol 43:137, 1986.
29. McPhee SJ: Secondary syphilis: uncommon manifestations of a common disease. West J Med 140:35, 1984.
30. Ho DD, Sarngadharan MG, Resnick L, et al: Primary human T-lymphotropic virus type III infection. Ann Intern Med 103:880, 1985.
31. Ho DD, Rota TR, Schooley RT, et al: Isolation of HTLV-III from cerebrospinal fluid and neural tissues of patients with neurologic syndromes related to the acquired immunodeficiency syndrome. N Engl J Med 313:1493, 1985.
32. Resnick L, diMarzo-Veronese F, Schupbach J, et al: Intra-blood-brain-barrier synthesis of HTLV-III-specific IgG in patients with neurologic symptoms associated with AIDS or AIDS-related complex. N Engl J Med 313:1498, 1985.
33. Tenholder MF, Moser RJ III, Tellis CJ: Mycobacteria other than tuberculosis. Pulmonary involvement in patients with acquired immunodeficiency syndrome. Arch Intern Med 148:953, 1988.
34. Kovacs JA, Kovacs AA, Polis M, et al: Cryptococcosis in the acquired immunodeficiency syndrome. Ann Intern Med 103:533, 1985.
35. Pachner AR, Steere AC: The triad of neurologic manifestations of Lyme disease: meningitis, cranial neuritis, and radiculoneuritis. Neurology 35:47, 1985.

Selected Readings

Arends JP, Zanen HC: Meningitis caused by *Streptococcus suis* in humans. Rev Infect Dis 10:131, 1988.
Data from 30 patients in the Netherlands with Streptococcus suis *meningitis are reviewed and compared with patients outside the Netherlands. Hearing loss was the most frequent sequela in survivors. Pork industry workers appear at higher risk.*

Bamborschke S, Heiss WD: Cerebrospinal fluid and peripheral blood leukocyte subsets in acute inflammation of the CNS. J Neurol Sci 79:1, 1987.
Leukocyte subsets in cerebrospinal fluid (CSF) and peripheral blood were evaluated in 21 patients with acute inflammation of the CNS with monoclonal antibodies OKT3, OKT4, OKT8, Leu12, and OKM1 in an immunoperoxidase slide assay. Significant differences between acute aseptic and bacterial meningitis were found in CSF.

Beghi E, Nicolosi A, Kurland LT, et al: Encephalitis and

aseptic meningitis, Olmsted County, Minnesota, 1950–81. I. Epidemiology. Ann Neurol 16:283, 1984.

Cases of encephalitis and aseptic meningitis occurring in Olmsted County, Minnesota from 1950 to 1981 were reviewed. Incidence rates were 7.4 per 100,000 person-years for encephalitis and 10.9 per 100,000 person-years for aseptic meningitis. Most common agents identified were California and mumps viruses in cases of encephalitis and enterovirus and mumps virus in aseptic meningitis.

Benson CA, Harris AA: Acute neurologic infections. Med Clin North Am 70:987, 1986.

A discussion of acute bacterial, viral, toxin-mediated, and parasitic neurologic infections. Authors emphasize that those that are potentially treatable are also rapidly fatal if untreated and pose a significant risk of transmission.

Cabral DA, Flodmark O, Farrell K. Speert DP: Prospective study of computed tomography in acute bacterial meningitis. J Pediatr 111:201, 1987.

Serial CT scans on admission and discharge of children admitted with bacterial meningitis were performed on 60 patients. Etiologic infectious agents found in decreasing frequency were H. influenzae, N. meningitidis, and S. pneumoniae. CT abnormalities included subdural effusions in eight patients, focal infarction in five, pus in basal cisterns in one, and marked cerebral edema in two patients who died. Transient mild dilation of the subarachnoid space was a common finding.

Dougherty JM, Jones J: Cerebrospinal fluid cultures and analysis. Ann Emerg Med 15:317, 1986.

This paper reviews the current state of the art in CSF testing, discusses cost considerations, and offers an algorithm for efficient selection of tests.

Dougherty JM, Roth RM: Cerebral spinal fluid. Emerg Med Clin North Am 4:281, 1986.

Clinical review of state-of-the-art CSF testing. Some newer techniques reviewed include rapid agglutination tests, monoclonal antibodies, and modifications of enzyme immunoassays of bacterial antigens. Useful information and well referenced.

Feder HM Jr: *Bacteroides fragilis* meningitis. Rev Infect Dis 9:783, 1987.

Only 9 cases of Bacteroides *fragilis have been reported in the antibiotic era. Most occurred in premature infants and neonates. Neurologic sequelae occurred in four of seven patients. Predisposing conditions included sepsis, otitis media, and ventriculoatrial shunt infections.*

Gorse GJ, Thrupp LD, Nudleman KL, et al: Bacterial meningitis in the elderly. Arch Intern Med 144:1603, 1984.

Study indicating meningitis in the elderly is likely to be bacterial and is associated with higher morbidity and mortality.

Kaplan SL, Fishman MA: Update on bacterial meningitis. J Child Neurol 3:82, 1988.

Recommended review of recent advances in diagnosis, pathogenesis, and treatment of bacterial meningitis. Newer CSF examination techniques are considered, such as acridine orange staining, that help identify bacteria with partially treated meningitis when Gram stain fails, and the usefulness of monoclonal antibodies to detect meningococcus group B antigen. Clinical course, prognosis, and newer antibiotics are also reviewed.

Krasinski K, Nelson JD, Butler S, et al: Possible association of *Mycoplasma* and viral respiratory infections with bacterial meningitis. Am J Epidemiol 125:499, 1987.
One hundred sixty children older than 3 months who were hospitalized with bacterial meningitis were evaluated for viral infection. Twenty-nine of 131 patients with H. influenzae had evidence of recent adenovirus infection. Results of this study suggest to authors that primary infection with adenoviruses and possibly influenza B or Mycoplasma precedes bacterial meningitis in some patients and may be considered a predisposing factor.

Lukes SA, Posner JB, Nielsen S, et al: Bacterial infections of the CNS in neutropenic patients. Neurology 34:269, 1984.
A review of the difficult problem of diagnosing and managing bacterial infections of the CNS in neutropenic patients. In these patients, fever and mental status changes are frequently the primary clinical manifestations of CNS bacterial infection, whereas the common and expected manifestations of headache and meningeal signs found in bacterial CNS infections are exceptional.

Orren A, Potter PC, Cooper RC, du Toit E: Deficiency of the sixth component of complement and susceptibility to *Neisseria meningitidis* infections: studies in 10 families and five isolated cases. Immunology 62:249, 1987.
Complement component C6 deficiency (C6D) was found in 15 patients with recurrent meningococcal infection. Ten patients belonged to multiple families; family studies led to other cases of C6D. Authors suggest that their data indicate that C6D is an important risk factor for developing meningococcal infection in their region of Cape Town, South Africa.

Polk DB, Steele RW: Bacterial meningitis presenting with normal cerebrospinal fluid. Pediatr Infect Dis J 6:1040, 1987.
Cases of pediatric bacterial meningitis with normal initial cerebrospinal fluid other than culture or antigen detection assays were reviewed from a large children's hospital. During a 5-year period, 7 of 261 patients fulfilled this criterion. Laboratory parameters, such as blood counts, sedimentation rate, and C-reactive protein, were compared. No unique indicators for bacterial meningitis were revealed. Authors emphasize the importance of relying on clinical judgment in initiating empiric antimicrobial therapy.

Ponka A, Ojala K, Teppo AM, et al: The differential diagnosis of bacterial and aseptic meningitis using cerebrospinal fluid laboratory tests. Infection 11:129, 1983.
Study suggesting that the cerebrospinal fluid lactate level is most sensitive in the differential diagnosis of bacterial and aseptic meningitis.

Powers WJ: Cerebrospinal fluid lymphocytosis in acute bacterial meningitis. Am J Med 79:216, 1985.
A study of the occurrence of CSF lymphocytosis in cases of acute bacterial meningitis found CSF lymphocytosis in 14 of 104 cases of bacteriologically proven acute bacterial meningitis. Etiologic agents in decreasing frequency were S. pneumoniae, N. meningitidis, and H. influenzae. Author suggests that since CSF lymphocytosis is not uncommon in acute bacterial meningitis.

Quagliarello VJ, Scheld WM: Recent advances in the pathogenesis and pathophysiology of bacterial meningitis. Am J Med Sci 292:306, 1986.

Current concepts of pathogenesis and pathophysiology of bacterial meningitis related to recent understanding gained from studying animal models and basic research.

Sarwar M, Falkoff G, Naseem M: Radiologic techniques in the diagnosis of CNS infections. Neurol Clin 4:41, 1986.
A review of neuroradiographic findings in various CNS infections.

Swartz MN: Bacterial meningitis: more involved than just the meninges (editorial). N Engl J Med 311:912, 1984.
Pithy discussion of the pathogenesis and clinical manifestations of neurologic complications and sequelae of bacterial meningitis.

Sze G, Zimmerman RD: The magnetic resonance imaging of infections and inflammatory diseases. Radiol Clin North Am 26:839, 1988.
MRI of inflammatory lesions of the central nervous system are reviewed. Sensitivity and specificity of MRI and CT in identifying inflammatory lesions are compared.

Talan DA, Hoffman JR, Yoshikawa TT, Overturf GD: Role of empiric parenteral antibiotics prior to lumbar puncture in suspected bacterial meningitis: state of the art. Rev Infect Dis 10:365, 1988.
The question of need for empiric parenteral antibiotics in suspected meningitis patients who have delayed lumbar punctures (LP) was evaluated in this literature review. Authors conclude (1) existing data are inadequate to assess effect of a short delay of antibiotic therapy on mortality and morbidity; (2) short course of antibiotics does not change CSF white blood cell count, protein, or glucose; (3) yield of CSF Gram stain and culture may be reduced by even a short course of antibiotic therapy; and (4) adjunctive tests, such as blood cultures and CSF antigen tests, can often identify the bacterial pathogen. Authors recommend that if bacterial meningitis is suspected, even if LP is delayed, intravenous antibiotics are warranted.

Tallman RD, Kimbrough SM, O'Brien JF, et al: Assay for β-glucuronidase in cerebrospinal fluid: usefulness for the detection of neoplastic meningitis. Mayo Clin Proc 60:293, 1985.
Current concepts of specificity and sensitivity of the beta-glucuronidase assay.

Tenney JH: Bacterial infections of the central nervous system in neurosurgery. Neurol Clin 4:91, 1986.
A clinical review of CNS infections after neurosurgery, neurotrauma, and placement of CSF shunts and ventriculostomies. Diagnostic modalities and recommended therapies in this setting are reviewed.

Weinstein L: Bacterial meningitis. Specific etiologic diagnosis on the basis of distinctive epidemiologic, pathogenetic, and clinical features. Med Clin North Am 69:219, 1985.
A review with an emphasis on the clinical features most helpful in differentiating common bacterial meningitides.

Williams RG, Hart CA: Rapid identification of bacterial antigen in blood cultures and cerebrospinal fluid. J Clin Pathol 41:691, 1988.
The ability of antibody-coated latex particle suspensions to diagnose infectious agents in septicemia and meningitis was assessed in 272 blood culture sets and 85 cerebrospinal fluid specimens. Results of this study found this method 100% sensitive and 99% specific, with predictive values ranging from 63% to 100%.

72
Chronic Meningitis: Infectious and Noninfectious Causes

A variety of infectious and noninfectious disorders manifest and can mimic the clinical picture of chronic meningitis, which is characterized by a 4-week or longer history of headache, lethargy, confusion, nausea, vomiting, elevated cerebrospinal fluid (CSF) protein, and a CSF lymphocytic pleocytosis.[1,2]

Infectious Causes

It is often necessary to reculture the CSF several times for bacteria, acid-fast bacilli, and particularly fungi to establish the infectious etiology. In patients who have established infectious chronic meningitis without known risk factors, consider possible underlying immune compromise, such as undiagnosed lymphoma, leukemia, acquired immune deficiency syndrome (AIDS), and human immunodeficiency virus (HIV) infection.

Tuberculosis[3]: a deteriorating mental status, low CSF glucose, negative bacterial cultures, and negative India ink preparation should raise the consideration of mycobacterial meningitis.[4,5]

Cryptococcosis: serum and CSF serology for cryptococcal polysaccharide antigen helpful[6]

Other fungal infections: blastomycosis,[7] coccidioidomycosis,[8,9] histoplasmosis,[10] chromomycosis,[11] *Sporothrix schenckii*[12]

Syphilis: neurosyphilis occurs with increasing frequency in HIV-infected patients and may be a first manifestation of underlying HIV infection.[13,14]

Brucellosis: exposure to goats, cows, sheep and unpasteurized cheese; isolation of brucella from CSF is uncommon[15–17]; CT scan may have basal ganglia calcifications[18]

Leptospirosis

Toxoplasmosis: most common infectious cause of focal cerebral mass lesions in AIDS patients[19]

Actinomycosis[20]

Cysticercosis[21,22]

Nocardia asteroides

Cytomegalovirus[23]

Angiostrongylus cantonensis: most common cause of eosinophilic meningitis in the Pacific islands and Southeast Asia[24,25]

Listeria monocytogenes: usually associated with immunocompromise, but can occur without evidence of immune dysfunction[26,27]

HIV infection: can be associated with an acute meningitis at time of seroconversion and can also cause sporadic episodes of acute or chronic meningitis in HIV-infected patients with relatively preserved immune function[28]; common associated infections include various viral syndromes, *Toxoplasma gondii, Cryptococcus neoformans, Candida albicans,* mycobacteria; common central nervous system neoplasms include lymphoma and metastatic Kaposi's sarcoma.[29,30]

Lyme meningitis: characterized by erythema chronicum migrans, facial palsies, and lymphocytic meningitis[31-34]

Meningoradiculomyelitis (Bannwarth's syndrome): *Borrelia burgdorferi* is the infectious agent in some cases.[35-39]

Herpes simplex virus (HSV): Although it is usually an acute viral encephalitis, consider HSV in patients with a history of undiagnosed encephalitis causing chronic encephalopathy.[40,41]

Noninfectious Causes of Chronic Meningitis

Sarcoidosis: often basilar meningitis with associated systemic sarcoidosis[42]

Meningeal carcinomatosis: primary or metastatic; common associated primary neoplasms include lung, breast, stomach, pancreas, and melanoma; it is often difficult to distinguish superimposed infection from neoplastic meningitis[43-45]

Meningeal neoplasia: lymphoma, carcinoma, leukemia, sarcoma, glioma, and melanoma may infiltrate meninges to mimic chronic meningitis caused by fungi, mycobacteria, sarcoidosis, or syphilis.

Behçet's syndrome: in about 20% of patient's with Behçet's disease the CNS is affected, presenting as aseptic meningitis, a meningoencephalomyelitis, or intracranial hypertension.[46]

Chronic benign lymphocytic meningitis[47]

Vogt-Koyanagi-Harada syndrome: uveitis, aseptic meningitis and depigmentation[48]

Familial Mediterranean fever[49]

Granulomatous angiitis: disease of uncertain etiology; affects all ages, particularly patients with lymphomas[50]

Lymphomatoid granulomatosis: involves lung and nervous system, and may progress to lymphoma

Mollaret's meningitis[51,52]

Systemic lupus erythematosus[53]

Aseptic meningitis: consider HIV-infection in patients in high risk groups; can be drug related[54]

Rheumatoid meningitis[55]

Meningitis with Sjögren's syndrome[56]

Drug-induced meningitis: nonsteroidal anti-inflammatory drugs, azathioprine, isoniazid, sulfamethizole, trimethoprim[57,58]

Chemical meningitis: after intrathecal drug administration and foreign substances, such as antibiotics, steroids, isotopes, chemotherapy, air, spinal anesthetics, and metrizamide contrast medium[57,59]

Disorders That Mimic Chronic Meningitis

Partially treated infectious meningitis

Viral encephalitis: prolonged recovery period

Pyogenic or aseptic meningitis: prolonged recovery period

Parameningeal infections: meningeal irritation and CSF abnormalities caused by adjacent suppuration can mimic meningitis[57]

Abscess: cerebral, epidural, subdural, spinal; common initiating infections include osteomyelitis, sinusitis, and mastoiditis[60]

Otitis media with mastoid osteomyelitis[61]

Sinusitis[62,63]

Cyst rupture: epidermoid,[64] dermoid, and arachnoid; epidermoid and dermoid cysts are the most common tumors causing recurrent meningitis; they may cause bacterial meningitis in children and chemical meningitis in adults[65]

Spinal cord tumors[66]

Migraine with cerebrospinal fluid pleocytosis[67,68]

Craniopharyngioma: report of sterile persistent neutrophilic pleocytosis with normal glucose and protein presenting as chronic neutrophilic meningitis[69]

Subarachnoid hemorrhage: can present acutely with a severe headache, CSF pleocytosis, and sometimes a low CSF glucose

Postictal pleocytosis: generalized tonic-clonic seizures,[70] complex-partial seizures[71]

References

1. Ellner JJ, Bennett JE: Chronic meningitis. Medicine 55:341, 1976.
2. Wilhelm C, Ellner JJ: Chronic meningitis. Neurol Clin 4:115, 1986.
3. Sheller JR, Des Prez RM: CNS tuberculosis. Neurol Clin 4:143, 1986.
4. Klein NC, Damsker B, Hirschman SZ: Mycobacterial meningitis. Retrospective analysis from 1970 to 1983. Am J Med 79:29, 1985.
5. Traub M, Leake J, Scholtz C, Thakkar C: Chronic untreated tuberculous meningitis. J Neurol 233:254, 1986.
6. Sabetta JR, Andriole VT: Cryptococcal infection of the central nervous system. Med Clin North Am 69:333, 1985.
7. Benzel EC, King JW, Mirfakhraee M, et al: Blastomycotic meningitis. Surg Neurol 26:192, 1986.
8. Bouza E, Dreyer JS, Hewitt WL, et al: Coccidioidal meningitis. Medicine 60:139, 1981.
9. Shetter AG, Fischer DW, Flom RA: Computed tomography in cases of coccidioidal meningitis, with clinical correlation. West J Med 142:782, 1985.
10. Wheat J, French M, Batteiger B, et al: Cerebrospinal fluid histoplasma antibodies in central nervous system histoplasmosis. Arch Intern Med 145:1237, 1985.
11. Salem FA, Kannangara DW, Nachum R: Cerebral chromomycosis. Arch Neurol 40:173, 1983.
12. Scott EN, Kaufman L, Brown AC, Muchmore HG: Serologic studies in the diagnosis and management of meningitis due to *Sporothrix schenckii*. N Engl J Med 317:935, 1987.
13. Hotson JR: Modern neurosyphilis: a partially treated chronic meningitis. West J Med 135:191, 1981.
14. Johns DR, Tierney M, Felsenstein D: Alteration in the natural history of neurosyphilis by concurrent infection with the human immunodeficiency virus. N Engl J Med 316:1569, 1987.
15. Bouza E, Garcia de la Torre M, Parras F, et al: Brucellar meningitis. Rev Infect Dis 9:810, 1987.
16. Mousa AR, Koshy TS, Araj GF, et al: Brucella meningitis: presentation, diagnosis and treatment—a prospective study of ten cases. Q J Med 60:873, 1986.
17. Al Orainey IO, Laajam MA, Al Aska AK, Rajapakse CN: Brucella meningitis. J Infect 14:141, 1987.
18. Mousa AM, Muhtaseb SA, Reddy RR, et al: The high rate of prevalence of CT-detected basal ganglia calcification in neuropsychiatric (CNS) brucellosis. Acta Neurol Scand 76:448, 1987.
19. Elder GA, Sever JL: Neurologic disorders associated with AIDS retroviral infection. Rev Infect Dis 10:286, 1988.
20. Smego RA Jr: Actinomycosis of the central nervous system. Rev Infect Dis 9:855, 1987.
21. Nash TE, Neva FA: Recent advances in the diagnosis

and treatment of cerebral cysticercosis. N Engl J Med 311:1492, 1984.

22. Estanol B, Corona T, Abad P: A prognostic classification of cerebral cysticercosis: therapeutic implications. J Neurol Neurosurg Psychiatry 49:1131, 1986.

23. Bale JF Jr: Human cytomegalovirus infection and disorders of the nervous system. Arch Neurol 41:310, 1984.

24. Kuberski T, Wallace GD: Clinical manifestations of eosinophilic meningitis due to *Angiostrongylus cantonensis.* Neurology 29:1566, 1979.

25. Schmutzhard E, Boongird P, Vejjajiva A: Eosinophilic meningitis and radiculomyelitis in Thailand, caused by CNS invasion of *Gnathostoma spinigerum* and *Angiostrongylus cantonensis.* J Neurol Neurosurg Psychiatry 51:80, 1988.

26. Wilkinson JA, Keate RF: *Listeria monocytogenes* meningitis. Ann Emerg Med 13:474, 1984.

27. Bach MC, Davis KM: *Listeria* rhombencephalitis mimicking tuberculous meningitis. Rev Infect Dis 9:130, 1987.

28. Hollander H, Stringari S: Human immunodeficiency virus-associated meningitis. Clinical course and correlations. Am J Med 83:813, 1987.

29. Ho DD, Rota TR, Schooley RT, et al: Isolation of HTLV-III from cerebrospinal fluid and neural tissues of patients with neurologic syndromes related to the acquired immunodeficiency syndrome. N Engl J Med 313:1493, 1985.

30. Levy RM, Bredesen DE, Rosenblum ML: Neurological manifestations of the acquired immunodeficiency syndrome (AIDS): experience at UCSF and review of the literature. J Neurosurg 62:475, 1985.

31. Pachner AR, Steere AC: The triad of neurologic manifestations of Lyme disease: meningitis, cranial neuritis, and radiculoneuritis. Neurology 35:47, 1985.

32. Broderick JP, Sandok BA, Mertz LE: Focal encephalitis in a young woman 6 years after the onset of Lyme disease: tertiary Lyme disease? Mayo Clin Proc 62:313, 1987.

33. Razavi-Encha F, Fleury-Feith J, Gherardi R, Bernaudin JF: Cytologic features of cerebrospinal fluid in Lyme disease. Acta Cytol 31:439, 1987.

34. Pal GS, Baker JT, Humphrey PR: Lyme disease presenting as recurrent acute meningitis. Br Med J (Clin Res) 295:367, 1987.

35. Weder B, Wiedersheim P, Matter L, et al: Chronic progressive neurological involvement in *Borrelia burgdorferi* infection. J Neurol 234:40, 1987.

36. Wokke JH, van Gijn J, Elderson A, Stanek G: Chronic forms of *Borrelia burgdorferi* infection of the nervous system. Neurology 37:1031, 1987.

37. Hofstad H, Matre R, Nyland H, Ulvestad E: Bannwarth's syndrome: serum and CSF IgG antibodies against *Borrelia burgdorferi* examined by ELISA. Acta Neurol Scand 75:37, 1987.

38. Sindic CJ, Depre A, Bigaignon G, et al: Lymphocytic meningoradiculitis and encephalomyelitis due to *Borrelia burgdorferi:* a clinical and serological study of 18 cases. J Neurol Neurosurg Psychiatry 50:1565, 1987.

39. Henriksson A, Link H, Cruz M, Stiernstedt G: Immunoglobulin abnormalities in cerebrospinal fluid and blood over the course of lymphocytic meningoradiculitis (Bannwarth's syndrome). Ann Neurol 20:337, 1986.
40. Sage JI, Weinstein MP, Miller DC: Chronic encephalitis possibly due to herpes simplex virus: two cases. Neurology 35:1470, 1985.
41. Barnes DW, Whitley RJ: CNS diseases associated with varicella zoster virus and herpes simplex virus infection. Pathogenesis and current therapy. Neurol Clin 4:265, 1986.
42. Stern BJ, Krumholz A, Johns C, et al: Sarcoidosis and its neurological manifestations. Arch Neurol 42:909, 1985.
43. Ho K-L, Hoschner JA, Wolfe DE: Primary leptomeningeal gliomatosis. Symptoms suggestive of meningitis. Arch Neurol 38:662, 1981.
44. Trump DL, Grossman SA, Thompson G, et al: CSF infections complicating the management of neoplastic meningitis. Arch Intern Med 142:583, 1982.
45. Csako G, Chandra P: Bronchioloalveolar carcinoma presenting with meningeal carcinomatosis. Cytologic diagnosis in cerebrospinal fluid. Acta Cytol 30:653, 1986.
46. Mas JL, Louarn F, Degos JD: Non-specific angiitis and the central nervous system. Rev Neurol (Paris) 139:467, 1983.
47. Hopkins AP, Harvey PKP: Chronic benign lymphocytic meningitis. J Neurol Sci 18:443, 1973.
48. Perry HD, Font RL: Clinical and histopathologic observations in severe Vogt-Koyanagi-Harada syndrome. Am J Ophthalmol 83:242, 1977.
49. Vilaseca J, Tor J, Guardia J, et al: Periodic meningitis and familial Mediterranean fever. Arch Intern Med 142:378, 1982.
50. Reik L Jr, Grunnet ML, Spencer RP, et al: Granulomatous angiitis presenting as chronic meningitis and ventriculitis. Nuerology 33:1609, 1983.
51. Tyler KL, Adler D: Twenty-eight years of benign recurrent Mollaret meningitis. Arch Neurol 40:42, 1983.
52. Barakat MH, Mustafa HT, Shakir RA: Mollaret's meningitis. A variant of recurrent hereditary polyserositis, both provoked by metaraminol. Arch Neurol 45:926, 1988.
53. Sergent JS, Lockshin MD, Klempner MS, et al: Central nervous system disease in systemic lupus erythematosus. Am J Med 58:644, 1975.
54. Levy RM, Bredesen DE: Central nervous system dysfunction in acquired immunodeficiency syndrome. p. 29. In Rosenblum ML, Levy RM, Bredesen DE (eds): AIDS and the Nervous System. Raven Press, New York, 1988.
55. Spurlock RG, Richman AV: Rheumatoid meningitis. Arch Pathol Lab Med 107:129, 1983.
56. Alexander EL, Alexander GE: Aseptic meningoencephalitis in primary Sjögren's syndrome. Neurology 33:593, 1983.
57. Reik L Jr: Disorders that mimic CNS infections. Neurol Clin 4:223, 1986.

58. Jensen S, Glud TK, Bacher T, Ersgaard H: Ibuprofen-induced meningitis in a male with systemic lupus erythematosus. Acta Med Scand 221:509, 1987.
59. White WB: Metrizamide meningitis. South Med J 77:88, 1984.
60. Lechtenberg R, Sierra MF, Pringle GF, et al: *Listeria monocytogenes:* brain abscess or meningoencephalitis? Neurology 29:86, 1979.
61. Schwarz GA, Blumenkrantz MJ, Sundmaker WLH: Neurologic complications of malignant external otitis. Neurology 21:1077, 1971.
62. Kaufman DM, Litman N, Miller MH: Sinusitis: induced subdural empyema. Neurology 33:123, 1983.
63. Finkelstein R, Honigman S, Doron Y, et al: Sphenoid sinusitis presenting as chronic meningitis. Eur Neurol 25:183, 1986.
64. Becker WJ, Watters GV, de Chadarevian JP, Vanasse M: Recurrent aseptic meningitis secondary to intracranial epidermoids. Can J Neurol Sci 11:387, 1984.
65. Roach ES, Laster DW: Prolonged course of meningitis due to an arachnoid cyst. Arch Neurol 38:720, 1981.
66. Okawara S: Ruptured spinal ependymoma simulating bacterial meningitis. Arch Neurol 40:54, 1983.
67. Bruyn GW, Gerrari M, De Beer FC: Migraine, Tolosa-Hunt syndrome and pleocytosis. Clin Neurol Neurosurg 86:33, 1984.
68. Fitzsimmons RB, Wolfenden WH: Migraine coma. Meningitic migraine with cerebral oedema associated with a new form of autosomal dominant cerebellar ataxia. Brain 108:555, 1985.
69. Krueger DW, Larson EB: Recurrent fever of unknown origin, coma, and meningismus due to a leaking craniopharyngioma. Am J Med 84:543, 1988.
70. Edwards R, Schmidley JW, Simon RP: How often does a CSF pleocytosis follow generalized convulsions? Ann Neurol 13:460, 1983.
71. Devinsky O, Nadi S, Theodore WH, Porter RJ: Cerebrospinal fluid pleocytosis following simple, complex partial, and generalized tonic-clonic seizures. Ann Neurol 23:402, 1988.

Selected Readings

Anderson NE, Willoughby EW: Chronic meningitis without predisposing illness—a review of 83 cases. Q J Med 63:283, 1987.
Eighty-three cases of chronic meningitis that appeared in previously healthy adults are described. Etiologies in decreasing frequency included tuberculosis (40%), unknown (34%), malignancy (8%), and cryptococcus (7%). Tuberculous and neoplastic meningitis presented with the most characteristic clinical pictures. The study also identified a subgroup of patients with idiopathic chronic meningitis who were steroid responsive.

Body BA, Oneson RH, Herold DA: Use of cerebrospinal fluid lactic acid concentration in the diagnosis of fungal meningitis. Ann Clin Lab Sci 17:429, 1987.
This interesting study, review, and case report suggests that elevated lactic acid in CSF may be a useful nonspecific marker for cryptococcal infection in patients who have clinical pictures consis-

tent with cryptococcal meningitis, but have negative CSF stains and cultures.

Conrad KA, Gross JL, Trojanowski JQ: Leptomeningeal carcinomatosis presenting as eosinophilic meningitis. Acta Cytol 30:29, 1986.
A case report of a 67-year-old man with carcinomatous meningitis who presented with meningismus and eosinophilic CSF. Authors underscore the need to consider the clinical possibility of coincident meningeal carcinomatosis in cases of CSF eosinophilia that cannot be explained by the usual causative agents, such as bacterial, fungal, and parasitic agents.

Conti DJ, Rubin RH: Infection of the central nervous system in organ transplant recipients. Neurol Clin 6:241, 1988.
Central nervous system infection in organ transplant recipients is a significant cause of morbidity and mortality. This article reviews diagnostic and management approaches, with a particular emphasis on clinical features associated with the three most commonly involved organisms: L. monocytogens, Aspergillus fumigatus, *and* Cryptococcus neoformans.

Dougherty JM, Jones J: Cerebrospinal fluid cultures and analysis. Ann Emerg Med 15:317, 1986.
This review considers state-of-the-art CSF testing. Authors review cost considerations and present an algorithm for efficient selection of tests.

Gabuzda DH, Hirsch MS: Neurologic manifestations of infection with human immunodeficiency virus. Clinical features and pathogenesis. Ann Intern Med 107:383, 1987.
Important review of neurologic disease in HIV infection, which can be the only manifestation of HIV infection.

Graman PS, Trupei MA, Reichman RC: Evaluation of cerebrospinal fluid in asymptomatic late syphilis. Sex Transm Dis 14:205, 1987.
The role of lumbar puncture in the evaluation of asymptomatic late syphilis was studied by reviewing CSF from 47 asymptomatic patients with syphilis, which was either of unknown duration or of duration longer than 1 year. Thirty-two percent of subjects had abnormalities including elevated protein and pleocytosis of uncertain etiology. CSF-reactive VDRL was present in three patients; three of eight patients with rapid plasma reagin titers greater or equal to 1:128 had neurosyphilis. Authors suggest that lumbar puncture is indicated in patients with asymptomatic late syphilis of unknown duration.

Hayward RA, Shapiro MF, Oye RK: Laboratory testing on cerebrospinal fluid. A reappraisal. Lancet 1:1, 1987.
Five hundred fifty-five consecutive samples of CSF were reviewed to determine which CSF tests were most helpful diagnostically. In most cases if the CSF opening pressure, cell count, and protein are normal (except in cases of clinically suspected acute childhood meningitis, multiple sclerosis, or immune compromise), further CSF tests are rarely helpful.

Henry K, Crossley K: Meningitis. Principles of diagnosis, advances in treatment. Postgrad Med 80 (3):59, 1986.
A clinical review of the current state-of-the-art approach to patients with suspected and proven meningitis.

Kadival GV, Samuel AM, Mazarelo TB, Chaparas SD: Radioimmunoassay for detecting *Mycobacterium tuberculosis* antigen in cerebrospinal fluids of patients with tuberculous meningitis. J Infect Dis 155:608, 1987.

This paper describes a biotin-avidin radioimmunoassay for detecting Mycobacterium tuberculosis *antigen, which authors suggest may help in the early diagnosis of tuberculous meningitis.*

Lyons RW, Andriole VT: Fungal infections of the CNS. Neurol Clin 4:159, 1986.

This useful review of CNS fungal infections is organized into clinical presentations of those occurring in normal hosts and those occurring in immunosuppressed hosts. Cryptococcal infection is common in both groups.

Marton KI, Gean AD: The spinal tap: a new look at an old test. Ann Intern Med 104:840, 1986.

An important review of indications, technique, and usefulness of the lumbar puncture in light of newer neurodiagnostic procedures. A probability analysis is provided.

McGinnis MR: Detection of fungi in cerebrospinal fluid. Proceedings of a symposium: body fluids and infectious diseases. Clinical and microbiologic advances. Am J Med 75(Suppl 1B):129, 1983.

A review of CSF findings and clinical presentations of various fungi that were isolated or observed, or both in cerebrospinal specimens. Useful review.

Peacock JE Jr, McGinnis MR, Cohen MS: Persistent neutrophilic meningitis. Report of four cases and review of the literature. Medicine 63:379, 1984.

Comprehensive review of persistent neutrophilic meningitis, a poorly described variant of chronic meningitis characterized by persistence of neutrophils in the CSF greater than 1 week or extended periods in association with meningeal inflammation and negative CSF cultures. Diagnostic considerations, including indications for brain biopsy, are discussed.

Petito CK: Review of central nervous system pathology in human immunodeficiency virus infection. Ann Neurol 23 (Suppl):S54, 1988.

This article reviews the pathology and pathogenesis of the three major manifestations of HIV central nervous system infection: aseptic meningitis, subacute encephalitis, and vacuolar myelopathy.

Rubin SJ: Detection of viruses in spinal fluid. Proceedings of a symposium: body fluids and infectious diseases. Clinical and microbiologic advances. Am J Med 75(Suppl 1B):124, 1983.

Discussion of continued use of viral culture as means of diagnosing the origin of aseptic meningitis.

Salaki JS, Louria DB, Chmel H: Fungal and yeast infections of the central nervous system. A clinical review. Medicine 63:108, 1984.

Comprehensive, extensively referenced clinical review of central nervous system fungal and yeast infections. This review summarizes cases reported through 1982 with an emphasis on clinical manifestations.

Simon RP: Neurosyphilis. Arch Neurol 42:606, 1985.

This useful, state-of-the-art discussion of the diagnosis and management of neurosyphilis emphasizes that the diagnosis of all forms of neurosyphilis still relies on evidence of reactivity reflected by spinal fluid pleocytosis and increased protein content associated with reactive serology.

Steele RW, Marmer DJ, O'Brien MD, et al: Leukocyte

survival in cerebrospinal fluid. J Clin Microbiol 23:965, 1986.

A study designed to evaluate changes in cerebrospinal fluid leukocyte counts relative to time elapsed before analysis found that lymphocyte and monocyte numbers were not significantly altered until 3 hours have elapsed.

Tallman RD, Kimbrough SM, O'Brien JF, et al: Assay for β-glucuronidase in cerebrospinal fluid: usefulness for the detection of neoplastic meningitis. Mayo Clin Proc 60:293, 1985.

The assay for beta-glucuronidase in CSF was evaluated in CSF from 30 patients with cytology positive or suggestive for malignancy and compared with CSF from 131 patients with various disorders. Elevated beta-glucuronidase occurred most frequently in patients with neoplastic meningitis. Patients with adenocarcinoma and myelogenous leukemia had the highest levels.

van Zanten AP, Twijnstra A, Ongerboer de Visser BW: Routine investigations of the CSF with special reference to meningeal malignancy and infectious meningitis. Acta Neurol Scand 77:210, 1988.

Cerebrospinal fluid from patients with meningeal malignancies was compared with CSF with pleocytosis from patients with disorders other than meningeal malignancies. Usefulness of cell count, glucose concentrations, and total protein was evaluated. Authors concluded that these routine tests are of limited value in distinguishing viral, bacterial, or neoplastic causes and that the most consistently helpful finding was a significantly increased number of polymorphonuclear leukocytes, which often reflected acute bacterial meningitis.

73

Low Cerebrospinal Fluid Glucose (Hypoglycorrhachia): Associated Disorders

Hypoglycorrhachia, or low cerebrospinal fluid (CSF) glucose, exists when CSF glucose falls significantly below 60 to 80% of the blood glucose. Since there is a lag time of 30 to 60 minutes between changes in

CSF and serum glucose levels, an optimal CSF glucose level is obtained simultaneously with serum glucose after 4 hours of fasting. The most significant drops in CSF glucose are seen in acute bacterial meningitis with marked pleocytosis.[1]

Acute bacterial meningitis[2]: usually associated with predominantly granulocytic pleocytosis with greater than 1,000/mm[3]

Tuberculous meningitis: consider in patients with history of tuberculosis, the homeless, and in human immunodeficiency virus (HIV)-infected patients[3,4]

Mycobacterium other than tuberculosis: *M. avium-intracellulare* is common in acquired immune deficiency syndrome (AIDS)[5-9]

Fungal meningitis[10]: cryptococcosis,[11] blastomycosis,[12] coccidioidomycosis,[13,14] histoplasmosis,[15] chromomycosis,[16] *Sporothrix schenckii*[17]

Viral meningitis: mumps, herpes simplex,[18] herpes zoster

Carcinomatous meningitis[19]

Sarcoidosis: meningeal involvement[20,21]

Parasitic meningitis: Naegleria, trichinosis, cysticercosis[22]

Syphilitic meningitis: may be resistant to conventional therapy and more aggressive in HIV-infected patients[23-26]

Metrizamide lumbar myelography[27,28]

Central nervous system leukemia

Rheumatoid meningitis[29]

Subarachnoid hemorrhage[30]

Hypoglycemia

Partially treated meningitis with subdural empyema[31]

Leptomeningeal gliomatosis: normal or low CSF glucose[32]

Listeria monocytogenes meningitis: can mimic tuberculous meningitis[33,34]

Reticulum cell sarcoma[35]

Stroke: in young stroke victims with a history of intravenous drug use or other risk for HIV infection, consider underlying endocarditis, meningosyphilis, cryptococcus, and other fungal infections[36,37]

References

1. Fishman RA: Composition of cerebrospinal fluid. p. 208. In Cerebrospinal Fluid in Diseases of the Nervous System. WB Saunders, Philadelphia, 1980.

2. Martin WJ: Rapid and reliable techniques for the laboratory detection of bacterial meningitis. Proceedings of a symposium: body fluids and infectious diseases. Clinical and microbiologic advances. Am J Med 75(Suppl 1B):119, 1983.
3. Sheller JR, DesPrez RM: CNS tuberculosis. Neurol Clin 4:143, 1986.
4. Hamrick RM III, Yeager H Jr: Tuberculosis update. Am Fam Physician 38 (4):205, 1988.
5. Klein NC, Damsker B, Hirschman SZ: Mycobacterial meningitis. Retrospective analysis from 1970 to 1983. Am J Med 79:29, 1985.
6. Woolsey RM, Chambers TJ, Chung HD, McGarry JD: Mycobacterial meningomyelitis associated with human immunodeficiency virus infection. Arch Neurol 45:691, 1988.
7. Tenholder MF, Moser RJ III, Tellis CJ: Mycobacteria other than tuberculosis. Pulmonary involvement in patients with acquired immunodeficiency syndrome. Arch Intern Med 148:953, 1988.
8. Levy RM, Bredesen DE, Rosenblum ML: Opportunistic central nervous system pathology in patients with AIDS. Ann Neurol 23 (Suppl):S7, 1988.
9. Fournier AM, Dickinson GM, Erdfrocht IR, et al: Tuberculosis and nontuberculous mycobacteriosis in patients with AIDS. Chest 93:772, 1988.
10. Salaki JS, Louria DB, Chmel H: Fungal and yeast infections of the nervous system. Medicine 63:108, 1984.
11. Sabetta JR, Andriole VT: Cryptococcal infection of the central nervous system. Med Clin North Am 69:333, 1985.
12. Benzel EC, King JW, Mirfakhraee M, et al: Blastomycotic meningitis. Surg Neurol 26:192, 1986.
13. Bouza E, Dreyer JS, Hewitt WL, et al: Coccidioidal meningitis. Medicine 60:139, 1981.
14. Shetter AG, Fischer DW, Flom RA: Computed tomography in cases of coccidioidal meningitis, with clinical correlation. West J Med 142:782, 1985.
15. Wheat J, French M, Batteiger B, et al: Cerebrospinal fluid histoplasma antibodies in central nervous system histoplasmosis. Arch Intern Med 145:1237, 1985.
16. Salem FA, Kannangara DW, Nachum R: Cerebral chromomycosis. Arch Neurol 40:173, 1983.
17. Scott EN, Kaufman L, Brown AC, Muchmore HG: Serologic studies in the diagnosis and management of meningitis due to *Sporothrix schenckii*. N Engl J Med 317:935, 1987.
18. Mikati MA, Krishnamoorthy KS: Hypoglycorrhachia in neonatal herpes simplex virus meningoencephalitis. J Pediatr 107:746, 1985.
19. Heimann A, Merino MJ: Carcinomatous meningitis as the initial manifestation of breast cancer. Acta Cytol 30:25, 1986.
20. Douglas AC, Maloney AFJ: Sarcoidosis of the central nervous system. J Neurol Neurosurg Psychiatry 36:1024, 1973.
21. Atkinson R, Ghelman B, Tsairis P, et al: Sarcoidosis presenting as cervical radiculopathy: a case report and literature review. Spine 7:412, 1982.

22. Nash TE, Neva FA: Recent advances in the diagnosis and treatment of cerebral cysticercosis. N Engl J Med 311:1492, 1984.
23. Simon RP: Neurosyphilis. Arch Neurol 42:606, 1985.
24. Hotson JR: Modern neurosyphilis: a partially treated chronic meningitis. West J Med 135:191, 1981.
25. Johns DR, Tierney M, Felsenstein D: Alteration in the natural history of neurosyphilis by concurrent infection with the human immunodeficiency virus. N Engl J Med 316:1569, 1987.
26. Lanska MJ, Lanska DJ, Schmidley JW: Syphilitic polyradiculopathy in an HIV-positive man. Neurology 38:1297, 1988.
27. Kelley RE, Daroff RB, Sheremata WA, et al: Unusual effects of metrizamide lumbar myelography. Arch Neurol 37:588, 1980.
28. White WB: Metrizamide meningitis. South Med J 77:88, 1984.
29. Markenson JA, McDougal JS, Tsairis P, et al: Rheumatoid meningitis: a localized immune process. Ann Intern Med 90:786, 1979.
30. Pasquier F, Leys D, Vermersch P, Petit H: Severe hypoglycorrhachia after subarachnoid hemorrhage. Two cases with spontaneous recovery in adults. Acta Neurol Belg 87:76, 1987.
31. Kaufman DM, Miller MH, Steigbigel NH: Subdural empyema: analysis of 17 recent cases and review of the literature. Medicine 54:485, 1975.
32. Bailey P, Robitaille Y: Primary diffuse leptomeningeal gliomatosis. Can J Neurol Sci 12:278, 1985.
33. Bach MC, Davis KM: Listeria rhombencephalitis mimicking tuberculous meningitis. Rev Infect Dis 9:130, 1987.
34. Hansen PB, Jensen TH, Lykkegaard S, Kristensen HS: *Listeria monocytogenes* meningitis in adults. Sixteen consecutive cases 1973–1982. Scand J Infect Dis 19:55, 1987.
35. Wong MJ, Chan RM, Stordy SN: Reticulum cell sarcoma with unusual presenting features: fever and low cerebrospinal fluid glucose levels. Can Med Assoc J 131:905, 1984.
36. Kantor HL, Emsellem HA, Hogg JE, Simon GL: *Candida albicans* meningitis in a parenteral drug abuser. South Med J 77:404, 1984.
37. Saul RF, Gallagher JG, Mateer JE: Sudden hemiparesis as the presenting sign in cryptococcal meningoencephalitis. Stroke 17:753, 1986.

Selected Readings

Fishman R (ed): Composition of cerebrospinal fluid. p. 168. In Cerebrospinal Fluid in Diseases of the Nervous System. WB Saunders, Philadelphia, 1980.
Good general reference.

Leonard JM: Cerebrospinal fluid formula in patients with central nervous system infection. Neurol Clin 4:3, 1986.
Useful guidelines offered for the evaluation of the patient with meningitis of uncertain etiology with CSF suggestive of viral infection and with clinical signs suggestive of possible bacterial men-

ingitis. Such a presentation raises the clinical decision of whether to withhold antibiotics before the infectious agent is identified.

Martin WJ: Rapid and reliable techniques for the laboratory detection of bacterial meningitis. Proceedings of a symposium: body fluids and infectious diseases. Clinical and microbiologic advances. Am J Med 75(Suppl 1B):119, 1983. *State-of-the-art laboratory diagnosis of bacterial meningitis.*

See Selected Readings from Chapters 71 and 72.

74

Acquired Immune Deficiency Syndrome: Diagnostic Infections and Neoplasms

Acquired immune deficiency syndrome (AIDS) refers to patients infected with human immunodeficiency virus (HIV) who manifest profound immunosuppression and have developed those opportunistic infections which meet the current case definition of AIDS.[1] The following specified infections and neoplasms have been declared by the National Center for Health Statistics and Center for Infectious Diseases, Centers for Disease Control to constitute the first major category of the spectrum of HIV infection. The diagnosis of AIDS can be made when the following infections or malignant neoplasms are diagnosed in patients with HIV infection.[2] If patients present with the following infections or neoplasms without a history of HIV infection or other immune compromise, consider possible HIV infection, especially in the following high risk categories: homosexuals,[2-6] bisexuals, intravenous drug users,[7-10] blood product recipients[11,12] (particularly hemophiliacs[13-15]), infants of HIV-infected women,[16] sexual partners of

HIV seropositive individuals,[17-22] and members of certain endemic regions, such as found on the African continent.[23] Seroepidemiologic data suggest that many patients can be infected with HIV yet remain asymptomatic or manifest illnesses which are not associated with the detection of specific opportunistic pathogens. Although current data suggest 10 to 60% of patients infected with HIV may eventually develop AIDS, the exact number of HIV-infected patients who will progress to AIDS is unknown.

Specified Infections with HIV Infection[2]

Pneumocystosis: *Pneumocystis carinii* pneumonia
Toxoplasmosis[24-26]
Candidiasis of the lung
Coccidiosis
Cryptococcosis
Isosporiasis[27]
Progressive multifocal leukoencephalopathy (PML)[28,29]

Specified Malignant Neoplasms with HIV Infection[2]

Burkitt's tumor or lymphomas
Kaposi's sarcoma: particularly the disseminated, aggressive forms[30-35]
Primary lymphoma of the brain[36]
Immunoblastic sarcoma
Reticulosarcoma

References

1. Redfield RR, Burke DS: HIV infection: the clinical picture. Sci Am 259:90, 1988.
2. Centers for Disease Control: Revision of HIV classification codes. MMWR 36:821, 1988.
3. Gottlieb MS: Immunologic aspects of the acquired immunodeficiency syndrome and male homosexuality. Med Clin North Am 70:651, 1986.
4. Lui KJ, Darrow WW, Rutherford GW III: A model-based estimate of the mean incubation period for AIDS in homosexual men. Science 240:1333, 1988.
5. McDougal JS, Kennedy MS, Nicholson JK, et al: Antibody response to human immunodeficiency virus in homosexual men. Relation of antibody specificity, titer, and isotype to clinical status, severity of immunodeficiency, and disease progression. J Clin Invest 80:316, 1987.
6. Cooney TG, Ward TT (eds): AIDS and other medical problems in the male homosexual. Med Clin North Am 70:497, 1986.
7. Wong B, Gold JWM, Brown AE, et al: Central-nervous-

system toxoplasmosis in homosexual men and parenteral drug abusers. Ann Intern Med 100:36, 1984.

8. Des Jarlais DC, Friedman SR: HIV infection among intravenous drug users: epidemiology and risk reduction. AIDS 1:67, 1987.

9. DAquila RT, Williams AB: Epidemic human immunodeficiency virus (HIV) infection among intravenous drug users (IVDU). Yale J Biol Med 60:545, 1987.

10. Des Jarlais DC, Friedman SR, Stoneburner RL: HIV infection and intravenous drug use: critical issues in transmission dynamics, infection outcomes, and prevention. Rev Infect Dis 10:151, 1988.

11. Curran JW, Lawrence DN, Jaffe H, et al: Acquired immunodeficiency syndrome (AIDS) associated with transfusions. N Engl J Med 310:69, 1984.

12. Feorino PM, Jaffe HW, Palmer E, et al: Transfusion-associated acquired immunodeficiency syndrome. N Engl J Med 312:1293, 1985.

13. Kreiss JK, Kitchen LW, Prince HE, et al: Antibody to human T-lymphotropic virus type III in wives of hemophiliacs. Ann Intern Med 102:623, 1985.

14. McGrady GA, Jason JM, Evatt BL: The course of the epidemic of acquired immunodeficiency syndrome in the United States hemophilia population. Am J Epidemiol 126:25, 1987.

15. Stehr-Green JK, Holman RC, Jason JM, Evatt BL: Hemophilia-associated AIDS in the United States, 1981 to September 1987. Am J Public Health 78:439, 1988.

16. Scott GB, Buck BE, Leterman JG, et al: Acquired immunodeficiency syndrome in infants. N Engl J Med 310:76, 1984.

17. Johnson AM, Petherick A, Davidson SJ: Transmission of HIV to heterosexual partners of infected men and women. AIDS 3:367, 1989.

18. Chamberland ME, Dondero TJ Jr: Heterosexually acquired infection with human immunodeficiency virus (HIV). A view from the III International Conference on AIDS. Ann Intern Med 107:763, 1987.

19. Piot P, Kreiss JK, Mdinya-Achola JO, et al: Heterosexual transmission of HIV. AIDS 1:199, 1987.

20. Padian NS: Heterosexual transmission of acquired immunodeficiency syndrome: international perspectives and national projections. Rev Infect Dis 9:947, 1987.

21. Johnson AM: Heterosexual transmission of human immunodeficiency virus. Br Med J 296:1017, 1988.

22. DeGruttola V, Mayer KH: Assessing and modeling heterosexual spread of the human immunodeficiency virus in the United States. Rev Infect Dis 10:138, 1988.

23. Hrdy DB: Cultural practices contributing to the transmission of human immunodeficiency virus in Africa. Rev Infect Dis 9:1109, 1987.

24. Alonso R, Heiman-Patterson T, Mancall EL: Cerebral toxoplasmosis in acquired immune deficiency syndrome. Arch Neurol 41:321, 1984.

25. Snider WD, Simpson DM, Nielsen S, et al: Neurological complications of acquired immune deficiency syndrome: analysis of 50 patients. Ann Neurol 14:403, 1983.

26. Holliman RE: Toxoplasmosis and the acquired immune deficiency syndrome. J Infect 16:121, 1988.

27. Soave R, Johnson WD Jr: Cryptosporidium and *Isospora belli* infections. J Infect Dis 157:225, 1988.
28. Hseuh C, Reyes CV: Progressive multifocal leukoencephalopathy. Am Fam Physician 37(6):129, 1988.
29. Berger JR, Kaszovitz B, Post MJ, Dickinson G: Progressive multifocal leukoencephalopathy associated with human immunodeficiency virus infection. A review of the literature with a report of sixteen cases. Ann Intern Med 107:78, 1987.
30. Marmor M, Freidman-Kien AE, Zolla-Pazner S, et al: Kaposi's sarcoma in homosexual men. A seroepidemiologic case-control study. Ann Intern Med 100:809, 1984.
31. Groopman JE: AIDS-related Kaposi's sarcoma: therapeutic modalities. Semin Hematol 24(Suppl):5, 1987.
32. Krown SE: AIDS-associated Kaposi's sarcoma: pathogenesis, clinical course, and treatment. AIDS 2:71, 1988.
33. Nyberg DA, Federle MP: AIDS-related Kaposi sarcoma and lymphomas. Semin Roentgenol 22:54, 1987.
34. Mitsuyasu RT: Clinical variants and staging of Kaposi's sarcoma. Semin Oncol 14(Suppl):13, 1987.
35. Safai B: Pathophysiology and epidemiology of epidemic Kaposi's sarcoma. Semin Oncol 14(Suppl):7, 1987.
36. Hochberg FH, Miller DC: Primary central nervous system lymphoma. J Neurosurg 68:835, 1988.

Selected Readings

Armstrong D: Opportunistic infections in the acquired immune deficiency syndrome. Semin Oncol 14(Suppl 3):40, 1987.
From a major cancer center, a review of opportunistic infections in AIDS with a perspective on prognosis and management. Authors stress that the severity of the underlying immune deficit is the most significant prognostic factor and that opportunistic infection is currently the most common cause of death in AIDS patients.

Baker JL: What is the occupational risk to emergency care providers from the human immunodeficiency virus? Ann Emerg Med 17:700, 1988.
A focus on the risk of emergency room health care providers for HIV infection. Authors offer recommendations for prevention and management of certain HIV-related clinical problems that present in this setting.

Castro KG, Lifson AR, White CR, et al: Investigations of AIDS patients with no previously identified risk factors. JAMA 259:1338, 1988.
In 921 (45%) patients, the risk factor history was incomplete or unobtainable. Risk factors were identified in 825 (72%) of the remaining 1,138 patients.

Fauci AS: The human immunodeficiency virus: infectivity and mechanisms of pathogenesis. Science 239:617, 1988.
Important review of concepts of HIV infectivity. Clinical correlations relate to certain discussed HIV characteristics: HIV latent states, chronic forms of HIV infection, and possible HIV tropism for the brain causing neuropsychiatric abnormalities.

Health and Public Policy Committee, American College of Physicians; and the Infectious Diseases Society of America: The acquired immunodeficiency syndrome (AIDS) and infection with human immunodeficiency virus (HIV). Ann Intern Med 108:460, 1988.

A recent statement on AIDS and HIV infection from the Health and Public Policy Committee, American College of Physicians, and the Infecitous Diseases Society of America.

Ho DD, Pomerantz RJ, Kaplan JC: Pathogenesis of infection with human immunodeficiency virus. N Engl J Med 317:278, 1987.

Current concepts and state-of-the-art review of the pathogenesis of HIV infection.

Hopkins DR: AIDS in minority populations in the United States. Public Health Rep 102:677, 1987.

In black and Hispanic communities, intravenous drug abuse is the most frequent mode of transmission of HIV infection. Public health issues addressed toward infection prevention in the minority community are discussed.

Hsiung GD: Perspectives on retroviruses and the etiologic agent of AIDS. Yale J Biol Med 60:505, 1987.

Historical perspective of retrovirus infection and the emergence of HIV and AIDS. Understanding retrovirus infection and HIV emergency may provide important biologic clues toward successful isolation, identification, and control of the virus.

Leads from the MMWR. Quarterly report to the Domestic Policy Council on the prevalence and rate of spread of HIV and AIDS in the United States. JAMA 259:2657, 1988.

Current epidemiology data in the United States.

Levy JA: Mysteries of HIV: challenges for therapy and prevention. Nature 333:519, 1988.

A review of current problems toward developing antiviral therapy and vaccines against infection.

Osborn JE: The AIDS epidemic: six years. Annu Rev Public Health 9:551, 1988.

An AIDS epidemiology update.

Piel J (ed): What science knows about AIDS. A single topic issue. Sci Am 259:1988.

A single topic issue devoted to AIDS. Outstanding contributing authors review a wide range of current concepts of AIDS, usually within an historical perspective. Topics reviewed cover the molecular biology of the AIDS virus, clinical pictures, social issues, as well as current and proposed therapies. High-quality monograph.

Rosenberg MJ, Weiner JM: Prostitutes and AIDS: a health department priority? Am J Public Health 78:418, 1988.

Although prostitutes are considered as potential reservoirs for certain sexually transmitted diseases, a variety of studies suggest that HIV infection in prostitutes follows a different pattern from other sexually transmitted diseases. HIV infection in nondrug-using prostitutes is low or absent, which suggests that sexual activity without intravenous drug use results in a lower rate of HIV transmission, particularly when compared to rates of infection of other sexually transmitted diseases.

Ward JW, Holmberg SD, Allen JR, et al: Transmission of human immunodeficiency virus (HIV) by blood transfusions screened as negative for HIV antibody. N Engl J Med 318:473, 1988.

To identify instances of HIV transmission by antibody-negative blood donations, 13 persons seropositive for HIV who had received blood from 7 screened donors were evaluated. No risk factors wre found in the recipients, and all seven donors were ultimately found to be infected with HIV. The apparent seronegativity of the screened blood was caused by recent HIV infection of the donors.

75

HIV Infection and AIDS: Clinical Manifestations

Patients with acquired immune deficiency syndrome (AIDS) are infected with the human immunodeficiency virus (HIV), manifest profound immunosuppression, and develop opportunistic infections which meet the current case definition of AIDS. AIDS is only one stage of HIV infection. It is important to be familiar with common manifestations of HIV in the early stages. Many manifestations of HIV infection, such as certain opportunistic infections, are treatable. Early detection of HIV infection before late symptoms of HIV infection occur can help prolong and improve the quality of life of patients with HIV. Patients presenting with focal or generalized lymphadenopathy, particularly if they belong to a high risk category (see Ch. 74, Specified Infections with HIV Infection), present special problems in diagnosis (see Section X, Hematology; Ch. 112).

Disorders of the Nervous System Caused by HIV Infection

HIV-related disorders of the nervous system can be due to direct HIV infection, opportunistic infection, or malignant neoplasms. It is not uncommon for several of these disorders to occur simultaneously, especially in end-stage AIDS patients. Clinical manifestations virtually encompass the entire spectrum of neurologic signs, symptoms, and syndromes with common manifestations including dementia, encephalopathy, meningitis, seizures, peripheral neuropathy, myelopathy, acute confusional states, and strokes.[1-6]

HIV subacute encephalitis: often manifests as a dementia, or the "AIDS dementia complex"[7,8]

HIV myelopathy: often present in patients with subacute encephalitis; rarely can mimic spinal cord compression at onset

HIV meningitis: self-limited condition during which HIV can sometimes be isolated from the cerebral spinal fluid[9]

Toxoplasmosis of the central nervous system: *Toxoplasma* granulomas and primary lymphoma are the most common causes of focal brain lesions in patients with AIDS[10,11]

Cryptococcus neoformans meningitis: most common fungal infection of the brain in AIDS and nonimmunosuppressed patients[12]

Cytomegalovirus: although cytomegalovirus encephalitis is common in AIDS, it is not usually the immediate cause of death.[13,14]

Lymphoma: often presents as multifocal intraparenchymal masses[15]

Mycobacterial infection: *Mycobacterium avium-intracellulare* infection or *Mycobacterium tuberculosis*[16]

Progressive multifocal leukoencephalopathy: papovavirus

Other common opportunistic infections: herpes simplex 1 and 2, *Candida albicans*, coccidioidomycosis, *Nocardia steroides, Treponema pallidum*, Epstein-Barr virus, and varicella zoster[17]

Other neuromuscular disorders: multiple types of polyneuropathy, ranging from a characteristic distal sensory neuropathy to acute Guillain-Barré syndrome, and inflammatory myopathies[18,19]

Ocular Manifestations and Disorders Associated with HIV Infection

Ophthalmologic manifestations of AIDS and HIV infection include primary and secondary infections and neoplasms known to occur more frequently in this patient population, such as viral infection, particularly cytomegalovirus chorioretinitis. Neuro-ophthalmologic manifestations and retinal vascular abnormalities, such as cotton-wool spots and vasculitis, are common in AIDS patients.[20]

Cytomegalovirus chorioretinitis

Other ocular viral infections: varicella zoster, herpes simplex, HIV
Ocular fungal infections: candidiasis, *Cryptococcus neoformans*
Ocular mycobacterial infections: *M. tuberculosis, M. avium-intracellulare*
Kaposi's sarcoma
Retinal vascular changes: i.e., cotton wool exudates, which can be manifestations of pneumocystis infection or vasculitis.

Oral Manifestations and Disorders Associated with HIV Infection

Opportunistic infections and neoplasms associated with HIV infection occur as primary and secondary oral lesions. Even benign-appearing oral lesions, such as warts, leukoplakia, and severe periodontal disease can be initial manifestations of underlying HIV infection.[21]

Oral candidiasis: viral leukoplakia may mimic Candida-like lesions.[22,23]
Viral infections: herpes simplex, herpes zoster, hairy leukoplakia, warts
Kaposi's sarcoma
Periodontal disease: both common forms and a particularly aggressive form of necrotizing gingivitis
Angular stomatitis
Aphthosis

Pulmonary Manifestations and Disorders Caused by HIV Infection

Respiratory disorders are the most common mode of presentation of AIDS. An acute pulmonary infection often superimposed on a chronic wasting disease is a common initial presentation. A wide range of opportunistic and nonopportunisitc infections, as well as neoplastic processes, such as Kaposi's sarcoma, present as respiratory manifestations of underlying HIV infection.[24-28]

Pneumocystis carinii pneumonia: the most common life-threatening infection, occurring in 65 to 80% of AIDS patients[29-32]
Cytomegalovirus pneumonia: can be severe with fatal interstitial pneumonitis[33,34]
M. avium-intracellulare pneumonia: often widely disseminated and resistant to treatment; patients may have persistent mycobacterial bacteremia[35,36]
M. tuberculosis: although pulmonary infection is the

most frequent site, extra pulmonary sites of tuberculosis are common in the AIDS population.[37]

Disseminated histoplasmosis, coccidioidomycosis, and cryptococcosis: particularly in endemic areas[38]

Kaposi's sarcoma of the lung[39]

Toxoplasma gondii pneumonia[40]

Gastrointestinal Manifestations and Disorders Associated with HIV Infection

Diarrhea in patients with AIDS or risk factors for HIV infection is a frequent gastrointestinal manifestation of underlying problems relating to HIV infection (see Section III, Gastroenterology; Ch. 30). Other common manifestations such as esophagitis, malabsorption syndromes, and hepatic dysfunction frequently uncover primary and secondary gastrointestinal involvement of underlying HIV-related infection or neoplasm.[41,42]

Candida esophagitis[43]

Herpes simplex esophagitis

Cytomegalovirus esophagitis and colitis[44–49]

Small intestinal coccidiosis[50]: isosporiasis

Kaposi's sarcoma: primary and secondary infiltration[51–53]

Protozoa, helminth, other parasites

Viral infections[54]

Cryptosporidiosis[55,56]

Malabsorption syndrome with weight loss and chronic diarrhea[57–59]

Multiple diarrhea-causing organism infections (see Section III, Gastroenterology; Ch. 30).[60]

Gastrointestinal histoplasmosis[61]

Hepatobiliary dysfunction: viral, multiple secondary complications, and nonspecific changes[62–65]

Primary gastrointestinal lymphoma[66,67]

M. avium complex: can infect small intestine and lymph nodes mimicking Whipple's disease[68,69]

M. tuberculosis: extrapulmonary tuberculous sites are common in AIDS[70,71]

Skin, Mucosal, and Lymphatic Manifestations and Disorders Associated with HIV Infection

The multiple focal and diffuse lymphatic changes reported in patients at high risk for HIV infection have been described and categorized with various AIDS-related syndromes or complexes[72,73] (see Section X, Hematology; Ch. 112). Mucosal and various cutaneous manifestations of underlying HIV infection can be either primary or, more often, secondary manifestations of infection or neoplasm associated with HIV infection.[74-77]

Enlarged lymph nodes: focal and diffuse (see Section X, Hematology; Ch. 112)

Anogenital viral infections: herpes simplex, papillomavirus[78]

Fungal and yeast infections: candidiasis, coccidioidomycosis, histoplasmosis, dermatophytosis, tinea versicolor

Kaposi's infiltration

Other neoplasms: lymphoma, squamous cell carcinoma, basal cell carcinoma, melanoma

Viral infections: cytomegalovirus, herpes simplex, varicella, herpes zoster, Epstein-Barr virus, molluscum contagiosum, common warts, condyloma acuminatum

Drug rashes: particularly with trimethoprim-sulfamethoxazole[79]

Dermatologic manifestations, infection, and dermatoses known to be exacerbated with HIV infection: syphilis, scabies, psoriasis[77]

Miscellaneous

Myocarditis: a frequent finding at necropsy of AIDS patients and usually of idiopathic etiology[80]

Autoimmune laboratory findings: hypergammaglobulinemia circulating immune complexes, autoantibodies[81]

Salmonellosis: in AIDS patients, a recurrent bacteremia can occur despite treatment and/or paucity of gastrointestinal symptoms.[82,83]

Macroamylasemia[84]

References

1. Booss J, Harris SA: Neurology of AIDS virus infection: a clinical classification. Yale J Biol Med 60:537, 1987.
2. Gabuzda DH, Hirsch MS: Neurologic manifestations of infection with human immunodeficiency virus. Clinical features and pathogenesis. Ann Intern Med 107:383, 1987.
3. Petito CK: Review of central nervous system pathology in human immunodeficiency virus infection. Ann Neurol 23(Suppl):S54, 1988.
4. Elder GA, Sever JL: Neurologic disorders associated with AIDS retroviral infection. Rev Infect Dis 10:286, 1988.
5. Berger JR: The neurological complications of HIV infection. Acta Neurol Scand 116(Suppl):40, 1988.

6. McArthur JC: Neurologic manifestations of AIDS. Medicine 66:407, 1987.
7. Shaw GM, Harper ME, Hahn BH, et al: HTLV-III infection in brains of children and adults with AIDS encephalopathy. Science 227:177, 1985.
8. Price RW, Brew B, Sidtis J, et al: The brain in AIDS: central nervous system HIV-1 infection and AIDS dementia complex. Science 239:586, 1988.
9. Ho DD, Rota TR, Schooley RT, et al: Isolation of HTLV-III from cerebrospinal fluid and neural tissues of patients with neurologic syndromes related to the acquired immunodeficiency syndrome. N Engl J Med 313:1493, 1985.
10. Wong B, Gold JW, Brown AE, et al: Central-nervous-system toxoplasmosis in homosexual men and parenteral drug abusers. Ann Intern Med 100:36, 1984.
11. Alonso R, Heiman-Patterson T, Mancall EL: Cerebral toxoplasmosis in acquired immune deficiency syndrome. Arch Neurol 41:321, 1984.
12. Kovacs JA, Kovacs AA, Polis M, et al: Cryptococcosis in the acquired immunodeficiency syndrome. Ann Intern Med 103:533, 1985.
13. Morgello S, Cho ES, Nielsen S, et al: Cytomegalovirus encephalitis in patients with acquired immunodeficiency syndrome: an autopsy study of 30 cases and a review of the literature. Hum Pathol 18:289, 1987.
14. Koppel BS, Wormser GP, Tuchman AJ, et al: Central nervous system involvement in patients with acquired immune deficiency syndrome (AIDS). Acta Neurol Scand 71:337, 1985.
15. Snider WD, Simpson DM, Nielsen S, et al: Neurological complications of acquired immune deficiency syndrome: analysis of 50 patients. Ann Neurol 14:403, 1983.
16. Young LS: *Mycobacterium avium* complex infection. J Infect Dis 157:863, 1988.
17. Lechtenberg R, Sher JH: AIDS in the Nervous System. p. 64. Churchill Livingstone, New York, 1988.
18. Dalakas MC, Pezeshkpour GH: Neuromuscular diseases associated with human immunodeficiency virus infection. Ann Neurol 23(Suppl):S38, 1988.
19. Cornblath DR: Treatment of the neuromuscular complications of human immunodeficiency virus infection. Ann Neurol 23(Suppl):S88, 1988.
20. Schuman JS, Orellana J, Friedman AH, Teich SA: Acquired immunodeficiency syndrome (AIDS). Surv Ophthalmol 31:384, 1987.
21. Greenspan D, Greenspan JS: Oral mucosal manifestations of AIDS? Dermatol Clin 5:733, 1987.
22. Klein RS, Harris CA, Small CB, et al: Oral candidiasis in high-risk patients as the initial manifestation of the acquired immunodeficiency syndrome. N Engl J Med 311:354, 1984.
23. Greenspan JS, Greenspan D, Lennette ET, et al: Replication of Epstein-Barr virus within the epithelial cells of oral "hairy" leukoplakia, an AIDS-associated lesion. N Engl J Med 313:1564, 1985.
24. Rankin JA, Collman R, Daniele RP: Acquired immune deficiency syndrome and the lung. Chest 94:155, 1988.

25. Donath J, Khan FA: Pulmonary infections in AIDS. Compr Ther 13:49, 1987.
26. Millar AB: Respiratory manifestations of AIDS. Br J Hosp Med 39:204, 1988.
27. Murray JF, Garay SM, Hopewell PC, et al: NHLBI workshop summary. Pulmonary complications of the acquired immunodeficiency syndrome: an update. Report of the second National Heart, Lung and Blood Institute workshop. Am Rev Respir Dis 135:504, 1987.
28. Suster B, Akerman M, Orenstein M, et al: Pulmonary manifestations of AIDS: review of 106 episodes. Radiology 161:87, 1986.
29. Fauci AS (moderator): Acquired immunodeficiency syndrome: epidemiologic, clinical, immunologic, and therapeutic considerations. Ann Intern Med 100:92, 1984.
30. Broaddus C, Dake MD, Stulbarg MS, et al: Bronchoalveolar lavage and transbronchial biopsy for the diagnosis of pulmonary infections in the acquired immunodeficiency syndrome. Ann Intern Med 102:747, 1985.
31. Peters SG, Prakash UB: Pneumocystis carinii pneumonia. Review of 53 cases. Am J Med 82:73, 1987.
32. Brenner M, Ognibene FP, Lack EE, et al: Prognostic factors and life expectancy of patients with acquired immunodeficiency syndrome and Pneumocystis carinii pneumonia. Am Rev Respir Dis 136:1199, 1987.
33. Klotman ME, Hamilton JD: Cytomegalovirus pneumonia. Semin Respir Infect 2:95, 1987.
34. Drew WL: Cytomegalovirus infection in patients with AIDS. J Infect Dis 158:449, 1988.
35. Centers for Disease Control: Diagnosis and management of mycobacterial infection and disease in persons with human immunodeficiency virus infection. Ann Intern Med 106:254, 1987.
36. American Thoracic Society and Centers for Disease Control: Mycobacterioses and the acquired immunodeficiency syndrome. Am Rev Respir Dis 136:492, 1987.
37. Goldman KP: AIDS and tuberculosis. Br Med J 295:511, 1987.
38. Bronnimann DA, Adam RD, Galgiani JN, et al: Coccidioidomycosis in the acquired immunodeficiency syndrome. Ann Intern Med 106:372, 1987.
39. Sivit CJ, Schwartz AM, Rockoff SD: Kaposi's sarcoma of the lung in AIDS: radiologic-pathologic analysis. AJR 148:25, 1987.
40. Berk SL, Verghese A: Parasitic pneumonia. Semin Respir Infect 3:172, 1988.
41. Smith PD, Lane HC, Gill VJ, et al: Intestinal infections in patients with the acquired immunodeficiency syndrome (AIDS). Etiology and response to therapy. Ann Intern Med 108:328, 1988.
42. Rodgers VD, Kagnoff MF: Gastrointestinal manifestations of the acquired immunodeficiency syndrome. West J Med 146:57, 1987.
43. Walsh TJ, Hamilton SR, Belitsos N: Esophageal candidiasis. Managing an increasingly prevalent infection. Postgrad Med 84(2):193, 1988.
44. Balthazar EJ, Megibow AJ, Hulnick D, et al: Cytomegalovirus esophagitis in AIDS: radiographic features in 16 patients. AJR 149:919, 1987.

45. Jacobson MA, Mills J: Serious cytomegalovirus disease in the acquired immunodeficiency syndrome (AIDS). Clinical findings, diagnosis, and treatment. Ann Intern Med 108:585, 1988.
46. Rene E, Marche C, Chevalier T, et al: Cytomegalovirus colitis in patients with acquired immunodeficiency syndrome. Dig Dis Sci 33:741, 1988.
47. Cunningham AL, Grohman GS, Harkness J, et al: Gastrointestinal viral infections in homosexual men who were symptomatic and seropositive for human immunodeficiency virus. J Infect Dis 158:386, 1988.
48. Weber JN, Thom S, Barrison I, et al: Cytomegalovirus colitis and esophageal ulceration in the context of AIDS: clinical manifestations and preliminary report of treatment with Foscarnet (phosphonoformate). Gut 28:482, 1987.
49. Teixidor HS, Honig CL, Norsoph E, et al: Cytomegalovirus infection of the alimentary canal: radiologic findings with pathologic correlation. Radiology 163:317, 1987.
50. Cook GC: Small-intestinal coccidiosis: an emergent clinical problem. J Infect 16:213, 1988.
51. Lustbader I, Sherman A: Primary gastrointestinal Kaposi's sarcoma in a patient with acquired immune deficiency syndrome. Am J Gastroenterol 82:894, 1987.
52. Biggs BA, Crowe SM, Lucas CR, et al: AIDS related Kaposi's sarcoma presenting as ulcerative colitis and complicated by toxic megacolon. Gut 28:1302, 1987.
53. Bieluch VM, Wagner S, Kim K, Freimer EH: Unusual manifestations of gastrointestinal Kaposi's sarcoma in acquired immunodeficiency syndrome. Arch Dermatol 124:652, 1988.
54. Nelson JA, Wiley CA, Reynolds-Kohler C, et al: Human immunodeficiency virus detected in bowel epithelium from patients with gastrointestinal symptoms. Lancet 1:259, 1988.
55. Tzipori S: Cryptosporidiosis in perspective. Adv Parasitol 27:63, 1988.
56. Soave R, Armstrong D: Cryptosporidium and cryptosporidiosis. Rev Infect Dis 8:1012, 1986.
57. Gillin JS, Shike M, Alcock N, et al: Malabsorption and mucosal abnormalities of the small intestine in the acquired immunodeficiency syndrome. Ann Intern Med 102:619, 1985.
58. Feczko PJ: Malignancy complicating inflammatory bowel disease. Radiol Clin North Am 25:157, 1987.
59. Budhraja M, Levendoglu H, Kocka F, et al: Duodenal mucosal T cell subpopulation and bacterial cultures in acquired immune deficiency syndrome. Am J Gastroenterol 82:427, 1987.
60. Laughon BE, Druckman DA, Vernon A, et al: Prevalence of enteric pathogens in homosexual men with and without acquired immunodeficiency syndrome. Gastroenterology 94:984, 1988.
61. Cappell MS, Mandell W, Grimes MM, Neu HC: Gastrointestinal histoplasmosis. Dig Dis Sci 33:353, 1988.
62. Roulot D, Valla D, Brun-Vezinet F, et al: Cholangitis in the acquired immunodeficiency syndrome: report of cases and review of the literature. Gut 28:1653, 1987.

63. Palmer M, Braly LF, Schaffner F: The liver in acquired immune deficiency disease. Semin Liver Dis 7:192, 1987.
64. Lebovics E, Dworkin BM, Heier SK, Rosenthal WS: The hepatobiliary manifestations of human immunodeficiency virus infection. Am J Gastroenterol 83:1, 1988.
65. Aaron JS, Wynter CD, Kirton OC, Simko V: Cytomegalovirus associated with acalculous cholecystitis in a patient with acquired immune deficiency syndrome. Am J Gastroenterol 83:879, 1988.
66. Haber DA, Mayer RJ: Primary gastrointestinal lymphoma. Semin Oncol 15:154, 1988.
67. Ioachim HL, Weinstein MA, Robbins RD, et al: Primary anorectal lymphoma. A new manifestation of the acquired immune deficiency syndrome (AIDS). Cancer 60:1449, 1987.
68. Schneebaum CW, Novick DM, Chabon AB, et al: Terminal ileitis associated with *Mycobacterium avium-intracellulare* infection in a homosexual man with acquired immune deficiency syndrome. Gastroenterology 92:1127, 1987.
69. Joint Position Paper of the American Thoracic Society and the Centers for Disease Control: Mycobacterioses and the acquired immunodeficiency syndrome. Am Rev Respir Dis 136:492, 1987.
70. Lax JD, Haroutiounian G, Attia A, et al: Tuberculosis of the rectum in a patient with acquired immune deficiency syndrome. Report of a case. Dis Colon Rectum 31:394, 1988.
71. Chaisson RE, Schecter GF, Theuer CP, et al: Tuberculosis in patients with the acquired immunodeficiency syndrome. Clinical features, response to therapy, and survival. Am Rev Respir Dis 136:570, 1987.
72. Pallesen G, Gerstoft J, Mathiesen L: Stages in LAV/HTLV-III lymphadenitis. 1. Histological and immunohistological classification. Scand J Immunol 25:83, 1987.
73. Gold JWM, Weikel CS, Godbold J, et al: Unexplained persistent lymphadenopathy in homosexual men and the acquired immune deficiency syndrome. Medicine 64:203, 1985.
74. Wexler PS, Phelps RG, Novick NL: Mucous membrane manifestations of the acquired immunodeficiency syndrome. Clin Dermatol 5:182, 1987.
75. Kaplan MH, Sadick N, McNutt NS, et al: Dermatologic findings and manifestations of acquired immunodeficiency syndrome (AIDS). J Am Acad Dermatol 16:485, 1987.
76. Libman H: Generalized lymphadenopathy. J Gen Intern Med 2:48, 1987.
77. Fisher BK, Warner LC: Cutaneous manifestations of the acquired immunodeficiency syndrome. Update 1987. Int J Dermatol 26:615, 1987.
78. Sillman FH, Sedlis A: Anogenital papillomavirus infection and neoplasia in immunodeficient women. Obstet Gynecol Clin North Am 14:537, 1987.
79. Gordin FM, Simon GL, Wofsy CB, et al: Adverse reactions to trimethoprim-sulfamethoxazole in patients with the acquired immunodeficiency syndrome. Ann Intern Med 100:495, 1984.

80. Anderson DW, Virmani R, Reilly JM, et al: Prevalent myocarditis at necropsy in the acquired immunodeficiency syndrome. J Am Coll Cardiol 11:792, 1988.
81. Calabrese LH: Autoimmune manifestations of human immunodeficiency virus (HIV) infection. Clin Lab Med 8:269, 1988.
82. Profeta F, Forrester C, Eng RH, et al: Salmonella infections in patients with acquired immunodeficiency syndrome. Arch Intern Med 145:670, 1985.
83. Sperber SJ, Schleupner CJ: Salmonellosis during infection with human immunodeficiency virus. Rev Infect Dis 9:925, 1987.
84. Greenberg RE, Bank S, Singer C: Macroamylasemia in association with the acquired immunodeficiency syndrome. Postgrad Med J 63:677, 1987.

Selected Readings

Clever LH, Omenn GS: Hazards for health care workers. Annu Rev Public Health 9:273, 1988.
Important considerations with growing numbers of health care workers involved in caring for HIV-infected patients.

Faulstich ME: Psychiatric aspects of AIDS. Am J Psychiatry 144:551, 1987.
AIDS patients exhibit significant neuropsychiatric complications including anxiety, depression, suicidal ideation, and anger toward ineffective medical care and public discrimination. Central nervous system dysfunction and subsequent neuropsychiatric impairment complicate both evaluation and reasonable management. Case management and research activity in these areas are discussed.

Feinkind L, Minkoff HL: HIV in pregnancy. Clin Perinatol 15:189, 1988.
Information particularly important for obstetricians who will increasingly face social, ethical, and medical dilemmas occurring in HIV-infected pregnant women.

Glatt AE, Chirgwin K, Landesman SH: Current concepts. Treatment of infections associated with human immunodeficiency virus. N Engl J Med 318:1439, 1988.
State-of-the-art review of infection associated with HIV infection.

Gray F, Gherardi R, Scaravilli F: The neuropathology of the acquired immune deficiency syndrome (AIDS). A review. Brain 111:245, 1988.
Major review of the neuropathology of AIDS. Opportunistic infection is the major pathologic process, commonly including toxoplasmosis, cytomegalovirus, progressive multifocal leukoencephalopathy, and mycoses, primarily cryptococcosis. Primary lymphoma is three times as common as secondary lymphoma. Kaposi's sarcoma is usually metastatic from the lungs. Neuropathologic findings of direct HIV infection in central and peripheral nervous system do not always correlate with clinical symptoms.

Guinan ME, Hardy A: Epidemiology of AIDS in women in the United States. 1981 through 1986. JAMA 257:2039, 1987.
A review of 1,819 cases of AIDS in women reported from 1981 through 1986. Most women were infected with HIV through intravenous drug use, followed in frequency by heterosexual contact with a person in the high-risk group.

Humphreys MH, Schoenfeld PY: Renal complications in patients with the acquired immune deficiency syndrome (AIDS). Am J Nephrol 7:1, 1987.

Although the kidney is not a major target organ for AIDS and is usually only transiently or secondarily complicated, several major renal complications have been identified with AIDS in this review. Authors group general types of renal involvement into three categories: (1) occurrence of glomerular lesions and proteinuria, (2) acute renal insufficiency, and (3) a variety of fluid and electrolyte disorders.

Lechtenberg R, Sher JH: AIDS in the Nervous System. Churchill Livingstone, New York, 1988.

Highly recommended text, particularly to neurologists, for a readable, well-documented, current review of the character, epidemiology, clinical, and pathologic aspects of AIDS as it affects the nervous system. A successful, combined effort of a clinician and a neuropathologist.

Levine AM: Non-Hodgkin's lymphomas and other malignancies in the acquired immune deficiency syndrome. Semin Oncol 14(Suppl 3):34, 1987.

The great majority of neoplasms in AIDS patients are comprised of either Kaposi's sarcoma or non-Hodgkin's malignant lymphoma, with Kaposi's sarcoma by far the most prevalent reported malignancy. A review of current conceptsof Epstein-Barr vbirus (EBV) infection and high incidence of lymphomas. Other possible cofactors, such as cytomegalovirus and nitrites, involved in the induction of B cell lymphomas or Kaposi's sarcoma in AIDS patients are also discussed.

Levine AM, Gill PS, Muggia F: Malignancies in the acquired immunodeficiency syndrome. Curr Probl Cancer 11:209, 1987.

Clinical and pathologic features of AIDS-related Kaposi's sarcoma and other neoplasms are reviewed. Discussions of management and prognosis are helpful.

Levy JA: The transmission of AIDS: the case of the infected cell. JAMA 259:3037, 1988.

Current concepts of the pathogenesis of HIV transmission.

Lifson AR: Do alternate modes for transmission of human immunodeficiency virus exist? A review. JAMA 259:1353, 1988.

Review addressing continued questions of possible HIV transmission through alternate modes in light of the fact that HIV has been isolated from saliva, tears, and urine. No evidence emerges from this review that HIV infection is transmitted through casual contact.

Lipsett P, Allo MD: AIDS and the surgeon. Surg Clin North Am 68:73, 1988.

Clinical review from a surgical perspective that reviews common presentations of AIDS that require surgical intervention, as well as alternatives to surgical procedures for diagnosis. Precautions necessary for handling tissue and body secretions are stressed.

Ostrow D, Grant I, Atkinson H: Assessment and management of the AIDS patient with neuropsychiatric disturbances. J Clin Psychiatry 49(Suppl):14, 1988.

Recommended review outlining psychiatric aspects of AIDS patients. Focus is on practical management issues, including dose and drug suggestions appropriate in the complicated setting of psychotic episodes and depression in this patient group. Authors include useful information regarding drug-related adverse reactions in immuno-compromised patients.

Penn I: Tumors of the immunocompromised patient. Annu Rev Med 39:63, 1988.
Review of a surgical experience of tumor patterns in AIDS patients and clinical contrasts with similar tumors in non-HIV-infected patients.

Piel J (ed): What science knows about AIDS. A single-topic issue. Sci Am 259:1988.
A single topic issue devoted to AIDS. Outstanding contributing authors review a wide range of current concepts of AIDS, usually within an historical perspective. Topics reviewed cover the molecular biology of the AIDS virus, clinical presentations, social issues as well as current and proposed therapies. High-quality monograph.

Ramsey RG, Geremia GK: CNS complications of AIDS: CT and MR findings. AJR 151:449, 1988.
Cranial imaging features of cerebral complications in AIDS patients on CT and MRI from a large metropolitan center are reviewed. Useful descriptions of probability patterns, although not pathognomonic, are helpful, particularly in initial management decision-making. When MRI is used initially, contrast-enhanced CT may still be necessary to further characterize the lesions. Gadolinium-DTPA contrast-enhanced MRI may be a particularly useful imaging method in these patients.

Seligmann M, Pinching AJ, Rosen FS, et al: Immunology of human immunodeficiency virus infection and the acquired immunodeficiency syndrome. An update. Ann Intern Med 107:234, 1987.
Current concepts of the pathogenesis of HIV infection. Factors and markers considered significant to prognosis, such as genetic markers, environmental and nutritional status, concurrent sexually transmitted diseases, and degree of immunologic impairment as measured by antibody titers and CD4 lymphocyte number and function are discussed.

Steis RG, Longo DL: Clinical, biologic, and therapeutic aspects of malignancies associated with the acquired immunodeficiency syndrome. Part I and Part II. Ann Allergy 60:310, 1988.
Current concepts and management recommendations of malignancies related to HIV infection from the National Cancer Institute, Maryland.

Sze G, Brant-Zawadzki MN, Norman D, Newton TH: The neuroradiology of AIDS. Semin Roentgenol 22:42, 1987.
Well-referenced review of neuroradiology experience in AIDS patients from the University of California, San Francisco.

Sze G, Zimmerman RD: The magnetic resonance imaging of infections and inflammatory diseases. Radiol Clin North Am 26:839, 1988.
Magnetic resonance imaging features of inflammatory lesions of the central nervous system are reviewed. MRI and CT sensitivities and specificities are compared.

76
Fever and Pulmonary Infiltrates in a Compromised Host: Infectious and Non-infectious Causes

Appropriate management of fever and pulmonary infiltrates in the compromised host is best approached by considering a differential diagnosis weighted by the type of immunocompromise. Each patient's immune defect should be classified as humoral, phagocytic, or cellular; commonly a combination of defects is present.[1] Other major historical factors to consider are chronicity of symptoms, exposure to granulomatous disease, risk factors for aspiration, and community or nosocomial exposure. Pulmonary nodules most often represent fungal, nocardia, legionella, cytomegalovirus, or pneumocystis infection. Chest radiograph pattern-recognition in immunocompromised hosts is often of limited value because any infection can cause several different patterns. Noninfectious causes must be considered.[2,3]

Common Causes of Infection with Humoral and Phagocytic Immune Dysfunction

In patients with humoral immune dysfunction, such as occurs with hypogammaglobulinemia, multiple myeloma, and asplenia, bacterial infection with Pneumococcus, *Haemophilus influenzae*, and Meningococcus are common. Neutropenia predisposes the patient to bacterial and fungal infection. Even with significant infection, patients with neutropenia sometimes produce only minimal sputum and fail to mount the expected amount of pulmonary consolidation.

Bacteria
  Pneumococcus

Haemophilus influenzae
Meningococcus
Gram-negative bacteria
Staphylococcus aureus: may present with cavity lesion.
Fungi
  Aspergillus: invasive pulmonary aspergillus[4] can mimic acute pneumonia or a pulmonary embolus. A more chronic form of necrotizing aspergillosis[5] occurs in mild immunocompromise and is often associated with indolent upper lobe infiltrates and/or fungus balls seen on radiograph.
  Candida
Abscess: sometimes a cavitary lesion, often with mixed organisms

Common Causes of Infection in non-AIDS Cellular-Mediated Dysfunction

Examples of patients with non-HIV-related disorders of cellular-mediated dysfunction include those with Hodgkin's disease, patients who are status-post organ transplant, and patients receiving steroids or cytotoxic agents.

Bacteria
  Gram-negative bacilli[6]
  S. aureus
  Legionella: infections are most commonly associated with cell-mediated dysfunction than with other immune defects. In contrast to *Legionella pneumophila*, which commonly occurs in noncompromised patients, *L. micdadei* (Pittsburgh pneumonia agent) is thought by some to occur predominantly in the immunocompromised patient.[7-11]
Fungi[12]
  Actinomycetes: Nocardia; may cavitate[13]
  Aspergillus: may cavitate
  Candida
  Cryptococcus
  Histoplasmosis: in patients with disseminated histoplasmosis, antigenuria is often detected by radioimmunoassay[14,15]
  Coccidioidomycosis: reactivation of old diseases
  Mucormycosis[16]
Mycobacteria: tuberculosis and atypical mycobacteria[17]
Viruses[18,19]
  Cytomegalovirus: monoclonal antibody studies of

bronchoalveolar lavage fluid have promise of being rapid, highly sensitive, screening tests[20–22]

Herpes simplex I and II: hematogenous spread of herpes simplex I and II can cause diffuse infiltrates; contiguous spread of herpes simplex I from the oropharynx is associated with focal infiltrates[23,24]

Herpes zoster: zoster pneumonia is usually preceded or accompanied by skin lesions[25]

Varicella-zoster

Adenovirus[26]

Epstein-Barr virus[27]

Parasitic pneumonia[28]

Pneumocystis carinii: widely variable chest radiographic findings include (1) no abnormality, (2) an ARDS-like pattern, (3) pulmonary infiltrates, and (4) pulmonary nodules[29–31]

Toxoplasma gondii: most commonly seen in HIV-infected patients

Strongyloides: uncommon cause

Ascaris

Hookworm

Dirofilaria

Paragonimus

Entamoeba histolytica

Cat-scratch fever[32]

Common Causes of Pulmonary Infiltrates in AIDS

Greater than 50% of patients with AIDS have pulmonary disease.[33] Cell-mediated immune deficiency makes these patients at high risk for opportunistic pathogens, with *P. carinii* the most common infectious agent, followed by *M. avium-intracellulare*, cytomegalovirus, and *Cryptococcus neoformans*.[34] Nonopportunistic agents occur with increasing frequency such as *M. tuberculosis*, *Histoplasma capsulatum*, *L. pneumophila*, and *Coccidioides immitis*.[34] Kaposi's sarcoma is also an important diagnostic consideration in this population.[35]

P. carinii pneumonia (PCP): PCP is the most common life-threatening opportunistic infection among patients with AIDS.[36] However, even when infection is significant, usual screening tests, such as blood gases and chest radiographs, can be normal.[30,37]

Cytomegalovirus pneumonia[38]

M. avium-intracellulare[39] diagnosis often made by blood culture; important consideration in HIV-infected and HIV-high risk patients

C. neoformans
M. tuberculosis
H. capsulatum
C. immitis
Legionella pneumonia.
Respiratory syncytial virus[40]
Cryptosporidium: usually found in HIV-infected patients with other infectious agents; pathologic role is unclear[41]
Kaposi's pulmonary infiltrate: mimics infection with fever, dyspnea, hypoxemia, and diffuse interstitial or alveolar infiltrates; cutaneous involvement and pleural effusions are not uncommon[42]

Noninfectious Causes of Pulmonary Infiltrates in the Compromised Host

Fever is often associated with noninfectious pulmonary disease in the immunocompromised patient.[2]

Pulmonary emboli or infarction: commonly associated with pleural effusion
Pulmonary edema
Pulmonary hemorrhage: thrombocytopenia and invasive fungal infections have been associated with severe pulmonary hemorrhage in compromised hosts.[43]
Neoplasm: bronchogenic carcinoma, lymphoma, or leukemic infiltration[44,45]
Radiation pneumonitis: occurs 6 weeks to 6 months after radiation therapy and can occur up to 6 years postirradiation in association with steroid withdrawal. Clinical manifestations vary from asymptomatic to clinical pictures that mimic pulmonary infection.[46–48]
Drug-induced pneumonitis: busulfan, bleomycin, BCNU, methotrexate, and mitomycin are agents commonly associated with pulmonary toxicity; cyclophosphamide has been implicated as contributory in conjunction with other agents.[49,50]
Leukoagglutin reaction
Nonspecific interstitial pneumonitis: diagnosis of diffuse infiltrates often seen in compromised hosts at open lung biopsy[51] and in bone marrow transplant patients
Adult respiratory distress syndrome (ARDS)
Wegener's granulomatosis
Fat embolization[52]

References

1. Fanta CH, Pennington JE: Fever and new lung infiltrates in the immunocompromised host. Clin Chest Med 2:19, 1981.
2. Rosenow EC, Wilson WR, Cockerill FR III: Pulmonary disease in the immunocompromised host (first of two parts). Mayo Clin Proc 60:473, 1985.
3. Ognibene FP, Pass HI, Roth JA, et al: Role of imaging and interventional techniques in the diagnosis of respiratory disease in the immunocompromised host. J Thorac Imaging 3:1, 1988.
4. Rinaldi MG: Invasive aspergillosis. Rev Infect Dis 5:1061, 1983.
5. Binder RE, Faling LJ, Pugatch RD, et al: Chronic necrotizing pulmonary aspergillosis: a discrete clinical entity. Medicine 61:109, 1982.
6. Pennington JE: Gram-negative bacterial pneumonia in the immunocompromised host. Semin Respir Infect 1:145, 1986.
7. Muder RR, Yu VL, Zuravieff JJ: Pneumonia due to the Pittsburgh pneumonia agent: new clinical perspective with a review of the literature. Medicine 62:120, 1983.
8. Muder RR, Reddy SC, Yu VL, et al: Pneumonia caused by Pittsburgh pneumonia agent: radiologic manifestations. Radiology 150:633, 1984.
9. Jaeger TM, Atkinson PP, Adams BA, et al: *Legionella bozemanii* pneumonia in an immunocompromised patient. Mayo Clin Proc 63:72, 1988.
10. Gump DW, Keegan M: Pulmonary infections due to *Legionella* in immunocompromised patients. Semin Respir Infect 1:151, 1986.
11. Muder RR, Yu VL, Parry MF: The radiologic manifestations of Legionella pneumonia. Semin Respir Infect 2:242, 1987.
12. Davies SF: An overview of pulmonary fungal infections. Clin Chest Med 8:495, 1987.
13. Chazen G: Nocardia. Infect Control 8:260, 1987.
14. Wheat LJ, Kohler RB, Tewari RP: Diagnosis of disseminated histoplasmosis by detection of *Histoplasma capsulatum* antigen in serum and urine specimens. N Engl J Med 314:83, 1986.
15. Wheat LJ, Slama TG, Zeckel ML: Histoplasmosis in the acquired immune deficiency syndrome. Am J Med 78:203, 1985.
16. Bigby TD, Serota ML, Tierney LM Jr, Matthay MA: Clinical spectrum of pulmonary mucormycosis. Chest 89:435, 1986.
17. Maloney JM, Gregg CR, Stephens DS, et al: Infections caused by *Mycobacterium szulgai* in humans. Rev Infect Dis 9:1120, 1987.
18. Sullivan CJ, Jordan MC: Diagnosis of viral pneumonia. Semin Respir Infect 3:148, 1988.
19. Shanley JD, Jordan MC: Viral pneumonia in the immunocompromised patient. Semin Respir Infect 1:193, 1986.
20. Emanuel D, Peppard J, Stover D, et al: Rapid immunodiagnosis of cytomegalovirus pneumonia by bronchoalveolar lavage using human and murine monoclonal antibodies. Ann Intern Med 104:476, 1986.

21. Meyers JD: Management of cytomegalovirus infection. Am J Med 85:102, 1988.
22. Klotman ME, Hamilton JD: Cytomegalovirus pneumonia. Semin Respir Infect 2:95, 1987.
23. Wong KK, Hirsch MS: Herpes virus infections in patients with neoplastic disease. Am J Med 76:464, 1984.
24. Saral R: Management of mucocutaneous herpes simplex virus infections in immunocompromised patients. Am J Med 85:57, 1988.
25. Balfour HH Jr: Varicella zoster virus infections in immunocompromised hosts. A review of the natural history and management. Am J Med 85:68, 1988.
26. Zahradnik JM: Adenovirus pneumonia. Semin Respir Infect 2:104, 1987.
27. List AF, Greco FA, Vogler LB: Lymphoproliferative diseases in immunocompromised hosts: the role of Epstein-Barr virus. J Clin Oncol 5:1673, 1987.
28. Berk SL, Verghese A: Parasitic pneumonia. Semin Respir Infect 3:172, 1988.
29. Doppman JL, Geelhoed GW, De Vita VT: Atypical radiographic features in *Pneumocystis carinii* pneumonia. Radiology 114:39, 1975.
30. Levine SJ, White DA: *Pneumocystis carinii.* Clin Chest Med 9:395, 1988.
31. Hopewell PC: *Pneumocystis carinii* pneumonia: diagnosis. J Infect Dis 157:1115, 1988.
32. Black JR, Herrington DA, Hadfield TL, et al: Life-threatening cat-scratch disease in an immunocompromised host. Arch Intern Med 146:394, 1986.
33. Rankin JA, Collman R, Daniele RP: Acquired immune deficiency syndrome and the lung. Chest 94:155, 1988.
34. Hopewell PC, Luce JM: Pulmonary involvement in the acquired immunodeficiency syndrome. Chest 87:111, 1985.
35. Gill PS, Akil B, Colletti P, et al: Pulmonary Kaposi's sarcoma: clinical findings and results of therapy. Am J Med 87:57, 1989.
36. Golden JA, Hollander H, Stulbarg MS, et al: Bronchoalveolar lavage as the exclusive diagnostic modality for *Pneumocystis carinii* pneumonia. Chest 90:18, 1986.
37. Kelly AR, Sutker WL: *Pneumocystis* pneumonia in a patient with normal chest roentgenograms and normal arterial blood gas values. South Med J 79:1315, 1986.
38. Shuster EA, Beneke JS, Tegtmeier GE, et al: Monoclonal antibody for rapid laboratory detection of cytomegalovirus infections: characterization and diagnostic application. Mayo Clin Proc 60:577, 1985.
39. Hawkins CC, Gold JWM, Whimbey E, et al: *Mycobacterium avium* complex infections in patients with the acquired immunodeficiency syndrome. Ann Intern Med 105:184, 1986.
40. Englund JA, Sullivan CJ, Jordan MC, et al: Respiratory syncytial virus infection in immunocompromised adults. Ann Intern Med 109:203, 1988.
41. Ma P, Villanueva TG, Kaufman D, et al: Respiratory cryptosporidiosis in the acquired immune deficiency syndrome. JAMA 252:1298, 1984.
42. Ognibene FP, Steis RG, Macher AM, et al: Kaposi's

sarcoma causing pulmonary infiltrates and respiratory failure in the acquired immunodeficiency syndrome. Ann Intern Med 102:471, 1985.

43. Kahn FW, Jones JM, England DM: Diagnosis of pulmonary hemorrhage in the immunocompromised host. Am Rev Respir Dis 136:155, 1987.
44. Weingarten NM, Fred HL: Pneumonia simulating tumor of the lung. Am Fam Physician 26(6):117, 1982.
45. Penn I: Tumors of the immunocompromised patient. Annu Rev Med 39:63, 1988.
46. Gross NJ: Pulmonary effects of radiation therapy. Ann Intern Med 86:81, 1977.
47. Ikezoe J, Takashima S, Morimoto S, et al: CT appearance of acute radiation-induced injury in the lung. AJR 150:765, 1988.
48. Mah K, Poon PY, Van Dyk J, et al: Assessment of acute radiation-induced pulmonary changes using computed tomography. J Comput Assist Tomogr 10:736, 1986.
49. Batist G, Andrews JL Jr: Pulmonary toxicity of antineoplastic drugs. JAMA 246:1449, 1981.
50. Ginsberg SJ, Comis RL: The pulmonary toxicity of antineoplastic agents. Semin Oncol 9:34, 1982.
51. Chung MT, Raskin J, Krellenstein DJ, Teirstein AS: Bronchoscopy in diffuse lung disease: evaluation by open lung biopsy in nondiagnostic transbronchial lung biopsy. Ann Otol Rhinol Laryngol 96:654, 1987.
52. Rosen JM, Braman SS, Hasan FM, Teplitz C: Nontraumatic fat embolization. A rare cause of new pulmonary infiltrates in an immunocompromised patient. Am Rev Respir Dis 134:805, 1986.

Selected Readings

Bamberger DM: Diagnosis of nosocomial pneumonia. Semin Respir Infect 3:140, 1988.
A review of causes of nosocomial pneumonia found the usual causative agents—gram-negative bacilli, Staphylococcus aureus, Streptococcus pneumoniae, *and anaerobic bacteria—and the following causative agents in immunocompromised hosts: fungi, mycobacteria, viruses,* Nocardia, *and* P. carinii. *Selection of current diagnostic techniques is discussed.*

Deitch EA: Infection in the compromised host. Surg Clin North Am 68:181, 1988.
Good general clinical review of problems of infection in the immunocompromised host.

Garay SM, Plottel CS: Pulmonary effects of AIDS: nosocomial transmission. Clin Chest Med 9:519, 1988.
An overview of the risk of nosocomial infection in the "AIDS era" suggests that airborne spread of M. tuberculosis *from hospitalized patients has reemerged as a hazard to hospital personnel. Infection control is discussed.*

Hopewell PC, Luce JM: Pulmonary involvement in the acquired immunodeficiency syndrome. Chest 87:104, 1985.
Epidemiology, prognosis, and infection control.

Klotz SA, Penn RL, George RB: Antigen detection in the diagnosis of fungal respiratory infections. Semin Respir Infect 1:16, 1986.

The often difficult diagnosis of fungal infections, which frequently indicates invasive diagnostic procedures, stimulates interest in the development of noninvasive diagnostic techniques. This article reviews newer methods for the detection of fungal antigens in body fluids such as serum, pleural fluid, and bronchoalveolar lavage.

Linder J, Vaughan WP, Armitage JO, et al: Cytopathology of opportunistic infection in bronchoalveolar lavage. Am J Clin Pathol 88:421, 1987.

The usefulness of bronchoalveolar lavage for determination of opportunistic infection was examined in this clinical study. Papanicolaou-stained slides from 604 lavage specimens and 344 patients were evaluated for fungal, parasitic, and viral organisms. In 155 specimens (25.7%), yeast, pseudohyphae, or hyphae were found. Candida was the most frequent opportunistic fungus identified in immunocompromised hosts. Other pathogens identified included P. carinii, herpes simplex, and cytomegalovirus.

Maxfield RA, Sorkin IB, Fazzini EP, et al: Respiratory failure in patients with acquired immunodeficiency syndrome and *Pneumocystis carinii* pneumonia. Crit Care Med 14:443, 1986.

Results of a study to define the pathophysiology of respiratory failure of patients with AIDS and P. carinii pneumonia.

McCabe RE: Diagnosis of pulmonary infections in immunocompromised patients. Med Clin North Am 72:1067, 1988.

Good general review of clinical presentations and state-of-the-art laboratory, noninvasive, and invasive diagnostic techniques.

McCabe RE, Brooks RG, Mark JBD, et al: Open lung biopsy in patients with acute leukemia. Am J Med 78:609, 1985.

Review of a series of patients with acute leukemia, pulmonary infiltrates, neutropenia, and fever who underwent open lung biopsy.

Ognibene FP, Pass HI, Roth JA, et al: Role of imaging and interventional techniques in the diagnosis of respiratory disease in the immunocompromised host. J Thorac Imaging 3:1, 1988.

Clinical review covering probabilities of certain pulmonary infections and other causes of pulmonary infiltrates occurring in association with several types of immunosuppression.

Pass HI, Potter D, Shelhammer J, et al: Indications for and diagnostic efficacy of open-lung biopsy in the patient with acquired immunodeficiency syndrome (AIDS). Ann Thorac Surg 41:307, 1986.

Criteria for use of open-lung biopsy in patients with AIDS.

Poe RH, Wahl GW, Qazi R, et al: Predictors of mortality in the immunocompromised patient with pulmonary infiltrates. Arch Intern Med 146:1304, 1986.

A study to determine predictors of mortality in immunocompromised patients with pulmonary infiltrates was performed by a record review of all immunocompromised patients who underwent a lung biopsy and were admitted to two community teaching hospitals during a 10-year period. Major clinical factors associated with poor prognosis were hypoxia, corticosteroid-induced immunosuppression, and indications for mechanical ventilation within the first 72 hours of hospitalization.

Rosenow EC III, Wilson WR, Cockerill FR III: Pulmonary

disease in the immunocompromised host (first of two parts). Mayo Clin Proc 60:473, 1985.
Well-referenced clinical review.

Springmeyer SC, Hackman RC, Holle R, et al: Use of bronchoalveolar lavage to diagnose acute diffuse pneumonia in the immunocompromised host. J Infect Dis 154:604, 1986.
Authors compared diagnostic information from bronchoscopy and needle aspiration of the lung with open lung biopsy in 15 marrow transplant recipients. Diagnostic sensitivity of bronchoscopy was 89% compared with 17% for needle aspiration.

Thomas JH, Farek PE, Hermreck AS, Pierce GE: Diagnostic value of open lung biopsy in immunocompromised patients. Am J Surg 154:692, 1987.
The role of open lung biopsy was evaluated in a retrospective review of 46 immunocompromised patients with diffuse pulmonary infiltrates who underwent open lung biopsy. Specific diagnosis was made in 30 of 46 patients (65%). Infectious diagnoses were made in 15 patients; nonspecific diagnoses were made in 16 patients. Authors conclude that open lung biopsy is an important technique in evaluating the immunocompromised patient with diffuse pulmonary infiltrates.

Thorpe JE, Baughman RP, Frame PT, et al: Bronchoalveolar lavage for diagnosing acute bacterial pneumonia. J Infect Dis 155:855, 1987.
This clinical study evaluated the usefulness of bronchoalveolar lavage in the diagnoses of acute bacterial pneumonia, first in 92 patients without known immunocompromise and then in 59 immunocompromised patients presenting with pulmonary infiltrates. Eight (21%) of the 39 patients presenting with microbial-related infiltrates were found to have acute bacterial pneumonia by bronchoalveolar lavage culture.

Williams D, Yungbluth M, Adams G, et al: The role of fiberoptic bronchoscopy in the evaluation of immunocompromised hosts with diffuse pulmonary infiltrates. Am Rev Respir Dis 131:880, 1985.
This study found fiberoptic bronchoscopy to be highly sensitive for diagnosing pulmonary infections.

Wilson WR, Cockerill FR III, Rowenow EC III: Pulmonary disease in the immunocompromised host (second of two parts). Mayo Clin Proc 60:610, 1985.
A review of infections associated with pulmonary infiltrates in the immunocompromised host and the diagnostic approaches for both infectious and noninfectious conditions. Outstanding clinical review.

77
Major Infectious Disease Risks for Travelers: The United States and Other Countries

Air travel allows many travelers to return home in the incubation phase of many communicable diseases; important examples are malaria, typhoid fever, and intestinal infections[1] (see Section III, Gastroenterology; Ch. 31). Some important considerations when evaluating recent travelers include place and duration of travel, type of accommodations, ingested food and liquid, pretravel immunizations, and prophylactic measures taken during travel.

United States

Plague: especially New Mexico
Rabies: none in Hawaii[2]
Rocky Mountain spotted fever: especially mid-Atlantic, Rocky Mountains from spring to autumn
Tularemia
Arboviral encephalitis: summer months
Babesia: especially Nantucket, Martha's Vineyard, Long Island, Shelter Islands
Lyme disease[3]
Coccidioidomycosis: California (particularly San Joaquin Valley), Arizona, west Texas, New Mexico
Histoplasmosis: Missouri and Mississippi river valleys
Blastomycosis: midwestern and eastern United States
Vibrio parahaemolyticus: especially Gulf states
Echinococcosis: especially Alaska
Trichinosis: especially Alaska
Fire ants: southeastern United States
Jellyfish
Trypanosomiasis: Texas border area
Amebiasis
Acquired immune deficiency syndrome (AIDS)[4,5]

Giardiasis[6]
Chlamydial infections[7]

Northern Europe

Travelers' diarrhea: USSR[8]
Giardiasis: especially western USSR[6]
Malaria: southern USSR
Leishmaniasis: southern USSR
Tick-borne typhus: east and central USSR
Tick-borne encephalitis: USSR
Tick-borne hemorrhagic fever: USSR
Taeniasis
Trichinosis
Diphyllobothriasis: from freshwater fish in Baltic Sea
    area
Rabies

Southern Europe

Travelers' diarrhea: especially during summer and
    autumn in southeastern and southwestern areas[8]
Typhoid: particularly during summer and autumn
    in southeastern and southwestern areas[9]
Hepatitis A: not destroyed by many methods of water
    purification[1]
Murine and tick-borne typhus: or boutonneuse fever,
    particularly along Mediterranean shores
West Nile fever: Mediterranean shores
Leishmaniasis
Tick-borne encephalitis: eastern areas
Hemorrhagic fever: eastern areas
Brucellosis: southwest and southeast
Echinococcosis: southeast
Rabies: except Portugal and Spain

**Australia, New
Zealand, Antartic**

Viral encephalitis: particularly some rural areas of
    Australia
Mosquito-borne epidemic polyarthritis: some rural
    areas of Australia
Ross River fever: some rural areas of Australia
Dengue: in parts of northern Queensland and the
    Torres Strait Islands
Amebic meningoencephalitis

**Mexico and Central
America**

Travelers' diarrhea[10]
Malaria
Amebiasis
Giardiasis[6]
Typhoid[9]
Hepatitis A

Leishmaniasis
Onchocerciasis
Chagas' disease
Dengue[11]
Venezuelan equine encephalitis
Helminths
Paragonimiasis: Costa Rica, Panama
Brucellosis
Polio: except Costa Rica, Panama
Coccidioidomycosis: areas of northern Mexico
Cysticercosis: increasing numbers of neurocysticercosis, most often presenting with seizures, seen in the United States in immigrants from Mexico[12]
Plague[13]

Tropical South America

Travelers' diarrhea[14]
Malaria
Typhoid[9]
Amebiasis
Hepatitis A
Yellow fever[15]
Dengue
Arboviral encephalitis
Chagas' disease
Leishmaniasis
Onchocerciasis
Bancroft's filariasis: parts of Brazil, French Guiana, Guyana, Surinam, possibly Venezuela
Plague: Bolivia
Bartonellosis: arid river valleys on western slopes of Andes up to 3,000 meters
Louse-borne typhus: mountain areas of Peru and Columbia
Schistosomiasis: Brazil, Surinam, northcentral Venezuela
Paragonimiasis: Ecuador, Peru
Brucellosis
Echinococcosis
Polio
Rabies[16]
Pentastomiasis: parasitic zoonosis generally limited to tropics and subtropics[17]

Temperate South America

Travelers' diarrhea[14]
Giardiasis[6]
Malaria: northwestern Argentina

Amebiasis
Leishmaniasis: northeastern Argentina
Typhoid fever[9]
Intestinal helminths
Hepatitis A
Taeniasis
Echinococcosis
Anthrax
Rabies
Trachoma: northeastern Argentina
Hemorrhagic fever: Argentinean pampas and central
    area
Yaws[18]

Eastern South Asia   Travelers' diarrhea[19]
Typhoid[9]
Malaria
Amebiasis
Giardiasis[6]
Hepatitis
Cholera
Filariasis
Leishmaniasis: Burma
Plague: Burma, Vietnam
Japanese encephalitis
Dengue
Mite-borne typhus
Schistosomiasis: Philippines, Central Sulawesi in In-
    donesia, Mekong Delta
Intestinal helminths
Fasciolopsiasis
Clonorchiasis: Indochina peninsula, Malaysia, Phil-
    ippines, Thailand
Paragonimiasis: Philippines
Melioidosis
Polio: infrequent in Brunei, Malaysia
Trachoma: Burma, Thailand, Indonesia, Vietnam
Rabies

Middle South Asia   Travelers' diarrhea[19]
Malaria
Amebiasis
Hepatitis
Intestinal helminths
Giardiasis[6]

Cholera
Filariasis: especially India, Bangladesh
Leishmaniasis
Sandfly fever
Tick-borne relapsing fever: Afghanistan, India, Iran
Tick-borne typhus: Afghanistan, India, Iran
Dengue: especially Bangladesh, India, Pakistan, Sri Lanka
Japanese encephalitis: eastern area
Crimean-Congo hemorrhagic fever: western area
Schistosomiasis: southwestern Iran
Dracunculiasis: India, Sri Lanka
Brucellosis
Echinococcosis
Polio
Trachoma: especially Afghanistan, India, Iran, Nepal, Pakistan
Rabies

Western South Asia

Travelers' diarrhea[19]
Typhoid
Giardiasis[6]
Amebiasis
Hepatitis
Cholera
Malaria
Leishmaniasis
Murine and tick-borne typhus
Tick-borne relapsing fever
Crimean-Congo hemorrhagic fever: Iraq
Schistosomiasis: South Yemen, Iraq, Saudi Arabia, Syria, Yemen
Dracunculiasis
Taeniasis
Brucellosis
Echinococcosis
Polio
Trachoma
Rabies

East Asia

Travelers' diarrhea: hygienic conditions in Japan and most of Hong Kong are such that intestinal infections appear to occur at frequencies similar to that in the United States.
Amebiasis

Hepatitis
Giardiasis[6]
Malaria: China, especially southern provinces
Bancroft's filariasis: China, Japan
Malayan filariasis: China, Republic of Korea
Leishmaniasis: China *
Plague: China
Dengue
Hemorrhagic fever with renal syndrome[20]
Japanese encephalitis
Tick-borne encephalitis: China, Republic of Korea
Mite-borne or scrub typhus: southern China, areas
    of Japan, Republic of Korea
Schistosomiasis: southeastern and eastern China
Clonorchiasis: China, Japan, Republic of Korea
Paragonimiasis: China, Japan, Republic of Korea
Fasciolopsiasis: China
Polio: infrequent
Trachoma: China
Brucellosis: China
Leptospirosis: China

Sub-Sahara Africa

Travelers' diarrhea
Malaria[21]
Amebiasis
Typhoid
Hepatitis A
Yellow fever and other arthropod-borne viruses[15]
Meningococcal meningitis
Filariasis: loiasis[22]
Onchocerciasis: major blinding disease[23]
Leishmaniasis
Trypanosomiasis
Relapsing fever
Typhus: louse, flea, tick-borne
Plague
Tungiasis
Polio
Trachoma
Arenavirus: including Lassa fever virus[24,25]
Echinococcosis
Diphtheria
AIDS[26-29]

North Africa

Travelers' diarrhea
Malaria[21]

Typhoid
Hepatitis A
Amebiasis
Schistosomiasis
Alimentary helminths
Giardiasis[6]
Brucellosis
Echinococcosis
Polio
Trachoma
Rabies
Dengue
Filariasis: Nile delta
Leishmaniasis
Relapsing fever
Rift Valley fever: eastern area
Sandfly fever
Typhus
Mediterranean spotted fever

Southern Africa

Travelers' diarrhea
Malaria[21]
Typhoid
Amebiasis
Hepatitis A
Schistosomiasis: northern and eastern areas
Plague
Relapsing fever
Tick-bite fever
Typhus
Trypanosomiasis: Botswana, Namibia, northern
    Transvaal

Melanesia,
Micronesia, Polynesia

Travelers' diarrhea
Typhoid
Hepatitis A
Malaria
Filariasis
Mite-borne typhus: Papua, New Guinea
Dengue
Japanese encephalitis
Intestinal helminths
Polio: Papua, New Guinea
Trachoma: parts of Melanesia

Caribbean

Travelers' diarrhea
Malaria: Haiti, western Dominican Republic

Giardiasis[6]
Typhoid
Amebiasis
Hepatitis A
Filariasis: especially Haiti
Dengue
Tularemia: Haiti
Yellow fever: Trinidad, Tobago[15]
Schistosomiasis: Dominican Republic, Guadeloupe, Martinique, Puerto Rico, Saint Lucia
Polio: Haiti and Dominican Republic
Rabies

References

1. Walker E, Williams G: ABC of healthy travel. Br Med J 286:543, 1983.
2. Fishbein DB, Dobbins JG, Bryson JH, et al: Rabies surveillance, United States, 1987. MMWR CDC Surveill Summ 37:1, 1988.
3. Stechenberg BW: Lyme disease: the latest great imitator. Pediatr Infect Dis J 7:402, 1988.
4. Padian NS: Heterosexual transmission of acquired immunodeficiency syndrome: international perspectives and national projections. Rev Infect Dis 9:947, 1987.
5. The acquired immunodeficiency syndrome (AIDS) and infection with the human immunodeficiency virus (HIV). Health and Public Policy Committee, American College of Physicians; and the Infectious Diseases Society of America. Ann Intern Med 108:460, 1988.
6. Pickering LK, Engelkirk PG: *Giardia lamblia*. Pediatr Clin North Am 35:565, 1988.
7. Lisby SM, Nahata MC: Recognition and treatment of chlamydial infections. Clin Pharm 6:25, 1987.
8. MacDonald KL, Cohen ML: Epidemiology of travelers' diarrhea: current perspectives. Rev Infect Dis 8(Suppl 1):S117, 1986.
9. Keusch GT: Antimicrobial therapy for enteric infections and typhoid fever: state of the art. Rev Infect Dis 10(Suppl 1):S199, 1988.
10. Steffen R, Mathewson JJ, Ericsson CD, et al: Travelers' diarrhea in West Africa and Mexico: fecal transport systems and liquid bismuth subsalicylate for self-therapy. J Infect Dis 157:1008, 1988.
11. Morens DM, Rigau-Perez JG, Lopez-Correa RH, et al: Dengue in Puerto Rico, 1977: public health response to characterize and control an epidemic of multiple serotypes. Am J Trop Med Hyg 35:197, 1986.
12. Earnest MP, Reller LB, Filley CM, Grek AJ: Neurocysticercosis in the United States: 35 cases and a review. Rev Infect Dis 9:961, 1987.
13. Hull HF, Montes JM, Mann JM: Septicemic plague in New Mexico. J Infect Dis 155:113, 1987.
14. Black RE: Pathogens that cause travelers' diarrhea in Latin America and Africa. Rev Infect Dis 8(Suppl 2):S131, 1986.

15. Monath TP: Yellow fever: a medically neglected disease. Report on a seminar. Rev Infect Dis 9:165, 1987.
16. Symposium on rabies and brucellosis in Mediterranean countries and the Arab peninsula. Montpellier, 4-6 November 1985. Abstracts. Comp Immunol Microbiol Infect Dis 9:1, 1986.
17. Drabick JJ: Pentastomiasis. Rev Infect Dis 9:1087, 1987.
18. St. John RK: Yaws in the Americas. Rev Infect Dis 7(Suppl 2):S266, 1985.
19. Taylor DN, Echeverria P: Etiology and epidemiology of travelers' diarrhea in Asia. Rev Infect Dis 8(Suppl 2):S136, 1986.
20. Takada T, Miyanga O, Ishibashi H, et al: Clinical analysis of 17 cases of Japanese encephalitis experienced in the ten years. Kansenshogaku Zasshi 63:494, 1989.
21. Lobel HO, Campbell CC, Schwartz IK, Roberts JM: Recent trends in the importation of malaria caused by *Plasmodium falciparum* into the United States from Africa. J Infect Dis 152:613, 1985.
22. Nutman TB, Miller KD, Mulligan M, Ottesen EA: Loa loa infection in temporary residents of endemic regions: recognition of a hyperresponsive syndrome with characteristic clinical manifestations. J Infect Dis 154:10, 1986.
23. Taylor HR: Global priorities in the control of onchocerciasis. Rev Infect Dis 7:844, 1985.
24. Monath TP: Lassa fever—new issues raised by field studies in West Africa. J Infect Dis 155:433, 1987.
25. McCormick JB, Webb PA, Krebs JW, et al: A prospective study of the epidemiology and ecology of Lassa fever. J Infect Dis 155:437, 1987.
26. Getchell JP, Hicks DR, Svinivasan A, et al: Human immunodeficiency virus isolated from a serum sample collected in 1976 in Central Africa. J Infect Dis 156:833, 1987.
27. Hrdy DB: Cultural practices contributing to the transmission of human immunodeficiency virus in Africa. Rev Infect Dis 9:1109, 1987.
28. Vittecoq D, May T, Roue RT, et al: Acquired immunodeficiency syndrome after travelling in Africa: an epidemiological study in seventeen Caucasian patients. Lancet 1:612, 1987.
29. Ebbesen P: The global epidemic of AIDS. AIDS Res 2(Suppl 1):S23, 1986.

Selected Readings

Antal GM, Causse G: The control of endemic treponematoses. Rev Infect Dis 7(Suppl 2):S220, 1985.
A review of the prevalence of endemic treponematosis that discusses reasons for the resurgence of yaws and endemic syphilis in some areas. Although yaws and pinta continue to decline in the Americas, yaws and endemic syphilis have returned to high levels in west Africa.

Burgdorfer W: The enlarging spectrum of tick-borne spirochetoses: R.R. Parker Memorial Address. Rev Infect Dis 8:932, 1986.
A review of tick-borne spirochetoses from the perspective of a medical entomologist in the Public Health Service's Rocky Mountain Laboratory. The tick-borne agent Borelia burgdorferi, *which*

causes Lyme disease, and other tick-borne spirochetoses-related diseases are discussed.

Ellner PD: Diagnostic laboratory procedures in infectious diseases. Med Clin North Am 71:1065, 1987.
Useful review of state-of-the-art microbiology diagnostic techniques available to identify a variety of infectious diseases.

Helmick CG, Tauxe RV, Vernon AA: Is there a risk to contacts of patients with rabies? Rev Infect Dis 9:511, 1987.
This paper examined records of the Centers for Disease Control and reviewed the literature to evaluate current concepts of indications for prophylaxis in persons in contact with rabid humans. Authors point out that, although rabies virus is present in several human fluids and tissues during the first 5 weeks of illness, there are only 4 well-documented reports of human-to-human transmission, all via corneal transplant recipients.

Hill DR, Pearson RD: Health advice for international travel. Ann Intern Med 108:839, 1988.
Important current review for travelers and clinicians with current concepts of vaccine-prophylaxis, pretravel advice, and immunizations required in certain countries.

Levin S, Goodman LJ, Fuhrer J: Fulminant community-acquired infectious diseases: diagnostic problems. Med Clin North Am 70:967, 1986.
Interesting, useful clinical discussion of some less common, but potentially catastrophic infectious syndromes, which, if recognized earlier, may lead to early life-saving management. Diseases are discussed, such as meningitis due to Naegleria fowleri, *a free-living ameba in brackish water, and hemorrhagic mediastinitis due to inhalation of* Bacillus anthracis, *which occurs during occupational exposure to goat's hair, wool, or other animals.*

Neill MA, Hightower AW, Broome CV: Leprosy in the United States, 1971–1981. J Infect Dis 152:1064, 1985.
The current state of leprosy in the United States as reviewed from cases reported during 1971 through 1981. An increase in the number of cases reflects the increased number of refugees and immigrants from areas endemic for leprosy.

Stansfield SK: Acute respiratory infections in the developing world: strategies for prevention, treatment, and control. Pediatr Infect Dis J 6:622, 1987.
Current concepts of acute respiratory infection in developing countries. Interesting data and review covering epidemiology, etiology, and risk factors. Useful discussion of current recommendations for chemoprophylaxis and vaccines. Well referenced.

Steffen R, Rickenbach M, Wilhelm U, et al: Health problems after travel to developing countries. J Infect Dis 156:84, 1987.
A clinical study comprised of travelers to Greek or Canary Islands to evaluate health risks associated with short visits to these nations was conducted, with 10,524 participants completing questionnaires. Incidence of infections per month abroad was as follows: giardiasis 7/1,000; amebiasis 4/1,000; hepatitis 4/1,000; gonorrhea 3/1,000; malaria, helminthiasis, or syphilis, less than 1/1,000. No cases of typhoid fever or cholera were reported.

U.S. Department of Health and Human Services: Health Information for International Travel. U.S. Government Printing Office, Washington, DC, 1985.

A yearly updated monograph that provides information regarding disease risks and vaccine recommendations. Available from Superintendent of Documents, U.S. Government Printing Office, Washington, DC 20402.

Walker E, Willliams G: ABC of healthy travel. Br Med J 286:541, 629, 703, 865, 930, 1039, 1133, 1423, 1983.
Series of articles covering topics pertaining to travel abroad.

Warren KS, Mahmoud AAF (eds): Tropical and Geographical Medicine. McGraw-Hill, New York, 1984.
Monograph detailing clinical and biologic aspects of tropical medicine.

Wolfe MS: Diseases of travelers. Clin Symp 36:2, 1984.
Detailed discussion of disorders frequently seen in travelers.

VIII

DERMATOLOGY

78
Generalized Pruritus: Common and Uncommon Causes

Pruritus, or itching, is a cutaneous sensation that provokes the urge to scratch. It is the most common symptom of dermatologic disease.[1] A wide variety of underlying systemic disorders are found in patients with generalized pruritus; renal, hepatic, hematopoietic, and endocrine disorders are most common.[1] Several environmental, physiologic, and psychological factors appear to lower the threshold for itching. Itching may be more noticeable when a patient is unoccupied.

Environmental, Physiologic, and Psychological Causes

Cold weather
Aging: itching in the elderly is commonly caused by dry skin.[2]
Low humidity
Sunburn
Excessive bathing: especially with alkaline soaps and detergents[3–5]
Psychoneurosis[6–8]
Delusions of parasitosis[9]
Pregnancy: most common in the third trimester[10–13]
Transitory periods of emotional stress

Dermatologic Disorders Causing Pruritus

Atopic dermatitis[14,15]
Contact dermatitis[16]
Xerosis (dry skin)
Urticaria[17]
Infectious and parasitic dermatoses: pediculosis, mite infestation (scabies), hookworm, roundworm, onchocerciasis, filariasis
Pyogenic infections and fungal infections
Psoriasis
Bullous pemphigoid[18]
Lichen planus

Dermatitis herpetiformis
Miliaria
Toxic eruptions: drug
Fiberglass dermatitis
Cat-scratch disease[19]

**Common Underlying
Systemic Disorders
Causing Pruritus**

Diabetes: evidence anecdotal[20,21]
Chronic renal failure: uremia,[22,23] hemodialysis[24,25]
Blood diseases, reticuloendothelioses and other ma-
lignancies: lymphoma, leukemia,[26,27] mycosis fun-
goides,[28] Hodgkin's disease,[29] carcinoid,[30] oat cell
carcinoma of the bronchus,[31] polycythemia vera,[32–34] mast cell disease,[35] visceral carcinoma
Liver disease: obstructive jaundice,[36] biliary cirrhosis,
viral hepatitis
Acquired immune deficiency syndrome (AIDS):
AIDS dermatosis[37,38]
Iron deficiency anemia: anecdotal evidence[39,40]
Multiple sclerosis[41]
Hyperthyroidism[42,43]
Hypothyroidism: associated with dry skin
Asthma[44]: Atopic diathesis
Hypercalcemia: usually due to hyperparathyroidism
Brain abscesses[45]
Central nervous system infarcts[46]

**Drugs and Toxins
Causing Pruritus**

Urticaria may be present with pruritus caused by
drugs and toxins.[47]

Hypervitaminosis A
Barbiturates
PUVA: psoralen + UVA phototherapy
Heroin, opium alkaloids, and narcotic anesthesia[48]
Oral contraceptives[49,50]
Belladonna alkaloids
Drug allergies
Arthropod bites
Chloroquine: in treatment of malaria[51]
Cocaine
Antidepressants
Hepatotoxic drugs (often with cholestasis): pheno-
thiazines, tolbutamide, erythromycin ethyl succi-
nate, anabolic hormones, estrogens, progestins
Histamine-releasing drugs: D-tubocurarine, poly-
mixin, radiopaque dyes, thiamine[52]

Vancomycin[53]
Immunotherapy: interleukin-2[54]

References

1. Gilchrest BA: Pruritus: pathogenesis, therapy and significance in systemic disease states. Arch Intern Med 142:101, 1982.
2. Thorne EG: Coping with pruritus: a common geriatric complaint. Geriatrics 33(7):47, 1978.
3. Behrman HT, Labow TA, Rozen JH: Itching in Common Skin Diseases. Diagnosis and Treatment. p. 63. 3rd Ed. Grune & Stratton, New York, 1978.
4. Steinman HK: Water-induced pruritus. Clin Dermatol 5:41, 1987.
5. Bircher AJ, Meier-Ruge W: Aquagenic pruritus. Water-induced activation of acetylcholinesterase. Arch Dermatol 124:84, 1988.
6. Fruensgaard K, Hjortshoj A: Diagnosis of neurotic excoriations. Int J Dermatol 21:148, 1982.
7. Laihinen A: Psychosomatic aspects in dermatoses. Ann Clin Res 19:147, 1987.
8. Fjellner B, Arnetz BB: Psychological predictors of pruritus during mental stress. Acta Derm Venereol 65:504, 1985.
9. Gould WM, Gragg TM: Delusions of parasitosis. An approach to the problem. Arch Dermatol 112:1745, 1976.
10. Wong RC, Ellis CN: Physiologic skin changes in pregnancy. J Am Acad Dermatol 10:929, 1984.
11. Alcalay J, Ingber A, David M, et al: Pruritic urticarial papules and plaques of pregnancy. A review of 21 cases. J Reprod Med 32:315, 1987.
12. Alcalay J, Ingber A, Kafri B, et al: Hormonal evaluation and autoimmune background in pruritic urticarial papules and plaques of pregnancy. Am J Obstet Gynecol 158:417, 1988.
13. Dacus JV, Muram D: Pruritus in pregnancy. South Med J 80:614, 1987.
14. Hanifin JM: Atopic dermatitis. J Am Acad Dermatol 6:1, 1982.
15. Rajka G: Natural history and clinical manifestations of atopic dermatitis. Clin Rev Allergy 4:3, 1986.
16. Bendsoe N, Bjornberg A, Asnes H: Itching from wool fibres in atopic dermatitis. Contact Dermatitis 17:21, 1987.
17. Kaplan AP: Chronic urticaria. Possible causes, suggested treatment alternatives. Postgrad Med 74(3):209, 1983.
18. Bingham EA, Burrows D, Sandford JC: Prolonged pruritus and bullous pemphigoid. Clin Exp Dermatol 9:564, 1984.
19. Daye S, McHenry JA, Roscelli JD: Pruritic rash associated with cat scratch disease. Pediatrics 81:559, 1988.
20. Stawiski MA, Voorhees JJ: Cutaneous signs of diabetes mellitus. Cutis 18:415, 1976.
21. Neilly JB, Martin A, Simpson N, MacCuish AC: Pruritus in diabetes mellitus: investigation of prevalence and correlation with diabetes control. Diabetes Care 9:273, 1986.

22. Massry SG, Popovtzer MM, Coburn JW, et al: Intractable pruritus as a manifestation of secondary hyperparathyroidism in uremia. N Engl J Med 279:697, 1968.
23. Bencini PL, Montagnino G, Citterio A, et al: Cutaneous abnormalities in uremic patients. Nephron 40:316, 1985.
24. Gilchrest BA, Stern RS, Steinman TI, et al: Clinical features of pruritus among patients undergoing maintenance hemodialysis. Arch Dermatol 118:154, 1982.
25. Bousquet J, Maurice F, Rivory JP, et al: Allergy in long-term hemodialysis. II. Allergic and atopic patterns of a population of patients undergoing long-term hemodialysis. J Allergy Clin Immunol 81:605, 1988.
26. Czarnecki DB, Downes NP, O'Brien T: Pruritic specific cutaneous infiltrates in leukemia and lymphoma. Arch Dermatol 118:119, 1982.
27. Chan HL, Su IJ, Kuo TT, et al: Cutaneous manifestations of adult T cell leukemia/lymphoma. Report of three different forms. J Am Acad Dermatol 13:213, 1985.
28. Lamberg SI, Green SB, Byar DP, et al: Status report of 376 mycosis fungoides patients at four years: mycosis fungoides cooperative group. Cancer Treat Rep 63:701, 1979.
29. Gobbi PG, Attardo-Parrinello G, Lattanzio G, et al: Severe pruritus should be a B-symptom in Hodgkin's disease. Cancer 51:1934, 1983.
30. Mengel CE: Cutaneous manifestations of the malignant carcinoid syndrome. Severe pruritus and orange blotches. Ann Intern Med 58:989, 1963.
31. Thomas S, Harrington CI: Intractable pruritus as the presenting symptom of carcinoma of the bronchus: a case report and review of the literature. Clin Exp Dermatol 8:459, 1983.
32. Salem HH, Van Der Weyden MB, Young IF, et al: Pruritus and severe iron deficiency in polycythemia vera. Br Med J 285:91, 1982.
33. Berk PD, Goldberg JD, Donovan PB, et al: Therapeutic recommendations in polycythemia vera based on Polycythemia Vera Study Group protocols. Semin Hematol 23:132, 1986.
34. Jackson N, Burt D, Crocker J, Boughton B: Skin mast cells in polycythaemia vera: relationship to the pathogenesis and treatment of pruritus. Br J Dermatol 116:21, 1987.
35. Parks A, Camisa C: Reddish-brown macules with telangiectasia and pruritus. Urticaria pigmentosa-telangiectasia macularis eruptiva perstans (TMEP) variant, with systemic mastocytosis. Arch Dermatol 124:429, 432, 1988.
36. Goldman RD, Rea TH, Cinque J: The "butterfly" sign. A clue to generalized pruritus in a patient with chronic obstructive hepatobiliary disease. Arch Dermatol 119:183, 1983.
37. Berk MA, Medenica M, Laumann A: Tubuloreticular structures in a papular eruption associated with human immunodeficiency virus disease. J Am Acad Dermatol 18:452, 1988.
38. Shapiro RS, Samorodin C, Hood AF: Pruritus as a

presenting sign of acquired immunodeficiency syndrome. J Am Acad Dermatol 16:1115, 1987.
39. Lewiecki EM, Rahman F: Pruritus: a manifestation of iron deficiency. JAMA 236:2319, 1976.
40. Rector WG Jr, Fortuin NJ, Conley CL: Non-hematologic effects of chronic iron deficiency. A study of patients with polycythemia vera treated solely with venesections. Medicine 61:382, 1982.
41. Osterman PO: Paraoxysmal itching in multiple sclerosis. Br J Dermatol 95:555, 1976.
42. Isaacs NJ, Ertel NH: Urticaria and pruritus: uncommon manifestations of hyperthyroidism. J Allergy Clin Immunol 48:73, 1971.
43. Mullin GE, Eastern JS: Cutaneous signs of thyroid disease. Am Fam Physician 34(4):93, 1986.
44. David TJ, Wybrew M, Hennessen U: Prodromal itching in childhood asthma. Lancet 2:154, 1984.
45. Sullivan MJ, Drake ME Jr: Unilateral pruritus and *Nocardia* brain abscess. Neurology 34:828, 1984.
46. Massey EW: Unilateral neurogenic pruritus following stroke. Stroke 15:901, 1984.
47. Dunagin WG, Millikan LE: Drug eruptions. Med Clin North Am 64:983, 1980.
48. Young AW Jr, Sweeney EW: Cutaneous clues to heroin addiction. Am Fam Physician 7(2):79, 1973.
49. Drill VA: Benign cholestatic jaundice of pregnancy and benign cholestatic jaundice from oral contraceptives. Am J Obstet Gynecol 119:165, 1974.
50. Diffey BL: Use of UV-A sunbeds for cosmetic tanning. Br J Dermatol 115:67, 1986.
51. Osifo NG: Chloroquine-induced pruritus among patients with malaria. Arch Dermatol 120:80, 1984.
52. Herndon JH Jr: Pruritus. p. 2. In Demis DJ (ed): Clinical Dermatology. Vol. 4, Unit 29-2. Harper & Row, Philadelphia, 1985.
53. Polk RE, Healy DP, Schwartz LB, et al: Vancomycin and the red-man syndrome: pharmacodynamics of histamine release. J Infect Dis 157:502, 1988.
54. Gaspari AA, Lotze MT, Rosenberg SA, et al: Dermatologic changes associated with interleukin-2 administration. JAMA 258:1624, 1987.

Selected Readings

Arnold HL Jr: Paroxysmal pruritus. Its clinical characterization and a hypothesis of its pathogenesis. J Am Acad Dermatol 11:322, 1984.

This interesting paper proposes a hypothesis of pathogenesis and a clinical distinction between certain underlying disorders that cause pruritus. The author makes a clinical distinction between pruritus caused by skin disorders, such as insect bites and ringworm, which do not provoke scratching to the point of bleeding or lichenification and disorders which do provoke scratching that results in bleeding, scarring, or lichenification.

Beauregard S, Gilchrest BA: A survey of skin problems and skin care regimens in the elderly. Arch Dermatol 123:1638, 1987.

A study of dermatologic disease and skin care needs in the elderly examined 68 noninstitutionalized volunteers 50 to 91 years of age and found that pruritus was their most frequent complaint. In decreasing order of prevalence, disorders included actinic keratoses, tinea pedis, contact dermatitis, seborrheic dermatitis, stasis dermatitis, and skin cancer.

Bigby M, Jick S, Jick H, Arndt K: Drug-induced cutaneous reactions. A report from the Boston Collaborative Drug Surveillance Program on 15,438 consecutive inpatients, 1975 to 1982. JAMA 256:3358, 1986.
An analysis of data on 15,438 consecutive medical inpatients monitored from 1975 to 1982 provides quantitative data helpful in clinical decision making when drug-induced exanthems, urticaria, or generalized pruritus occurs.

Denman ST: A review of pruritus. J Am Acad Dermatol 14:375, 1986.
This article reviews concepts of neurophysiology of pruritus with clinical correlations.

Fjellner B, Arnetz BB, Eneroth P, Kallner A: Pruritus during standardized mental stress. Relationship to psychoneuroendocrine and metabolic parameters. Acta Derm Venereol 65:199, 1985.
Experimentally-induced emotional stress on pruritic response of human skin was studied in healthy subjects. Physiologic, endocrine, and metabolic parameters were measured. The individual cutaneous reactions to stress exposure appeared most related to the adrenaline response pattern.

Jorizzo JL: The itchy patient. A practical approach. Primary Care 10:339, 1983.
An overview of the practical approach to the evaluation of the itchy patient.

Kantor GR, Lookingbill DP: Generalized pruritus and systemic disease. J Am Acad Dermatol 9:375, 1983.
A study of generalized pruritus in an outpatient population with recommendations for workup.

Lawrence CM, Strange RC, Scriven AJ, et al: Plasma bile salt levels in patients presenting with generalized pruritus: an improved indicator of occult liver disease. Ann Clin Biochem 22:232, 1985.
Fasting bile salt concentrations and conventional liver function tests were measured in 26 patients presenting with generalized pruritus without primary skin disease. Since fasting plasma-conjugated-cholate measurements identified all patients with hepatobiliary disease, authors suggest plasma bile salt concentrations may be a useful screening test for hepatobiliary disease in patients with generalized pruritus.

Paul R, Paul R, Jansen CT: Itch and malignancy prognosis in generalized pruritus: a 6 year follow-up of 125 patients. J Am Acad Dermatol 16:1179, 1987.
One hundred twenty-five patients with generalized pruritus were followed for 6 years. In four patients, a malignancy was identified at initial examination. In four patients, malignancies developed during follow-up.

Rubenstein R: Pruritus: a new look at an old problem. J Fam Pract 24 (6):625, 1987.
Clinical review of problems related to evaluating and treating pruritus, with a focus on patients as they present in general practice.

79
Urticaria: Major Causes of Acute and Chronic Urticaria

Urticaria, or hives, is a skin reaction characterized by transient, pruritic, edematous, sometimes lightly erythematous papules or wheals, occasionally with central clearing.[1] Although acute urticaria can rarely proceed to life-threatening laryngeal edema or anaphylactic shock, most underlying causes of urticaria are not serious and can be determined by taking a history to determine use of pharmaceutical agents, food, infection, physical agents, psychogenic factors, inhalants, insect bites, internal diseases, immune complex diseases, contactants, and even genetic factors.[2] Chronic urticaria (recurrent urticaria of at least 6 weeks duration with no known cause) often has no known etiology and must be a diagnosis of exclusion after underlying disease, drug reactions, and food allergies are ruled out.[3]

Drugs Causing Urticaria

Drugs and chemicals, ingested or injected, are among the most common causes of acute urticaria.[1] Almost any drug can cause urticaria; antibiotics are among the most frequent offenders.

Antibiotics: sulfonamides; penicillin is a common cause of allergic drug-induced urticaria.[4]
Aspirin: chronic urticaria in 20 to 40% of patients is exacerbated by aspirin[5,6]
Nonsteroidal anti-inflammatory agents
Histamine-releasing drugs[7]
Morphine and codeine
D-tubocurarine
Polymyxin
Sedatives: barbiturates, anesthesia[8]
Analgesics: aspirin, phenacetin
Diuretics: cross reactions with sulfonamides
Neuromuscular blocking agents: cholinergic urticaria[9]

Phenothiazines
Allopurinol

**Foods Commonly
Causing Urticaria**

Foods are a common cause of acute urticaria. Protein and additives are often responsible, including tartrazine-azo dyes, benzoic acid derivatives, and yeasts.[10-12]

Nuts
Shellfish
Fish
Eggs
Berries
Tomatoes
Chocolate
Milk: pencillin residues may be a potential precipitant of urticaria.[13]
Pork
Caffeine[14]

**Toxins, Chemicals,
and Physical Agents
Causing Urticaria**

Transfusion reactions[15]
Insect stings
Arthropod bites
Physical agents[16]: cold,[17] heat,[18] sun,[19,20] pressure,[21,22] water,[23] vibration, contact,[24-26] (which usually occurs on the hands and around the mouth)
Inhalants: pollens, mold spores, animal danders, dust, grass
Exercise[27,28]
Animal proteins: immune globulins, vaccines, animal-derived insulin
Epoxy resins[29]
Plants: contact urticaria[30,31]

**Infections Causing
Urticaria**

Urticaria can be the presenting sign of a viral prodrome, such as hepatitis, or rarely, it can be the only sign of occult infection, such as parasitic infestation.

Chronic focal bacterial infections: sinusitis,[32] gallbladder, dental infections,[33] urinary tract infections
Systemic viral infections: hepatitis (serum hepatitis),[34] mononucleosis (cold urticaria),[35] coxsackievirus
Fungal: candidiasis, dermatophytosis

Parasites: amebiasis, giardiasis,[36] trichomoniasis, malaria, scabies,[37] helminth infestations[38]
Tertiary syphilis: rare

Systemic Diseases Causing Urticaria

Chronic urticaria can be a manifestation of an underlying disease such as carcinoma, vasculitis, or collagen vascular disease.[1]

Collagen vascular diseases with vasculitis[39]: lupus erythematosus,[40,41] polymyositis[42]
Neoplasms[43]: lymphoma, leukemias, carcinomas
Cryoglobulinemia, cryoproteinemia
Polycythemia vera
Amyloidosis
Urticaria pigmentosa: systemic mastocytosis[44]
Bullous pemphigoid
Dermatitis herpetiformis: most commonly presents with vesicles[45]
Immune complex processes: serum sickness, monoclonal IgM[46]
Complement activation processes
Hyperthyroidism: uncommon[47,48]

Physiologic Causes of Urticaria

Pregnancy[49-52]
Premenstrual: probably a progesterone effect[53]

Genetic Causes of Urticaria

Hereditary angioedema[54,55]
Erythropoietic protoporphyria: urticaria is a rare manifestation
Atopy[56]
Syndrome of urticaria, deafness, amyloidosis: Muckle-Wells syndrome[57]
C3b inactivator deficiency
Familial urticaria pigmentosa[58]

References

1. Monroe EW: Urticaria and urticarial vasculitis. Med Clin North Am 64:867, 1980.
2. Synkowski DR: Urticaria. Emerg Med Clin North Am 3:737, 1985.
3. Kaplan AP: Chronic urticaria. Possible causes, suggested treatment alternatives. Postgrad Med 74(3):209, 1983.
4. Boonk WJ, Van Ketel WG: The role of penicillin in the pathogenesis of chronic urticaria. Br J Dermatol 106:183, 1982.

5. James J, Warin RP: Chronic urticaria: the effect of aspirin (letter). Br J Dermatol 82:204, 1970.
6. Szczeklik A: Adverse reactions to aspirin and nonsteroidal anti-inflammatory drugs. Ann Allergy 59:113, 1987.
7. Paton WDM: Histamine release by compounds of simple chemical structure. Pharmacol Rev 9:269, 1957.
8. Smith GB, Shribman AJ: Anesthesia and severe skin disease. Anaesthesia 39:443, 1984
9. Wolf R: Cholinergic urticaria and neuromuscular blocking agents. Cutis 28:448, 1981.
10. Brown EB: Urticaria and angioedema can be caused by food additives and dyes (letter). Ann Allergy 52:200, 1984.
11. Hannuksela M, Haahtela T: Hypersensitivity reactions to food additives. Allergy 42:561, 1987.
12. Juhlin L: Additives and chronic urticaria. Ann Allergy 59:119, 1987.
13. Ormerod AD, Reid TM, Main RA: Penicillin in milk— its importance in urticaria. Clin Allergy 17:229, 1987.
14. Pola J, Subiza J, Armentia A, et al: Urticaria caused by caffeine. Ann Allergy 60:207, 1988.
15. Schmidt PJ: Transfusion reactions. Status in 1982. Clin Lab Med 2:221, 1982.
16. Sibbald RG: Physical urticaria. Dermatol Clin 3:57, 1984.
17. Lin RY, Krysickajanniger C, Schwartz RA, et al: Cold urticaria. Am Fam Physician 33(2):145, 1986.
18. Michaëlsson G, Ros AM: Familial localized heat urticaria of delayed type. Acta Dermatovener 51:279, 1971.
19. Armstrong RB: Solar urticaria. Dermatol Clin 4:253, 1986.
20. Norris PG, Murphy GM, Hawk JL, Winkelmann RK: A histological study of the evolution of solar urticaria. Arch Dermatol 124:80, 1988.
21. Czarnetzki BM, Cap HP, Forck G: Late cutaneous reactions to common allergens in patients with delayed pressure urticaria. Br J Dermatol 117:695, 1987.
22. Mekori YA, Dobozin BS, Schocket AL, et al: Delayed pressure urticaria histologically resembles cutaneous late-phase reactions. Arch Dermatol 124:230, 1988.
23. Panconesi E, Lotti T: Aquagenic urticaria. Clin Dermatol 5:49, 1987.
24. Turjanmaa K, Reunala T: Condoms as a source of latex allergen and cause of contact urticaria. Contact Dermatitis 20:360, 1989
25. Burdick AE, Mathias CG: The contact urticaria syndrome. Dermatol Clin 3:71, 1985.
26. Estlander T, Jolanki R, Kanerva L: Contact urticaria from rubber gloves: a detailed description of four cases. Acta Derm Venereol (Suppl) 134:98, 1987.
27. Kaplan AP: Exercise-induced hives. J Allergy Clin Immunol 73:704, 1984.
28. Casale TB, Keahey TM, Kaliner M: Exercise-induced anaphylactic syndromes. Insights into diagnostic and pathophysiologic features. JAMA 255:2049, 1986.
29. Jolanki R, Estlander T, Kanerva L: Occupational contact dermatitis and contact urticaria caused by epoxy resins. Acta Derm Venereol (Suppl) 134:90, 1987.
30. Webster GL: Plant dermatitis. Irritant plants in the

Urticaria **583**

spurge family (Euphorbiaceae). Clin Dermatol 4:36, 1986.

31. Lahti A: Contact urticaria to plants. Clin Dermatol 4:127, 1986.
32. Nelson HS: Routine sinus roentgenograms and chronic urticaria (letter). JAMA 251:1680, 1984.
33. Thyagarajan K, Kamalam A: Chronic urticaria due to abscessed teeth roots. Int J Dermatol 21:606, 1982.
34. Vaida GA, Goldman MA, Bloch KJ: Testing for hepatitis B virus in patients with chronic urticaria and angioedema. J Allergy Clin Immunol 72:193, 1983.
35. Wu LYF, Mesko JW, Petersen BH: Cold urticaria associated with infectious mononucleosis. Ann Allergy 50:271, 1983.
36. Veronesi S, Palmerio B, Negosanti M, et al: Urticaria and giardiasis. Dermatologica 166:42, 1983.
37. Witkowski JA, Parish LC: Scabies: a cause of generalized urticaria. Cutis 33:277, 1984.
38. Corsini AC: Strongyloidiasis and chronic urticaria. Postgrad Med J 58:247, 1982.
39. Jones RR, Bhogal B, Dash A, et al: Urticaria and vasculitis: a continuum of histological and immunopathological changes. Br J Dermatol 108:695, 1983.
40. Horvath A, Kramer M, Ablonczy E: Clinical evaluation and pathomechanism of urticaria-like skin eruption in systemic lupus erythematosus. Acta Dermatovener 62:253, 1982.
41. Matarredona J, Sendagorta E, Rocamora A, et al: Systemic lupus erythematosus appearing as an urticarial vasculitis. Int J Dermatol 25:446, 1986.
42. Callen JP, Dubin HV: Urticaria and polymyositis. Arch Dermatol 114:1545, 1978.
43. Dreizen S, McCredie KB, Bodey GP, Keating MJ: External expressions of internal malignancy. Postgrad Med 82(5):91, 1987.
44. Burklow SL, Marney SR Jr: Mastocytosis: one year's experience. South Med J 80:51, 1987.
45. Katz SI, Hall RP III, Lawley TJ, et al: Dermatitis herpetiformis: the skin and the gut. Ann Intern Med 93:857, 1980.
46. Doutre MS, Beylot C, Bioulac P, Bezian JH: Monoclonal IgM and chronic urticaria: two cases. Ann Allergy 58:413, 1987.
47. Isaacs NJ, Ertel NH: Urticaria and pruritus: uncommon manifestations of hyperthyroidism. J Allergy Clin Immunol 48:73, 1971.
48. Mullin GE, Eastern JS: Cutaneous signs of thyroid disease. Am Fam Physician 34(4):93, 1986.
49. Winton GB, Lewis CW: Dermatoses of pregnancy. J Am Acad Dermatol 6:977, 1982.
50. Fox GN: Pruritic urticarial papules and plaques of pregnancy. Am Fam Physician 34(3):191, 1986.
51. Alcalay J, Ingber A, Kafri B, et al: Hormonal evaluation and autoimmune background in pruritic urticarial papules and plaques of pregnancy. Am J Obstet Gynecol 158:417, 1988.
52. Alcalay J, Ingber A, David M, et al: Pruritic urticarial papules and plaques of pregnancy. A review of 21 cases. J Reprod Med 32:315, 1987.

53. Hart R: Autoimmune progesterone dermatitis. Arch Dermatol 113:426, 1977.
54. Frank MM, Gelfand JA, Atkinson JP: Hereditary angioedema: the clinical syndrome and its management. Ann Intern Med 84:580, 1976.
55. Warin RP, Cunliffe WJ, Greaves MW, Wallington TB: Recurrent angioedema: familial and oestrogen-induced. Br J Dermatol 115:731, 1986.
56. Hanifin JM: Atopic dermatitis. Special clinical complications. Postgrad Med 74(3):188, 1983.
57. Muckle TJ, Wells M: Urticaria, deafness, and amyloidosis: a new heredo-familial syndrome. Q J Med 31:235, 1962.
58. Fowler JF Jr, Parsley WM, Cotter PG: Familial urticaria pigmentosa. Arch Dermatol 122:80, 1986.

Selected Readings

Burrall BA, Huntley AC: Urticaria and angioedema. Clin Rev Allergy 3:95, 1985.
A clinical review of current concepts of angioneurotic edema and urticaria.

Fineman SM: Urticaria and angioedema. Prim Care 14:503, 1987.
This article offers a practical approach to both differential diagnosis and therapeutic modalities important when confronted with urticaria and angioedema.

Guin JD: The evaluation of patients with urticaria. Dermatol Clin 3:29, 1985.
Authors discuss current methods found clinically useful in the evaluation of urticaria which include compressed printed history forms and certain laboratory tests.

Hirschmann JV, Lawlor F, English JS, et al: Cholinergic urticaria. A clinical and histologic study. Arch Dermatol 123:462, 1987.
A clinical study of the natural history of atopy and systemic symptoms during attacks of cholinergic urticaria in 35 patients. Symptoms usually began between the ages of 10 and 30 years and caused patients to modify certain contributing factors, particularly provoking factors involving exercise, emotion, and heat.

Wagner WO: Urticaria—a challenge in diagnosis and treatment. Postgrad Med 83(5):321, 329, 1988.
The wide variety of internal and external causes of urticaria seen in clinical practice is discussed. Clinical tests, such as skin testing, ice-cube testing, skin biopsy, and food challenges, are some of the helpful methods of evaluation suggested.

Wintroub BU, Stern R: Cutaneous drug reactions: pathogenesis and clinical classification. J Am Acad Dermatol 13:167, 1985.
A clinically useful classification of drug-induced cutaneous reactions, with a focus on pathogenesis and clinical morphology. Urticaria, photosensitivity eruptions, erythema multiforme, pigmentation disturbances, and drug-induced cutaneous reactions are discussed.

80
Alopecia: Common and Less Common Causes

Hair loss (alopecia) is most commonly physiologic. Less common and acquired causes are multiple, such as underlying systemic illnesses, metabolic-toxic causes, trauma, and physical agents. Alopecia can be classified by pattern of hair loss: diffuse or localized, scarring and nonscarring.

Physiologic Causes of Hair Loss

Male pattern hair loss: normal male hair loss begins frontally and continues until a horsehoe-shaped rim of hair remains on the scalp before final baldness.[1,2]
Female pattern hair loss: thinning over the vertex, parietal, and temporal areas[3]
Postpartum

Alopecia Areata: Common Associations

Alopecia areata is a hair disorder of localized or patchy hair loss on the scalp, eyebrows, and beard without known cause, but often considered an autoimmune phenomenon[4] because of the following commonly identified associations[5-7]:

Emotional stress
Down syndrome
Thyroid disease: Hashimoto's thyroiditis, Graves' disease
Pernicious anemia
Atopic dermatitis
Addison's disease
Vogt-Koyanagi syndrome
Collagen vascular disorders
Vitiligo

Drug and Chemical Causes of Hair Loss

Almost any drug can cause hair loss; some more commonly used drugs causing alopecia are

Chemotherapy[8,9] (anagen effluvium): alkylating

585

agents, antimetabolites, cytotoxic agents, alkaloid cytostatics

Anticonvulsants: phenytoin

Androgenic hormones: birth control pills, exogenous and endogenous testosterone[10–13]

Anticoagulants: heparin, coumadin, phenindione

Miscellaneous drugs: indomethacin, allopurinol, methyldopa, levodopa, phenothiazines, amphetamines, danazol,[14] metoprolol[15]

Hypervitaminosis A and retinoids: isotretinoin[16]

Sodium borate

Chemicals: selenium, bismuth, thallium,[17] iodides

Thyreostatics: carbimazole, thiouracil

Lipid-lowering agents: clofibrate

Colchicine

Zinc deficiency[18,19]

Traumatic Causes of Hair Loss

Tight winding or braiding: traction alopecia

Neurotic plucking of hair: trichotillomania[20]

Hot combs: hot comb alopecia

Prolonged pressure on scalp: i.e., during general anesthesia or prolonged bed rest[21]

Stress-Related Causes of Hair Loss

Febrile illnesses: postfebrile effluvium

Childbirth: Postpartum telogen effluvium

Surgery[22]

Weight loss[23]

Psychic shock: psychogenic telogen effluvium[24]

Radiation therapy

Severe acute or traumatic illness: spinal cord injury[24]

Systemic Disorders Associated with Alopecia

Severe chronic illness: renal, cardiovascular, hepatic, pulmonary insufficiency, neoplasia

Nutritional deficiency: kwashiorkor, marasmus, protein deficiency states, hyperalimentation-induced deficiencies, i.e., zinc and iron deficiencies, inflammatory bowel disease

Sarcoidosis[25]

Amyloidosis[26]

Secondary syphilis: moth-eaten appearance[27,28]

Leprosy

Collagen vascular diseases: discoid and systemic lupus, scleroderma, dermatomyositis[29,30]

Endocrinopathies: hypopituitarism, hypothyroidism,

hyperthyroidism, diabetes mellitus, hypoparathyroidism, oophorectomy

Scarring Alopecia: Common Causes

Scalp infections, trauma, and some dermatologic diseases are common causes of scarring alopecia.[31,32]

Hereditary disorders and congenital defects[33-35]: Hutchinson-Gilford progeria syndrome,[36] congenital triangular alopecia[37]
Physical injuries: mechanical trauma, burns,[38] radiodermatitis
Scalp infections
Fungal: dermatophyte focus
Bacterial: lupus vulgaris, leprosy, tertiary lues, yaws, carbuncles, furuncles, folliculitis
Viral: varicella, zoster, variola
Protozoal: *Leishmania*
Tick bite alopecia[39]
Neoplasms: morphea basal cell carcinoma,[40] metastatic carcinoma, epidermal nevi, nevus sebaceous, nerve sheath myxoma[41]
Dermatologic diseases: lichen planus and lichenoid drug eruptions, lupus erythematosus (discoid), alopecia mucinosa,[42] morphea, bullous or mucosal pemphigoid, acne keloidalis nuchae

References

1. Cervia M, Rebora A: Age-related severity of male-pattern alopecia. Dermatologica 166:81, 1983.
2. Pitts RL: Serum elevation of dehydroepiandrosterone sulfate associated with male pattern baldness in young men. J Am Acad Dermatol 16:571, 1987.
3. Dawber RPR: Common baldness in women. Int J Dermatol 20:647, 1981.
4. Alopecia areata—an autoimmune disease? (editorial). Lancet 1:1335, 1984.
5. Mikesell JF, Bergfeld WF, Braun WE: HLA-DR antigens in alopecia areata. Preliminary report. Cleve Clin Q 53:189, 1986.
6. Mitchell AJ, Balle MR: Alopecia areata. Dermatol Clin 5:553, 1987.
7. Orecchia G, Belvedere MC, Martinetti M, et al: Human leukocyte antigen region involvement in the genetic predisposition to alopecia areata. Dermatologica 175:10, 1987.
8. Cancer, cancer therapy and hair (editorial). Lancet 2:1177, 1983.
9. Hood AF: Cutaneous side effects of cancer chemotherapy. Med Clin North Am 70:187, 1986.
10. Kasick JM, Bergfeld WF, Steck WD, et al: Adrenal

androgenic female-pattern alopecia: sex hormones and the balding woman. Cleve Clin Q 50:111, 1983.

11. Bergfeld WF, Redmond GP: Androgenic alopecia. Dermatol Clin 5:491, 1987.

12. Georgala G, Papasotiriou V, Stavropoulos P: Serum testosterone and sex hormone binding globulin levels in women with androgenetic alopecia. Acta Derm Venereol (Stockh) 66:532, 1986.

13. DeVillez RL, Dunn J: Female androgenic alopecia. The 3 alpha, 17 beta-androstanediol glucuronide/sex hormone binding globulin ratio as a possible marker for female pattern baldness. Arch Dermatol 122:1011, 1986.

14. Duff P, Mayer AR: Generalized alopecia: an unusual complication of danazol therapy. Am J Obstet Gynecol 141:349, 1981.

15. Graeber CW, Lapkin RA: Metoprolol and alopecia. Cutis 28:633, 1981.

16. Inkeles SB, Connor WE, Illingworth DR: Hepatic and dermatologic manifestations of chronic hypervitaminosis A in adults. Report of two cases. Am J Med 80:491, 1986.

17. Insley BM, Grufferman S, Ayliffe HE: Thallium poisoning in cocaine abusers. Am J Emerg Med 4:545, 1986.

18. Evans GW: Zinc and its deficiency diseases. Clin Physiol Biochem 4:94, 1986.

19. Prasad AS: Clinical, endocrinological, and biochemical effects of zinc deficiency. Clin Endocrinol Metab 14:567, 1985.

20. Muller SA: Trichotillomania. Dermatol Clin 5:595, 1987.

21. Kosanin RM, Riefkohl R, Barwick WJ: Postoperative alopecia in a woman after a lengthy plastic surgical procedure. Plast Reconstr Surg 73:308, 1984.

22. Desai SP, Roaf ER: Telogen effluvium after anesthesia and surgery. Anesth Analg 63:83, 1984.

23. Goette DK, Odom RB: Alopecia in crash dieters. JAMA 235:2622, 1976.

24. Dahlin PA, George J, Nerette JC: Telogen effluvium: hair loss after spinal cord injury. Arch Phys Med Rehabil 65:485, 1984.

25. Smith SR, Kendall MJ, Kondratowicz GM: Sarcoidosis—a cause of steroid responsive total alopecia. Postgrad Med J 62:205, 1986.

26. Wheeler GE, Barrows GH: Alopecia universalis. A manifestation of occult amyloidosis and multiple myeloma. Arch Dermatol 117:815, 1981.

27. Hira SK, Patel JS, Bhat SG, et al: Clinical manifestations of secondary syphilis. Int J Dermatol 26:103, 1987.

28. van der Willigen AH, Peereboom-Wynia JD, van der Hoek JC, et al: Hair root studies in patients suffering from primary and secondary syphilis. Acta Derm Venereol (Stockh) 67:250, 1987.

29. Tsokos GC, Gorden P, Antonovych T, et al: Lupus nephritis and other autoimmune features in patients with diabetes mellitus due to autoantibody to insulin receptors. Ann Intern Med 102:176, 1985.

30. Koh HK, Laub DA, Tahan SR, Gonzalez E: Alopecia, photosensitivity, and arthritis. Arch Dermatol 122:1435, 1986.
31. Newton RC, Hebert AA, Freese TW, Solomon AR: Scarring alopecia. Dermatol Clin 5:603, 1987.
32. Gibson V, Tschen JA, Bean SF: Localized cicatricial pemphigoid (Brunsting-Perry syndrome). Cutis 38:252, 1986.
33. Birnbaum PS, Baden HP: Heritable disorders of hair. Dermatol Clin 5:137, 1987.
34. Appell ML, Sherertz EF: A kindred with alopecia, keratosis, pilaris, cataracts, and psoriasis. J Am Acad Dermatol 16:89, 1987.
35. Headington JT, Astle N: Familial focal alopecia. A new disorder of hair growth clinically resembling pseudopelade. Arch Dermatol 123:234, 1987.
36. Ogihara T, Hata T, Tanaka K, et al: Hutchinson-Gilford progeria syndrome in a 45-year-old man. Am J Med 81:135, 1986.
37. Tosti A: Congenital triangular alopecia. Report of fourteen cases. J Am Acad Dermatol 16:991, 1987.
38. Buckland R, Wilson GR, Sully L: Effect of scalp burns on common male pattern baldness. Br Med J (Clin Res) 293:1645, 1986.
39. Heyl T: Tick bite alopecia. Clin Exp Dermatol 7:537, 1982.
40. Labareda JM, Garcia e Silva L: Basil cell carcinomas of the scalp. Review of 77 patients with 81 tumors. Med Cutan Ibero Lat Am 16:367, 1988.
41. Burket JM: Alopecia associated with underlying nerve sheath myxoma. J Am Acad Dermatol 16:209, 1987.
42. Snyder RA, Crain WR, McNutt NS: Alopecia mucinosa. Report of a case with diffuse alopecia and normal-appearing scalp skin. Arch Dermatol 120:496, 1984.

Selected Readings

Birnbaum PS, Arndt KA: Alopecia: common and uncommon. Hosp Practice 21(5A):19, 1986.
General clinical review of a half dozen of the most common causes of alopecia.

Ebling FJ: The biology of hair. Dermatol Clin 5:467, 1987.
A review of current concepts of hair biology. The focus on structural and endocrinologic aspects of hair growth and hair loss offer interesting basic concepts helpful to understand both normal physiologic changes, as well as disorders involving hair loss.

Fenske NA, Lober CW: Structural and functional changes of normal aging skin. J Am Acad Dermatol 15:571, 1986.
Extensive informative review covering the multitude of problems related to aging skin. Both environmental factors, such as solar-induced cutaneous changes, and structural and functional alterations caused by the intrinsic aging process are discussed. Hair changes in the elderly are among the interesting changes reviewed.

Gibbons RD, Fiedler-Weiss VC: Computer-aided quantification of scalp hair. Dermatol Clin 4:627, 1986.
A statistical model applied with image analysis technology to quantify two-component visual fields is described, with applications suggested for the quantification of hair density in patients with hair loss disorders.

Hordinsky MK: General evaluation of the patient with alopecia. Dermatol Clin 5:483, 1987.
Clinical review of the evaluation of the patient with alopecia, with a particular emphasis on how to examine cut and plucked hair, perform scalp biopsies, and current helpful laboratory studies.

Kemmett D: ABC of dermatology. Diseases of the hair and scalp. Br Med J (Clin Res) 296:552, 1988.
Clinical approach to evaluation of diseases of the hair and scalp. Scalp dermatoses, alopecia, and hirsutism are reviewed.

Messenger AG, Slater DN, Bleehen SS: Alopecia areata: alterations in the hair growth cycle and correlation with the follicular pathology. Br J Dermatol 114:337, 1986.
A histopathologic study of 17 patients with alopecia areata was performed with a focus on hair cycle dynamics. Authors review current concepts of pathogenesis and suggest a new pathogenic hypothesis relating alterations in hair cycle dynamics to pathologic changes within the anagen follicle.

Mitchell AJ, Krull EA: Alopecia areata: pathogenesis and treatment. J Am Acad Dermatol 11:763, 1984.
Review of etiology of alopecia areata and summarization of immunologic data. Well referenced.

Nelson DA, Spielvogel RL: Alopecia areata. Int J Dermatol 24:26, 1985.
Current, informative, well-referenced review.

Phillips JH III, Smith SL, Storer JS: Hair loss. Common congenital and acquired causes. Postgrad Med 79(5):207, 1986.
Clinical review suggesting a perspective for the clinical practitioner. Authors state that the most frequent causes of hair loss in pediatric patients include tinea capitis, alopecia areata, traction alopecia, and trichotillomania. Most frequent causes of alopecia in the adult population include alopecia areata and hair loss associated with systemic and endocrine disorders. Primary dermatologic conditions should be distinguished.

Rebora A: Alopecia areata incognita: a hypothesis. Dermatologica 174:214, 1987.
Author proposes that the restricted zone of hair loss in alopecia areata occurs to a group of hair that is simultaneously in the early anagen VI subphase of the hair cycle. Further conclusions are drawn with pathogenetic implications for hair loss of Kligman's telogen effluvium or alopecia areata incognita.

Spencer LV, Callen JP: Hair loss in systemic disease. Dermatol Clin 5:565, 1987.
Alopecia in the adult can reflect underlying systemic processes. Telogen effluvium is preceded by severe stress usually 2 months before loss of normal club hairs. Clues to other causes of hair loss can often be found by careful histories including drug ingestion, nutritional compromise, or concurrent symptoms, particularly if they suggest genetic, endocrinologic, collagen vascular, or infectious processes.

Stroud JD: Diagnosis and management of the hair loss patient. Cutis 40:272, 1987.

Useful information written from a practicing dermatologist's view-point. Hair loss presenting to a dermatologist is more than 90% accounted for by the following disorders: telogen effluvium, alopecia areata, traction/chemical alopecia, and androgenetic alopecia. These hair diseases are discussed.

Tosti A, Colombati S, DePadova MP, et al: Retinal pigment epithelium function in alopecia areata. J Invest Dermatol 86:553, 1986.

Electroretinography (ERG) and electro-oculography (EOG) were performed in 98 patients with alopecia areata and in 40 controls to evaluate potential bioelectrical changes in retinal pigment epithelium of patients with alopecia areata. ERG was normal; however, EOG showed bioelectrical changes in the alopecia areata group. Authors suggest that melanocytes may be significant in the pathogenesis of alopecia areata.

81
Hirsutism and Hypertrichosis: Common and Uncommon Associations

The distinction between hirsutism and hypertrichosis is not always possible because of clinical overlap. Hirsutism is excessive hair growth in females in a male distribution pattern, sometimes associated with virilization. Hypertrichosis is an excessive growth of hair that is longer and coarser than normal. Hirsutism is most commonly idiopathic; other common causes of hirsutism and hypertrichosis include endocrine dysfunction, usually ovarian or adrenal, drugs, physiologic states, and congenital syndromes.

Physiologic and Congenital Causes

Idiopathic hirsutism is the most common cause of hirsutism and is often associated with a family history.[1]

Pregnancy

Precocious puberty
Menopause
Ethnic background: particularly Middle Eastern and
Mediterranean populations
Hypertrichosis lanuginosa: congenital and acquired;
acquired form associated with malignancy
Cornelia de Lange's syndrome
Hurler syndrome
Porphyria cutanea tarda

Drugs Associated with Hirsutism

Dilantin[2]
Androgen therapy
Diazoxide
Corticosteroids: ACTH
Minoxidil[3]
Phenothiazines: Mellaril[4]
Testosterone ingestion
Oral contraceptives: hirsutism is an occasional side
effect, probably associated with progestin.[5]
Diethylstilbestrol: in utero[6]
Danazol[7]

Endocrine Causes

Excessive androgen and androgen-precursor steroids
secreted by ovaries or adrenal glands are the most
common endocrine causes of hirsutism with or without virilization.

Adrenal virilizing syndromes[8-12]
  Adrenal rest tumors[13]
  Adrenal adenomas and hyperplasia[14]
  Adrenal carcinoma
  Congenital and adult adrenogenital syndromes: 21-
    hydroxylase deficiency most common[15-17]
  Cushing's syndrome
Ovarian disorders: polycystic-ovary disease and hy-
  perthecosis are the most common disorders causing
  hirsutism[18,19]
  Polycystic ovary: Stein-Leventhal syndrome with
    hirsutism, amenorrhea, ovulatory failure,
    obesity[20-23]
  Hyperthecosis: often with marked virilization[24]
  Ovarian tumors: most masculinizing tumors are
    benign.[25]
  Metastatic tumors
  Hilar-cell tumors and hyperplasia: occur in older
    women[26]
  Arrhenoblastomas[27]

Luteomas: pregnancy luteoma[28]
Pituitary tumors: acromegaly[29]

Other Endocrine Causes

Archard-Thiers' syndrome
Male pseudohermaphroditism[30]
Turner syndrome
Hypothyroidism: seen in children[31]
Hyperthyroidism: coarse hair seen over pretibial plaques
Berardinelli syndrome

Miscellaneous Associations

Anorexia nervosa[32]
Hepatoblastoma[33]
Malnutrition: primary or secondary malabsorptive conditions, severe infections
Dermatomyositis
Head injury
Viral encephalitis
Acrodynia
Malignancy: hypertrichosis lanuginosa appears to be associated with a variety of malignancies without a definite hormonal stimulus.[34–36]

References

1. Moore A, Magee F, Cunningham S, et al: Adrenal abnormalities in idiopathic hirsutism. Clin Endocrinol 18:391, 1983.
2. Livingston S, Petersen D, Boks LL: Hypertrichosis occurring in association with Dilantin therapy. J Pediatr 47:351, 1955.
3. Kaler SG, Patrinos MF, Lambert GH, et al: Hypertrichosis and congenital anomalies associated with maternal use of minoxidil. Pediatrics 79:434, 1987.
4. Phillips P, Shraberg D, Weitzel WD: Hirsutism associated with long-term phenothiazine neuroleptic therapy. JAMA 241:920, 1979.
5. Wild RA, Umstot ES, Andersen RN, et al: Adrenal function in hirsutism. II. Effect of an oral contraceptive. J Clin Endocrinol Metab 54:676, 1982.
6. Peress MR, Tsai CC, Mathur RS, et al: Hirsutism and menstrual patterns in women exposed to diethylstilbestrol in utero. Am J Obstet Gynecol 144:135, 1982.
7. Meldrum DR, Pardridge WM, Karow WG, et al: Hormonal effects of danazol and medical oophorectomy in endometriosis. Obstet Gynecol 62:480, 1983.
8. McKenna TJ, Cunningham SK, Loughlin T: The adrenal cortex and virilization. Clin Endocrinol Metab 14:997, 1985.
9. Molta L, Schwartz U: Gonadal and adrenal androgen

secretion in hirsute females. Clin Endocrinol Metab 15:229, 1986.

10. Mauvais-Jarvis P: Regulation of androgen receptor and 5 alpha-reductase in the skin of normal and hirsute women. Clin Endocrinol Metab 15:307, 1986.
11. Ebling FJ: Hair follicles and associated glands as androgen targets. Clin Endocrinol Metab 15:319, 1986.
12. London DR: The consequences of hyperandrogenism in young women. J R Soc Med 80:741, 1987.
13. Wallace EZ, Leonidas JR, Stanek AE, et al: Endocrine studies in a patient with functioning adrenal rest tumor of the liver. Am J Med 70:1122, 1981.
14. Kamilaris TC, DeBold CR, Manolas KJ, et al: Testosterone-secreting adrenal adenoma in a peripubertal girl. JAMA 258:2558, 1987.
15. Chrousos GP, Loriaux DL, Mann DL, et al: Late-onset 21-hydroxylase deficiency mimicking idiopathic hirsutism or polycystic ovarian disease. Ann Intern Med 96:143, 1982.
16. Lucky AW, Rosenfield RL, McGuire J, et al: Adrenal androgen hyperresponsiveness to adrenocorticotropin in women with acne and/or hirsutism: adrenal enzyme defects and exaggerated adrenarche. J Clin Endocrinol Metab 62:840, 1986.
17. Baskin HJ: Screening for late-onset congenital adrenal hyperplasia in hirsutism or amenorrhea. Arch Intern Med 147:847, 1987.
18. Longcope C, Robboy SJ: A 29-year-old woman with amenorrhea and hirsutism. N Engl J Med 302:621, 1980.
19. Morris DV, Adams J, Jacobs HS: The investigation of female gonadal dysfunction. Clin Endocrinol Metab 14:125, 1985.
20. Lobo RA, Goebelsmann U, Horton R: Evidence for the importance of peripheral tissue events in the development of hirsutism in polycystic ovary syndrome. J Clin Endocrinol Metab 57:393, 1983.
21. Gindoff PR, Jewelewicz R: Polycystic ovarian disease. Obstet Gynecol Clin North Am 14:931, 1987.
22. Lobo RA: Disturbances of androgen secretion and metabolism in polycystic ovary syndrome. Clin Obstet Gynaecol 12:633, 1985.
23. Pang SY, Softness B, Sweeney WJ III, New MI: Hirsutism, polycystic ovarian disease, and ovarian 17-ketosteroid reductase deficiency. N Engl J Med 316:1295, 1987.
24. Bardin CW, Lipsett MB, Edgcomb JH, et al: Studies of testosterone metabolism in a patient with masculinization due to stromal hyperthecosis. N Engl J Med 277:399, 1967.
25. Maguire HC Jr, Hanno R: Diseases of the hair. p. 1369. In Moschella SL, Hurley HJ (eds): Dermatology. 2nd Ed. WB Saunders, Philadelphia, 1985.
26. MacRae DJ, Willmott MP, Ismail AAA, et al: Androgen patterns in a case of hilar cell hyperplasia of the ovary. J Obstet Gynaecol Br Commonweath 78:741, 1971.
27. Lunde O, Djoseland O: Hirsutism caused by an androgen-producing ovarian tumor. A case of arrhenoblastoma. J Endocrinol Invest 9:513, 1986.

28. Patterson R: Hirsutism in pregnancy. Obstet Gynecol 66:738, 1985.
29. Nabarro JD: Acromegaly. Clin Endocrinol 26:481, 1987.
30. Rosen GF, Vermesh M, d'Ablaing G III, et al: The endocrinologic evaluation of a 45,X true hermaphrodite. Am J Obstet Gynecol 157:1272, 1987.
31. Stern SR, Kelnar CJ: Hypertrichosis due to primary hypothyroidism. Arch Dis Child 60:763, 1985.
32. Lacey JH: Anorexia nervosa and a bearded female saint. Br Med J 285:1816, 1982.
33. Behrle FC, Mantz FA Jr, Olson RL, et al: Virilization accompanying hepatoblastoma. Pediatrics 32:265, 1963.
34. Hovenden AL: Acquired hypertrichosis lanuginosa associated with malignancy. Arch Intern Med 147:2013, 1987.
35. Sindhuphak W, Vibhagool A: Acquired hypertrichosis lanuginosa. Int J Dermatol 21:599, 1982.
36. Jemec GB: Hypertrichosis lanuginosa acquisita. Report of a case and review of the literature. Arch Dermatol 122:805, 1986.

Selected Readings

Badawy SZ: Diagnosis and management of hirsute women. Int J Fertil 32:349, 1987.
A clinical overview of the workup of the hirsute woman with an emphasis on adrenal and ovarian evaluations.

Bergfeld WF, Redmond GP: Hirsutism. Dermatol Clin 5:501, 1987.
The evaluation of the hirsute patient is discussed from the perspective of physicians in a department of dermatology who see large numbers of tertiary referral hirsute patients. The overlap between dermatologic and endocrinologic perspectives is addressed.

Hauner H, Ditschuneit HH, Pal SB, et al: Fat distribution, endocrine and metabolic profile in obese women with and without hirsutism. Metabolism 37:281, 1988.
Twenty hirsute women were compared with 20 nonhirsute women to ascertain the relationship between adipose tissue distribution, androgen levels, and metabolic complications of obesity. This study found an upper body type of obesity and higher serum levels of testosterone in their hirsute patients compared to their nonhirsute patients.

Kvedar JC, Gibson M, Krusinski PA: Hirsutism: evaluation and treatment. J Am Acad Dermatol 12:215, 1985.
Well referenced.

Leshin M: Hirsutism. Am J Med Sci 294:369, 1987.
Current concept of the pathogenesis of hirsutism in women. Review of characteristic endocrinologic findings in patients troubled with this common problem. Well referenced.

Maguire HC Jr, Hanno R: Diseases of the hair. p. 1369. In Moschella SL, Hurley HJ (eds): Dermatology. 2nd Ed. WB Saunders, Philadelphia, 1985.
Current textbook discussion of hirsutism and other diseases of hair.

Morris DV: Hirsutism. Clin Obstet Gynaecol 12:649, 1985.
Informative, well-referenced review of current concepts of evaluation and management of hirsutism as approached by gynecologists.

A protocol of investigation, including pelvic ultrasonography, is presented.

Rittmaster RS, Loriaux DL: Hirsutism. Ann Intern Med 106:95, 1987.
State-of-the-art, well-referenced, clinical overview of hirsutism. Androgen-mediated hirsutism is often caused by dysfunctional adrenals, ovaries, or problems with conversion in peripheral tissues of precursor steroids from these organs. Adrenal causes, such as Cushing's disease, adrenal tumors, congenital adrenal hyperplasia, as well as ovarian disorders, are among diagnostic possibilities discussed. Valuable review.

Rosen GF, Kaplan B, Lobo RA: Menstrual function and hirsutism in patients with gonadal dysgenesis. Obstet Gynecol 71:677, 1988.
Thirty adult patients with gonadal dysgenesis were evaluated, and chromosome analysis revealed several karyotypes. Within this group, patients with hirsutism as their primary complaint had karyotypes of 45,X/46,XY; 45X/46X,i(Yq) and 45,X. Management is discussed.

82

Acne: Acne Vulgaris and Acne-like Eruptions

Acne vulgaris is a disorder of the pilosebaceous unit, a cosmetic plague of youth, causing comedones, nodules, pustules, and cysts, usually on the face, neck, and back of a young adult. Not all acne-like lesions are acne vulgaris; acneiform eruptions can be caused by drugs or chemicals, and acne-like diseases have been defined with distinct etiologic and therapeutic implications.

Drugs and Chemicals Causing Acneiform Eruptions

Steroids and anticonvulsants are medications commonly causing acne-like eruptions. Specific foods are not believed to cause acne.[1]

Corticosteroids (ACTH): lesions are often most prominent on the back and chest.

Oral contraceptives

Endogenous and exogenous androgenic hormones in men and women[2-6]
Halogens: iodides, bromides, chlorides, halothane
Phenobarbital
Trimethadione
Chloral hydrate
Disulfiram
Lithium carbonate[7]
Ethambutol
Ethionamide
Isoniazide
Cyanocobalamin: vitamin B_{12}
Actinomycin D: folliculitis associated

Topical Agents Producing Acneiform Eruptions

Topical corticosteroids
Coal tar derivatives
Chlorinated hydrocarbons[8]
Industrial oils[9]
Cosmetics and hair care products: particularly pomades[10,11]
Radiation therapy[12]
Sunscreen[13]
Mechanical: occlusive

Acne-Like Diseases

Adult onset acne may be secondary to endogenous androgens or androgen-receptor hypersensitivity.[14]

Acne conglobata: usually in males, nodulocystic lesions and multiple comedones found on buttocks, thighs, face, and upper arms[15]
Acne neonatorum
Infantile acne: if virilization is present, consider an underlying endocrinopathy
Tropical acne: severe form of acne vulgaris occurring in tropical climates, probably with secondary staphylococcal infection[16]
Excoriated acne: secondary lesions of acne vulgaris caused by excessive picking of the face
Rosacea: may be associated with rhinophyma in males[17]; rarely rosacea may mask carcinoma[18,19]
Perioral dermatitis[20]
Folliculitis of the beard area
Pseudofolliculitis of the beard area: foreign body reaction to ingrown hairs
Acneiform eruption of Apert syndrome[21]

Adenoma sebaceum of tuberous sclerosis: angio-fibromas[22]
Folliculitis: bacterial, pityrosporon[23,24]
Familial dyskeratotic comedones[25]
Familial acne conglobata: more widespread severe than ordinary acne conglobata[26,27]
Acne keloidalis nuchae[28]
Acne necrotica: varioliformis[29]

References

1. Rasmussen JE: Diet and acne. Int J Dermatol 16:488, 1977.
2. Held BL, Nader S, Rodriguez-Rigau LJ, et al: Acne and hyperandrogenism. J Am Acad Dermatol 10:223, 1984.
3. van der Meeren HLM, Thijssen JHH: Circulating androgens in male acne. Br J Dermatol 110:609, 1984.
4. Darley CR, Moore JW, Besser GM, et al: Androgen status in women with late onset or persistent acne vulgaris. Clin Exp Dermatol 9:28, 1984.
5. Traupe H, von Muhlendahl KE, Bramswig J, Happle R: Acne of the fulminans type following testosterone therapy in three excessively tall boys. Arch Dermatol 124:414, 1988.
6. Asscheman H, Gooren LJ, Eklund PL: Mortality and morbidity in transsexual patients with cross-gender hormone treatment. Metabolism 38:869, 1989.
7. Heng MCY: Lithium carbonate toxicity. Acneform eruption and other manifestations. Arch Dermatol 118:246, 1982.
8. Tindall JP: Chloracne and chloracnegens. J Am Acad Dermatol 13:539, 1985.
9. Farkas J: Oil acne from mineral oil among workers making prefabricated concrete panels. Contact Dermatitis 8:141, 1982.
10. Epinette WW, Greist MC, Ozols II: The role of cosmetics in postadolescent acne. Cutis 29:500, 1982.
11. Andersen KE: Testing of cosmetics and toiletries. Acta Physiol Scand (Suppl) 554:180, 1986.
12. Aversa AJ, Nagy R: Localized comedones following radiation therapy. Cutis 31:296, 1983.
13. Mills OH Jr, Kligman AM: Comedogenicity of sunscreens. Arch Dermatol 118:417, 1982.
14. Marynick SP, Chakmakjian ZH, McCaffree DL, et al: Androgen excess in cystic acne. N Engl J Med 308:981, 1983.
15. Camisa C: Squamous cell carcinoma arising in acne conglobata. Cutis 33:185, 1984.
16. Tucker SB: Occupational tropical acne. Cutis 31:79, 1983.
17. Wiemer DR: Rhinophyma. Clin Plast Surg 14:357, 1987.
18. Law TH, Jackson IT, Muller SA: Nasal septal carcinoma masquerading as acne rosacea. J Dermatol Surg Oncol 13:1021, 1987.
19. Rosen T, Stone MS: Acne rosacea in blacks. J Am Acad Dermatol 17:70, 1987.

20. Wilkinson DS, Kirton V, Wilkinson JD: Perioral dermatitis: a 12-year review. Br J Dermatol 101:245, 1979.
21. Steffen C: The acneform eruption of Apert's syndrome is not acne vulgaris. Am J Dermatopathol 6:213, 1984.
22. Cassidy SB, Pagon RA, Pepin M, et al: Family studies in tuberous sclerosis. Evaluation of apparently unaffected parents. JAMA 249:1302, 1983.
23. Ford G: Pityrosporon folliculitis. Int J Dermatol 23:320, 1984.
24. Piamphongsant T: Pustular acne. Int J Dermatol 24:441, 1985.
25. Hall JR, Holder W, Knox JM, et al: Familial dyskeratotic comedones. A report of three cases and review of the literature. J Am Acad Dermatol 17:808, 1987.
26. Quintal D, Jackson R: Aggressive squamous cell carcinoma arising in familial acne conglobata. J Am Acad Dermatol 14:207, 1986.
27. Fitzsimmons JS, Fitzsimmons EM, Gilbert G: Familial hidradenitis suppurativa: evidence in favour of single gene transmission. J Med Genet 21:281, 1984.
28. Goette DK, Berger TG: Acne keloidalis nuchae. A transepithelial elimination disorder. Int J Dermatol 26:442, 1987.
29. Kossard S, Collins A, McCrossin I: Necrotizing lymphocytic folliculitis: the early lesion of acne necrotica (varioliformis). J Am Acad Dermatol 16:1007, 1987.

Selected Readings

Bruinsma W: A Guide to Drug Eruptions. 3rd Ed. De-Zwaluw, Oosthuizem, The Netherlands, 1982.
Well-organized and easy-to-use handy reference.

Darley CR: Recent advances in hormonal aspects of acne vulgaris. Int J Dermatol 23:539, 1984.
Current concepts relating acne, hormones, and end-organ sensitivity.

Downing DT, Stewart ME, Wertz PW, Strauss JS: Essential fatty acids and acne. J Am Acad Dermatol 14:221, 1986.
Current concepts and a review of known and proposed mechanisms involving sebum secretion, hyperkeratosis of the follicular epithelium and subsequent comedone formation, with an emphasis on the role of essential fatty acids.

Eady EA, Cove JH, Blake J, et al: Recalcitrant acne vulgaris. Clinical, biochemical and microbiological investigation of patients not responding to antibiotic treatment. Br J Dermatol 118:415, 1988.
In this study, 49 of 610 patients who were considered treatment failures were compared with age and sex-matched untreated controls. The mean sebum excretion rate was significantly higher in patients with recalcitrant acne. Authors conclude that a nonmicrobiologic explanation should be considered in patients with recalcitrant acne.

Engel A, Johnson ML, Haynes SG: Health effects of sunlight exposure in the United States. Results from the first National Health and Nutrition Examination Survey, 1971–1974. Arch Dermatol 124:72, 1988.
Extensive review of dermatologic consequences of sunlight exposure, including hypomelanism, hypermelanism, seborrheic kera-

toses, senile lentigines, freckles, acne, rosacea, spider nevi, and a variety of oral and buccal mucosal lesions.

Jillson OF: Doctor, do I have acne? Cutis 34:27, 1984.
Concepts of acne from a perspective of 17 years of dermatology practice.

Lookingbill DP, Horton R, Demers LM, et al: Tissue production of androgens in women with acne. J Am Acad Dermatol 12:481, 1985.
This study supports the concept that target tissue androgen production plays a dominant hormonal role in the pathogenesis of mild and moderate acne in females.

Lucky AW: Endocrine aspects of acne. Pediatr Clin North Am 30:495, 1983.
Clinical summary of diagnostic methods available to determine whether elevated androgens underlie selected cases of acne vulgaris.

Rasmussen JE, Smith SB: Patient concepts and misconceptions about acne. Arch Dermatol 119:570, 1983.
Useful information for patient education.

Schaefer DG, Wolf JE: Common dermatologic disorders. Clin Plast Surg 14:209, 1987.
Clinical summary of the most common dermatologic disorders encountered by plastic surgeons. Helpful diagnostic features and characteristic photographs are included.

Yonkosky DM, Pochi PE; Acne vulgaris in childhood. Pathogenesis and management. Dermatol Clin 4:127, 1986.
Good general clinical review of acne, with an emphasis on acne vulgaris of mid to late childhood. Both pathogenesis and treatment are discussed.

83

Splinter Hemorrhages of the Nail Bed: Common Causes

Splinter hemorrhages are a common finding in normal and hospitalized patients. Although an occasional splinter hemorrhage is most likely due to trauma, multiple splinter hemorrhages on more than one digit, without a history of trauma, should raise the possibility of an underlying illness. Common clinical associations include infection, cardiovascular disease, vasculitis, increased capillary fragility, and immune complex diseases.[1]

Traumatic Causes

Normal population[2]
Occupational or athletic hazards[3]
Radial artery puncture
Radial artery indwelling catheter[4]
Elderly: nail trauma from walking aids is the usual cause; therefore, it is an unhelpful clue to medical illness in the elderly population[5]

Cardiovascular Disease

Endocarditis: splinter hemorrhages are of little value as an isolated finding in the diagnosis of endocarditis because fewer than 15% of patients with endocarditis have splinter hemorrhages.[6,7]
Mitral stenosis: high incidence of splinter hemorrhages in one hospital study in patients with mitral stenosis without endocarditis[8]
Hypertension
Thromboangitis obliterans[9]
Radial artery thrombosis[10]

Infectious Causes

Endocarditis
Rheumatic fever
Septicemia
Trichinosis: usually horizontal
Psittacosis[11]

Dermatologic Diseases

Psoriasis
Dermatitis
Onychomycosis: fungal nail infections
Darier's disease

Systemic Illness

Vasculitic syndromes
Rheumatoid arthritis
Collagen vascular diseases: systemic lupus erythematosus, Behçet's disease, dermatomyositis[12]
Raynaud's disease
Neoplasm
Cryoglobulinemia
Eosinophilic polymyositis[13]

Hemodialysis[14]
Peritoneal dialysis
Glomerulonephritis
Pityriasis rubra pilaris[15]: adult type I
Blood dyscrasias
Thyrotoxicosis
Drug reactions
Hepatic disease: cirrhosis
Scurvy
Peptic ulceration
Sarcoidosis
Pulmonary disease

References

1. Shearn MA: Nails and systemic disease. West J Med 129:358, 1978.
2. Robertson JC, Braune ML: Splinter hemorrhages, pitting, and other findings in fingernails of healthy adults. Br Med J 4:279, 1974.
3. Mortimer PS, Dawber RP: Trauma to the nail unit including occupational sports injuries. Dermatol Clin 3:415, 1985.
4. Tobi M, Kobrin I: Splinter hemorrhages associated with an indwelling brachial artery cannula (letter). Chest 80:767, 1981.
5. Young J, Mulley G: Splinter hemorrhages in the elderly. Age Ageing 16:101, 1987.
6. Pelletier LL Jr, Petersdorf RG: Infective endocarditis: a review of 125 cases from the University of Washington hospitals, 1963–72. Medicine 56:287, 1977.
7. Suhge-d'Aubermont PC, Honig PJ, Wood MG: Subacute bacterial endocarditis presenting with necrotic skin lesions. Int J Dermatol 22:295, 1983.
8. Kilpatrick ZM, Greenberg PA, Sanford JP: Splinter hemorrhages—their clinical significance. Arch Intern Med 115:730, 1965.
9. Quenneville JG, Prat A, Gossard D: Subungueal-splinter hemorrhage an early sign of thromboangiitis obliterans. Angiology 32:424, 1981.
10. Richards RR, Urbaniak JR: Spontaneous retrocarpal radial artery thrombosis: a report of two cases. J Hand Surg (Am) 9:823, 1984.
11. Semel JD: Cutaneous findings in a case of psittacosis. Arch Dermatol 120:1227, 1984.
12. Samitz MH: Cuticular changes in dermatomyositis. A clinical sign. Arch Dermatol 110:866, 1974.
13. Layzer RB, Shearn MA, Satya-Murti S: Eosinophilic polymyositis. Ann Neurol 1:65, 1977.
14. Blum M, Aviram A: Splinter hemorrhages in patients receiving regular hemodialysis. JAMA 239:47, 1978.
15. Sonnex TS, Dawber RP, Zachary CB, et al: The nails in adult type I pityriasis rubra pilaris. A comparison with Sezary syndrome and psoriasis. J Am Acad Dermatol 15:956, 1986.

Selected Readings

Bureau H, Baran R, Haneke E: Nail surgery and traumatic abnormalities. p.347. In Baran R, Dawber RPR (eds): Disease of the Nails and Their Management. Blackwell Scientific Publications, Oxford, 1984.
Well-referenced review of the pathophysiology and disorders associated with splinter hemorrhages.

Daniel CR III, Sams WM Jr, Scher RK: Nails in systemic disease. Dermatol Clin 3:465, 1985.
This article reviews nail signs and classifies them into findings that may signal systemic disease. Useful information for general physical diagnosis.

Gunnoe RE: Diseases of the nails. How to recognize and treat them. Postgrad Med 74(3):357, 1983.
A concise and practical discussion of color changes, nail dystrophy, and inflammation of subungual and periungual tissues.

Kabongo ML, Bedell AW: Nail signs of systemic conditions. Am Fam Physician 36(4):109, 1987.
Nail signs including color variations, swelling, abnormal blood vessels, and separation of nail plates—all potential clinical clues to underlying systemic illness—are presented for the general physician.

Samman PD: The Nails in Disease. 4th Ed. Year Book Medical Publishers, Chicago, 1986.
Good general reference.

84
Palmar Erythema: Common Associations

An exaggeration of the normal mottled erythema of the palms is a common finding in the general population. New onset palmar erythema, however, may be the first objective skin response to a systemic or local irritant.[1]

Normal
Idiopathic
Anxiety: vasomotor lability and may be associated with hyperhydrosis

Pregnancy[2]
Familial predisposition: erythema palmare hereditarium
Hepatic insufficiency[3,4]: cirrhosis, infectious and toxic hepatitis, biliary obstruction, hepatoma, hemochromatosis, and hepatic metastases
Hyperthyroidism
Rheumatoid arthritis[5]
Collagen vascular diseases: systemic lupus erythematosus, dermatomyositis, and scleroderma—fingers and nail beds may also be involved
Polycythemia
Thiamine deficiency: beriberi
Pancreatic carcinoma
Secondary syphilis: ham-colored macular lesions may be seen with scaling papular lesions.[6]
Arsenic poisoning
Drug reactions: especially with chemotherapeutic agents[7]; cytarabine,[8] doxorubicin, 5-fluorouracil,[9] methotrexate, bleomycin, mercaptopurine[10]
Food allergies
Dermatologic diseases: contact dermatitis, psoriasis, pityriasis rubra pilaris, certain genodermatoses—usually associated with other skin changes
Reflex dystrophies
Constrictive pericarditis
Chronic pulmonary disease

References

1. Domonkos AN, Arnold HL Jr, Odom RB: Erythema and urticaria. p.144. In Andrews' Diseases of the Skin. 7th Ed. WB Saunders, Philadelphia, 1982.
2. Sodhi VK, Sausker WF: Dermatoses of pregnancy. Am Fam Physician 37(1):131, 1988.
3. Bean WB: Acquired palmar erythema and cutaneous vascular "spiders." Arch Intern Med 134:846, 1974.
4. Tarao K, Sakurai A, Hayashi K, et al: The incidence of palmar erythema in patients with alcoholic fatty liver—a comparative study with fatty liver of other origins. Nippon Shokakibyo Gakkai Zasshi 83:2365, 1986.
5. Saario R, Kalliomaki JL: Palmar erythema in rheumatoid arthritis. Clin Rheumatol 4:449, 1985.
6. Drusin LM: Syphilis: clinical manifestations, diagnosis, and treatment. Urol Clin North Am 11:121, 1984.
7. Seyfer AE, Solimando DA Jr: Toxic lesions of the hand associated with chemotherapy. J Hand Surg 8:39, 1983.
8. Walker IR, Wilson WEC, Sauder DN, et al: Cytarabine-induced palmar-plantar erythema (letter). Arch Dermatol 121:1240, 1985.
9. Cantrell JE Jr, Hart RD, Taylor RF, Harvey JH Jr: Pilot trial of prolonged continuous-infusion 5-fluorouracil

and weekly cisplatin in advanced colorectal cancer. Cancer Treat Rep 71:615, 1987.
10. Cox GJ, Robertson DB: Toxic erythema of palms and soles associated with high-dose mercaptopurine chemotherapy. Arch Dermatol 122:1413, 1986.

Selected Readings

Domonkos AN, Arnold HL Jr, Odom RB: Erythema and urticaria. p.144. In Andrews' Diseases of the Skin. 7th Ed. WB Saunders, Philadephia, 1982.
A good discussion of the pathophysiology of hyperemia, with a description of patterns and causes of focal and generalized erythema.

King LE Jr, Dufresne RG Jr, Lovett GL, Rosin MA: Erythroderma: review of 82 cases. South Med J 79:1210, 1986.
Clinical, laboratory, and biopsy material of 82 cases of erythroderma provide informative data. Diseases most commonly associated with erythroderma included drug eruptions, preexisting dermatoses, and lymphoreticular neoplasms, particularly cutaneous T-cell lymphoma.

Rapini RP: Dermatologic emergencies. Am Fam Physician 34 (5):159, 1986.
Clinical review of dermatologic emergencies covering blistering diseases, exfoliative erythroderma, reactive erythemas, and other dermatologic manifestations seen in the emergency setting. Practical clinical concepts.

85
Transient Erythema (Flushing): Causes and Associated Disorders

Transient erythema, also called flushing, is a visible manifestation of vasodilation and may be caused by a number of physiologic and pharmacologic reactions. It appears usually on the face, but may include other areas, such as the neck, chest, and abdomen. If initial evaluation excludes purely emotional factors, ethnic predilection, association with alcohol ingestion, medications, menopausal or postoophorectomy state, angioedema, cold urticaria, and rosacea, a search for more obscure causes is warranted.

Anatomic Causes of Flushing

Mesenteric traction[1]

Rovsing syndrome[2]: flushing since an early age, relieved by anteflexed posture; nausea and abdominal pain, in patients with a horseshoe kidney

Physiologic, Endogenous, and Hormonal Flushing

Emotional

Postmenopausal: brought on by hot foods, alcohol, emotional upsets, or warm room[3]

Postoophorectomy

Hereditary vibratory angioedema[4]: may have flushes with episodes of vibratory angioedema

Cold urticaria: may have flushing and nausea after prolonged generalized cold exposure

Thermal induced: commonly associated with rosacea, fever flush, and with hot liquids

Diabetes: facial redness

Histamine[5]

Prostaglandin E1,[6] D2, F2 alpha, and I2

Substance P[7]

Postorchidectomy: postorchidectomy testicular failure may be associated with vascular disturbances analogous to menopausal hot flashes.[8]

Enkephalin and enkephalin analogs

Vasoactive intestinal polypeptide (VIP)[9,10]

Growth hormone-releasing factor[11]

Calcitonin: postulated[12-14]

Leutenizing hormone secretion

Pituitary insufficiency[15]

Alcohol-Induced Flushing

This is perhaps the most common type and may be due to alcohol alone or due to alcohol in conjunction with a chemical. The cause is thought to be elevated acetaldehyde levels. Alcohol may precipitate flushing in patients with other causes of flushing, i.e., tumors, medications, menopause.[16,17]

Alcohol alone: especially seen in Asians[18]; may also have increased heart rate, cardiac output, rate and depth of respiration, and decreased blood pressure. Certain fermented alcoholic beverages, e.g., beer and sherry, contain large amounts of histamine and may cause flushing independent of ethnic background.

Alcohol and chemicals: trichloroethylene, carbon disulfide, dimethylformamide, xylene, cyanamide, thiuram derivatives, N-butyraldoxine, and certain chemicals in mushrooms

Alcohol and medications: disulfiram, calcium carbimide, phentolamine, griseofulvin, metronidazole, quinacrine, antidiabetic drugs (chlorpropamide),[19] cephalosporins, furazolidone, benadryl

Alcohol and neoplasia: carcinoid, mastocytosis, medullary carcinoma of thyroid, lymphoid tumors

Toxic or Drug-Induced Flushing

Mahimahi: scombroid fish poisoning[20,21]

Chlorpropamide: with and without alcohol

Nicotinic acid and derivatives: perhaps via prostaglandins[22]

Histamine and histamine-releasing drugs: morphine, meperidine, some muscle relaxants, compound 48/80, polymixin B

Monosodium glutamate: postulated cause of Chinese restaurant syndrome[23]

Mithramycin: seen in 35% of patients; begins as erythema and skin becomes coarser with time

Vancomycin[24]

Sorbic acid[25]

Calcium channel blockers[26]

Neoplasia Causes of Flushing

Amine precursor uptake decarboxylation (APUD) tumors

Carcinoid: syndrome usually includes flushing, diarrhea, tachycardia, and hypotension. Associated with elevated urinary 5-hydroxyindole acetic acid (5-HIAA)[27,28]

Other APUD tumors: pheochromocytoma,[29] pancreatic tumors with Zollinger-Ellison syndrome, medullary carcinoma of thyroid,[30,31] bronchogenic carcinoma; mediators vary

Malignant histiocytoma, neuroblastoma, ganglioneuroma (VIP may be mediator)

Mastocytosis[32,33]: syndrome usually includes flushing, diarrhea, tachycardia, and hypotension; associated with elevated histamine in blood and urine

Basophilic chronic granulocytic leukemia (via histamine)[34]

Renal cell carcinoma[35]

Neurologic and Miscellaneous Conditions with Facial Flushing as a Symptom

Familial dysautonomia: Riley-Day syndrome[36]
Ciliary neuralgia: unilateral paroxysmal headaches with lacrimation, nasal congestion, and unilateral flushing
Sphenopalatine syndrome
Autonomic epilepsy[37]
Hypertensive diencephalic syndrome
Hypertension: paroxysmal hypertension after brain surgery; autonomic hyperreflexia[38]
Brain stem stroke: paroxysmal facial flushing, paroxysmal hypertension, and diaphoresis can occur after brain stem injury or spinal cord lesions above the level of sympathetic outflow.[39]

Dermatologic Disorders

Rosacea[40,41]

References

1. Seltzer JL, Ritter DE, Starsnic MA, et al: The hemodynamic response to traction on the abdominal mesentery. Anesthesiology 63:96, 1985.
2. Kissane JM: Urinary system. p. 581. In Kissane JM (ed): Pathology of Infancy and Childhood. 2nd Ed. CV Mosby, St. Louis, 1975.
3. Tulandi T, Lal S, Guyda H: Effect of estrogen on the growth hormone response to the alpha-adrenergic agonist clonidine in women with menopausal flushing. J Clin Endocrinol Metab 65:6, 1987.
4. Metzger WJ, Kaplan AP, Beaven MA, et al: Hereditary vibratory angioedema: confirmation of histamine release in a type of physical hypersensitivity. J Allergy Clin Immunol 57:605, 1976.
5. Kaliner M, Shelhamer JH, Ottesen EA: Effects of infused histamine: correlation of plasma histamine levels and symptoms. J Allergy Clin Immunol 69:283, 1982.
6. Phillips WS, Lightman SL: Is cutaneous flushing prostaglandin mediated? Lancet 1:754, 1981.
7. Schaffalitzky De Muckadell OB, Aggestrup S, Stentoft P: Flushing and plasma substance P concentration during infusion of synthetic substance P in normal man. Scand J Gastroenterol 21:498, 1986.
8. Ginsburg J, O'Reilly B: Climacteric flushing in a man. Br Med J 287:262, 1983.
9. Kane MG, O'Dorisio TM, Krejs GJ: Production of secretory diarrhea by intravenous infusion of vasoactive intestinal polypeptide. N Engl J Med 309:1482, 1983.
10. Frase LL, Gaffney FA, Lane LD, et al: Cardiovascular effects of vasoactive intestinal peptide in healthy subjects. Am J Cardiol 60:1356, 1987.
11. Gelato MC, Pescovitz O, Cassorla F, et al: Effects of a growth hormone releasing factor in man. J Clin Endocrinol Metab 57:674, 1983.

12. Cunliffe WJ, Black MM, Hall R, et al: A calcitonin-secreting thyroid carcinoma. Lancet 2:63, 1968.
13. Brain SD, Tipins JR, Morris HR, et al: Potent vasodilator activity of calcitonin gene-related peptide in human skin. J Invest Dermatol 87:533, 1986.
14. Howden CW, Logue C, Gavin K, et al: Hemodynamic effects of intravenous human calcitonin-gene-related peptide in man. Clin Sci 74:413, 1988.
15. Meldrum DR, Erlik Y, Lu JKH, et al: Objectively recorded hot flushes in patients with pituitary insufficiency. J Clin Endocrinol Metab 52:684, 1981.
16. Mooney E: The flushing patient. Int J Dermatol 24:549, 1985.
17. Wilkin JK: Quantitative assessment of alcohol-provoked flushing. Arch Dermatol 122:63, 1986.
18. Goedde HW, Agarwal DP: Polymorphism of aldehyde dehydrogenase and alcohol sensitivity. Enzyme 37:29, 1987.
19. Hoskins PJ, Wiles PG, Volkmann HP, Pyke DA: Chlorpropamide alcohol flushing: a normal response? Clin Sci 73:77, 1987.
20. Kim R: Flushing syndrome due to mahimahi (scombroid fish) poisoning. Arch Dermatol 115:963, 1979.
21. Bartholomew BA, Berry PR, Rodhouse JC, et al: Scombrotoxic fish poisoning in Britain: features of over 250 suspected incidents from 1976 to 1986. Epidemiol Infect 99:775, 1987.
22. Knodel LC, Talbert RL: Adverse effects of hypolipidemic drugs. Med Toxicol 2:10, 1987.
23. Wilkin JK: Does monosodium glutamate cause flushing (or merely "glutamania")? J Am Acad Dermatol 15:225, 1986.
24. Southorn PA, Plevak DJ, Wright AJ, Wilson WR: Adverse effects of vancomycin administered in the perioperative period. Mayo Clin Proc 61:721, 1986.
25. Soschin D, Leyden JJ: Sorbic acid-induced erythema and edema. J Am Acad Dermatol 14:234, 1986.
26. Russell RP: Side effects of calcium channel blockers. Hypertension 11:1142, 1988.
27. Lucas KJ, Feldman JM: Flushing in the carcinoid syndrome and plasma kallikrein. Cancer 58:2290, 1986.
28. Norheim I, Oberg K, Theodorsson-Norheim E, et al: Malignant carcinoid tumors. An analysis of 103 patients with regard to tumor localization, hormone production, and survival. Ann Surg 206:115, 1987.
29. Case records of the Massachusetts General Hospital. Weekly clinicopathological exercises. Case 6-1986. A 34 year-old man with hypertension and episodes of flushing, nausea, and vomiting. N Engl J Med 314:431, 1986.
30. Hollenberg CH: Medullary carcinoma of the thyroid. Arch Otolaryngol 109:103, 1983.
31. Jerkins TW, Sacks HS, O'Dorisio TM, et al: Medullary carcinoma of the thyroid, pancreatic nesidioblastosis and microadenosis, and pancreatic polypeptide hypersecretion: a new association and clinical and hormonal responses to long-acting somatostatin analog SMS 201-995. J Clin Endocrinol Metab 64:1313, 1987.
32. Korenblat PE, Wedner HJ, Whyte MP, et al: Systemic mastocytosis. Arch Intern Med 144:2249, 1984.

33. Kirshenbaum AS, Kettelhut BV, Metcalfe DD, Garriga MM: Mastocytosis in infants and children: recognition of patterns of skin disease. Allergy Proc 10:17, 1989.
34. Rosenthal S, Schwartz JH, Canellos GP: Basophilic chronic granulocytic leukaemia with hyperhistaminemia. Br J Haematol 36:367, 1977.
35. Plaksin J, Landau Z, Coslovsky R: A carcinoid-like syndrome caused by a prostaglandin-secreting renal cell carcinoma. Arch Intern Med 140:1095, 1980.
36. Cunliffe WJ: The skin and the nervous system. p. 2016. In Rook A, Wilkinson DS, Ebling FJG (eds): Textbook of Dermatology. 3rd Ed. Blackwell Scientific Publications, London, 1979.
37. Metz SA, Halter JB, Porte D Jr, et al: Autonomic epilepsy: clonidine blockage of paroxysmal catecholamine release and flushing. Ann Intern Med 88:189, 1978.
38. Sandel ME, Abrams PL, Horn LJ: Hypertension after brain injury: case report. Arch Phys Med Rehabil 67:469, 1986.
39. Gandhavadi B: Hypertension after brainstem stroke. Arch Phys Med Rehabil 69:130, 1988.
40. Wilkin JK: Epigastric rosacea. Arch Dermatol 116:584, 1980.
41. Guarrera M, Parodi A, Cipriani C, et al: Flushing in rosacea: a possible mechanism. Arch Dermatol Res 272:311, 1982.

Selected Readings

Drummond PD, Lance JW: Facial flushing and sweating mediated by the sympathetic nervous system. Brain 110:793, 1987.

Sweating and facial flushing in response to body heating, embarrassment, and gustatory stimulation were investigated in 23 patients with unilateral lesions in the sympathetic pathway to the face. Authors conclude that cervical sympathetic outflow is the main pathway for thermoregulatory flushing and emotional blushing. Interesting data and projections regarding the pathophysiology of flushing and blushing.

Mooney E: The flushing patient. Int J Dermatol 24:549, 1985.

Informative current clinical review incorporating differential diagnosis, pathophysiology, and a literature review of the many causes of flushing.

Vinik AI, Strodel WE, Eckhauser FE, et al: Somatostatinomas, PPomas, neurotensinomas. Semin Oncol 14:263, 1987.

A review of the tumor syndromes that occur with overproduction of certain peptide hormones. The possibility of a neurotensin-secreting tumor should be considered in patients with edema, hypotension, cyanosis, and flushing.

Wilkin JK: Flushing reactions: consequences and mechanisms. Ann Intern Med 95:468, 1981.

Extensively referenced review of the subject, with an excellent discussion of the mechanisms of flushing.

86

Hypopigmented Macules (White Spots): Congenital and Acquired Causes

Less common than hyperpigmented macules, hypopigmented macules can be congenital or acquired and provide the earliest clues to disease in other organ systems or represent an end stage of epidermal injury by physical, chemical, infectious, or inflammatory events.

Localized or Patterned Hypomelanosis Due to Genetic and Nevoid Factors

X-linked ocular albinism: reduced ocular pigment and hypomelanotic macules

Congenital leukoderma: partial albinism, piebaldism associated with a white forelock[1]

Waardenburg's syndrome: increased interpupillary distance, white forelock, hypertrophy of nasal root, and hyperplastic eyebrows; may also have deafness

Ziprkowski-Margolis syndrome[2]: congenital patterned leukoderma and deafness

Xeroderma pigmentosum: 1 to 5 mm hypopigmented macules in 45%[3]

Ataxia telangiectasia: congenital, stable hypomelanotic macules in about 30%[4]

Hypopigmented macules of tuberous sclerosis: "ash leaf macules"[5-8]

Nevus depigmentosus

Incontinentia pigmenti achromians (Ito) with ectodermal and central nervous system abnormalities[9-12]

Vitiligo (localized and generalized): associated with autoimmune disorders, thyroiditis, pernicious anemia, Addison's disease, diabetes mellitus, alopecia areata, morphea, halo nevus, and melanoma

Nevus anemicus: pale, but not hypomelanotic[13,14]

Dyschromatosis symmetrica hereditaria: pigmented and hypopigmented spots on the extremities[15]

Chemical, Physical, and Environmental Causes[16]	Monobenzyl ether of hydroquinone
	P-tertiary butyl phenol
	P-tertiary amyl phenol
	Cinnamic aldehyde[17]
	Arsenic
	Sulfhydryl compounds
	4-Isopropylcatechol
	Butylated hydroxytoluene
	Corticosteroids: tape or intralesional
	Burns: thermal, ultraviolet, ionizing
	Trauma: dermabrasion[18]
	Liquid nitrogen
	Chloroquine sulfate[19]

Postinflammatory and Infectious Causes

Postinflammatory: eczema, psoriasis, pityriasis lichenoides chronica, scarring discoid lupus erythematosus, actinic reticuloid, atrophic lichen planus, lichen sclerosus et atrophicus, atopic dermatitis, postexanthem
Pityriasis alba
Morphea, scleroderma: vitiligo-like macules[20]
Sarcoidosis[21,22]
Vagabond's leukoderma: Hypopigmentation and hyperpigmentation of skin in older ill-kempt men with poor nutrition, poor hygiene, and chronic alcohol abuse
Tinea versicolor
Pinta, syphilis, yaws
Lupus vulgaris
Leprosy
Post-kala-azar: geographic maplike appearance with chronic untreated kala-azar
Onchocerciasis: leopard appearance, late feature

Neoplastic Causes

Halo nevus
Melanoma: hypopigmentation may be associated with a better prognosis in malignant melanoma[23,24]
Mycosis fungoides: hypopigmentation and hyperpigmentation are reported.[25–29]

Miscellaneous or Idiopathic Causes

Leukoderma punctata: possible relationship among idiopathic guttate hypomelanosis, leukoderma punctata, and vitiligo[30]
Vogt-Koyanagi syndrome: vitiligo, poliosis, alopecia, uveitis, and deafness after a febrile illness

Idiopathic guttate hypomelanosis[31]
Alezzandrini's syndrome: facial vitiligo, poliosis, deafness, and unilateral tapetoretinal degeneration

References

1. Hayashibe K, Mishima Y: Tyrosinase-positive melanocyte distribution and induction of pigmentation in human piebald skin. Arch Dermatol 124:381, 1988.
2. Ziprkowski L, Krakowski A, Adam A, et al: Partial albinism and deaf mutism. Arch Dermatol 86:530, 1962.
3. Nishigori C, Miyachi Y, Takebe H, Imamura S: A case of xeroderma pigmentosum with clinical appearance of dyschromatosis symmetrica hereditaria. Pediatr Dermatol 3:410, 1986.
4. Cohen LE, Tanner DJ, Schaefer HG, Levis WR: Common and uncommon cutaneous findings in patients with ataxia-telangiectasia. J Am Acad Dermatol 10:431, 1984.
5. Hurwitz S, Braverman IM: White spots in tuberous sclerosis. J Pediatr 77:587, 1970.
6. Wiederholt WC, Gomez MR, Kurland LT: Incidence and prevalence of tuberous sclerosis in Rochester, Minnesota, 1950 through 1982. Neurology 35:600, 1985.
7. Oppenheimer EY, Rosman NP, Dooling EC: The late appearance of hypopigmented maculae in tuberous sclerosis. Am J Dis Child 139:408, 1985.
8. Hausser I, Anton-Lamprecht I: Electron microscopy as a means for carrier detection and genetic counselling in families at risk of tuberous sclerosis. Hum Genet 76:73, 1987.
9. Takematsu H, Sato S, Igarashi M, et al: Incontinentia pigmenti achromians (Ito). Arch Dermatol 119:391, 1983.
10. Fleury P, Dingemans K, de Groot WP, et al: Ito's hypomelanosis (incontinentia pigmenti achromians). A review of four cases. Clin Neurol Neurosurg 88:39, 1986.
11. Turleau C, Taillard F, Doussau de Bazignan M, et al: Hypomelanosis of Ito (incontinentia pigmenti achromians) and mosaicism for a microdeletion of 15q1. Hum Genet 74:185, 1986.
12. Bartholomew DW, Jabs EW, Levin LS, Ribovich R: Single maxillary central incisor and coloboma in hypomelanosis of Ito. Clin Genet 31:370, 1987.
13. Fleisher TL, Zeligman I: Nevus anemicus. Arch Dermatol 100:750, 1969.
14. Mountcastle EA, Diestelmeier MR, Lupton GP: Nevus anemicus. J Am Acad Dermatol 14:628, 1986.
15. Hata S, Yokomi I: Density of dopa-positive melanocytes in dyschromatosis symmetrica hereditaria. Dermatologica 171:27, 1985.
16. Mosher DB, Fitzpatrick TB, Ortonne JP, Hori Y: Disorders of pigmentation. p. 794. In Fitzpatrick TB, Eisen AZ, Wolff K, et al (eds): Dermatology in General Medicine. McGraw-Hill, New York, 1986.
17. Mathias CGT, Maibach HI, Conant MA: Perioral leukoderma simulating vitiligo from use of a toothpaste

containing cinnamic aldehyde. Arch Dermatol 116: 1172, 1980.

18. Ship AG, Weiss PR: Pigmentation after dermabrasion: an avoidable complication. Plast Reconstr Surg 75:528, 1985.

19. Dupre A, Ortonne JP, Viraben R, Arfeux F: Chloroquine-induced hypopigmentation of hair and freckles. Association with congenital renal failure. Arch Dermatol 121:1164, 1985.

20. Sanchez JL, Vazquez M, Sanchez NP: Vitiligolike macules in systemic scleroderma. Arch Dermatol 119:129, 1983.

21. Hubler WR Jr: Hypomelanotic canopy of sarcoidosis. Cutis 19:86, 1977.

22. Mitchell IC, Sweatman MC, Rustin MH, Wilson R: Ulcerative and hypopigmented sarcoidosis. J Am Acad Dermatol 15:1062, 1986.

23. Nordlund JJ: Hypopigmentation, vitiligo, and melanoma. New data, more enigmas. Arch Dermatol 123:1005, 1987.

24. Bystryn JC, Rigel D, Friedman RJ, Kopf A: Prognostic significance of hypopigmentation in malignant melanoma. Arch Dermatol 123:1053, 1987.

25. Zackheim HS, Epstein EH Jr, Grekin DA, et al: Mycosis fungoides presenting as areas of hypopigmentation. J Am Acad Dermatol 6:340, 1982.

26. Goldberg DJ, Schinella RS, Kechijian P: Hypopigmented mycosis fungoides. Speculations about the mechanism of hypopigmentation. Am J Dermatopathol 8:326, 1986.

27. David M, Shanon A, Hazaz B, Sandbank M: Diffuse, progressive hyperpigmentation: an unusual skin manifestation of mycosis fungoides. J Am Acad Dermatol 16:257, 1987.

28. Rustin MH, Griffiths M, Ridley CM: The immunopathology of hypopigmented mycosis fungoides. Clin Exp Dermatol 11:332, 1986.

29. Misch KJ, Maclennan KA, Marsden RA: Hypopigmented mycosis fungoides. Clin Exp Dermatol 12:53, 1987.

30. Falabella R, Escobar CE, Carrascal E, Arroyave JA: Leukoderma punctata. J Am Acad Dermatol 18:485, 1988.

31. Falabella R, Escobar C, Giraldo N, et al: On the pathogenesis of idiopathic guttate hypomelanosis. J Am Acad Dermatol 16:35, 1987.

Selected Readings

Alper JC: The genodermatoses and their significance in pediatric dermatology. Dermatol Clin 4:45, 1986.

Six genetic disorders, related genetic principles, and their major cutaneous manifestations are reviewed: neurofibromatosis, tuberous sclerosis, xeroderma pigmentosum, incontinentia pigmenti, incontinentia pigmenti achromians, and Down syndrome. Genetic counseling is discussed.

Cowan CL Jr, Halder RM, Grimes PE, et al: Ocular disturbances in vitiligo. J Am Acad Dermatol 15:17, 1986.

This article documents ocular findings in patients with vitiligo;

however, ocular inflammation (uveitis, as reported by others) was not a prominent feature.

Goldman L, Moraites RS, Kitzmiller KW: White spots in biblical times. Arch Dermatol 93:744, 1966.
Interesting discussion of biblical references to a variety of skin disorders characterized by white spots, loosely translated by many scholars as leprosy.

Klein LE, Nordlund JJ: Genetic basis of pigmentation and its disorders. Int J Dermatol 20:621, 1981.
Complete review of the topic from embryogenesis and physiology to clinical expressions of pigment disorders. The thrust of the review is biology of the melanocyte.

Lucky PA, Nordlund JJ: The biology of the pigmentary system and its disorders. Dermatol Clin 3:197, 1985.
Information review of current concepts of melanin biology and abnormalities and diseases affecting pigmentation. Diseases presenting with hyperpigmentation and hypopigmentation are discussed.

Vici CD, Sabetta G, Gambarara M, et al: Agenesis of the corpus callosum, combined immunodeficiency, bilateral cataract, and hypopigmentation in two brothers. Am J Med Genet 29:1, 1988.
Case report of two brothers with a malformation syndrome consisting of agenesis of the corpus callosum, cutaneous hypopigmentation, bilateral cataracts, and immunodeficiency. Authors suggest that the clinical and pathologic findings indicate a pathogenetic mechanism involving the embryonic organization of the central nervous system as well as the immune system.

Witkop CJ Jr: Inherited disorders of pigmentation. Clin Dermatol 3:70, 1985.
A clinical summary of basic clinical skills needed to diagnose and manage most commonly and some uncommonly encountered inherited disorders of pigmentation.

87

Hyperpigmented Macules (Brown Spots): Congenital and Acquired Causes

Disorders of hyperpigmentation are multiple. Most are due to increased numbers of melanocytes or increased melanin pigment in the skin, but other substances or chemicals deposited in the skin may impart a "pigmented" appearance. Hyperpigmented macules are frequently congenital and are associated with other cutaneous or systemic abnormalities. They may also be acquired and associated with environmental factors, inflammatory skin conditions, and hormonal, chemical, or neoplastic conditions.

Circumscribed Hyperpigmentation Due to Genetic and Nevoid Factors	Café-au-lait macules: prominent in neurofibromatosis,[1] Albright's syndrome, and Watson's syndrome. Also found in Russell-Silver dwarfism, multiple lentigines syndrome,[2] ataxia telangiectasia,[3,4] tuberous sclerosis, Westerhoff's syndrome, Leschke's disease, Cowden's disease, basal cell nevus syndrome, epidermal nevus,[5] Gaucher's syndrome, Hunter syndrome, and Turner syndrome[5]

Nevocellular nevi: NAME syndrome,[6] LAMB syndrome[7]

Dermal melanocytosis: nevus of Ota, nevus of Ito, mongolian spot, blue nevus

Lentigines: lentigo simplex, lentiginosis perigenito axillaris, lentiginous mosaicism, centrofacial lentiginosis, periorificial lentiginosis (Peutz-Jeghers syndrome), lentiginosis profusa (LEOPARD syndrome)[8]

Freckles: ephelides

Nevus spilus

Becker's nevus[9,10]

Seborrheic keratosis: flat

Dyschromatosis universalis

Incontinentia pigmenti and clinical variants[11,12]:
Ment, Alimurung, Greither-Haensch
Freckle-like macules: neurofibromatosis, progeria,
Moynahan syndrome
Reticulate pigmentation syndromes
Acral pigmentation syndromes
Periorbital pigmentation[13]
Macular amyloidosis
Pachyonychia congenita: hyperpigmentation resembles macular amyloidosis around the neck and back.[14]

Localized Hypermelanosis Due to Environmental and Postinflammatory Causes

Postinflammatory: almost any inflammatory eruption may hyperpigment, especially in highly pigmented individuals. Hyperpigmentation is prominent in diabetic dermopathy, statis dermatitis, pigmented purpuric eruptions,[15,16] and graft-versus-host disease.[17]
Fixed drug eruption[18-20]
Erythema dyschromicum perstans: blue to gray-brown color[21]
Morphea: atrophoderma of Pasini and Pierini
Tar melanosis: pigmented cosmetic dermatitis
Phytophotodermatitis (plant photocontact dermatitis)[22]: parsnips, wild carrot, bergamot orange, lime, figs, gas plant, celery,[23] and perfumes containing oil of bergamot
PUVA-induced lentigines: psoralens, topical or systemic plus UVA
Coin rubbing,[24] cupping: ecchymotic initially, then possibly hyperpigmented
Thermal injury: heat, liquid nitrogen
Ionizing radiation[25]
Laser[26,27]
Erythem ab igne
Lentigo senilis
Earwig pigment[28]
Atopic dermatitis: ripple pigmentation of the neck may mimic macular amyloidosis[29]

Hormonal or Neoplastic Causes of Localized Hyperpigmentation

Melasma: oral contraceptives, pregnancy, idiopathic
Acanthosis nigricans: some cases show hypermelanosis
Melanoma in situ[30]
Brain tumors: melasma-like pigmentation[31]
Carcinoid: with increased ACTH levels[32]

Infectious Causes	Tinea versicolor[33] Pinta

Circumscribed Hyperpigmentation Due to Chemicals, Drugs or Systemic Cause

Hydantoin derivatives: melasma-like
Bleomycin: flagellate and linear[34]
Nitrosoureas: sites of application
Doxorubicin: palmar, plantar, nail[35]
5-Fluorouracil: sun-exposed sites, radiation portal, sites and overlying IV injection sites[36-38]
Cyclophosphamide: localized or widespread
Antimalarials: especially pretibial surfaces
Arsenic: guttate[39]
Triazinate: caused acanthosis nigricans-like picture in patients with brain tumor[40]
PUVA-induced lentigines[41,42]: psoralen[43] and UVA
Cronkhite-Canada syndrome: lentigo-like macules with multiple intestinal polyps[44]
Fanconi's anemia[45]
Nitroglycerin[46]
Quinidine[47]

Localized Non-melanotic Hyperpigmentation

Tattoos
Minocycline-induced macular hyperpigmentation[48,49]
Gold: especially periorbitally and at injection sites[50,51]
Ochronosis: circumscribed or diffuse
Acanthosis nigricans
Laugier-Hunziker syndrome[52]

References

1. Ishida O, Jimbow K: A computed image analyzing system for quantitation of melanocyte morphology in café-au-lait macules of neurofibromatosis. J Invest Dermatol 88:287, 1987.
2. Ortonne JP, Brocard E, Floret D, et al: Valeur diagnostique des taches café-au-lait (T.C.L.). Ann Dermatol Venereol 107:313, 1980.
3. Cohen LE, Tanner DJ, Schaefer HG, Levis WR: Common and uncommon cutaneous findings in patients with ataxia telangiectasia. J Am Acad Dermatol 10:431, 1984.
4. Tsukahara M, Masuda M, Ohshiro K, et al: Ataxia telangiectasia with generalized skin pigmentation and early death. Eur J Pediatr 145:121, 1986.
5. Rogers M, McCrossin I, Commens C: Epidermal nevi and the epidermal nevus syndrome. A review of 131 cases. J Am Acad Dermatol 20:476, 1989.
6. Atherton DJ, Pitcher DW, Wells RS, et al: A syndrome of various cutaneous pigmented lesions, myxoid neu-

rofibromata and atrial myxoma: the NAME syndrome. Br J Dermatol 103:421, 1980.

7. Rhodes AR, Silverman RA, Harrist TJ, et al: Mucocutaneous lentigines, cardiomucocutaneous myxomas, and multiple blue nevi: the "LAMB" syndrome. J Am Acad Dermatol 10:72, 1984.
8. Gorlin RJ, Anderson RC, Blaw M: Multiple lentigenes syndrome. Am J Dis Child 117:652, 1969.
9. Person JR, Longcope C: Becker's nevus: an androgen-mediated hyperplasia with increased androgen receptors. J Am Acad Dermatol 10:235, 1984.
10. Slifman NR, Harrist TJ, Rhodes AR: Congenital arrector pili hamartoma. A case report and review of the spectrum of Becker's melanosis and pilar smooth-muscle hamartoma. Arch Dermatol 121:1034, 1985.
11. Kegel MF: Dominant disorders with multiple organ involvement. Dermatol Clin 5:205, 1987.
12. Cohen BA: Incontinentia pigmenti. Neurol Clin 5:361, 1987.
13. Haddock N, Wilkin JK: Periorbital hyperpigmentation (letter). JAMA 246:835, 1981.
14. Tidman MJ, Wells RS, MacDonald DM: Pachyonychia congenita with cutaneous amyloidosis and hyperpigmentation—a distinct variant. J Am Acad Dermatol 16:935, 1987.
15. Newton RC, Raimer SS: Pigmented purpuric eruptions. Dermatol Clin 3:165, 1985.
16. Solomon AR Jr: The histologic spectrum of the reactive inflammatory vascular dermatoses. Dermatol Clin 3:171, 1985.
17. Basuk PJ, Scher RK: Onychomycosis in graft versus host disease. Cutis 40:237, 1987.
18. Masu S, Seiji M: Pigmentary incontinence in fixed drug eruptions. Histologic and electron microscopic findings. J Am Acad Dermatol 8:525, 1983.
19. Westerhof W, Wolters EC, Brookbakker JT, et al: Pigmented lesions of the tongue in heroin addicts—fixed drug eruption. Br J Dermatol 109:605, 1983.
20. Goolamali SK: Drug eruptions. Postgrad Med J 61:925, 1985.
21. Person JR, Rogers RS III: Ashy dermatosis. An apoptotic disease? Arch Dermatol 117:701, 1981.
22. Pathak MA: Phytophotodermatitis. Clin Dermatol 4:102, 1986.
23. Berkley SF, Hightower AW, Beier RC, et al: Dermatitis in grocery workers associated with high natural concentrations of furanocoumarins in celery. Ann Intern Med 105:351, 1986.
24. Yeatman GW: Cao Gio (coin rubbing). Vietnamese attitudes toward health care. JAMA 244:2748, 1980.
25. Fitzpatrick TB: Ultraviolet-induced pigmentary changes: benefits and hazards. Curr Probl Dermatol 15:25, 1986.
26. Wheeland RG, Walker NP: Lasers—25 years later. Int J Dermatol 25:209, 1986.
27. Bonafe JL, Laffitte F, Chavoin JP, et al: Hyperpigmentation induced by argon laser therapy of hemangiomas. Optical and electron microscope studies. Dermatologica 170:225, 1985.
28. Potter AR: An unusual case of non-malignant skin hyperpigmentation. Br Med J 2:1628, 1979.

29. Manabe T, Inagaki Y, Nakagawa S, et al: Ripple pigmentation of the neck in atopic dermatitis. Am J Dermatopathol 9:301, 1987.
30. Steiner A, Pehamberger H, Wolff K: In vivo epiluminescence microscopy of pigmented skin lesions. II. Diagnosis of small pigmented skin lesions and early detection of malignant melanoma. J Am Acad Dermatol 17:584, 1987.
31. Andreev VC, Petkov I: Skin manifestations associated with tumors of the brain. Br J Dermatol 92:675, 1975.
32. Rodriguez-Vaca MD, Angel M, Halperin I, et al: Diagnosis of lung carcinoid with cutaneous hyperpigmentation eight years after bilateral adrenalectomy. J Endocrinol Invest 10:537, 1987.
33. Allen HB, Charles CR, Johnson BL: Hyperpigmented tinea versicolor. Arch Dermatol 112:1110, 1976.
34. Fernandez-Obregon AC, Hogan KP, Bibro MK: Flagellate pigmentation from intrapleural bleomycin. A light microscopy and electron microscopy study. J Am Acad Dermatol 13:464, 1985.
35. Kelly TM, Fishman LM, Lessner HE: Hyperpigmentation with daunorubicin therapy. Arch Dermatol 120:262, 1984.
36. Baran R, Laugier P: Melanonychia induced by topical 5-fluorouracil. Br J Dermatol 112:621, 1985.
37. Hood AF: Cutaneous side effects of cancer chemotherapy. Med Clin North Am 70:187, 1986.
38. Seyfer AE, Solimando DA Jr: Toxic lesions of the hand associated with chemotherapy. J Hand Surg (Am) 8:39, 1983.
39. Granstein RD, Sober AJ: Drug- and heavy metal-induced hyperpigmentation. J Am Acad Dermatol 5:1, 1981.
40. Greenspan AH, Shupack JL, Foo SH, et al: Acanthosis nigricans-like hyperpigmentation secondary to triazinate therapy. Arch Dermatol 121:232, 1985.
41. Bruce DR, Berger TG: PUVA-induced pigmented macules: a case involving palmoplantar skin. J Am Acad Dermatol 16:1087, 1987.
42. Kanerva L, Lauharanta J, Niemi KM, et al: Persistent ashen-gray maculae and freckles induced by long-term PUVA treatment. Dermatologica 166:281, 1983.
43. Honigsmann H: Psoralen photochemotherapy—mechanisms, drugs, toxicity. Curr Probl Dermatol 15:52, 1986.
44. Cronkhite LW Jr, Canada WJ: Generalized gastrointestinal polyposis. An unusual syndrome of polyposis, pigmentation, alopecia and onychotrophia. N Engl J Med 252:1011, 1955.
45. Johansson E, Niemi KM, Siimes M, et al: Fanconi's anemia. Tumor-like warts, hyperpigmentation associated with deranged keratinocytes, and depressed cell-mediated immunity. Arch Dermatol 118:249, 1982.
46. Harari Z, Sommer I, Knobel B: Multifocal contact dermatitis to nitroderm TTS 5 with extensive postinflammatory hypermelanosis. Dermatologica 174:249, 1987.
47. Mahler R, Sissons W, Watters K: Pigmentation induced by quinidine therapy. Arch Dermatol 122:1062, 1986.

48. Basler RSW: Minocycline-related hyperpigmentation. Arch Dermatol 121:606, 1985.
49. Argenyi ZB, Finelli L, Bergfeld WF, et al: Minocycline-related cutaneous hyperpigmentation as demonstrated by light microscopy, electron microscopy, and x-ray energy spectroscopy. J Cutan Pathol 14:176, 1987.
50. Leonard PA, Moatamed F, Ward JR, et al: Chrysiasis: the role of sun exposure in dermal hyperpigmentation secondary to gold therapy. J Rheumatol 13:58, 1986.
51. Bailin PL, Matkaluk RM: Cutaneous reactions to rheumatological drugs. Clin Rheum Dis 8:493, 1982.
52. Koch SE, LeBoit PE, Odom RB: Laugier-Hunziker syndrome. J Am Acad Dermatol 16:431, 1987.

Selected Readings

Advances in pigment cell research. Proceedings of symposia and lectures from the Thirteenth International Pigment Cell Conference. Tucson, Arizona, October 5–9, 1986. Prog Clin Biol Res 256:1, 1988.
A collection of basic research papers presenting advances in pigment cell research.

Alper J, Holmes LB, Mihm MC Jr: Birthmarks with serious medical significance: nevocellular nevi, sebaceous nevi, and multiple café au lait spots. J Pediatr 95:696, 1979.
Discussion of common birthmarks and their significance.

Buxton PK, Kemmett D: ABC of dermatology. Black spots in the skin. Br Med J (Clin Res) 296:703, 1988.
Practical clinical review of pigmented nevi and other pigmented disorders, with an emphasis on distinguishing cutaneous neoplasms.

David M, Shanon A, Hazaz B, Sandbank M: Diffuse, progressive hyperpigmentation: an unusual skin manifestation of mycosis fungoides. J Am Acad Dermatol 16:257, 1987.
Interesting case report of mycosis fungoides presenting with pruritic, diffuse macular hyperpigmentation of the skin. This case contrasts with previous case reports of hypopigmented mycosis fungoides.

Fulk CS: Primary disorders of hyperpigmentation. J Am Acad Dermatol 10:1, 1984.
A good classification of pigmentary disorders, including diffuse and localized types. Fair amount of emphasis on case reports and unusual genetic syndromes.

Iijima S, Naito Y, Naito S, Uyeno K: Reticulate hyperpigmentation distributed in a zosteriform fashion: a new clinical type of hyperpigmentation. Br J Dermatol 117:503, 1987.
Two cases of hyperpigmentation in children that was reticulate and distributed in a zosteriform pattern are described with a review of similar case reports. Authors suggest that these cases may represent a new clinical entity.

Lucky PA, Nordlund JJ: The biology of the pigmentary system and its disorders. Dermatol Clin 3:197, 1985.
Review of current concepts of the pathophysiology of melanin and the pathogenesis of diseases of hyperpigmentation and hypopigmentation.

McGavran MH: Cutaneous pigmentation. Clin Plast Surg 14:301, 1987.
Clinical paper that discusses skin color and briefly reviews a few pigmentary anomalies, such as melanoderma, ceruloderma, and leukoderma.

Nordlund JJ, Abdel-Malek ZA: Mechanisms for postinflammatory hyperpigmentation and hypopigmentation. Prog Clin Biol Res 256:219, 1988.
Current concepts of mediators of inflammation and biochemical pathways thought to result in postinflammatory hyperpigmentation and hypopigmentation. Interesting ideas that may help clinical understanding of pigmentation disorders of the epidermis, with a focus on the role of the melanocyte.

Pehamberger H, Steiner A, Wolff K: In vivo epiluminescence microscopy of the pigmented skin lesions. I. Pattern analysis of pigmented skin lesions. J Am Acad Dermatol 17:571, 1987.
A study of the usefulness of epiluminescence microscopy in diagnosing skin lesions, with an emphasis on melanoma, looked at more than 3,000 pigmented skin lesions, and defined morphologic criteria. Authors suggest that such pattern analysis can be helpful in the sometimes difficult distinction between benign and malignant hyperpigmented lesions.

Vazquez M, Maldonado H, Benmaman C, Sanchez JL: Melasma in men. A clinical and histologic study. Int J Dermatol 27:25, 1988.
Melasma is usually characterized as a facial hypermelanosis more common in Hispanic females. This study evaluated 27 males with melasma and compared clinical and histologic features to previous studies. Sunlight exposure and familial predisposition were the two major etiologic factors.

Wintroub BU, Stern R: Cutaneous drug reactions: pathogenesis and clinical classification. J Am Acad Dermatol 13:167, 1985.
Cutaneous drug reactions classified with pathogenesis and clinical morphology presenting a useful clinical structure to the clinician. Cutaneous drug reactions discussed include urticaria, photosensitivity eruptions, erythema multiforma, disturbances of pigmentation, fixed drug reactions, and others.

Witkop CJ Jr: Inherited disorders of pigmentation. Clin Dermatol 3:70, 1985.
Useful review of inherited pigmentation disorders. Clinical disorders highlighted include acanthosis nigricans, neurofibromatosis, xeroderma pigmentosum, and melanoma.

88
Blisters (Vesicles and Bullae): Causes and Associated Disorders

Vesicles and bullae are clear, fluid-filled blisters differing only in their size: vesicles are less than 1 cm, bullae are greater than 1 cm. Because there is tremendous overlap in their causes, they are discussed together. Mechanisms of blister formation are also variable from epidermal edema (as in contact dermatitis) to upper dermal edema (as in bullous erythema multiforme) to immunologically mediated attack on structural components of the skin (as in pemphigus and pemphigoid).

Infectious Causes

Viral: H simplex,[1,2] H zoster, varicella,[3] variola, coxsackievirus A16 (hand-foot-and-mouth-disease), coxsackievirus B2,[4] cytomegalovirus (rare)[5,6]
Bacterial: bullous impetigo, ecthyma gangrenosum, sepsis (*Escherichi coli*)[7,8] (controversial), blistering distal dactylitis,[9,10] necrotic bullous erysipelas[11]
Spirochetal: congenital syphilis
Fungal: *Candida* (usually pustular), dermatophytosis

Genetically Determined, Congenital Causes

Bullous mastocytosis: urticaria pigmentosa[12]
Bullous congenital ichthyosiform erythroderma
Epidermolysis bullosa: all variants except epidermolysis bullosa acquisita[13-16]
Benign familial pemphigus: Hailey-Hailey disease[53]
Incontinentia pigmenti: first stage
Hereditary callosities with blisters[17]
Tyrosinemia: rare[18]
Darier's disease: bullous variant[19]
Porphyria: all except acute intermittent porphyria[55-57]

Physical Agents and Foreign Substances

Snake bites
Insect bite reactions (papular urticaria): mites, insects, arachnids, ticks, mosquitoes[20,21]
Electromagnetic radiation: UVB, PUVA (especially

topical psoralen and UVA), electrical burns, sun lamps[22–24]
Ionizing radiation[25]
Photodermatosis: hydroa estivale, polymorphous light eruption[26,27]
Pressure urticaria
Friction: enhanced by retinoids
Miliaria crystallina: sweat duct occlusion
Pressure: pressure-induced ischemia and anoxia with a variety of neurologic diseases[28]
Suction blisters
Thermal: heat,[29] frostbite,[30] pernio, cryoproteins[31]

Toxic or Drug Induced[32]

Bullae in (drug-induced) coma: reported with coma due to accident, illness (hypoglycemic coma, neurologic disease), or suicidal dose of drugs (narcotics, barbiturates, carbon monoxide,[33] amitriptyline, clorazepate dipotassium,[34] and nitrazepam)
Drugs: azapropazone,[35] captopril, clonidine, cytostatics,[36] diclofenac, furosemide, gold salts, minoxidil, penicillamine, psoralens (especially topical), and rifampicin
Erythema multiforme: many implicated drugs, but most commonly sulfonamides, hydantoins, rifampicin, pyrazolon derivatives, barbiturates, penicillins, carbamazepine,[37] and gold salts
Bullous fixed drug: large number implicated, but most commonly barbiturates, phenolphthalein, pyrazolon derivatives (phenylbutazone, oxyphenbutazone, phenazone), sulfonamides, tetracyclines
Pseudoporphyria: nalidixic acid, furosemide (dialysis patients), tetracycline, naproxen
Pemphigus: penicillamine, captopril, gold salts, rifampicin
Toxic epidermal necrolysis: most commonly barbiturates, pyrazolon derivatives, hydantoin derivatives, sulfonamides, monsteroidal anti-inflammatory drugs[38]
Bullous photodermatosis (phototoxic and photoallergic)[39]: most commonly tetracyclines, phenothiazines, nalidixic acid, benzothiadiazines, protriptyline, cis-retinoic acid, psoralens, and cytostatics
Staphylococcal scalded skin syndrome
Bullous toxic shock syndrome[40]

Neoplastic or Paraneoplastic Causes

Bullous pyoderma gangrenosum
Mycosis fungoides[41]
Kaposi's sarcoma[42]

Lymphangiomas
Atypical bullous pyoderma gangrenosum[43]
Malignant melanoma[44]
Chronic lymphocytis leukemia[45]

Primary Dermatologic and Autoimmune Blistering Disorders[47]

Bullous erythema multiforme[46]
Toxic epidermal necrolysis: large sheets of wet tissue-like denudation of skin
Dermatitis herpetiformis: intensely pruritic small blisters on extensor surfaces of extremities and mid-back
Pemphigus vulgaris (and variants): frequent oral lesions and flaccid blisters, widespread distribution[49]
Bullous pemphigoid (and variants): especially seen in older people, large tense blisters on erythematous or normal skin[48–53]
Mixed bullous disease: possible transitional cases[54]
Herpes gestationis: starts on abdomen, especially in second and third trimesters
Epidermolysis bullosa acquisita: immunologically mediated and late onset; similar clinical lesions as porphyria cutanea tarda, but negative porphyrin studies[55–58]
Bullous dermatosis of childhood
Intracutaneous bulla formation[59]

Dermatologic and Autoimmune Disorders That May Have Blisters

Bullous Grover's disease
Bullous lichen planus
Bullous lichen sclerosus et atrophicus
Bullous morphea
Bullous graft-versus-host disease[60]
Bullous erythema elevatum diutinum
Bullous acute dermatitis[61]: especially contact dermatitis, dyshidrosiform and id dermatitis
Bullous amyloidosis[62]
Acquired immune deficiency syndrome (AIDS)[63]

Dermatologic and Autoimmune Systemic Associations

Bullous pyoderma gangrenosum[64]
Erythema multiforme: associated with drugs, infections, neoplasia,[65] radiation therapy
Toxic epidermal necrolysis: associated with drugs, infections, neoplasia, radiation therapy
Sweet's syndrome: acute febrile neutrophilic dermatosis; rarely bullous[66]
Graft-versus-host disease[67]

Bullosis of renal failure: possibly drug related[68]
Bullosis diabeticorum[69]
Bullous lupus erythematosus[70,71]
Behçet's syndrome: rare bullous variant

**Miscellaneous
Associations**

Erythema toxicum neonatorum
Subcorneal pustular dermatosis: rare vesicles, usually
pustules

References

1. Orkin FK: Herpetic whitlow—occupational hazard to the anesthesiologist. Anesthesiology 33:671, 1970.
2. Jones JG: Herpetic whitlow: an infectious occupational hazard. J Occup Med 27:725, 1985.
3. Melish ME: Bullous varicella: its association with the staphylococcal scalded skin syndrome. J Pediatr 83:1019, 1973.
4. Barson WJ, Reiner CB: Coxsackievirus B2 infection in a neonate with incontinentia pigmenti. Pediatrics 77:897, 1986.
5. Blatt J, Kastner O, Hodes DS: Cutaneous vesicles in congenital cytomegalovirus infection. J Pediatr 92:509, 1978.
6. Bhawan J, Gellis S, Ucci A, Chang TW: Vesiculobullous lesions caused by cytomegalovirus infection in an immunocompromised adult. J Am Acad Dermatol 11:743, 1984.
7. Fisher K, Berger BW, Keusch GT: Subepidermal bullae secondary to *Escherichia coli* septicemia. Arch Dermatol 110:105, 1974.
8. Voron DA: Bullae due to pressure (letter). Arch Dermatol 111:528, 1975.
9. McCray MK, Esterly NB: Blistering distal dactylitis. J Am Acad Dermatol 5:592, 1981.
10. Parras F, Ezpeleta C, Romero J, et al: Blistering distal dactylitis in an adult. Cutis 41:127, 1988.
11. Agnholt J, Andersen I, Sndergaard G: Necrotic bullous erysipelas. Acta Med Scand 223:191, 1988.
12. Fenske NA, Lober CW, Pautler SE: Congenital bullous urticaria pigmentosa. Treatment with concomitant use of H1- and H2-receptor antagonists. Arch Dermatol 121:115, 1985.
13. Cooper TW, Bauer EA: Epidermolysis bullosa: a review. Pediatr Dermatol 1:181, 1984.
14. Fine JD: Changing clinical and laboratory concepts in inherited epidermolysis bullosa. Arch Dermatol 124:523, 1988.
15. Pearson RW: Clinicopathologic types of epidermolysis bullosa and their nondermatological complications. Arch Dermatol 124:718, 1988.
16. Holbrook KA: Extracutaneous epithelial involvement in inherited epidermolysis bullosa. Arch Dermatol 124:726, 1988.
17. Baden HP, Bronstein BR, Rand RE: Hereditary callos-

ities with blisters. Report of a family and review. J Am Acad Dermatol 11:409, 1984.

18. Buist NRM, Kennaway NG, Burns RP: Eye and skin lesions in tyrosinaemia (letter). Lancet 1:620, 1973.
19. Hori Y, Tsuru N, Niimura N: Bullous Darier's disease. Arch Dermatol 118:278, 1982.
20. Hoogstraal H, Gallagher MD: Blisters, pruritus, and fever after bites by the Arabian tick ornithodoros (alectorobius) muesebecki. Lancet 2:288, 1982.
21. Walker GB, Harrison PV: Seasonal bullous eruption due to mosquitoes. Clin Exp Dermatol 10:127, 1985.
22. Petrozzi JW, Kaidbey KM, Kligman AM: Topical methoxsalen and blacklight in the treatment of psoriasis. Arch Dermatol 113:292, 1977.
23. Patterson JW, Ali M, Murray JC, Hazra TA: Bullous pemphigoid. Occurrence in a patient with mycosis fungoides receiving PUVA and topical nitrogen mustard therapy. Int J Dermatol 24:173, 1985.
24. Drijkoningen M, DeWolf-Peeters C, Roelandts R, et al: A morphological and immunohistochemical study of phytophotodermatitis-like bullae induced by PUVA. Photodermatology 3:199, 1986.
25. Duschet P, Schwarz T, Gschnait F: Bullous pemphigoid after radiation therapy. J Am Acad Dermatol 18:441, 1988.
26. Holzle E, Plewig G, von Kries R, Lehmann P: Polymorphous light eruption. J Invest Dermatol 88(Suppl 3):32s, 1987.
27. Elpern DJ, Morison WL, Hood AF: Papulovesicular light eruption. A defined subset of polymorphous light eruption. Arch Dermatol 121:1286, 1985.
28. Arndt KA, Mihm MC Jr, Parrish JA: Bullae: a cutaneous sign of a variety of neurologic diseases. J Invest Dermatol 60:312, 1973.
29. Poh-Fitzpatrick MB, Ellis DL: Porphyrialike bullous dermatosis after chronic intense tanning bed and/or sunlight exposure. Arch Dermatol 125:1236, 1989.
30. Ward M: Frostbite. Br Med J 1:67, 1974.
31. Ireland TA, Werner DA, Rietschel RL, et al: Cutaneous lesions in cryofibrinogenemia. J Pediatr 105:67, 1984.
32. Bruinsma W: A Guide to Drug Eruptions. The File of Adverse Reactions to the Skin. 3rd Ed. DeZwaluw, Oosthuizen, The Netherlands, 1982.
33. Myers RAM, Snyder SK, Majerus TC: Cutaneous blisters and carbon monoxide poisoning. Ann Emerg Med 14:603, 1985.
34. Herschthal D, Robinson MJ: Blisters of the skin in coma induced by amitriptyline and clorazepate dipotassium. Arch Dermatol 115:499, 1979.
35. Barker DJ, Cotterill JA: Skin eruptions due to azapropazone (letter). Lancet 1:90, 1977.
36. Hood AF: Cutaneous side effects of cancer chemotherapy. Med Clin North Am 70:187, 1986.
37. Godden DJ, McPhie JL: Bullous skin eruption associated with carbamazepine overdosage. Postgrad Med J 59:336, 1983.
38. Roujeau JC: Clinical aspects of skin reactions to NSAIDs. Scand J Rheumatol (Suppl) 65:131, 1987.
39. Azulay RD, Abulafia LA, Azulay DR: A new classifica-

tion of photodermatoses. Med Cutan Ibero Lat Am 17:22, 1989.

40. Elbaum DJ, Wood C, Abuabara F, et al: Bullae in a patient with toxic shock syndrome. J Am Acad Dermatol 10:267, 1984.

41. Roenigk HH Jr, Castrovinci AJ: Mycosis fungoides bullosa. Arch Dermatol 104:402, 1971.

42. Recht B, Nickoloff BJ, Wood GS: A bullous variant of Kaposi's sarcoma in an elderly female. J Dermatol Surg Oncol 12:1192, 1986.

43. Hay CR, Messenger AG, Cotton DW, et al: Atypical bullous pyoderma gangrenosum associated with myeloid malignancies. J Clin Pathol 40:387, 1987.

44. Wagner RF Jr, Nathanson L: Paraneoplastic syndromes, tumor markers, and other unusual features of malignant melanoma. J Am Acad Dermatol 14:249, 1986.

45. Rosen LB, Frank BL, Rywlin AM: A characteristic vesiculobullous eruption in patients with chronic lymphocytic leukemia. J Am Acad Dermatol 15:943, 1986.

46. Huff JC, Weston WL, Tonnesen MG: Erythema multiforme: a critical review of characteristics, diagnostic criteria, and causes. J Am Acad Dermatol 8:763, 1983.

47. Millikan LE: Vesiculobullous skin disease with prominent immunologic feature. JAMA 258:2910, 1987.

48. Korman N: Bullous pemphigoid. J Am Acad Dermatol 16:907, 1987.

49. Kaplan RP, Callen JP: Pemphigus associated diseases and induced pemphigus. Clin Dermatol 1:42, 1983.

50. Salomon RJ, Briggaman RA, Wernikoff SY, Kayne AL: Localized bullous pemphigoid. A mimic of acute contact dermatitis. Arch Dermatol 123:389, 1987.

51. Ahmed AR, Newcomer VD: Bullous pemphigoid. Clinical features. Clin Dermatol 5:6, 1987.

52. Dahl MV: Bullous pemphigoid: associated diseases. Clin Dermatol 5:64, 1987.

53. Michel B: "Familial benign chronic pemphigus" by Hailey and Hailey, April 1939. Commentary: Hailey-Hailey disease, familial benign chronic pemphigus. Arch Dermatol 118:774, 1982.

54. Barranco VP: Mixed bullous disease. Arch Dermatol 110:221, 1974.

55. Sekula SA, Tschen JA, Rosen T: The porphyrias. Am Fam Physician 33(3):219, 1986.

56. Grossman ME, Poh-Fitzpatrick MB: Porphyria cutanea tarda. Diagnosis, management, and differentiation from other hepatic porphyrias. Dermatol Clin 4:297, 1986.

57. Lefer LG, Wenner N: Vesicles on the dorsa of the fingers. Porphyria cutanea tarda (PCT). Arch Dermatol 123:107, 1987.

58. McCuaig CC, Chan LS, Woodley DT, et al: Epidermolysis bullosa acquisita in childhood. Differentiation from hereditary epidermolysis bullosa. Arch Dermatol 125:944, 1989.

59. Devine DC, Milne JA: Intracutaneous bulla formation. ("Polythene bag bullae"). Br J Dermatol 76:362, 1964.

60. De Dobbeleer GD, Ledoux-Corbusier MH, Achten GA: Graft versus host reaction. An ultrastructural study. Arch Dermatol 11:1597, 1975.

61. Wollina U, Funfstuck V, Hipler C, Knopf B: Alterations

of epidermal lectin binding sites in acute contact dermatitis. Contact Dermatitis 19:109, 1988.

62. Beacham BE, Greer KE, Andrews BS, et al: Bullous amyloidosis. J Am Acad Dermatol 3:506, 1980.
63. Warner LC, Fisher BK: Cutaneous manifestations of the acquired immunodeficiency syndrome. Int J Dermatol 25:337, 1986.
64. Perry HO, Winkelmann RK: Bullous pyoderma gangrenosum and leukemia. Arch Dermatol 106:901, 1972.
65. Schwartz BK, Clendenning WE: Bullous erythema multiforme associated with *Haemophilus influenzae* pneumonia. Cutis 36:255, 1985.
66. Callen JP: Acute febrile neutrophilic dermatosis (Sweet's syndrome) and the related conditions of "bowel bypass" syndrome and bullous pyoderma gangrenosum. Dermatol Clin 3:153, 1985.
67. Hymes SR, Farmer ER, Burns WH, et al: Bullous sclerodermalike changes in chronic graft-vs-host disease. Arch Dermatol 121:1189, 1985.
68. Gilchrest B, Rowe JW, Mihm MC Jr: Bullous dermatosis of hemodialysis. Ann Intern Med 83:480, 1975.
69. Huntley AC: The cutaneous manifestations of diabetes mellitus. J Am Acad Dermatol 7:427, 1982.
70. Barton DD, Fine JD, Gammon WR, Sams WM Jr: Bullous systemic lupus erythematosus: an unusual clinical course and detectable circulating autoantibodies to the epidermolysis bullosa acquisita antigen. J Am Acad Dermatol 15:369, 1986.
71. Camisa C, Sharma HM: Vesiculobullous systemic lupus erythematosus. Report of two cases and a review of the literature. J Am Acad Dermatol 9:924, 1983.

Selected Readings

Alcalay J, David M, Ingber A, et al: Bullous pemphigoid mimicking bullous erythema multiforme: an untoward side effect of penicillins. J Am Acad Dermatol 18:345, 1988.
Case report of three young and middle-aged patients who developed severe bullous eruptions after receiving penicillins. Authors describe cutaneous manifestations in detail and suggest that drug-induced bullous pemphigoid is a different entity from the classic bullous pemphigoid.

Buxton PK: ABC of dermatology. Blisters and pustules. Br Med J (Clin Res) 295:1399, 1987.
Clinical overview of dermatologic disorders manifesting with blisters and pustules.

Flowers FP, Sherertz EF: Immunologic disorders of the skin and mucous membranes. Med Clin North Am 69:657, 1985.
A clinical dermatologic approach to dermatologic disorders in which immunologic mechanisms are involved. Dermatologic disorders with autoimmune and other immune mechanisms are emphasized.

Ganderup G, Newburger AE, Barr RJ, Riley RJ: A rapid immunoperoxidase technique to distinguish herpetic types. Int J Dermatol 25:369, 1986.
Authors describe their experience with using a rapid test for the often difficult diagnosis and differentiation of herpes simplex and

herpes zoster infections. The test uses scrapings from viral vesicles and employs standard immunoperoxidase techniques.

Goldberg GI, Eisen AZ, Bauer EA: Tissue stress and tumor promotion. Possible relevance to epidermolysis bullosa. Arch Dermatol 124:737, 1988.

In severe epidermolysis bullosa or other cutaneous ulcers, cutaneous carcinomas have been reported to arise. Authors suggest that chronic tissue stress may promote carcinogenesis in preexisting somatic mutants in a stem cell population.

Nethercott JR, Choi BC: Erythema multiforme (Stevens-Johnson syndrome)—chart review of 123 hospitalized patients. Dermatologica 171:383, 1985.

One hundred twenty-three hospitalized patients with erythema multiforme were reviewed. Bullous skin lesions appeared associated with longer hospital stays. Use and implications of steroid therapy are discussed.

Razzaque AA: Diagnosis of bullous disease and studies in the pathogenesis of blister formation using immunopathological techniques. J Cutan Pathol 11:237, 1984.

Useful review of bullous diseases that discusses current concepts of pathogenesis and suggests application of current immunopathologic techniques to diagnosis. Techniques were found particularly helpful in differentiating pemphigus, bullous pemphigoid, cicatrical pemphigoid, herpes gestationis, dermatitis herpetiformis, linear IgA dermatotsis, and porphyria.

Roujeau JC, Bracq C, Huyn NT, et al: HLA phenotypes and bullous cutaneous reactions to drugs. Tissue Antigens 28:251, 1986.

Interesting discussion linking HLA phenotypes and bullous cutaneous reactions to drugs; that is, drug-induced toxic epidermal necrolysis and Stevens-Johnson syndrome are weakly associated with HLA-B12. Other stronger links to sulphonamides, such as HLA-A29, B12, and DR7, may provide clinicians with helpful prognostic information for using certain drugs in defined phenotypes.

Weston WL: Blistering diseases in children. How to recognize and treat the most common. Postgrad Med 80 (2):241, 1986.

Brief overview of the most common causes of blisters in childhood.

Wintroub BU, Stern R: Cutaneous drug reactions: pathogenesis and clinical classification. J Am Acad Dermatol 13:167, 1985.

Informative, general review of cutaneous drug reactions that are classified with respect to pathogenesis and clinical morphology. Current concepts of immunologic and nonimmunologic mechanisms are reviewed. Cutaneous drug reactions reviewed include urticaria, photosensitivity eruptions, erythema multiforme, pigmentation disorders, erythema nodosum, bullous reactions, and others. Criteria for evaluation of possible drug reactions are presented.

89
Leg Ulcers: Common and Less Common Associations

Ulceration of the lower extremity is fairly common, especially in older patients. The major types are venous stasis ulcers, ischemic ulcers due to occlusive arterial and arteriolar disease, neurotropic ulcers, and pressure ulcers. There are myriad other causes that a thorough history, physical examination, and some laboratory testing may help to identify.[1]

Environmental, Traumatic, and External Causes

Burns: chemical, thermal, electrical, and ionizing radiation

Pressure: prolonged pressure over small body areas, especially in bedridden patients

Injury: may initiate ulcers in skin damaged or thinned by other processes

Self-inflicted

Poststeroid injections

Pernio (chilblains): localized inflammatory lesions that arise as an abnormal reaction to cold; may ulcerate in severe cases

Erythrocyanosis: dusky discoloration of the skin, worse in winter. After cold exposure, chilblain-like lesions may occur.

Infections, Infestations, and Bites

Bacterial

Desert sore: multifactorial, including trauma, poor nutrition, staphylococci, and streptococci

Gas gangrene: *Clostridium*[2,3]

Bacterial synergistic gangrene (Meleney's ulcer): *Peptostreptococcus* plus *Staphylococcus aureus* or Enterobacteriaceae

Ecthyma: *Streptococcus*

Rare causes: tularemia, anthrax, brucellosis, cat-scratch fever, glanders

Spirochetal: syphilis,[4] yaws

Mycobacterial
Swimming pool granuloma: *Mycobacterium marinum*
Buruli ulcer: *Mycobacterium ulcerans*
Tuberculosis
Leprosy[5]
Leishmania
Mycotic (superficial and deep fungal infections): coccidioidomycosis, histoplasmosis, blastomycosis, mucormycosis,[6] cryptococcosis,[7] sporotrichosis, *Candida albicans*, Madura foot (mycetoma—a localized skin infection with a variety of fungi)[8]
Bites: spider,[9] scorpion, snake

**Systemic and
Metabolic Causes**

Diabetes: vascular damage with or without neuropathy[10]
Prolidase deficiency[11–13]
Hyperparathyroidism: associated with renal disease
Werner's disease
Underlying bone disease: Paget's disease
Overlying cutaneous calcinosis of any cause
Hematologic causes: sickle cell anemia (shins),[14,15] thalassemia,[16,17] spherocytosis, paroxysmal nocturnal hemoglobinuria,[18] polycythemia, macroglobulinemia,[19] dysglobulinemia, paraproteinemia, cryoproteinemia, Cooley's anemia,[20] thrombocythemia, and also coagulation and platelet disorders
Granulomatous processes: ulcerated rheumatoid nodule, necrobiosis lipoidica diabeticorum, sarcoid,[21] Crohn's disease[22]

Vascular Causes

Venous[23–25]: stasis dermatitis with ulceration, postphlebitic, congenital absence of veins
Arterial/arteriolar: hypertension (lateral malleolus—Martorell's ulcer),[26] atherosclerosis, Buerger's disease (thromboangiitis obliterans), septic emboli, cholesterol emboli, atrophie blanche (segmental hyalinizing vasculitis),[27] Takayasu's arteritis[28]
Arteriovenous malformations: congenital or acquired[29]
Vasculitis[30]: Collagen vascular disease–rheumatoid arthritis,[31,32] Felty's syndrome, scleroderma,[33] lupus; immune complex deposition,[34] pyoderma gangrenosum,[35] livedoid vasculitis,[36] erythema induratum (Bazin's disease), periarteritis nodosa,[37] livedo reticularis with ulcerations

**Neuropathic Causes
"Mal Perforans"**

Diabetes: decreased vascular supply
Leprosy
Tabes dorsalis
Other conditions with cutaneous anesthesia: spinal
cord injury, syringomyelia, peripheral nerve injury

**Neoplastic, Drug-
Induced, and
Miscellaneous**

Epitheliomata: rare causes, usually exophytic; squamous cell carcinoma, basal cell carcinoma, metastatic carcinoma
Kaposi's sarcoma
Mycosis fungoides
Leukemia and reticuloses: if blood vessel involvement
is present[38]
Other neoplasms: melanoma, angiosarcoma, metastatic carcinoma
Halogen-induced lesions: iododerma, bromoderma
Barbiturate intoxication: after bullae rupture
Rupture of any bullous process involving the legs
Acrodermatitis chronica atrophicans
Klinefelter's syndrome: venous and arterial leg ulcers
reported[39]
Lupus anticoagulant: certain cutaneous symptoms,
including leg ulcers, are associated with the presence of lupus anticoagulant.[40]

References

1. Ryan TJ, Wilkinson DS: Diseases of arteries. p. 1059. In Rook A, Wilkinson DS, Ebling FJG (eds): Textbook of Dermatology. 3rd Ed. Blackwell Scientific Publications, Oxford, 1979.
2. Feingold DS: Gangrenous and crepitant cellulitis. J Am Acad Dermatol 6:289, 1982.
3. Vo NM, Watson S, Bryant LR: Infections of the lower extremities due to gas-forming and non-gas-forming organisms. South Med J 79:1493, 1986.
4. Walzman M, Wade AA, Drake SM, Thomas AM: Rest pain and leg ulceration due to syphilitic osteomyelitis of the tibia. Br Med J (Clin Res) 293:804, 1986.
5. Sane SB, Mehta JM: Malignant transformation in trophic ulcers in leprosy: a study of 12 cases. Indian J Lepr 60:93, 1988.
6. Rothburn MM, Chambers DK, Roberts C, Downie RJ: Cutaneous mucormycosis: a rare cause of leg ulceration. J Infect 13:175, 1986.
7. Lerner EA, Kibbi AG, Haas A: Calf ulcer in an immunocompromised host. Cryptococcosis. Arch Dermatol 124:430, 1988.
8. Dennis KJ, Harkless LB, Fetchik R, Heckman JD: Madura foot. A case presentation. J Am Podiatr Med Assoc 79:36, 1989.
9. Gutowicz M, Fritz RA, Sonoga AL: Brown recluse spider

bite. A literature review and case report. J Am Podiatr Med Assoc 79:142, 1989.

10. Huntley AC: The cutaneous manifestations of diabetes mellitus. J Am Acad Dermatol 7:427, 1982.

11. Ogata A, Tanaka S, Tomoda T, et al: Autosomal recessive prolidase deficiency. Arch Dermatol 117:689, 1981.

12. Leoni A, Cetta G, Tenni R, et al: Prolidase deficiency in two siblings with chronic leg ulcerations. Clinical, biochemical, and morphologic aspects. Arch Dermatol 123:493, 1987.

13. Freij BJ, Der Kaloustian VM: Prolidase deficiency. A metabolic disorder presenting with dermatologic signs. Int J Dermatol 25:431, 1986.

14. Ofosu MD, Castro O, Alarif L: Sickle cell leg ulcers are associated with HLA-B35 and Cw4. Arch Dermatol 123:482, 1987.

15. Keidan AJ, Stuart J: Rheological effects of bed rest in sickle cell disease. J Clin Pathol 40:1187, 1987.

16. Gimmon Z, Wexler MR, Rachmilewitz EA: Juvenile leg ulceration in β-thalassemia major and intermedia. Plast Reconstr Surg 69:320, 1982.

17. Steinberg MH, Rosenstock W, Coleman MB, et al: Effects of thalassemia and microcytosis on the hematologic and vasoocclusive severity of sickle cell anemia. Blood 63:1353, 1984.

18. Rietschel RL, Lewis CW, Simmons RA, et al: Skin lesions in paroxysmal nocturnal hemoglobinuria. Arch Dermatol 114:560, 1978.

19. Nishijima S, Hosokawa H, Yanase K, et al: Primary macroglobulinemia presenting as multiple ulcers of the legs. Acta Derm Venereol (Stockh) 63:173, 1983.

20. Pascher F, Keen R: Ulcers of the leg in Cooley's anemia. N Engl J Med 256:1220, 1957.

21. Saxe N, Benatar SR, Bok L, et al: Sarcoidosis with leg ulcers and annular facial lesions. Arch Dermatol 120:93, 1984.

22. Perret CM, Bahmer FA: Extensive necrobiosis in metastatic Crohn's disease. Dermatologica 175:208, 1987.

23. Eriksson G, Eklund AE, Kallings LO: The clinical significance of bacterial growth in venous leg ulcers. Scand J Infect Dis 16:175, 1984.

24. Heng MC: Venous leg ulcers. The post-phlebitic syndrome. Int J Dermatol 26:14, 1987.

25. Sindrup JH, Avnstorp C, Steenfos HH, Kristensen JK: Transcutaneous PO2 and laser Doppler blood flow measurements in 40 patients with venous leg ulcers. Acta Derm Venereol (Stockh) 67:160, 1987.

26. Duncan HJ, Faris IB: Martorell's hypertensive ischemic leg ulcers are secondary to an increase in the local vascular resistance. J Vasc Surg 2:581, 1985.

27. Shornick JK, Nicholes BK, Bergstresser PR, et al: Idiopathic atrophie blanche. J Am Acad Dermatol 8:792, 1983.

28. Perniciaro CV, Winkelmann RK, Hunder GG: Cutaneous manifestations of Takayasu's arteritis. A clinicopathologic correlation. J Am Acad Dermatol 17:998, 1987.

29. Lee EB, Dubin HV: Ulcers associated with congenital arteriovenous fistulas. Arch Dermatol 119:949, 1983.

30. Fauci AS, Haynes BF, Katz P: The spectrum of vasculitis. Clinical, pathologic, immunologic, and therapeutic considerations. Ann Intern Med 89:660, 1978.
31. Schneider HA, Yonker RA, Katz P, et al: Rheumatoid vasculitis: experience with 13 patients and review of the literature. Semin Arthritis Rheum 14:280, 1985.
32. Jorizzo JL, Daniels JC: Dermatologic conditions reported in patients with rheumatoid arthritis. J Am Acad Dermatol 8:439, 1983.
33. Thomas JR III, Winkelmann RK: Vascular ulcers in scleroderma. Arch Dermatol 119:803, 1983.
34. Braverman IM: The angiitides. p. 378. In Braverman IM (ed): Skin Signs of Systemic Disease. 2nd Ed. WB Saunders, Philadelphia, 1981.
35. Newell LM, Malkinson FD: Commentary: pyoderma gangrenosum. Arch Dermatol 118:769, 1982.
36. Cabbabe EB, Clift SD: Leg ulcerations in livedoid vasculitis. Plast Reconstr Surg 75:888, 1985.
37. Horan RF, Tahan SR, Margolis RJ, Haynes HA: Atypical angiomatosis in polyarteritis nodosa. Br J Dermatol 115:611, 1986.
38. Stahl RL, Silber R: Vasculitic leg ulcers in chronic myelogenous leukemia. Am J Med 78:869, 1985.
39. Downham TF II, Mitek FV: Chronic leg ulcers and Klinefelter's syndrome. Cutis 38:110, 1986.
40. Grob JJ, Bonerandi JJ: Cutaneous manifestations associated with the presence of the lupus anticoagulant. A report of two cases and a review of the literature. J Am Acad Dermatol 15:211, 1986.

Selected Readings

Agren MS, Stromberg HE, Rindby A, Hallmans G: Selenium, zinc, iron and copper levels in serum of patients with arterial and venous leg ulcers. Acta Derm Venereol (Stockh) 66:237, 1986.

Interesting clinical study that compared total serum concentrations of selenium, zinc, iron, and copper in geriatric patients with leg ulcers to controls. Authors found that levels of selenium, zinc, and iron were significantly lower in patients with leg ulcers and that ratios of copper to zinc were significantly higher in the leg ulcer group.

Buxton PK: ABC of dermatology. Leg ulcers. Br Med J (Clin Res) 295:1542, 1987.

Helpful clinical summary of basics needed to evaluate and manage leg ulcers.

Callam MJ, Harper DR, Dale JJ, Ruckley CV: Arterial disease in chronic leg ulceration: an underestimated hazard? Lothian and Forth Valley leg ulcer study. Br Med J (Clin Res) 294:929, 1987.

Six hundred patients with chronic leg ulcers were evaluated for arterial dysfunction. Risk factors for arterial impairment and subsequent foot ulceration included claudication symptoms, ischemic heart disease, cerebrovascular disease, and signs of chronic venous insufficiency.

Cole GW: The measurement of the volume of leg ulcers. J Dermatol Surg Oncol 14:421, 1988.

A new technique for measuring the volume of cutaneous ulcers using silicon rubber dental material is described and compared with conventional methods of image analysis.

Edmondson RS, Flowers MW: Intensive care in tetanus: management, complications, and mortality in 100 cases. Br Med J 1:1401, 1979.
An interesting article showing that in 5% of tetanus cases, the portal of entry was probably a stasis ulcer.

Hansson C, Andersson E, Swanbeck G: A follow-up study of leg and foot ulcer patients. Acta Derm Venereol (Stockh) 67:496, 1987.
Three hundred fifty patients with leg and foot ulcers were evaluated, followed, and compared with an age-matched population. Both mortality rate and incidence of ischemic heart disease were found to be significantly higher in patients with leg ulcers compared to controls.

Robinson DC, Adriaans B, Hay RJ, Yesudian P: The clinical and epidemiologic features of tropical ulcer (tropical phagedenic ulcer). Int J Dermatol 27:49, 1988.
A comparative study of patients with tropical ulcers in Zambia, Gambia, southern India, and Papua, New Guinea compared clinical features, socioeconomic backgrounds, and nutritional correlates in 170 patients. No correlation between nutritional status and leg ulcers was found; however, a strong association between the development of tropical ulcers and exposure to mud or slow-moving fresh water was made.

Spittell JA Jr: Diagnosis and management of leg ulcer. Geriatrics 38 (6):57, 1983.
General review of leg ulcers with a geriatric focus.

Young JR: Differential diagnosis of leg ulcers. Cardiovasc Clin 13:171, 1983.
General clinical review of differential diagnosis of leg ulcers, with an emphasis on vascular causes such as arteriosclerosis obliterans.

90
Leukocytoclastic Vasculitis: Causes of LCV and Conditions That Can Mimic LCV

Leukocytoclastic vasculitis (LCV) is also known as hypersensitivity vasculitis, allergic vasculitis, or cutaneous necrotizing vasculitis and presents typically as palpable purpuric lesions in symmetric distribution on dependent areas. The spectrum of skin lesions includes erythematous papules or plaques, livedo reticularis, vesiculobullous lesions, urticarial lesions, or ulcerations. Systemic symptoms of fever, arthralgias, myalgias, or kidney and gastrointestinal involvement may also occur. Characteristic pathologic features of LCV include infiltration of postcapillary venules and arterioles with leukocytes, presence of nuclear dust resulting from neutrophil degranulation and fibrinoid necrosis of vessel wall, and perivascular connective tissue.

Subclasses of LCV include (1) Henoch-Schönlein purpura (HSP) or anaphylactoid purpura, which typically occurs in children after upper respiratory infection and has palpable purpura with associated arthritis, abdominal pain, gastrointestinal bleeding, and a tendency toward renal disease[1]; (2) urticarial vasculitis, which is characterized by persistence of urticaria for longer than 24 hours, typical LCV lesions on biopsy, and may be associated with hypocomplementemia[2]; and (3) erythema elevatum diutinum, which is an uncommon chronic disease characterized by persistent firm papules, plaques, or nodules over extensor surfaces that typically show LCV on biopsy.[3,4]

Causes of LCV

LCV can be triggered by many factors including infections, drugs, toxins, and various diseases. In many cases, no precipitating factor can be identified.

Infections

Streptococcal infection: especially beta-hemolytic group A variety

Staphylococcus aureus infection

Bacterial endocarditis[5]

Escherichia coli infection

Yersiniosis[6]

Malaria

Schistosomiasis

Acute viral hepatitis: hepatitis A, B or non-A, non-B virus leads to variable skin manifestations, including urticarial lesions, and may be seen in absence of clinically overt liver disease.[7,8]

Epstein-Barr viral infections: infectious mononucleosis may also be associated with urticarial vasculitis.[9]

Cytomegalovirus

Influenza

Varicella[10]

Acquired immune deficiency syndrome (AIDS)[11,12]

Mycobacterial infections

Histoplasmosis

Candidiasis

Drugs and Toxins

Drug exposure or drug allergy are the most likely causes of HSP if physical findings are limited to the skin and there are no significant systemic features.[13]

Antibiotics: including penicillin, streptomycin, tetracycline, erythromycin, chloramphenicol, cephalosporins, sulfonamides, vancomycin[14]

Aspirin

Phenylbutazone

Phenytoin

Barbiturates

Carbamazepine[15]

Phenothiazines

Amphetamines

Quinidine[16]

Procainamide

Busulfan

Methotrexate[17]

Gold compounds

Allopurinol

Levamisole

Propylthiouracil: characteristic skin findings include recurrent, self-limited, tender, symmetric palpable purpuric eruption that can involve the face or ear lobes with LCV pattern on biopsy[18]

Iodides
Phenacetin
Captopril[19]
Griseofulvin
Intracoronary streptokinase: serum sickness-like illness after intracoronary streptokinase characterized by skin rash (proven LCV by biopsy in two patients), pretibial edema, and polyarthralgia-arthritis[20]
Vaccines[21]
Animal serum
Petroleum products
Insecticides and herbicides: several environmental chemicals including thiram, a thiocarbamate used as rubber accelerator, fungicide, and insecticide have been associated with development of LCV.[22]
Azo dyes and benzoates: ingestion of food and drug additives such as azo dyes and benzoates[23]
Heat-activated photocopy paper: exposure to heat-activated photocopy paper containing behenic acid while using microfilm copying machines[24]

Connective Tissue and Immunologic Diseases

LCV is commonly associated with connective tissue diseases in adults, but not in children, and visceral or extracutaneous involvement may be more common in LCV associated with these diseases.[25]

Systemic lupus erythematosus: ten to 20% of these patients develop dermal vasculitis during the course of their disease, which is manifested as cutaneous infarcts or purpuric papules. LCV may coexist with larger vessel vasculitis and lead to digital infarcts, ulcerations, and distal gangrene.[26]
Rheumatoid arthritis: rheumatoid vasculitis can be seen as LCV, cutaneous gangrene, mononeuritis multiplex, petechiae, or ulcerations and may involve small to large vessels with systemic involvement of nervous system, gastrointestinal tract, lungs, or kidneys.[27]
Mixed connective tissue disease
Sjögren's syndrome: frequently associated with LCV as palpable purpura or urticarial lesions. These patients have high titers of Ro (SS-A) and La (SS-B) autoantibodies. Approximately 70% of Sjögren patients with cutaneous vasculitis also develop peripheral and/or CNS disease.[28]

Scleroderma: vascular changes are prominent, but necrotizing vasculitis is uncommon.[29]

Dermatomyositis: the childhood form of this disease is occasionally accompanied by vasculitis of the skin, gastrointestinal tract, muscle, and nerves, which is not seen in the adult form.[30]

Behçet's syndrome: may include various cutaneous lesions such as pustules, nodules, erythema nodosum-like eruptions, skin hyperreactivity or hyperirritability (pathergy), and ulcerations, which are all secondary to small vessel vasculitis[31]

Goodpasture's syndrome[32]

Rheumatic fever

Familial Mediterranean fever (FMF): FMF and HSP have remarkable clinical similarities, and it is speculated that pathogenesis of both are related to immune complexes; HSP in FMF patients has occurred after penicillin injections.[33]

Essential mixed cryoglobulinemia: syndrome of purpura, arthralgia, and weakness with widespread vasculitis and often severe glomerulonephritis as well as typical LCV on skin biopsy[26]; hepatitis B antigenemia may be present.[34]

Complement deficiencies: particularly C1r, C2, or C3 deficiencies[35]

Selective immunoglobulin A deficiency

Serum sickness

Gastrointestinal Disease

Inflammatory bowel disease: either regional enteritis or ulcerative colitis

Chronic active hepatitis: either non-A non-B or hepatitis B related and often associated with cryoglobulins[7]

Primary biliary cirrhosis

Intestinal bypass syndrome: occurs in patients after jejunoileostomies performed to treat morbid obesity and is characterized by arthralgias or arthritis, fever, and erythematous skin lesions often with pustular centers, which most often demonstrate LCV on biopsy.[36]

Neoplastic Disease

LCV may precede the appearance of the tumor and its course may not parallel the malignancy.[25]

Multiple myeloma[37]: IgA myeloma has been associated with LCV and erythema elevatum diutinum.[38,39]

Leukemia: LCV is seen in chronic lymphocytic leukemia[40] and particularly in hairy cell leukemia.[41]

Lymphoma[42,43]

Lymphosarcoma

Myeloproliferative disorders

Macroglobulinemia of Waldenström

Miscellaneous

Benign hypergammaglobulinemic purpura: may be a subset of LCV with polyclonal elevation of gamma globulin levels, elevated sedimentation rate, mild anemia, and recurrent purpura and has been associated with various diseases[44]

Cystic fibrosis

Thyroiditis

Ventriculoatrial shunt[35]

Disseminated intravascular coagulation

Serous otitis media

Insect bite: has been reported to lead to Henoch-Schönlein purpura[45]

Dermatitis herpetiformis

Retroperitoneal fibrosis[46]

Sarcoidosis[47]

Conditions that Can Mimic LCV

Several diseases have clinical presentations similar to LCV and some even have histologic similarities, such as polyarteritis nodosa, Wegener's granulomatosis, Churg-Strauss allergic granulomatosis and leprosy; whereas, others have very different histology.

Similar Histology to LCV

Polyarteritis nodosa (PAN): a multisystem disease of small and medium-sized vessels in which the skin is involved in 40 to 50% of patients with classic PAN. The skin lesions may be histologically identical to LCV if only a superficial skin biopsy is examined. Constitutional and systemic features clue the physician to search for other organ involvement to make a diagnosis of PAN.[36] A unique chronic cutaneous vasculitis called cutaneous PAN has been described, which has the pathology of PAN and a benign chronic course with inflammatory nodules developing into livedo reticularis.[48]

Wegener's granulomatosis: skin involvement occurs in 40 to 50% of patients and commonly presents as papules with necrotic centers, pyoderma grangrenosum-like lesions, and ulcerations. Typical changes of LCV may be present in the upper dermis, but pallisading granulomas and granulomatous vasculitis can be found if the deep dermis and subcutaneous tissue are examined.[9]

Churg-Strauss allergic granulomatosis: approximately two-thirds of patients have skin involvement, which is about equally divided between purpuric and nodular skin lesions. The purpuric lesions may demonstrate LCV on biopsy, but nodular lesions typically reveal necrotizing pallisading granulomas with eosinophils.[36]

Leprosy: the reactional states of leprosy are characterized by acute inflammatory changes in skin lesions and include erythema nodosum leprosum (development of tender, erythematous, cutaneous nodules) or the Lucio phenomenon (severe, necrotizing cutaneous ulcerations in diffuse non-nodular leprosy). Both of these reactions can reveal LCV on skin biopsy along with the features of lepromatous leprosy of foamy histiocytes and acid-fast bacilli.[49]

Histology Different from LCV

Septic vasculitis: mixture of papular, purpuric, vesicular, and pustular discrete lesions can be seen in streptococcal, gonococcal, or meningococcal disease.[48] These septicemias may mimic LCV or Henoch-Schönlein purpura.[50]

Syphilis: may also present with various skin lesions including purpuric papules[48]

Rocky Mountain spotted fever: characteristic exanthem is macular rash, which begins on palms, soles, and distal extremities and spreads centripetally evolving into maculopapular then purpuric lesions that could be mistaken for LCV.[9]

Viral disease exanthems[9]: often purpuric

Thrombocytopenic purpura[9]: typically does not demonstrate palpable purpura and is associated with low platelet counts

Sweet's syndrome: acute or recurrent symptom complex of erythematous plaques, fever, arthralgia, leukocytosis, and biopsy reveals neutrophilic infiltration without vascular damage.[36]

Erythema multiforme: LCV may mimic this skin lesion if it is in the vesiculobullous form.[13]

Vietnamese folk medicine: the Vietnamese lay practice of dermabrasion (called Cao Gao) has been misdiagnosed in children as Henoch-Schönlein purpura.[51]

References

1. Fink CW: Vasculitis. Pediatr Clin North Am 33:1203, 1986.
2. Gammon WR, Wheeler CE Jr: Urticarial vasculitis: report of a case and review of the literature. Arch Dermatol 115:76, 1979.
3. Gammon R: Leukocytoclastic vasculitis. Clin Rheum Dis 8:397, 1982.
4. Le Boit PE, Yen TS, Wintroub B: The evolution of lesions in erythema elevatum diutinum. Am J Dermatopathol 8:392, 1986.
5. Horwitz LD, Silber R: Subacute bacterial endocarditis presenting as purpura. Arch Intern Med 120:483, 1967.
6. Rasmussen NH: Henoch-Schönlein purpura after yersiniosis (letter). Arch Dis Child 57:322, 1982.
7. Popp JW, Harrist TJ, Dienstag JL, et al: Cutaneous vasculitis associated with acute and chronic hepatitis. Arch Intern Med 141:623, 1981.
8. Inman RD, Hodge M, Johnston MEA, et al: Arthritis, vasculitis, and cryoglobulinemia associated with relapsing hepatitis A virus infection. Ann Intern Med 105:700, 1986.
9. Mackel SE: Treatment of vasculitis. Med Clin North Am 66:941, 1982.
10. Ashkenazi S, Mimouni M, Varsano I: Henoch-Schönlein vasculitis following varicella (letter). Am J Dis Child 139:440, 1985.
11. Velji AM: Leukocytoclastic vasculitis associated with positive HTLV-III serological findings (letter). JAMA 256:2196, 1986.
12. Schulhafer EP, Grossman ME, Fagin G, et al: Steroid-induced Kaposi's sarcoma in a patient with pre-AIDS. Am J Med 82:313, 1987.
13. Nusinow SR, Izuno GT, Curd JG: The dermal manifestations of vasculitis: a clinical approach to diagnosis and treatment. Postgrad Med 78(3):122, 1985.
14. Rawlinson WD, George CR: Vancomycin-induced vasculitis (letter). Med J Aust 147:470, 1987.
15. Harats N, Shalit M: Carbamazepine induced vasculitis (letter). J Neurol Neurosurg Psychiatry 50:1241, 1987.

16. Shalit M, Flugelman MY, Harats N, et al: Quinidine-induced vasculitis. Arch Intern Med 145:2051, 1985.
17. Navarro M, Pedragosa R, Lafuerza A, et al: Leukocytoclastic vasculitis after high-dose methotrexate (letter). Ann Intern Med 105:471, 1986.
18. Carrasco MD, Riera C, Clotet B: Cutaneous vasculitis associated with propylthiouracil therapy. Arch Intern Med 147:1677, 1987.
19. Laaban J, Marie J-P, Wallach D, et al: Necrotizing vasculitis associated with captopril therapy (letter). Eur Heart J 8:319, 1987.
20. Noel J, Rosenbaum LH, Gangadharan V, et al: Serum sickness-like illness and leukocytoclastic vasculitis following intracoronary streptokinase. Am Heart J 113:395, 1987.
21. Warrington RJ, Martens CJ, Rubin M, et al: Immunologic studies in subjects with a serum sickness-like illness after immunization with human diploid cell rabies vaccine. J Allergy Clin Immunol 79:605, 1987.
22. Duell PB, Morton WE: Henoch-Schönlein purpura following thiram exposure. Arch Intern Med 147:778, 1987.
23. Michaelsson G, Pettersson L, Juhlin L, et al: Purpura caused by food and drug additives. Arch Dermatol 109:49, 1974.
24. Tencati JR, Novey HS: Hypersensitivity angiitis caused by fumes from heat-activated photocopy paper. Ann Intern Med 98:320, 1983.
25. Katz P: Hypersensitivity vasculitis. Am Fam Physician 26(1):171, 1982.
26. Gilliam JN, Smiley JD: Cutaneous necrotizing vasculitis and related disorders. Ann Allergy 37:328, 1976.
27. Vollertsen RS, Conn DL, Ballard DJ, et al: Rheumatoid vasculitis: survival and associated risk factors. Medicine 65:365, 1986.
28. Alexander E, Provost TT: Sjögren's syndrome: association of cutaneous vasculitis with central nervous system disease. Arch Dermatol 123:801, 1987.
29. Alarcon-Segovia D: The necrotizing vasculitides: a new pathogenetic classification. Med Clin North Am 61:241, 1977.
30. Sams WM Jr: Necrotizing vasculitis. J Am Acad Dermatol 3:1, 1980.
31. Plotkin GR, Patel BR, Shah VN: Behçet's syndrome complicated by cutaneous leukocytoclastic vasculitis. Arch Intern Med 145:1913, 1985.
32. Tucker RM, Brown AL Jr: Clinicopathologic conference. Goodpasture's syndrome. Mayo Clin Proc 43:449, 1968.
33. Flatau E, Kohn D, Schiller D, et al: Schönlein-Henoch syndrome in patients with familial Mediterranean fever. Arthritis Rheum 25:42, 1982.
34. Levo Y, Gorevic PD, Kassab HJ, et al: Association between hepatitis B virus and essential mixed cryoglobulinemia. N Engl J Med 296:1501, 1977.
35. Sloane PD, Tardell R: Palpable purpura in leukocytoclastic vasculitis. Am Fam Physician 33(4):197, 1986.
36. Callen JP: Cutaneous vasculitis and its relationship to systemic disease. DM 28:1, 1981.
37. Raper RF, Ibels LS: Osteosclerotic myeloma complicated

by diffuse arteritis, vascular calcification, and extensive cutaneous necrosis. Nephron 39:389, 1985.

38. McMillen JJ, Krueger SK, Dyer GA: Leukocytoclastic vasculitis in association with immunoglobulin A myeloma. Ann Intern Med 105:709, 1986.

39. Means RT Jr, Greer JP, Sergent JS, McCurley TL: Leukocytoclastic vasculitis and multiple myeloma (letter). Ann Intern Med 106:329, 1987.

40. Fauci AS, Haynes BF, Katz P: The spectrum of vasculitis: clinical, pathologic, immunologic, and therapeutic considerations. Ann Intern Med 89:660, 1978.

41. Spann CR, Callen JP, Yam LT: Cutaneous leukocytoclastic vasculitis complicating hairy cell leukemia (leukemic reticuloendotheliosis). Arch Dermatol 122:1057, 1986.

42. Kesseler ME, Slater DN: Cutaneous vasculitis: a presenting feature in Hodgkin's disease. J R Soc Med 79:485, 1986.

43. Mor F, Leibovici L, Wysenbeek AJ: Leukocytoclastic vasculitis in malignant lymphoma. Isr J Med Sci 23:829, 1987.

44. Hudson CP, Callen JP: Cutaneous leukocytoclastic vasculitis with hyperglobulinemia and splenomegaly: a variant of hyperglobulinemic purpura of Waldenström. Arch Dermatol 120:1224, 1984.

45. Sharan G, Anand RK, Sinha KP: Schönlein-Henoch syndrome after insect bite. Br Med J 1:656, 1966.

46. Hellstrom HR, Perez-Stable EC: Retroperitoneal fibrosis with disseminated vasculitis and intrahepatic sclerosing cholangitis. Am J Med 40:184, 1966.

47. Hodge SJ, Callen JP, Ekenstam E: Cutaneous leukocytoclastic vasculitis: correlation of histopathological changes with clinical severity and course. J Cutan Pathol 14:279, 1987.

48. Winkelmann RK: The spectrum of cutaneous vasculitis. Clin Rheum Dis 6:413, 1980.

49. Pursley TV, Jacobson RR, Apisarnthanarax P: Lucio's phenomenon. Arch Dermatol 116:201, 1980.

50. Rosenberg H, Bortolussi R, Gatien JB: Rash resembling anaphylactoid purpura as the initial manifestation of meningococcemia. Can Med Assoc J 125:179, 1981.

51. Golden SM, Duster MC: Hazards of misdiagnosis due to Vietnamese folk medicine. Clin Pediatr 16:949, 1977.

Selected Readings

Callen JP: Cutaneous vasculitis and its relationship to systemic disease. DM 28:1, 1981.
Complete review of cutaneous vasculitis from classification to therapy, with particular attention to its association with systemic diseases.

Ekenstam E, Callen JP: Cutaneous leukocytoclastic vasculitis: clinical and laboratory features of 82 patients seen in private practice. Arch Dermatol 120:484, 1984.
Analysis of patients with LCV from private dermatology offices with supporting data of good prognosis despite frequent systemic symptoms or findings.

Gammon R: Leucocytoclastic vasculitis. Clin Rheum Dis 8:397, 1982.

Concise general review of LCV.

Nusinow SR, Izuno GT, Curd JG: The dermal manifestations of vasculitis: a clinical approach to diagnosis and treatment. Postgrad Med 78(3):122, 1985.
Excellent review with emphasis on guidelines for clinical evaluation of cutaneous vasculitis.

Winkelmann RK: The spectrum of cutaneous vasculitis. Clin Rheum Dis 6:413, 1980.
Thorough well-referenced review of cutaneous vasculitis, with excellent illustrations and photomicrographs.

91
Scleroderma-like Disorders: Diseases Featuring Hardening of the Skin

The hallmark of scleroderma and its variants is hardening or sclerosis of the skin. Firm skin, however, is a feature of other dermatologic, metabolic, immunologic, oncologic, and inherited disorders. It can also be induced by drugs, chemicals, and other environmental agents. This section lists those entities that give the appearance or feel of hardening of the skin. Many of the disorders are associated with internal organ manifestations, but others are limited to cutaneous and subcutaneous changes.

Scleroderma:
Generalized

Diffuse scleroderma (progessive systemic sclerosis)[1]: symmetric fibrous thickening and hardening (sclerosis) of the skin combined with fibrous and degenerative changes in synovium, digital arteries, and certain internal organs, most notably esophagus, intestinal tract, heart, lungs, and kidneys.[2]

CREST syndrome (calcinosis, Raynaud's phenomenon, esophageal dysmotility, sclerodactyly, telangiectasia)[1]: skin changes are restricted to the fingers and face.

Overlap syndrome[1,3]: mixed connective tissue disease, systemic lupus erythematosus, dermatomyositis, rheumatoid arthritis, Sjögren's syndrome, and primary biliary cirrhosis can all be associated with sclerodermatous features.

Scleroderma: Localized

Morphea[4,5]: circumscribed, ivory-colored sclerotic plaques with erythematous or violaceous borders ranging in diameter from 1 to 30 cm. They can range from a few to many in number.

Linear scleroderma[4-6]: bandlike hypopigmentation and sclerosis, most commonly on the legs and less commonly on the arms, the frontal region of the head (*en coup de sabre*), and the anterior thorax.

Scleroderma-like Disorders

Fasciitis with eosinophilia (eosinophilic fasciitis, Shulman's syndrome)[7]: inflammation and sclerosis of the deep fascia, subcutis, and dermis, primarily involving the extremities. This widespread condition occurs with a rapid onset, usually after significant exertion, and is often associated with peripheral eosinophilia. Raynaud's phenomenon is rare.

Dermatologic

Scleredema[1,8]: diffuse, firm, painless, nonpitting swelling and induration of the skin; often follows a recent febrile illness and may also be associated with diabetes mellitus

Scleromyxedema (lichen myxedematosus, papular mucinosis)[9]: asymptomatic pale red or yellowish papules associated with diffuse thickening of the skin that is not bound down to underlying structures

Acrodermatitis chronica atrophicans[10]: cutaneous inflammation followed by atrophy

Atrophoderma[8]: centrally depressed, irregular sharply demarcated, indurated, slate-gray plaques measuring 1 to 10 cm in diameter on the trunk

Keloids and hypertrophic scars[8]

Lichen sclerosus et atrophicus[1,8]: small, ivory plaques showing atrophy that develop most commonly in the anogenital region, but may also develop on the trunk, neck, axillae, and flexor surfaces of the extremities; may be difficult to clinically differentiate from morphea

Lipoatrophy[10]

Pseudosclerodermatous artifact[8]: a skin biopsy can have the histologic appearance of scleroderma if the deep portion of a punch biopsy specimen is squeezed by forceps.

Metabolic

Acromegaly[10]: considerable thickening of the skin and subcutaneous tissue may appear in acromegaly as the result of connective tissue hyperplasia.

Amyloidosis[11]: diffuse deposition of amyloid in the skin can produce physical findings of the fingers, hands, and face that may mimic scleroderma.

Diabetes mellitus, type I (juvenile onset diabetes mellitus)[12,13]: digital sclerosis and mild finger contractures occur in one-third of patients with type I diabetes mellitus.

Glycogen storage disease[14]: can be associated with scleroderma-like induration of the skin

Myxedema

Phenylketonuria[15]: scleroderma-like skin changes and muscle induration occur in some cases.

Porphyria cutanea tarda[1,10]: hypopigmented plaquelike sclerodermatous indurations of the skin occur usually in sun-exposed areas in porphyria cutanea tarda. Congenital porphyrias can also cause scleroderma-like skin changes.

Immunologic

Graft-versus-host reaction[16]: can give scleroderma-like skin changes

Infectious

Lyme disease[17]: antibodies to *Borrelia burgdorferi*, the etiologic agent in Lyme disease, have been found in 50% of patients with morphea in Austria.

Inherited syndromes

Progeria (Hutchinson-Gilford syndrome)[1,10]: a rare pediatric autosomal recessive syndrome characterized by premature aging and shortened survival. Can have markedly thickened, bound-down skin on the abdomen, flanks, and proximal thighs.

Rothmund syndrome[10]: a recessive disorder in which atrophy of the skin, beginning in infancy, is associated with juvenile cataracts

Werner syndrome[18]: an autosomal recessive disorder marked by premature aging. Sclerodermatous skin changes are frequent.

Winchester's syndrome[8]: a rare inherited disorder characterized by dwarfism, small joint destruction, corneal opacities, hypertrichosis, hypertrophic lips and gingivae, and thickened skin

Etiology unknown

Melorheostosis[19]: a rare acquired disorder of bone with radiographs showing linear hyperostosis that may be associated with scleroderma-like skin lesions

Tumor associated

Breast cancer (*carcinoma en cuirasse*)[8]: a diffuse induration of the breast secondary to lymphatic metastases of breast cancer

Bronchogenic carcinoma (pachydermoperiostosis)[8]: thickened furrowed skin of the face and scalp can occur with digital clubbing and hyperplasia of the soft tissue of the forearms and legs secondary to bronchogenic carcinomas; may be associated with hypertrophic osteoarthropathy.[20]

Carcinoid syndrome[21]: scleroderma-like skin lesions on the legs, characterized by indurated, taut, and bound-down skin, usually differentiated from progressive scleroderma by the lack of Raynaud's phenomenon, visceral organ involvement, or proximal scleroderma.

Mycosis fungoides[22]: sclerodermatous changes of the skin of the hands and sclerodactyly of all digits.

POEMS syndrome[23]: a rare form of plasma cell dyscrasia characterized by the various association of polyneuropathy, organomegaly, endocrinopathy, monoclonal protein, and skin changes

Drug-induced

Bleomycin[24,25]: can cause thickened plaques, nodules, and bands on the hands of patients treated with this antitumor drug

Carbidopa[3,10]

Penicillamine[26]

Pentazocine[27]: nodular cutaneous sclerosis, often associated with ulceration, may occur at the site of an intramuscular injection of pentazocine.

Phytonadione[28]: subcutaneous sclerosis can occur at the site of an injection.

Tryptophan[3,10]

Environmental

Vinyl chloride[29]: workers exposed to vinyl chloride

may acquire an illness resembling systemic scleroderma, including nodular induration of the dorsum of the hands and forearms, clubbing, acro-osteolysis, synovial thickening of the proximal interphalangeal joints, hepatic portal fibrosis, splenomegaly, and pulmonary fibrosis.

Toxic oil syndrome[30]: adulterated rapeseed cooking oil in Spain associated with a chronic illness with symptoms including diffuse hard, taut, and shiny skin, dry eyes and mouth, motor weakness and muscle atrophy, alopecia, dysphagia, and pulmonary hypertension.

Epoxy resins[31]: can produce marked skin sclerosis and muscle weakness after only short-term exposure

Organic solvents (aromatic and aliphatic hydrocarbons)[32]: skin sclerosis may occur at site of direct contact with solvent

Perchlorpethylene[33]: produces skin lesions similar to those found with vinyl chloride exposure

Radiation dermatitis[8]

Silicone or paraffin implantation[34,35]: a scleroderma-like illness can follow cosmetic surgery such as mammoplasty and rhinoplasty.

Silicosis[36]: silica dust may act to induce scleroderma.

Trichloroethylene[37]: produces skin lesions similar to those found with vinyl chloride exposure

Urea formaldehyde[38]: scleroderma-like illness after exposure to urea formaldehyde foam insulation.

Vibration associated ("jackhammer disease")[39]

References

1. Rocco VK, Hurd ER: Scleroderma and scleroderma-like disorders. Semin Arthritis Rheum 16:22, 1986.
2. Rodnan GP: When is scleroderma not scleroderma? The differential diagnosis of progressive systemic sclerosis. Bull Rheum Dis 31(2):7, 1981.
3. Bennett RM: Mixed connective tissue disease and other overlap syndromes. p. 1147. In Kelley WN, Harris ED Jr, Ruddy S, Sledge CB (eds): Textbook of Rheumatology. 3rd Ed. WB Saunders, Philadelphia, 1989.
4. Jablonska S, Rodnan GP: Localized forms of scleroderma. Clin Rheum Dis 5:215, 1979.
5. Piette WW, Dorsey JK, Foucar E: Clinical and serologic expression of localized scleroderma: case report and review of the literature. J Am Acad Dermatol 13:342, 1985.
6. Falanga V, Medsger TA Jr, Reichlin M, et al: Linear scleroderma: clinical spectrum, prognosis, and laboratory abnormalities. Ann Intern Med 104:849, 1986.

7. Sibrack LA, Mazur EM, Hoffman R, Bollet AJ: Eosinophilic fasciitis. Clin Rheum Dis 8:443, 1982.
8. Young EM Jr, Barr RJ: Sclerosing dermatoses. J Cutan Pathol 12:426, 1985.
9. Gabriel SE, Perry HO, Oleson GB, Bowles CA: Scleromyxedema: a scleroderma-like disorder with systemic manifestations. Medicine 67:58, 1988.
10. Medsger TA Jr: Systemic sclerosis (scleroderma), eosinophilic fasciitis, and calcinosis. p.994. In McCarty DJ (ed): Arthritis and Allied Conditions: A Textbook of Rheumatology. 10th Ed. Lea & Febiger, Philadelphia, 1985.
11. Rubinow A, Cohen AS: Skin involvement in generalized amyloidosis. A study of clinically involved and uninvolved skin in 50 patients with primary and secondary amyloidosis. Ann Intern Med 88:781, 1978.
12. Seibold JR: Digital sclerosis in children with insulin-dependent diabetes mellitus. Arthritis Rheum 25:1357, 1982.
13. Garza-Elizondo MA, Diaz-Jouanen E, Franco-Casique JJ, Alarcon-Segovia D: Joint contractures and scleroderma-like skin changes in the hands of insulin-dependent juvenile diabetics. J Rheumatol 10:797, 1983.
14. Jablonska S, Stachow A: Pseudoscleroderma concomitant with a muscular glycogenosis of unknown enzymatic defect. Acta Derm Venereol 52:379, 1972.
15. Jablonska S, Stachow A, Suffczynska M: Skin and muscle indurations in phenylketonuria. Arch Dermatol 95:443, 1967.
16. Wick MR, Moore SB, Gastineau DA, Hoagland HC: Immunologic, clinical, and pathologic aspects of human graft-versus-host disease. Mayo Clin Proc 58:603, 1983.
17. Aberer E, Neumann R, Stanek G: Is localised scleroderma a borrelia infection? (letter). Lancet 2:278, 1985.
18. Fleischmajer R, Nedwich A: Werner's syndrome. Am J Med 54:111, 1973.
19. Soffa DJ, Sire DJ, Dodson JH: Melorheostosis with linear sclerodermatous skin changes. Radiology 114:577, 1975.
20. Gray RG, Gottlieb NL: Pseudoscleroderma in hypertrophic osteoarthropathy. JAMA 246:2062, 1981.
21. Fries JF, Lindgren JA, Bull JM: Scleroderma-like lesions and the carcinoid syndrome. Arch Intern Med 131:550, 1973.
22. Wei N, Foon KA: Sclerodactyly in a patient with mycosis fungoides. Arch Intern Med 145:139, 1985.
23. Viard JP, Lesavre P, Boitard C, et al: POEMS syndrome presenting as systemic sclerosis: clinical and pathologic study of a case with microangiopathic glomerular lesions. Am J Med 84:524, 1988.
24. Cohen IS, Mosher MB, O'Keefe EJ, et al: Cutaneous toxicity of bleomycin therapy. Arch Dermatol 107:553, 1973.
25. Finch WR, Rodnan GP, Buckingham RB, et al: Bleomycin-induced scleroderma. J Rheumatol 7:651, 1980.
26. Miyagawa S, Yoshioka A, Hatoko M, et al: Systemic sclerosis-like lesions during long-term penicillamine therapy for Wilson's disease. Br J Dermatol 116:95, 1987.

27. Palestine RF, Millns JL, Spigel GT, et al: Skin manifestations of pentazocine abuse. J Am Acad Dermatol 2:47, 1980.
28. Janin-Mercier A, Mosser C, Souteyrand P, et al: Subcutaneous sclerosis with fasciitis and eosinophilia after phytonadione injections. Arch Dermatol 121:1421, 1985.
29. Suciu I, Prodan L, Ilea E, et al: Clinical manifestations in vinyl chloride poisoning. Ann NY Acad Sci 246:53, 1975.
30. Alonso-Ruiz A, Zea-Mendoza AC, Salazar-Vallinas JM, et al: Toxic oil syndrome: a syndrome with features overlapping those of various forms of scleroderma. Semin Arthritis Rheum 15:200, 1986.
31. Yamakage A, Ishikawa H, Saito Y, et al: Occupational scleroderma-like disorder occurring in men engaged in the polymerization of epoxy resins. Dermatologica 161:33, 1980.
32. Walder BK: Do solverts cause scleroderma? Int J Dermatol 22:157, 1983.
33. Sparrow GP: A connective tissue disorder similar to vinyl chloride disease in a patient exposed to perchlorethylene. Clin Exp Dermatol 2:17, 1977.
34. Kumagai Y, Shiokawa Y, Medsger TA Jr, Rodnan GP: Clinical spectrum of connective tissue disease after cosmetic surgery. Observations on eighteen patients and a review of the Japanese literature. Arthritis Rheum 27:1, 1984.
35. Endo LP, Edwards NL, Longley S, et al: Silicone and rheumatic diseases. Semin Arthritis Rheum 17:112, 1987.
36. Haustein UF, Ziegler V: Environmentally induced systemic sclerosis-like disorders. Int J Dermatol 24:147, 1985.
37. Lockey JE, Kelly CR, Cannon GW, et al: Progressive systemic sclerosis associated with exposure to trichloroethylene. J Occup Med 29:493, 1987.
38. Rush PJ, Chaiton A: Scleroderma, renal failure, and death associated with exposure to urea formaldehyde foam insulation. J Rheumatol 13:475, 1986.
39. Siegel RC: Scleroderma. Med Clin North Am 61:283, 1977.

Selected Readings

Fleischmajer R, Pollock JL: Progressive systemic sclerosis: pseudoscleroderma. Clin Rheum Dis 5:243, 1979.
Review of several entities with manifestations similar to systemic scleroderma.

Haustein UF, Ziegler V: Environmentally induced systemic sclerosis-like disorders. Int J Dermatol 24:147, 1985.
Covers chemical agents implicated in causing scleroderma-like disorders.

Medsger TA Jr: Systemic sclerosis (scleroderma), eosinophilic fasciitis, and calcinosis. p.994. In McCarty DJ (ed): Arthritis and Allied Conditions: A Textbook of Rheumatology. 10th Ed. Lea & Febiger, Philadelphia, 1985.
Textbook chapter on scleroderma with review of entities simulating systemic sclerosis.

Rocco VK, Hurd ER: Scleroderma and scleroderma-like disorders. Semin Arthritis Rheum 16:22, 1986.
Comprehensive subject review.

Uitto J, Murray LW, Blumberg B, et al: Biochemistry of collagen in disease. Ann Intern Med 105:740, 1986.
A review of genetics and biochemistry of fibrotic skin diseases.

Young EM Jr, Barr RJ: Sclerosing dermatoses. J Cutan Pathol 12:426, 1985.
Subject review from a pathologic perspective.

IX

RENAL AND ELECTROLYTE

92

Acute Renal Failure: Causes of Oliguric and Nonoliguric Failure

Acute cessation of glomerular filtration is manifested by oliguric or nonoliguric renal insufficiency resulting in the retention of nitrogenous waste.[1] Both oliguric and nonoliguric acute renal failure occur in a wide spectrum of clinical situations and can be associated with potentially serious complications. Cessation of glomerular filtration is a common problem among critically ill patients. Early detection and treatment of acute renal failure may significantly decrease the high morbidity and mortality found among critically ill patients.[2] Initial diagnostic evaluation should distinguish among prerenal, renal, and postrenal causes of acute renal failure.[3]

Prerenal Hypoperfusion or Azotemia: Common Causes and Associations

Prerenal failure results from decreased kidney perfusion. Hospitalized patients in the surgical setting are at particular risk as multiple potential causes of decreased cardiac output and intravascular volume can result in prerenal azotemia, which, if severe and sustained, may result in acute tubular necrosis.[4] Elderly patients are at higher risk, particularly if they are receiving antibiotics, have congestive heart failure, are volume depleted, are in septic shock, or are diabetic.[5]

Cardiogenic shock[6]
Pericardial tamponade[7]
Cardiovascular surgery: aortic cross clamping
Aortic dissection[8]
Hemorrhage
Gastrointestinal loss
Volume sequestration: burn injuries,[9] pancreatitis[10]
Osmotic diuresis
Acute respiratory failure[11,12]
Alcoholic cirrhosis[13]

Postrenal Azotemia: Common Causes and Associations

Obstruction causing postrenal cessation of glomerular filtration is a potentially treatable form of acute renal failure. Although bladder outlet obstruction usually results in anuria or oliguria, partial urinary obstruction can actually present with polyuria. Prostatic carcinoma and pelvic cancer are common causes of obstruction.

Intraureteric obstruction: clot, stone, infection[14]
Extraureteric obstruction: tumor, fibrosis, ligature
Neoplasms: bladder, pelvis, metastatic disease[15-17]
Lower urinary tract obstruction: urethral occlusion, bladder lesions, prostatic disease[18]
Postobstructive diuresis[19]
Pregnancy: rare complication[20]

Renal Causes of Acute Renal Failure

When prerenal and postrenal causes of acute renal failure have been ruled out, it is helpful to consider various causes of acute renal parenchymal disorders affecting renal vasculature, interstitium, and tubules. A wide variety of physiopathologic mechanisms are proposed, that can trigger or perpetuate renal failure.[21] Some of the more common associations are the following:

Diffuse renal vascular disorders: severe hypertension,[22,23] scleroderma, thrombotic thrombocytopenic purpura,[24-26] malignant nephrosclerosis, vasculitis,[27] sickle-cell disease[28]
Primary and secondary renal arterial disorders: thrombosis; embolism; aneurysm; middle aortic syndrome—thoracic, visceral, aortic and renal arterial narrowing causing severe hypertension in young adults[29]; fibromuscular disease
Primary and secondary renal venous disorders: thrombosis, vena cava obstruction
Glomerular disease: membranoproliferative, focal sclerosis, Nil disease, postinfectious glomerulonephritis, diffuse proliferative crescentic, i.e., poststreptococcal glomerulonephritis, and multiple other causes
Renal tubular occlusion: stones, crystals, proteins, hemoglobin
Myeloma protein deposition[30]
Myoglobulin: rhabdomyolysis most commonly occurs acutely after trauma, such as with crush injuries[31]; less commonly, it may be quite delayed, i.e., after electrical injuries[32]

Miscellaneous neoplasm: renal neoplasms via mass effect can decrease glomerular filtration, such as renal cell carcinoma, lymphoma[33,34] and metastases
Septic shock
Pyelonephritis in renal transplant patients
Sarcoidosis: with hypercalcemia[35]
Renal trauma[36]: acute renal failure can develop insidiously with normal urine output and vital signs.[37]

Drug and Toxin-Induced Renal Injury Associated with Acute Renal Failure

A wide spectrum of nephrotoxic injury and functional change is associated with certain drug categories, such as nonsteroidal anti-inflammatory drugs (NSAIDs). Clinical factors, such as age, medical disorders, amount, and duration of taking drugs, may increase the risk of developing acute and chronic renal insufficiency.

Aminoglycosides: gentamicin and gram-negative bacterermia may be synergistically nephrotoxic.[38]
NSAIDs: an increased use of these drugs has resulted in an increased number of reports of renal pathologic and physiologic injuries, listed in decreasing order of frequency: unspecified renal failure, papillary necrosis, acute interstitial nephritis, poor perfusion, nephrotic syndrome, acute tubular necrosis, and acute glomerulitis or vasculitis.[39]
Fenoprofen: appears to be particularly nephrotoxic[41]
Suprofen: unique clinical syndrome of flank pain and acute renal failure reported with this drug[40]
Indomethacin: has been associated with acute suppression of prostaglandin synthesis
Cimetidine: acute interstitial nephritis associated with increased serum creatinine due to decreased tubular secretion of creatinine[41]
Allopurinol: acute interstitial nephritis[43]
Dyazide: has been associated with interstitial nephritis, as well as tubular occlusion injuries[42]
Sulfonamides
Phenacetin: in compound analgesics has been correlated with the incidence of analgesic nephropathy or tubular interstitial nephropathy with or without papillary necrosis[43]
Heavy metals: mercury[44]
Mercuric chloride[45]
Epsilon-aminocaproic acid: hemophiliacs may be

more susceptible to clot-induced urinary obstruction.[46]

Amphotericin[47]

References

1. Anderson RJ, Schrier RW: Clinical spectrum of oliguric and nonoliguric acute renal failure. p.1. In Brenner BM, Stein JH (eds): Acute Renal Failure, Churchill Livingstone, New York, 1980.
2. Mann HJ, Fuhs DW, Hemstrom CA: Acute renal failure. Drug Intell Clin Pharm 20 (6):421, 1986.
3. Corwin HL, Bonventre JV: Acute renal failure. Med Clin North Am 70:1037, 1986.
4. Cook HE, Yamada RK: Acute renal failure in the surgical patient: initial diagnosis and treatment. J Oral Maxillofac Surg 44 (9):719, 1986.
5. Shusterman N, Strom BL, Murray TG, et al: Risk factors and outcome of hospital-acquired acute renal failure. Clinical epidemiologic study. Am J Med 83:65, 1987.
6. Burke TJ, Burnier M, Langberg H, et al: Renal response to shock. Ann Emerg Med 15:1397, 1986.
7. Kron IL, Joob AW, Van Meter C: Acute renal failure in the cardiovascular surgical patient. Ann Thorac Surg 39:590, 1985.
8. Diehl JT, Moon B, LeClerc Y, et al: Acute type A dissection of the aorta: surgical management with the sutureless intraluminal prosthesis. Ann Thorac Surg 43:502, 1987.
9. Güechot J, Cynober L, Lioret N, et al: Rhabdomyolysis and acute renal failure in a patient with thermal injury. Intensive Care Med 12:159, 1986.
10. Thomson SR, Hendry WS, McFarlane GA, Davidson AI: Epidemiology and outcome of acute pancreatitis. Br J Surg 74:398, 1987.
11. Pingleton SK: Complications of acute respiratory failure. Med Clin North Am 67:725, 1983.
12. Gillespie DJ, Marsh HM, Divertie MB, Meadows JA III: Clinical outcome of respiratory failure in patients requiring prolonged (greater than 24 hours) mechanical ventilation. Chest 90:364, 1986.
13. Praga M, Costa JR, Shandas GJ, et al: Acute renal failure in cirrhosis associated with macroscopic hematuria of glomerular origin. Arch Intern Med 147:173, 1987.
14. Charton M, Lanne J, Veillon B, et al: Obstruction of the upper excretory tract associated with primary urinary infection. Diagnosis, treatment and course. Apropos of 196 cases. Ann Urol (Paris) 21:168, 1987.
15. Takeuchi T, Shinoda I, Kuriyama M, et al: Evaluation of urinary cytology for upper urinary tract disease. Hinyokika Kiyo 32 (2):177, 1986.
16. Mitty HA, Droller MJ, Dikman SH: Ureteral and renal pelvic metastases from renal cell carcinoma. Urol Radiol 9:16, 1987.
17. Akmal M, Kapstein EM, Bertram J, Massry SG: Acute renal failure due to bilateral ureteral obstruction by metastases from breast cancer. Nephron 42:23, 1986.

18. Juraschek F, Schoenahl C, Fernandez R, et al: Invasive cancer of the prostate. Reconstruction of the lower urinary tract by prostatic resection and ureteral reimplantation into the bladder vault. Ann Urol (Paris) 21:59, 1987.
19. Jones BF, Nanra RS: Post-obstructive diuresis. Aust NZ J Med 13:519, 1983.
20. Weiss Z, Shalev E, Zuckerman H, et al: Obstructive renal failure and pleural effusion caused by the gravid uterus. Acta Obstet Gynecol Scand 65:187, 1986.
21. Grünfeld JP: Physiopathology of acute renal insufficiency. Schweiz Med Wochenschr 116:527, 1986.
22. Leitschuh M, Chobanian A: Vascular changes in hypertension. Med Clin North Am 71:827, 1987.
23. Schwartz GL, Strong CG: Renal parenchymal involvement in essential hypertension. Med Clin North Am 71:843, 1987.
24. Byrnes JJ, Moake JL: Thrombotic thrombocytopenic purpura and the hemolytic-uremic syndrome: evolving concepts of pathogenesis and therapy. Clin Haematol 15:413, 1986.
25. Eknoyan G, Riggs SA: Renal involvement in patients with thrombotic thrombocytopenic purpura. Am J Nephrol 6:117, 1986.
26. Rose M, Eldor A: High incidence of relapses in thrombotic thrombocytopenic purpura. Clinical study of 38 patients. Am J Med 83:437, 1987.
27. Bodaghi E, Kheradpir KM, Maddah M: Vasculitis in acute streptococcal glomerulonephritis. Int J Pediatr Nephrol 8:69, 1987.
28. Kelly CJ, Singer I: Acute renal failure in sickle-cell diease. Am J Kidney Dis 8:146, 1986.
29. Messina LM, Reilly LM, Goldstone J, et al: Middle aortic syndrome. Effectiveness and durability of complex arterial revascularization techniques. Ann Surg 204:331, 1986.
30. Ludwig H: The clinical picture of multiple myeloma. Onkologie 9 (4):206, 1986.
31. Kikta MJ, Meyer JP, Bishara RA, et al: Crush syndrome due to limb compression. Arch Surg 122:1078, 1987.
32. Haberal M: Electrical burns: a five-year experience— 1985 Evans lecture. J Trauma 26:103, 1986.
33. Truong LD, Soroka S, Sheth AV, et al: Primary renal lymphoma presenting as acute renal failure. Am J Kidney Dis 9:502, 1987.
34. Glicklich D, Sung MW, Frey M: Renal failure due to lymphomatous infiltration of the kidneys. Report of three new cases and review of the literature. Cancer 58:748, 1986.
35. Singer DR, Evans DJ: Renal impairment in sarcoidosis: granulomatous nephritis as an isolated cause (two case reports and review of the literature). Clin Nephrol 26:250, 1986.
36. McGonigal MD, Lucas CE, Ledgerwood AM: The effects of treatment of renal trauma on renal function. J Trauma 27:471, 1987.
37. Shin B, Mackenzie CF, Helrich M: Creatinine clearance of early detection of posttraumatic renal dysfunction. Anesthesiology 64:605, 1986.

38. Zager RA, Prior RB: Gentamicin and gram-negative bacteremia. A synergism for the development of experimental nephrotoxic acute renal failure. J Clin Invest 78:196, 1986.
39. Carmichael J, Shankel SW: Effects of nonsteroidal anti-inflammatory drugs on prostaglandins and renal function. Am J Med 78:992, 1985.
40. Hart D, Ward M, Lifschitz MD: Suprofen-related nephrotoxicity. A distinct clinical syndrome. Ann Intern Med 106:235, 1987.
41. Handa SP: Drug-induced acute interstitial nephritis: report of 10 cases. Can Med Assoc J 135:1278, 1986.
42. Farge D, Turner MW, Roy DR, Jothy S: Dyazide-induced reversible acute renal failure associated with intracellular crystal deposition. Am J Kidney Dis 8:445, 1986.
43. Nanra RS: Renal effects of antipyretic analgesics. Am J Med 75:70, 1983.
44. Wolfert AI, Laveri LA, Reilly KM, et al: Glomerular hemodynamics in mercury-induced acute renal failure. Kidney Int 32:246, 1987.
45. Conger JD, Falk SA: Glomerular and tubular dynamics in mercuric chloride-induced acute renal failure. J Lab Clin Med 107:281, 1986.
46. Pitts TO, Spero JA, Bontempo FA, Greenberg A: Acute renal failure due to high-grade obstruction following therapy with epsilon-aminocaproic acid. Am J Kidney Dis 8:441, 1986.
47. Sacks P, Fellner SK: Recurrent reversible acute renal failure from amphotericin. Arch Intern Med 147:593, 1987.

Selected Readings

Anderson S, Brenner BM: Effects of aging on the renal glomerulus. Am J Med 80:435, 1986.
After the age of 30, glomerular filtration and renal blood flow rates decline in a linear fashion, so that values in octagenarians are only one-half to two-thirds those measured in young adults. The aging kidney is at high risk of eventual failure when the functioning nephron number is further reduced by acquired renal disease. Dietary protein restriction may postpone end-stage renal disease in patients with progressive renal insufficiency.

Hocking WG: Hematologic abnormalities in patients with renal diseases. Hematol Oncol Clin North Am 1:229, 1987.
Renal diseases are associated with a host of hematologic abnormalities affecting erythropoiesis, thrombopoiesis, platelet function, coagulation, fibrinolysis, and immune function. Many of the abnormalities described in acute or chronic renal failure appear to be directly related to accumulation of uremic toxins. Renal cell carcinoma is associated with a variety of unusual hematologic manifestations that may be confused with other diseases.

Jeffrey RB, Laing FC, Wing VW, Hoddick W: Sensitivity of sonography in pyonephrosis: a reevaluation. AJR 144:71, 1985.
Because of the consequences of misdiagnosis, sonographically guided diagnostic needle aspiration may be required in patients with urosepsis and significant hydronephrosis.

Jones DA, George NJ, O'Reilly PH: Postobstructive renal function. Semin Urol 5:176, 1987.
Useful clinical discussion of phases of renal function following postobstructive renal conditions.

Maillet PJ, Pelle-Francoz D, Laville M, et al: Nondilated obstructive acute renal failure: diagnostic procedures and therapeutic management. Radiology 160:659, 1986.
Even in the absence of dilatation, antegrade pyelography guided by real-time ultrasound is a possible diagnostic method and can be the first step in the performance of percutaneous nephrostomy.

Merigian KS, Roberts JR: Cocaine intoxication: hyperpyrexia, rhabdomyloysis, and acute renal failure. J Toxicol Clin Toxicol 25:135, 1987.
This is the first reported case of cocaine intoxication resulting in severe hyperthermia, bizarre behavior, rhabdomyolysis, and acute renal failure.

Myers BD, Moran SM: Hemodynamically mediated acute renal failure. N Engl J Med 314:97, 1986.
Current concepts of the physiology of acute renal failure.

Nies AS: Renal effects of nonsteroidal anti-inflammatory drugs. Agents Action 24 (Suppl):95, 1988.
Review of effects of NSAIDs on renal function and clinical consequences. Author describes a unique syndrome of flank pain and mild reversible renal dysfunction in healthy individuals receiving suprofen, a uricosuric NSAID, which may be due to uric acid crystal deposition in renal tubules.

Olsen S, Solez K: Acute renal failure in man: pathogenesis in light of new morphological data. Clin Nephrol 27:271, 1987.
A review of current concepts of light microscopic and ultrastructural changes in acute renal failure, with particular attention to renal pathology seen in acute tubular necrosis, acute interstitial nephritis, and transplant anuria.

Rao TK, Friedman EA, Nicastri AD: The types of renal disease in the acquired immunodeficiency syndrome. N Engl J Med 316:1062, 1987.
Among 750 patients with acquired immune deficiency syndrome (AIDS) who were treated at 2 adjacent hospitals in New York City, 78 (10.4%) needed evaluation for renal disorders. Reversible acute renal failure due to nephrotoxic injury, ischemic injury, or both was present in 23 patients (30%) (group I). The remaining 55 (70%) had massive proteinuria, azotemia, or both (AIDS-associated nephropathy, group II); and irreversible uremia developed in 43 patients.

Rhyner P, Federle MP, Jeffrey RB: CT of the trauma to the abnormal kidney. AJR 142:747, 1984.
Traumatic injuries to already abnormal kidneys are difficult to assess by excretory urography and clinical evaluation. CT provided specific and clinically useful information in each case that was not apparent on excretory urography.

Richards IM, Fraser SM, Capell HA, et al: A survey of renal function in outpatients with rheumatoid arthritis. Clin Rheumatol 7:267, 1988.
A study of acute renal side effects of NSAIDs in an unselected outpatient population with definite or classic rheumatoid arthritis to determine the prevalence of renal problems. Twenty percent of this patient group had abnormalities that were mostly transient. Au-

thors conclude that the long-term use of NSAIDs is associated with relatively few renal side effects.

Sacks P, Fellner SK: Recurrent reversible acute renal failure from amphotericin. Arch Intern Med 147:593, 1987.

Case report of a patient with cryptogenic cirrhosis and disseminated sporotrichosis who developed acute renal failure immediately after the administration of amphotericin B on four separate occasions. Authors propose that amphotericin, in the setting of reduced effective arterial volume, may activate tubuloglomerular feedback, thereby contributing to acute renal failure.

Wheeler DC, Feehally J, Walls J: High risk acute renal failure. Q J Med 61:977, 1986.

Acute renal failure carries a high mortality rate, and little change in survival rate over the last 3 decades has been seen. Patients requiring intensive care, most of whom have developed acute renal failure after trauma of surgery, have a worse prognosis.

Zipser RD, Henrich WL: Implications of nonsteroidal anti-inflammatory drug therapy. Am J Med 80:78, 1986.

The panel considered the clinical implications of nephrotoxicity due to NSAIDs. Although the clinical benefits and safety of these agents are well established, the drugs may adversely affect renal perfusion, electrolyte balance, and blood pressure in susceptible patients. The renal effects of these agents are directly related to their potency in inhibiting renal prostaglandins as reflected by inhibition of urinary prostaglandin excretion.

93
Polyuria: Diabetes Insipidus and Other Causes

The initial challenge in a patient with polyuria is to distinguish those patients with central or nephrogenic diabetes insipidus from those who are excreting large amounts of urine in response to osmolar loads, and from those with primary drinking disorders. Conditions causing polyuria in response to increased solute loads can usually be quickly identified and treated, such as the polyuria with glycosuria in diabetes mellitus and iatrogenic causes. It is sometimes difficult, however, to distinguish those patients with primary polydipsia from those with diabetes insipidus. Diabetes insipidus is characterized by chronic polyuria and polydipsia.[1]

Common Causes of Osmolar Loads Leading to Osmotic Diuresis and Polyuria

Glycosuria
Mannitol or urea administration
Sodium loads: high dietary sodium, IV or tube feedings of excessive salt and water, rapid reabsorption of edema fluid

Conditions Associated with Nephrogenic Diabetes Insipidus

Nephrogenic diabetes insipidus occurs when the renal concentrating mechanism has become unresponsive to vasopressin. It is manifested by polyuria with dilute urine in the presence of normal or increased serum osmolality. The three most common causes of nephrogenic diabetes insipidus are metabolic disorders, drugs, and intrinsic renal disease. Congenital causes are rarer.

Idiopathic nephrogenic diabetes insipidus[2]
Postobstructive uropathy: with medullary washout
Polycystic medullary cystic disease
Acute pyelonephritis
Hypercalcemia: calcium nephropathy
Hypokalemia: hypokalemic nephropathy
Sickle-cell anemia
Sarcoidosis
Multiple myeloma
Amyloid disease[3]
Drug-induced renal dysfunction: methoxyflurane anesthesia, lithium carbonate,[4,5] diuretics
Congenital tubular disorders, usually associated with renal tubular acidosis[6,7]
Pregnancy[8]
Primary hyperparathyroidism

Conditions Associated with Central Diabetes Insipidus

Central diabetes insipidus can be primary or secondary and occurs when there is a partial or complete failure of pituitary vasopressin secretion. Partial diabetes insipidus is the most common presentation manifested by polyuria, dilute urine, and mild serum hyperosmolality. Traumatic and surgical pituitary stalk lesions are the most common causes.

Primary diabetes insipidus: idiopathic,[9] familial central diabetes insipidus,[10,11] Wolfram or DIDMOAD syndrome[12]

Secondary diabetes insipidus

Head trauma: diabetes insipidus can occur acutely or several days after head trauma; most patients with a delayed onset of diabetes insipidus have permanent antidiuretic hormone deficiency[13] and should be evaluated for other signs of hypopituitarism.[14]

Neurosurgical procedures

Cerebrovascular disease: atherosclerotic thrombosis, subarachnoid hemorrhage

Pituitary infarction: Sheehan's syndrome[15,16]

Hypothalamic neoplasms: craniopharyngioma[17] and germ-cell[18] are two of the most common.

Intracranial tumors: diabetes insipidus may be the initial sign of occult intracranial tumors.[19]

Primary and metastatic neoplasms[20]: leukemia,[21] lymphoma, metastatic breast carcinoma,[22] bronchogenic carcinoma,[23] myeloid metaplasia[24]

Central nervous system infections: meningitis, encephalitis, syphilis

Granulomatous processes: tuberculosis, sarcoidosis, eosinophilic granuloma,[25] histiocytosis,[26] Wegener's granulomatosis[27]

Empty sella syndrome

Pancytopenia[28]

Preeclampsia[29]

Pregnancy[30]

Carbon monoxide poisoning[31]

Aortocoronary bypass surgery[32]

References

1. Robertson GL: Differential diagnosis of polyuria. Annu Rev Med 39:425, 1988.
2. Niaudet P, Dechaux M, Trivin C, et al: Nephrogenic diabetes insipidus: clinical and pathophysiological aspects. Adv Nephrol 13:247, 1984.
3. Neugarten J, Gallo GR, Buxbaum J, et al: Amyloidosis in subcutaneous heroin abusers ("skin poppers" amyloidosis). Am J Med 81 (4):635, 1986.
4. Cairns SR, Wolman R, Lewis JG, Thakker R: Persistent nephrogenic diabetes insipidus, hyperparathyroidism, and hypothyroidism after lithium treatment. Br Med J (Clin Res) 290 (6467):516, 1985.
5. Salata R, Klein I: Effects of lithium on the endocrine system: a review. J Lab Clin Med 110 (2):130, 1987.
6. Ohzeki T, Igarashi T, Okamoto A: Familial cases of congenital nephrogenic diabetes insipidus type II: re-

markable increment of urinary adenosine 31,51-mon-
ophosphate in response to antidiuretic hormone. J
Pediatr 104 (4):593, 1984.

7. Moses AM, Scheinman SJ, Oppenheim A: Marked
hypotonic polyuria resulting from nephrogenic diabetes
insipidus with partial sensitivity to vasopressin. J Clin
Endocrinol Metab 59 (6):1044, 1984.
8. Ford SM Jr, Lumpkin HL III: Transient nasopressin-
resistant diabetes insipidus of pregnancy. Obstet Gynecol 68 (5):726, 1986.
9. Czernichow P, Pomarede R, Basmaciogullari A, et al:
Diabetes insipidus in children. III. Anterior pituitary
dysfunction in idiopathic types. J Pediatr 106 (1):41,
1985.
10. Blackett PR, Seif SM, Altmiller DH, Robinson AG:
Familial central diabetes insipidus: vasopressin and nicotine stimulated neurophysin deficiency with subnormal
oxytocin and estrogen stimulated neurophysin. Am J
Med Sci 286 (3):42, 1983.
11. Toth EL, Bowen PA, Crockford PM: Hereditary central
diabetes insipidus: plasma levels of antidiuretic hormone in a family with a possible osmoreceptor defect.
Can Med Assoc J 131 (10):1237, 1984.
12. Najjar SS, Saikaly MG, Zaytoun GM, Abdelnoor A:
Association of diabetes insipidus, diabetes mellitus, optic
atrophy, and deafness. The Wolfram or DIDMOAD
syndrome. Arch Dis Child 60 (9):823, 1985.
13. Hadani M, Findler G, Shaked I, Sahar A: Unusual
delayed onset of diabetes insipidus following closed
head trauma. Case report. J Neurosurg 63 (3):456,
1985.
14. Edwards OM, Clark JD: Post-traumatic hypopituitarism.
Six cases and a review of the literature. Medicine 65
(5):281, 1986.
15. Jialal I, Desai RK, Rajput MC: An assessment of posterior pituitary function in patients with Sheehan's
syndrome. Clin Endocrinol 27 (1):91, 1987.
16. Bakiri F, Benmiloud M: Antidiuretic function in Sheehan's syndrome. Br Med J (Clin Res) 289 (6445):579,
1984.
17. Baskin DS, Wilson CB: Surgical management of cran-
iopharyngiomas. A review of 74 cases. J Neurosurg 65
(1):22, 1986.
18. Jennings MT, Gelman R, Hochberg R: Intracranial
germ-cell tumors: natural history and pathogenesis. J
Neurosurg 63 (2):155, 1985.
19. Sherwood MC, Stanhope R, Preece MA, Grant DB:
Diabetes insipidus and occult intracranial tumours. Arch
Dis Child 61 (12):1222, 1986.
20. Branch CL Jr, Laws ER Jr: Metastatic tumors of the
sella turcica masquerading as primary pituitary tumors.
J Clin Endocrinol Metab 65 (3):469, 1987.
21. Juan D, Hsu SD, Hunter J: Case report of vasopressin-
responsive diabetes insipidus associated with chronic
myelogenous leukemia. Cancer 56 (6):1468, 1985.
22. Yap H-Y, Tashima CK, Blumenschein GR, et al: Diabetes insipidus and breast cancer. Arch Intern Med
139:1009, 1979.
23. Krol TC, Wood WS: Bronchogenic carcinoma and
diabetes insipidus: case report and review. Cancer
49:596, 1982.

24. Badon SJ, Ansell J, Smith TW, et al: Diabetes insipidus caused by extramedullary hematopoiesis. Am J Clin Pathol 83 (4):509, 1985.
25. Hocking WG, Swanson M: Multifocal eosinophilic granuloma. Response of a patient to etoposide. Cancer 58 (4):840, 1986.
26. Dean HJ, Bishop A, Winter JS: Growth hormone deficiency in patients with histiocytosis X. J Pediatr 109 (4):615, 1986.
27. Hurst NP, Dunn NA, Chalmers TM: Wegener's granulomatosis complicated by diabetes insipidus. Ann Rheum Dis 42:600, 1983.
28. Zijlstra F, Killinger D, Volpe R: Diabetes insipidus associated with dysplastic pancytopenia. Am J Med 82 (2):339, 1987.
29. Katz VL, Bowes WA Jr: Transient diabetes insipidus and preeclampsia. South Med J 80 (4):524, 1987.
30. van der Weiden RM, Visser W, Peeters LL, et al: Transient diabetes insipidus of pregnancy. Eur J Obstet Gynecol Reprod Biol 25 (4):331, 1987.
31. Halebian P, Yurt R, Petito C, Shires GT: Diabetes insipidus after carbon monoxide poisoning and smoke inhalation. J Trauma 25 (7):662, 1985.
32. Kuan P, Messenger JC, Ellestad MH: Transient central diabetes insipidus after aortocoronary bypass operations. Am J Cardiol 52 (10):1181, 1983.

Selected Readings

Colombo N, Berry I, Kucharczyk J, et al: Posterior pituitary gland: appearance on MR images in normal and pathologic states. Radiology 165 (2):481, 1987.
High-resolution MRI studies of the sella turcica in 200 subjects with a normal or abnormal sella were analyzed. It was determined that the T_1-weighted high signal intensity region of the neurohypophysis is useful in evaluating the functional status of the hypothalamic-hypophyseal axis.

Durr JA: Diabetes insipidus in pregnancy. Am J Kidney Dis 9 (4):276, 1987.
Article reviews the different forms of diabetes insipidus peculiar to pregnancy.

Greger NG, Kirkland RT, Clayton GW, Kirkland JL: Central diabetes insipidus. 22 years' experience. Am J Dis Child 140 (6):551, 1986.
The etiology of diabetes insipidus was determined in 73 children evaluated from 1962 through 1983. Etiologies in descending order of frequency included preoperative and postoperative intracranial tumors, infection, histiocytosis, and idiopathic.

Meanock CI, Turner GF, Smythe PJ, et al: Fluid balance and secretion of antidiuretic hormone following transsphenoidal pituitary surgery. A preliminary series. J Neurosurg 63 (3):404, 1985.
Delayed hyponatremia appears to occur most often in patients with hypoadrenalism, as glucocorticoid coverage is decreased.

Milles JJ, Spruce B, Baylis PH: A comparison of diagnostic methods to differentiate diabetes insipidus from primary polyuria: a review of 21 patients. Acta Endocrinol 104:410, 1983.

Majority of polyuric patients can be diagnosed by properly performed dehydration tests outlined in this study.

Puig ML, Webb SM, Del Pozo C, et al: Endocrine aspects of pituitary stalk enlargement. Clin Endocrinol (Oxf) 27 (1):25, 1987.

Four patients with various endocrine deficiencies of a predominantly hypothalamic nature are described and in whom CT scans demonstrated pituitary stalk enlargement.

Seckl JR, Dunger DB, Lightman SL: Neurohypophyseal peptide function during early postoperative diabetes insipidus. Brain 110:737, 1987.

Early postoperative diabetes insipidus is not due to decreased levels of circulating arginine vasopressin, but may be related to the release of biologically inactive precursors from the damaged neurohypophysis.

94

Hypertension: Renovascular and Other Secondary Causes

Although essential or primary hypertension accounts for about 90% of all hypertension,[1] renal and endocrine disorders account for most of the secondary and potentially curable causes. Certain clinical factors present an increased probability of finding secondary causes, such as (1) patients of any age with accelerated or malignant hypertension, (2) hypertension resistant to treatment, (3) new onset hypertension in patients over 50 years of age, and (4) young patients under 35 years of age with severe hypertension.[2]

Renal Causes of Hypertension

Hypertension secondary to renal disease can be caused by renovascular or renal parenchymal disease. The renin-angiotensin system is also a significant factor in the pathogenesis of renovascular hypertension.[3] Renovascular hypertension is more common in hypertensive children than in hypertensive adults.[4] In most patients with a renal cause for hypertension, the initial evaluation will reveal abnormalities in the urine and/or rapid-sequence intravenous urography. The initial distinction is between renal parenchymal and occlusive renal arterial disease.[2]

Renovascular causes[5,6]: the diagnosis of renovascular hypertension not only may identify a curable source of hypertension, but also lead to the prevention of renal ischemia and preserve renal function.[3]
Atherosclerosis and thromboembolic disease
Fibromuscular dysplasia[7]
Ehlers-Danlos syndrome: renovascular hypertension due to renal arterial aneurysms[8]
Takayasu's disease: lesions of the thoracoabdominal aorta[9]
Neurofibromatosis: renal vascular lesions
Middle aortic syndrome: occurs as severe hypertension in young patients with diffuse narrowing of distal thoracic and abdominal aorta, which can involve visceral and renal arteries[10]
Turner syndrome
Glomerular and tubular dysfunction: glomerulonephritis,[11] chronic nephritis, connective tissue disease, diabetic glomerulosclerosis,[12] arteritis, polycystic kidney, interstitial nephritis, chronic renal failure
Renal collecting system dysfunction: hydronephrosis, reflux nephropathy[13]
Renal trauma
Renin-producing tumors[3]: renin oversecretion has been observed in malignant neoplasms, such as Wilms' tumor, renal carcinoma, pulmonary carcinoma, pancreatic adenocarcinoma; and in benign tumors, such as hemangiopericytomas[14] of the renin-producing juxtaglomerular cells and ovarian tumors.[15]
Renal infection: tuberculosis[16]

Endocrine Causes of Hypertension

There are distinct hypertensive syndromes related to excessive hormone production, most of which are related to excessive adrenal hormone production. Other endocrine disorders that have a higher incidence of hypertension are without well-defined mechanisms to explain the associated hypertension.

Adrenal disorders[17,18]: Cushing's syndrome,[19] primary aldosteronism, congenital adrenal hyperplasia, adrenal adenomas, pheochromocytoma,[20,21] adrenocortical carcinoma,[22] primary reninisms (see renin-producing tumors above).
Thyroid dysfunction: hyperthyroidism
Acromegaly
Hyperparathyroidism[23]

Drugs That Can Cause Hypertension

Corticosteroids: prolonged administration[24]
Mineralocorticoids[25]
Salt loading[26,27]
Sympathomimetics: albuterol, amphetamine, dobutamine, dopamine, epinephrine, phenylpropanolamine hydrochloride (in over-the-counter preparations for colds and appetite suppression), isoetharine, isoproterenol, methoxamine, norepinephrine, phenylephrine, terbutaline, and tyramine
Angiotensin
Antidiuretic hormone
Monoamine oxidase inhibitors and tyramine-containing foods, e.g., cheese, beer, or red wine
Anesthetics: local and general
Licorice[28]: causing pseudoaldosteronism
Oral contraceptive agents[29,30]
Alcohol[31]
Disulfiram[32]
Cyclosporine[33]
Nonsteroidal anti-inflammatory drugs (NSAIDs): associated with fluid retention
Abrupt discontinuation of antihypertensives: beta-blockers,[34,35] clondine

Miscellaneous Causes of Hypertension

Hyperdynamic circulation disorders: usually cause predominantly systolic hypertension, such as aortic insufficiency, arteriovenous fistula, patent ductus arteriosus, Paget's disease, beriberi, physiologic responses to noxious stimuli, and burns
Obesity[36,37]: when the sphygmomanometer cuff is too small for an obese arm, blood pressure measurements can be spuriously high; conversely, if the sphygmomanometer cuff is too large, blood pressure measurements can be spuriously low.
Aortic coarctation and other anomalies of the descending aorta

Pregnancy[38]: preeclampsia, eclampsia
Increased intracranial pressure: particularly posterior fossa masses, such as cerebellar tumors, basilar artery aneurysm, and cerebrovascular infarction with edema
Arterial rigidity[39]
Smoking[40,41]
Normal activities[42]: e.g., sleep, exercise
Renal transplantation[43]
Hemangioblastoma of the cervicomedullary junction: neurogenic hypertension produced by involving the tractus solitarius in the medulla[44]

References

1. Davidman M, Opsahl J: Mechanisms of elevated blood pressure in human essential hypertension. Med Clin North Am 68:301, 1984.
2. Bravo EL: Secondary hypertension. A streamlined approach to diagnosis. Postgrad Med 80 (1):139, 1986.
3. Bravo EL: Clinical aspects of endocrine hypertension. Med Clin North Am 71 (5):907, 1987.
4. Tapper D, Brand T, Hickman R: Early diagnosis and management of renovascular hypertension. Am J Surg 153:495, 1987.
5. Simon G, Limas CC, Miller RP: Renovascular hypertension with unilateral atherosclerotic renal artery occlusion: diagnostic use of renal vein renins. Angiology 33:728, 1982.
6. Mahler F, Probst P, Haertel M, et al: Lasting improvement of renovascular hypertension by transluminal dilatation of atherosclerotic and nonatherosclerotic renal artery stenoses. A follow-up study. Circulation 65:611, 1982.
7. Lüscher TF, Lie JT, Stanson AW, et al: Arterial fibromuscular dysplasia. Mayo Clin Proc 62:931, 1987.
8. Lüscher TF, Essandoh LK, Lie JT, et al: Renovascular hypertension: a rare cardiovascular manifestation of the Ehlers-Danlos syndrome. Mayo Clin Proc 62:223, 1987.
9. Lagneau P, Michel JB, Vuong PN: Surgical treatment of Takayasu's disease. Ann Surg 205 (2):157, 1987.
10. Messina LM, Reilly LM, Goldstone J, et al: Middle aortic syndrome. Effectiveness and durability of complex arterial revascularization techniques. Ann Surg 204 (3):331, 1986.
11. Danielson H, Kornerup HJ, Olsen S, et al: Arterial hypertension in chronic glomerulonephritis. An analysis of 310 cases. Clin Nephrol 19:284, 1983.
12. Hostetter TH, Rennke HG, Brenner BM: The case for intrarenal hypertension in the initiation and progression of diabetic and other glomerulopathies. Am J Med 72:375, 1982.
13. Savage JM, Koh CT, Shah V, et al: Five year prospective study of plasma renin activity and blood pressure in patients with longstanding reflux nephropathy. Arch Dis Child 62 (7):678, 1987.

14. Pedrinelli R, Graziadei L, Taddei S, et al: A renin-secreting tumor. Nephron 46 (4):380, 1987.
15. Korzets A, Nouriel H, Steiner Z, et al: Resistant hypertension associated with a renin-producing ovarian Sertoli cell tumor. Am J Clin Pathol 85 (2):242, 1986.
16. Kelly JF, Atkinson AB, Adgey AA: Renal tuberculosis and accelerated hypertension: the use of renal vein renin sampling to predict the outcome after nephrectomy. Int J Cardiol 16 (3):318, 1987.
17. Reid IA: The renin-angiotensin system and body function. Arch Intern Med 145:1475, 1985.
18. Hollenberg NK, Moore T, Shoback D, et al: Abnormal renal sodium handling in essential hypertension. Relation to failure of renal and adrenal modulation of responses to angiotensin II. Am J Med 81:412, 1986.
19. Saruta T, Suzuki H, Handa M, et al: Multiple factors contribute to the pathogenesis of hypertension in Cushing's syndrome. J Clin Endocrinol Metab 62:275, 1986.
20. Manger WM, Gifford RW Jr: Hypertension secondary to pheochromocytoma. Bull NY Acad Med 58:139, 1982.
21. Krane NK: Clinically unsuspected pheochromocytomas. Experience at Henry Ford Hospital and a review of the literature. Arch Intern Med 146 (1):54, 1986.
22. Hamper UM, Fishman EK, Hartman DS, et al: Primary adrenocortical carcinoma: sonographic evaluation with clinical and pathologic correlation in 26 patients. AJR 148 (5):915, 1987.
23. Daniels J, Goodman AD: Hypertension and hyperparathyroidism. Inverse relation of serum phosphate level and blood pressure. Am J Med 75:17, 1983.
24. Nashel DJ: Is atherosclerosis a complication of long-term corticosteroid treatment? Am J Med 80:925, 1986.
25. Holland OB, Gomez-Sanchez C: Mineralocorticoids and hypertension. Am J Nephrol 3:156, 1983.
26. Hunt JC: Sodium intake and hypertension: a cause for concern. Ann Intern Med 98:724, 1983.
27. Houston MC: Sodium and hypertension. A review. Arch Intern Med 146 (1):179, 1986.
28. Beretta-Piccoli C, Salvade G, Crivelli PL, et al: Body-sodium and blood volume in a patient with licorice-induced hypertension. J Hypertens 3:19, 1985.
29. Khaw KT, Peart WS: Blood pressure and contraceptive use. Br Med J 285:403, 1982.
30. Stadel BV: Oral contraceptives and cardiovascular disease. (Two parts). N Engl J Med 305:612; 305:672, 1981.
31. Friedman GD, Klatsky AL, Siegelaub AB: Alcohol intake and hypertension. Ann Intern Med 98:846, 1983.
32. Volicer L, Nelson KL: Development of reversible hypertension during disulfiram therapy. Arch Intern Med 144:1294, 1984.
33. Myers BD, Ross J, Newton L, et al: Cyclosporine-associated chronic nephropathy. N Engl J Med 311:699, 1984.
34. Shand DG, Wood AJJ: Propranolol withdrawal syndrome—why? (editorial). Circulation 58:202, 1978.
35. Rangno RE: Propranolol withdrawal. Practical considerations (editorial). Arch Intern Med 141:161, 1981.

36. Lavie CJ, Messerli FH: Cardiovascular adaptation to obesity and hypertension. Chest 90:275, 1986.
37. Havlik RJ, Hubert HB, Fabsitz RR, et al: Weight and hypertension. Ann Intern Med 98:855, 1983.
38. Lindheimer MD, Katz AI: Hypertension in pregnancy. N Engl J Med 313:675, 1985.
39. Kannel WB, Wolf PA, McGee DL, et al: Systolic blood pressure, arterial rigidity, and risk of stroke. The Framingham study. JAMA 245:1225, 1981.
40. Baer L, Radichevich I: Cigarette smoking in hypertensive patients. Blood pressure and endocrine responses. Am J Med 78:564, 1985.
41. Green MS, Jucha E, Luz Y: Blood pressure in smokers and nonsmokers: epidemiologic findings. Am Heart J 111:932, 1986.
42. Pickering TG, Harshfield GA, Kleinert HD, et al: Blood pressure during normal daily activities, sleep and exercise. Comparison of values in normal and hypertensive subjects. JAMA 247:992, 1982.
43. Curtis JJ, Luke RG, Jones PJ, et al: Hypertension after successful renal transplantation. Am J Med 79:193, 1985.
44. Sanford RA, Smith RA: Hemangioblastoma of the cervicomedullary junction. Report of three cases. J Neurosurg 64 (2):317, 1986.

Selected Readings

Breslau NA: Update on secondary forms of hyperparathyroidism. Am J Med Sci 294 (2):120, 1987.
Emerging evidence has suggested a role for secondary hyperparathyroidism in the development of certain forms of hypertension and osteoporosis.

Criqui MH: Epidemiology of atherosclerosis: an updated overview. Am J Cardiol 57 (5):18C, 1986.
Ongoing epidemiologic research continues to provide new insight into the multifactorial etiology of atherosclerosis and coronary artery disease.

Dzau VJ: Implications of local angiotensin production in cardiovascular physiology and pharmacology. Am J Cardiol 59 (2):59A, 1987.
The traditional concept of the renin-angiotensin system is a circulation-borne endocrine system whose components are secreted by different organs. Recent data, however, demonstrate that renin and angiotensin are synthesized locally in many tissues. This concept has important implications to our understanding of cardiovascular homeostasis.

Ferguson JJ III, Randall OS: Systolic, diastolic, and combined hypertension. Differences between groups. Arch Intern Med 146 (6):1090, 1986.
In a study involving 182 consecutive outpatients for whom no secondary cause of hypertension could be found, there were significant differences in age, with the systolic group being the oldest and the diastolic group the youngest, and differences in the prevalence of complications among the categories. Peripheral vascular disease, retinopathy, and coronary artery disease were more prevalent in the systolic and combined groups, whereas diabetes was more prevalent in the systolic group.

Genest J, Cantin M: Atrial natriuretic factor. Circulation 75:I118, 1987.

A short and up-to-date review on the great advances made in the field of the atrial natriuretic factor.

Houston M: Hypertensive emergencies and urgencies: pathophysiology and clinical aspects. Am Heart J 111:205, 1986.
Discussion of guidelines to assist clinicians in determining the most appropriate therapeutic approach for each patient.

Houston MC: Sodium and hypertension. A review. Arch Intern Med 146:179, 1986.
Abnormal sodium metabolism may play a critical role in the cause of certain types of hypertension, particularly salt-sensitive hypertension.

Kaplan NM, Meese RB: The calcium deficiency hypothesis of hypertension: a critique. Ann Intern Med 105:947, 1986.
A critique examining the hypothesis that primary hypertension is related to calcium deficiency.

McCarron DA, Morris CD, Bukoski R: The calcium paradox of essential hypertension. Am J Med 82 (1B):27, 1987.
The complex interrelationships between calcium metabolism and essential hypertension are discussed in this review.

McRae RP Jr, Liebson PR: Hypertensive crisis. Med Clin North Am 70:749, 1986.
The necessity of prompt recognition of hypertensive crisis is discussed.

Messerli FH, Garavaglia GE, Schmieder RE, et al: Disparate cardiovascular findings in men and women with essential hypertension. Ann Intern Med 107 (2):158, 1987.
This study found that any level of arterial pressure, total peripheral resistance, and, therefore, the risk of hypertensive cardiovascular disease was lower in women than in men. They conclude that premenopausal women are hemodynamically younger than men of the same chronologic age.

Pickering TG: Pathophysiology of systemic hypertension. Am J Cardiol 58:12D, 1986.
Review of the different mechanisms that cause hypertension.

Sinclair AM, Isles CG, Brown I, et al: Secondary hypertension in a blood pressure clinic. Arch Intern Med 147:1289, 1987.
This study concluded that an investigation of hypertension for an underlying cause is likely to yield occasional patients who can be cured of their hypertension and a moderate number with irreversible renal disease who are at particularly high risk for heart attack and stroke.

Tuck ML: The sympathetic nervous system in essential hypertension. Am Heart J 112:877, 1986.
Review of the postulate that enhanced activity of the sympathetic nervous system could contribute to essential hypertension.

95
Metabolic Acidosis: Primary Disturbances and Etiologic Agents

Metabolic acidosis is the result of excess acid or insufficient base. The clinical presentation of metabolic acidosis includes a wide spectrum of nonspecific signs and symptoms that range from asymptomatic or hyperventilation seen in mild acidosis to dramatic, deep, rapid, Kussmaul breathing, which can occur with stupor and coma in severe cases of metabolic acidosis. Laboratory values that reflect increased hydrogen ion production, such as decreased bicarbonate, decreased arterial pH, decreased arterial PCO_2 (reflecting compensatory hyperventilation) lead to the diagnosis. Both clinical and laboratory manifestations of metabolic acidosis may be masked by initial respiratory and renal compensatory mechanisms. Nonvolatile acid retention and excessive loss of bicarbonate are the most common pathophysiologic mechanisms that produce metabolic acidosis.

Hyperchloremic or Normal Anion Gap Metabolic Acidosis

Hyperchloremic acidosis results when bicarbonate wasting is accompanied by retention of chloride, such as can be seen in gastrointestinal loss of bicarbonate, advanced renal failure, and primary and drug-induced renal tubular acidosis.

Medical disorders
    Diarrhea: VIPoma syndrome[1]
    Ureterosigmoidostomy
    Small bowel[2] or pancreatic fistula
    Interstitial renal disease
    Renal tubular acidosis
    Dehydration
    Hyperalimentation[3]: concurrent use of potassium-sparing diuretics may increase the risk of developing acidosis.[4]
    Pseudohypoaldosteronism[5]
    Drug-induced

Arginine hydrochloride
Lysine hydrochloride
Ammonium chloride
Anion exchange resins
Carbonic anhydrase inhibitors: acetazolamide
Amphotericin B: causes renal tubular acidosis
Tetracycline: outdated
Mercaptopurine
Sulfanilamide
Potassium chloride during fasting state[6]

Increased Undetermined Anion Metabolic Acidosis

Endogenous and exogenous sources of hydrogen ion cause metabolic acidosis. Conditions that cause excessive lactic and ketoacid production are common associations, such as anoxic states and diabetic ketoacidosis. Drug associations are common, particularly the alcohols (ethanol, methanol, isopropanol, ethylene glycol), which are important causes of poisoning, reflecting the widespread availability in aftershave lotion, brake fluid, antifreeze fluid, model fuel, mouthwash, rubbing alcohol, and other products.[7]

Medical disorders
  Diabetic ketoacidosis: most common cause of death in juvenile-onset diabetics[8]
  Inborn errors of metabolism: galactosemia, hereditary fructose intolerance, hyperglobulinemia, cystinosis
  Acute and chronic renal: uremic acidosis
  Conditions associated with excessive lactic acidosis: hypoxemia, anemia, leukemia, pancreatitis, pregnancy, shock,[9] hepatic cirrhosis, Kearns-Sayre syndrome,[10] severe exercise[11]
  Starvation
  Cholera: hyperproteinemia, lactic acidemia, and hyperphosphatemia contribute to severe acidosis, with an increased anion gap in severe cholera.[12]
Drug-induced
  Alcoholic keotacidosis: frequently encountered metabolic disturbance after prolonged ethanol intake and a brief duration of abstinence.[13-15]
  Methanol: methanol poisoning is characterized by a latent period with subsequent blindness and metabolic acidosis with and without an anion gap.[16]

Ethylene glycol intoxication: serum and urine levels of glycolic acid correlate with clinical symptoms and mortality.[17-20]

Salicylate intoxication: salicylates can stimulate or depress respiratory centers, as well as impair oxidative metabolism, resulting in severe mixed acid-base disturbances and associated electrolyte abnormalities.[21]

Paraldehyde poisoning

Phenformin[22]

Hydrofluoric acid exposure[23]

Isoniazid overdose[24]

Ibuprofen overdose[25]

Sodium azide poisoning[26]

Sublimed (inorganic) sulfur ingestion: present in persistently used folk remedies[27]

Chloramphenicol toxicity[28]

References

1. Krejs GJ: VIPoma syndrome. Am J Med 82:37, 1987.
2. Caprilli R, Frieri G, Latella G, et al: Electrolyte and acid base imbalance in patients with rectosigmoid bladder. J Urol 135:148, 1986.
3. Kushner RF: Total parenteral nutrition-associated metabolic acidosis. J Parenter Enteral Nutr 10 (3):306, 1986.
4. Kushner RF, Sitrin MD: Metabolic acidosis. Development in two patients receiving a potassium-sparing diuretic and total parenteral nutrition. Arch Intern Med 146:343, 1986.
5. Travis PS, Cushner HM: Mineralocorticoid-induced kaliuresis in type-II pseudohypoaldosteronism. Am J Med Sci 292:235, 1986.
6. Leiter LA, Josse RG, West ML, Halperin ML: Severe metabolic acidosis induced in a patient during fasting by KCl administration. Clin Invest Med 11:266, 1988.
7. Litovitz T: The alcohols: ethanol, methanol, isopropanol, ethylene glycol. Pediatr Clin North Am 33:311, 1986.
8. Krane EJ: Diabetic ketoacidosis. Biochemistry, physiology, treatment, and prevention. Pediatr Clin North Am 34:935, 1987.
9. Vogel GE: The patient in shock—clinical picture and pathophysiology. Endoscopy 18 (Suppl 2):1, 1986.
10. Curless RG, Flynn J, Bachynski B, et al: Fatal metabolic acidosis, hyperglycemia, and coma after steroid therapy for Kearns-Sayre syndrome. Neurology 36:872, 1986.
11. Wasserman K: The anaerobic threshold: definition, physiological significance, and identification. Adv Cardiol 35:1, 1986.
12. Wang F, Butler T, Rabbani GH, Jones PK: The acidosis of cholera. Contributions of hyperproteinemia, lactic acidemia, and hyperphosphatemia to an increased serum anion gap. N Engl J Med 315:1591, 1986.

13. Duffens K, Marx JA: Alcoholic ketoacidosis—a review. J Emerg Med 5:399, 1987.
14. Eiser AR: The effects of alcohol on renal function and excretion. Alcoholism (NY) 11:127, 1987.
15. Bacq Y, Constans T, Lamisse F: Alcoholic acidoketosis. Gastroenterol Clin Biol 11:293, 1987.
16. Palmisano J, Gruver C, Adams ND: Absence of anion gap metabolic acidosis in severe methanol poisoning: a case report and review of the literature. Am J Kidney Dis 9:441, 1987.
17. Gabow PA, Clay K, Sullivan JB, Lepoff R: Organic acids in ethylene glycol intoxication. Ann Intern Med 105:16, 1986.
18. Hewlett TP, McMartin KE, Lauro AJ, Ragan FA Jr: Ethylene glycol poisoning. The value of glycolic acid determinations for diagnosis and treatment. J Toxicol Clin Toxicol 24:389, 1986.
19. Rambourg-Schepens MO, Buffet M, Bertault R, et al: Severe ethylene glycol butyl ether poisoning. Kinetics and metabolic pattern. Hum Toxicol 7:187, 1988.
20. Jacobsen D, Hewlett TP, Webb R, et al: Ethylene glycol intoxication: evaluation of kinetics and crystalluria. Am J Med 84:145, 1988.
21. Meredith TJ, Vale JA: Non-narcotic analgesics. Problems of overdosage. Drugs 32 (Suppl 4):177, 1986.
22. Misbin RI: Phenformin-associated lactic acidosis: pathogenesis and treatment. Ann Intern Med 87:591, 1977.
23. Chan KM, Svancarek WP, Creer M: Fatality due to acute hydrofluoric acid exposure. J Toxicol Clin Toxicol 25:333, 1987.
24. Blanchard PD, Yao JD, McAlpine DE, Hurt RD: Isoniazid overdose in the Cambodian population of Olmstead County, Minnesota. JAMA 256:3131, 1986.
25. Lee CY, Finkler A: Acute intoxication due to ibuprofen overdose. Arch Pathol Lab Med 110:747, 1986.
26. Albertson TE, Reed S, Siefkin A: A case of fatal sodium azide ingestion. J Toxicol Clin Toxicol 24:339, 1986.
27. Schwartz SM, Carroll HM, Scharschmidt LA: Sublimed (inorganic) sulfur ingestion. A cause of life-threatening metabolic acidosis with a high anion gap. Arch Intern Med 146:1437, 1986.
28. Evans LS, Kleiman MB: Acidosis as a presenting feature of chloramphenicol toxicity. J Pediatr 108:475, 1986.

Selected Readings

Atkinson DE, Bourke E: Metabolic aspects of the regulation of systemic pH. Am J Physiol 252:F947, 1987.
A review of current concepts.

Batlle DC, von Riotte A, Schlueter W: Urinary sodium in the evaluation of hyperchloremic metabolic acidosis. N Engl J Med 316:140, 1987.
Authors conclude that the diagnosis of distal renal tubular acidosis cannot be made solely on the basis of the urinary pH response to acidemia. The urinary sodium level should be known before this diagnosis is considered in patients with unexplained hyperchloremic metabolic acidosis.

Ebie N, Ryan W, Harris J: Metabolic emergencies in cancer medicine. Med Clin North Am 70:1151, 1986.

This article describes the many metabolic complications encountered in the management of cancer patients. Pathogenic mechanisms and therapy are discussed, with special emphasis on hypercalcemia, the most common of these disorders.

Goldstein MB, Bear R, Richardson RM, et al: The urine anion gap: a clinically useful index of ammonium excretion. Am J Med Sci 292:198, 1986.

In patients with a normal plasma anion gap type of metabolic acidosis, knowledge of the rate of ammonium excretion can provide valuable information to determine if there is a renal cause for the disorder. Data are presented that demonstrate a direct linear relationship between the urine anion gap and the urine ammonium concentration. The applications of this index of ammonium excretion are discussed.

Halperin ML, Margolis BL, Robinson LA, et al: The urine osmolal gap: a clue to estimate urine ammonium in "hybrid" types of metabolic acidosis. Clin Invest Med 11;198, 1988.

The urine osmolal gap defined as the difference between urine osmolality and the sum of the concentrations of sodium, potassium, chloride, bicarbonate, urea, and glucose is normally 80 to 100 mOsm/kg water. This article discusses the usefulness of the urine osmolal gap in ascertaining the etiology of metabolic acidosis, which is of the mixed wide and normal anion gap or hybrid type of metabolic acidosis.

Miller PJ, Wenzel RP: Etiologic organisms as independent predictors of death and morbidity associated with bloodstream infections. J Infect Dis 156:471, 1987.

Authors studied 385 episodes of nosocomial bloodstream infections occurring over 45 months to ascertain if the etiologic organisms were independent predictors of death and morbidity. Independent predictors of death included respiratory failure, oliguria, metabolic acidosis, hypotension, increased age, antibiotic therapy in cases where susceptibility data were unknown, and infection with Pseudomonas aeruginosa.

Perez GO, Oster JR, Rogers A: Acid-base disturbances in gastrointestinal disease. Dig Dis Sci 32:1033, 1987.

Authors review the most important types of metabolic alkalosis and metabolic acidosis associated with gastrointestinal disorders, excluding liver disease. Special emphasis is placed on pathophysiologic mechanisms.

Vale JA, Meredith TJ: Acute poisoning due to nonsteroidal anti-inflammatory drugs. Clinical features and management. Med Toxicol 1:12, 1986.

An increased incidence of acute poisoning from NSAIDs can be expected. Unless they are ingested in substantial overdose, acute poisoning does not usually result in significant morbidity or mortality. In most cases, the clinical features are mild and confined to the gastrointestinal and central nervous systems, although acute renal failure, hepatic dysfunction, respiratory depression, coma, convulsions, cardiovascular collapse, and cardiac arrest may complicate severe poisoning.

Ventriglia WJ: Arterial blood gases. Emerg Med Clin North Am 4:235, 1986.

This article discusses the physiology, analysis, and interpretation of arterial blood gas.

96
Metabolic Alkalosis: Primary Disturbances and Etiologic Agents

Metabolic alkalosis reflects a deficit of hydrogen ions and an excess of bicarbonate. Clinical signs are nonspecific and are more likely to reflect concurrent electrolyte abnormalities, particularly of sodium, potassium, and calcium. Neuromuscular irritability, weakness, and even tetany can be manifestations of metabolic alkalosis, particularly if hypocalcemia is also present.

Appropriate diagnosis and management of metabolic alkalosis begins by answering two questions: (1) what caused the alkalosis and (2) what renal mechanism maintains it?[1] Common generators of metabolic alkalosis include vomiting, diarrhea, hyperaldosteronism (exogenous and endogenous), diuretics, and other iatrogenic causes such as nasogastric suction. When normal kidneys receive a bicarbonate load, a bicarbonate diuresis results, which maintains a normal level of blood bicarbonate. However, under certain conditions, the kidney will retain bicarbonate and raise the serum bicarbonate. Examples of conditions that cause renal-bicarbonate retention include hypochloremia, hypokalemia, and hypermineralocorticoidism.

Medical Disorders

Vomiting: particularly with significant volume depletion

Surreptitious vomiting: severe hypokalemia and metabolic alkalosis can be seen in patients who practice self-induced vomiting as part of a weight reduction technique.[2]

Nasogastric suction

Chloride-wasting diarrhea

Villous adenoma of the colon

Posthypercapnia: compensatory hypoventilation[3]

Hyperaldosteronism

Cushing's syndrome: pituitary, adrenal or ectopic ACTH

Bartter's[4] and pseudo-Bartter's syndrome[5]

Refeeding alkalosis

Severe potassium deficit: it is uncertain whether a potassium deficit alone, without coexisting known alkalosis-producing conditions, can sustain metabolic alkalosis.[6]

Chloride deficit

Munchausen syndrome: surreptitious vomiting,[1] sodium bicarbonate abuse,[7] laxative abuse,[8] and diuretic abuse[4]

Hypoproteinemia: hypoproteinemia by itself can cause a metabolic alkalosis.[9]

Alcoholism: both respiratory and metabolic alkalosis are frequently seen in alcoholics.[10]

Cystic fibrosis[11,12]

Drug and Other Iatrogenic Causes

Diuretic therapy: patients with hepatic insufficiency and ascites are at risk for metabolic alkalosis, when ascites is treated with diuretics.[13]

Carbenicillin or penicillin

Glucocorticoid and mineralocorticoid administration: corticosteroid-induced metabolic alkalemia is particularly important to recognize in the intensive care units because many patients compensate with alveolar hypoventilation.[14]

Licorice ingestion: secondary to mineralocorticoid excess syndrome

Carbenoxolone

Capreomycin[15]

Alkali ingestion: may be in the form of antacids, such as aluminum hydroxide, magnesium hydroxide, neutral phosphates[16,17]

Intravenous phosphate or sulfate salts administration: sodium-depleted patients particularly at risk

Plasmapheresis: large sodium citrate loads, particularly in patients with decreased renal function, can cause metabolic alkalosis[18]

Hemodialysis: reported in two patients requiring high infusion rates of citrate while mechanically ventilated[19]

References

1. Cogan MG, Liu F-Y, Berger BE, et al: Metabolic alkalosis. Med Clin North Am 67:903, 1983.
2. Richardson RM, Forbath N, Karanicolas S: Hypoka-

lemic metabolic alkalosis caused by surreptitious vomiting: report of four cases. Can Med Assoc J 129:142, 1983.
3. Lavie CJ, Crocker EF Jr, Key KJ, Ferguson TG: Marked hypochloremic metabolic alkalosis with severe compensatory hypoventilation. South Med J 79:1296, 1986.
4. Yabe R, Mizuno K, Ojima M, et al: A case of 21-hydroxylase deficiency and Bartter's syndrome associated with a balanced 6-9 translocation. Nippon Naibunpi Gakkai Zasshi 62 (8):843, 1986.
5. Sasaki H, Kawasaki T, Yamamoto T, et al: Pseudo-Bartter's syndrome induced by surreptitious ingestion of furosemide to lose weight: a case report and possible pathophysiology. Nippon Naibunpi Gakkai Zasshi 62 (8):867, 1986.
6. Hernandez RE, Schambelan M, Cogan MG, et al: Dietary NaCl determines severity of potassium depletion-induced metabolic alkalosis. Kidney Int 31:1356, 1987.
7. Linford SM, James HD: Sodium bicarbonate abuse: a case report. Br J Psychiatry 149:502, 1986.
8. Adam O, Goebel FD: Secondary gout and pseudo-Bartter syndrome in females with laxative abuse. Klin Wochenschr 65:833, 1987.
9. McAuliffe JJ, Lind LJ, Leith DE, Fencl V: Hypoproteinemic alkalosis. Am J Med 81:86, 1986.
10. Pitts TO, Van Thiel DH: Disorders of the serum electrolytes, acid-base balance, and renal function in alcoholism. Recent Dev Alcohol 4:311, 1986.
11. Arnold WC, Warren RH: Clinical incidence and causes of metabolic alkalosis in children. J Arkansas Med Soc 80:186, 1983.
12. Munoz AI, Rodriguez A, Jimenez JF: Cystic fibrosis of the pancreas presenting as metabolic alkalosis. Bol Asoc Med PR 75:230, 1983.
13. Oster JR, Perez GO: Acid-base disturbances in liver disease. J Hepatol 2:299, 1986.
14. Chernow B, Vernoski BK, Zaloga GP, et al: Dexamethasone causes less steroid-induced alkalemia than methylprednisolone or hydrocortisone. Crit Care Med 12:384, 1984.
15. Steiner RW, Omachi AS: A Bartter's-like syndrome from capreomycin, and a similar gentamicin tubulopathy. Am J Kidney Dis 7:245, 1986.
16. Agarwal BN, Robertson FM: Metabolic alkalosis and hypermagnesemia following "non-absorbable" antacid therapy. Del Med J 58:531, 1986.
17. Madias NE, Levey AS: Metabolic alkalosis due to absorption of "nonabsorbable" antacids. Am J Med 74:155, 1983.
18. Pearl RG, Rosenthal MH: Metabolic alkalosis due to plasmapheresis. Am J Med 79:391, 1985.
19. Kelleher SP, Schulman G: Severe metabolic alkalosis complicating regional citrate hemodialysis. Am J Kidney Dis 9:235, 1987.

Selected Readings

Anderson LE, Henrich WL: Alkalemia-associated morbidity and mortality in medical and surgical patients. South Med J 80:729, 1987.

Alkalemia-associated illnesses are common in hospitalized patients and are associated with high mortality in both medical and surgical patients. Mixed respiratory and metabolic alkalosis appears to be associated with a particularly poor prognosis.

Baltarowich LL: Chloride. Emerg Med Clin North Am 4:175, 1986.

The clinical significance of chloride should place this ion on an equal basis with sodium, potassium, and bicarbonate in the evaluation of body fluid or acid-base status. The rationale for ordering serum chloride determinations includes basically all the indications for requesting the other three electrolytes, particularly when there is concern about a patient's fluid, electrolyte, and/or acid-base status.

DuBose TD Jr: Clinical approach to patients with acid-base disorders. Med Clin North Am 67:799, 1983.

Simple relationships that hold during compensation for metabolic or respiratory acid-base disturbances were emphasized, which should allow for the interpretation and diagnosis of both simple and mixed acid-base disturbances.

Galla JH, Luke RG: Pathophysiology of metabolic alkalosis. Hosp Pract 22 (10):123, 1987.

Useful clinical discussion outlining current concepts of workup, differential diagnosis, and management of metabolic alkalosis.

Javaheri S, Kazemi H: Metabolic alkalosis and hypoventilation in humans. Am Rev Respir Dis 136:1011, 1987.

Update of current concepts of pathophysiology of the respiratory response to metabolic alkalosis.

Jehle D, Harchelroad F: Bicarbonate. Emerg Med Clin North Am 4:145, 1986.

Useful clinical paper reviewing the significance of serum bicarbonate values in emergency care evaluation.

McKenzie DC, Coutts KD, Stirling DR, et al: Maximal work production following two levels of artificially induced metabolic alkalosis. J Sports Sci 4:35, 1986.

In conditions where artificial alkalosis had been achieved before exercise, there was a significant increase in the work produced, leading authors to suggest that augmentation of bicarbonate reserves has a significant positive effect on the energy metabolism in interval-type exercise, and thus, an increase in the work performed and in the time to fatigue.

Perez GO, Oster JR, Rogers A: Acid-base disturbances in gastrointestinal disease. Dig Dis Sci 32:1033, 1987.

Authors review the most important types of metabolic alkalosis and metabolic acidosis associated with gastrointestinal disorders, excluding liver disease. Special emphasis is placed on pathophysiologic mechanisms.

Ventriglia WJ: Arterial blood gases. Emerg Med Clin North Am 4:235, 1986.

This well-referenced article discusses the physiology, analysis, and interpretation of arterial blood gases.

97

Hypokalemia: Common Mechanisms and Associated Conditions

Hypokalemia can be acute or chronic, with mild or life-threatening consequences. Because only 2% of total body potassium is extracellular, a low serum potassium usually reflects a total body deficit.[1] When potassium losses are sufficient to cause hypokalemia, significant adverse effects on neuromuscular, cardiac, vascular, and renal tissues may occur.[2] Renal wasting and gastrointestinal wasting are the most common mechanisms of potassium loss. Acidosis, alkalosis, excessive mineralocorticoids, and drug effects are also common causes of hypokalemia. Less common causes include poor potassium intake and conditions characterized by extracellular to intracellular potassium shifts.

Causes of Renal Potassium Wasting

Renal wasting of potassium is most commonly associated with a history of diuretic use. Conditions that enhance renal wasting include alkalosis, excessive mineralocorticoids, polyuria, and increased distal tubule delivery of sodium and nonresorbable anions.

Primary aldosteronism

Primary deoxycorticoid overproduction

Renin-induced secondary hyperaldosteronism: juxtaglomerular hyperplasia, renal neoplasm

Ectopic ACTH syndrome[3]: hypokalemia frequently accompanies nonadrenal ACTH-dependent hypercortisolism; however, it is relatively rare in Cushing's disease or pituitary-dependent hypercortisolism.[4]

Liddle's syndrome: pseudohyperaldosteronism; hypertension, hypokalemic alkalosis, and suppressed plasma renin activity[5]

Bartter's syndrome: hypokalemia, hypochloremic metabolic alkalosis, and normal blood pressure, with hyperreninemia and hyperaldosteronism[6]

Renal tubular acidosis
Diabetic ketoacidosis[7]

**Causes of
Gastrointestinal
Potassium Wasting**

Most patients with gastrointestinal causes for potassium wasting have a history of nausea, vomiting, or diarrhea, with signs of hypotension.

Vomiting: large quantities of potassium can be lost early during protracted vomiting.
Nasogastric suction: hypokalemia is usually associated with alkalosis.
Fistulae: gastrocolic, duodenal-colic, ureterosigmoidostomy
Malabsorption syndromes: regional enteritis, sprue, Whipple's disease
Vasoactive intestinal polypeptide (VIP) syndrome: elevated VIP released by tumors of the pancreatic islets or neural crest origin cause severe secretory diarrhea.[8]
Cholera and cholera-like infections[9]
Villous adenomas of the large bowel
Laxative abuse: commonly associated with multiple and osmotic cathartics
Binge-purge syndrome: hypokalemia and alkalosis initially present can cause diagnostic confusion[10]
Carcinoid tumors[11,12]

**Drugs and Substances
That Cause
Hypokalemia**

Diuretics: although diuretics produce hypokalemia in a high percentage of patients, most cases are usually not severe enough to cause symptoms.[13]
Steroids: corticosteroids, nasal spray with alpha-fluoroprednisolone[14]
Antibiotics: carbenicillin, penicillin, tetracycline (outdated)
Carbonic anhydrase inhibitors
Licorice, licorice extracts: glycyrrhizic acid, carbenoxolone[15]
Amphotericin-B
Glucose
Mannitol
Insulin
Vitamin B_{12}
Laxatives (abuse)
Toluene inhalation: causes a renal tubular acidosis[16]
Catecholamines: beta-2 receptor stimulation required

for catecholamine compartmental shift-induced hypokalemia[17,18]
Barium poisoning[19]

Miscellaneous Causes of Hypokalemia

Poor potassium intake
Periodic paralysis: familial, sporadic hypokalemic periodic paralysis,[20] and thyrotoxic periodic paralysis[21]
Factitious
Hemodialysis[22]
Heatstroke[23]
Stress-induced hypokalemia[24]

References

1. Nardone DA, McDonald WJ, Girard DE: Mechanisms in hypokalemia: clinical correlation. Medicine 57 (5):435, 1978.
2. Linshaw MA: Potassium homeostasis and hypokalemia. Pediatr Clin North Am 34 (3):649, 1987.
3. Jex RK, van Heerden JA, Carpenter PC, Grant CS: Ectopic ACTH syndrome. Diagnostic and therapeutic aspects. Am J Surg 149 (2):276, 1985.
4. Findling JW, Tyrrell JB: Occult ectopic secretion of corticotropin. Arch Intern Med 146 (5):929, 1986.
5. Mutoh S, Hirayama H, Ueda S, et al: Pseudohyperaldosteronism (Liddle's syndrome): a case report. J Urol 135 (3):557, 1986.
6. Rodriquez Portales JA: Renal tubular reabsorption of chloride in Bartter's syndrome and other conditions with hypokalemia. Clin Nephrol 26:269, 1986.
7. Leventhal RI, Goldman JM: Immediate plasma potassium levels in treating diabetic ketoacidosis. Arch Intern Med 147 (8):1501, 1987.
8. Krejs GJ: VIPoma syndrome. Am J Med 82 (5B):37, 1987.
9. Morris JG Jr, Black BE: Cholera and other vibrioses in the United States. N Engl J Med 312:343, 1985.
10. Oster JR: The binge-purge syndrome: a common albeit unappreciated cause of acid-base and fluid-electrolyte disturbances. South Med J 80 (1):58, 1987.
11. Creutzfeldt W, Stockmann F: Carcinoids and carcinoid syndrome. Am J Med 82 (5B):4, 1987.
12. Lee CH, Ching KN, Lui WY, et al: Carcinoid tumor of the pancreas causing the diarrheogenic syndrome: report of a case combined with multiple endocrine neoplasia, type I. Surgery 99 (1):123, 1986.
13. Moser M: Diuretics in the management of hypertension. Med Clin North Am 71 (5):935, 1987.
14. Mantero F, Armanini D, Opocher G, et al: Mineralocorticoid hypertension due to a nasal spray containing 9 alpha-fluoroprednisolone. Am J Med 71 (3):352, 1981.
15. Colloredo G, Bertone V, Peci P, et al: Pseudoaldosteronism caused by licorice. Review of the literature and

description of 4 clinical cases. Minerva Med 78 (2):93, 1987.

16. Patel R, Benjamin J Jr: Renal disease associated with toluene inhalation. J Toxicol Clin Toxicol 24 (3):213, 1986.
17. Brown MJ: Hypokalemia from beta 2-receptor stimulation by circulating epinephrine. Am J Cardiol 56 (6):3D, 1985.
18. Reid JL, Whyte KF, Struthers AD: Epinephrine-induced hypokalemia: the role of beta adrenoceptors. Am J Cardiol 57 (12):23F, 1986.
19. Tenenbein M: Severe cardiac dysrhythmia from barium acetate ingestion. Pediatr Emerg Care 1 (1):34, 1985.
20. Umeki S, Ohga R, Ono S, et al: Angiotensin I level and sporadic hypokalemic periodic paralysis. Arch Intern Med 146 (10):1956, 1986.
21. Ferreiro JE, Arguelles DJ, Rams H Jr: Thyrotoxic periodic paralysis. Am J Med 80 (1):146, 1986.
22. Wiegand CF, Davin TD, Raij L, Kjellstrand CM: Severe hypokalemia induced by hemodialysis. Arch Intern Med 141:167, 1981.
23. Tucker LE, Stanford J, Graves B, et al: Classical heatstroke: clinical and laboratory assessment. South Med J 78 (1):20, 1985.
24. Valladares BK, Lemberg L: Catecholamines, potassium, and beta-blockade. Heart Lung 15 (1):105, 1986.

Selected Readings

Flamenbaum W: Diuretic use in the elderly: potential for diuretic-induced hypokalemia. Am J Cardiol 57 (2):38A, 1986.
A clinical review of diuretic-associated hypokalemia.

Gordon M: Differential diagnosis of weakness—a common geriatric symptom. Geriatrics 41 (4):75, 1986.
Weakness can result from diuretics causing azotemia and hypokalemia, whereas psychotropic drugs are often implicated as a cause of impaired emotional and physical drive.

Isner JM, Harten JT: Factitious lowering of the serum potassium level after cardiopulmonary resuscitation. Implications for evaluating the arrhythmogenicity of hypokalemia in acute myocardial infarction. Arch Intern Med 145 (1):161, 1985.
Hypokalemia has been suggested as a predisposing factor to the development of fatal arrhythmias in acute myocardial infarction. Serial determinations of serum potassium obtained fortuitously before and intentionally after sudden unexpected cardiac arrest in a hospitalized patient demonstrate that the prearrest serum potassium level cannot be inferred from electrolyte values obtained after cardiopulmonary resuscitation.

Jacob J, De Buono B, Buchbinder E, Rolla AR: Tetany induced by hypokalemia in the absence of alkalosis. Am J Med Sci 291 (4):284, 1986.
Interesting case of 36-year-old patient who developed tetany without hypocalcemia, hypomagnesemia, or alkalosis.

Roe DA: Drug-nutrient interactions in the elderly. Geriatrics 41 (3):57,63,74, 1986.

Elderly patients receiving long-term drug therapies that cause diarrhea, with or without steatorrhea, should be monitored for evidence of hypokalemia, folate deficiency, and deficiencies of vitamins A and D.

Sterns RH, Cox M, Feig PU, Singer I: Internal potassium balance and the control of the plasma potassium concentration. Medicine 60 (5):339, 1981.

Comprehensive, well-referenced review.

Thier SO: Potassium physiology. Am J Med 80 (4A):3, 1986.

Useful state-of-the-art physiology review.

Williams ME, Gervino EV, Rosa RM, et al: Catecholamine modulation of rapid potassium shifts during exercise. N Engl J Med 312:823, 1985.

Plasma potassium rises during muscular exercise and falls rapidly when exercise is stopped. Beta-adrenergic receptors appear to moderate the acute hyperkalemia of exercise, whereas alpha-adrenergic receptors act to enhance hyperkalemia and may protect against hypokalemia when exertion ceases.

98
Hyperkalemia: Common and Less Common Causes

Hyperkalemia can occur suddenly and cause neuromuscular irritability in both cardiac and skeletal muscle. Symptoms of muscle irritability, such as cardiac dysrhythmias or skeletal muscle weakness, can progress quickly to life-threatening situations, such as cardiac asystole and sudden severe muscle weakness. Pseudohyperkalemia is not uncommonly caused by hemolysis of blood samples; potassium can be spuriously elevated with poor blood-drawing techniques. Decreased renal excretion, acidosis, and drug effects are the most common causes of significant hyperkalemia.

Pseudohyperkalemia: Most Common Causes

Tourniquet method of drawing blood: can occur when blood is drawn near a tight tourniquet around an exercising extremity
Hemolyzed blood sample
Leukocytic disintegration in disorders with increased white cell counts, such as leukemia
Thrombocytosis and thrombocythemia[1]
Single unexplained serum values

Conditions Associated with Decreased Renal Excretion

Decreased renal excretion is the primary cause of hyperkalemia. Hyperkalemia usually does not occur until late in the course of chronic renal failure, unless the patient receives an excessive potassium load.

Chronic renal failure
Acute renal failure
Renal tubular defects in potassium handling
  Obstructive uropathy with renal tubular acidosis[2]
  Familial hyperkalemia[3]
Adrenal steroid deficiency
  Addison's disease
  Hyporeninemic hypoaldosteronism[4,5]
  Isolated corticotropin deficiency associated with hyporeninemic hypoaldosteronism[6]
  Acquired immune deficiency syndrome (AIDS) associated hyporeninemic hypoaldosteronism[7]
Diabetic hyperkalemia: diabetic patients with insulin and mineralocorticoid deficiency are at high risk for hyperkalemia, particularly those with renal insufficiency.[8]

Drugs and Toxins Commonly Associated with Hyperkalemia

A large number of drugs commonly used can produce hyperkalemia. Most drug-related hyperkalemic episodes occur in patients with compromised potassium regulation, such as renal insufficiency, diabetes mellitus, and metabolic acidosis.[9]

Captopril, enalapril, lisinopril
Nonsteroidal anti-inflammatory drugs (NSAIDs)[10]: indomethancin-induced hyperkalemia may result from an inhibition of prostaglandin synthesis causing hyporeninemic hypoaldosteronism.[11]
Potassium-sparing diuretics[12]
Sulfur ingestion: sulfur persists in many folk remedies.[13]

Beta-blockers[14]
Potassium penicillin
Insulin deficiency[15]
Fluoride intoxication[16]

**Potassium Loading:
Exogenous and
Endogenous Causes**

Although an increased intake of potassium can cause hyperkalemia, this rarely occurs with normal renal function.

Exogenous potassium loads
  Potassium salts: used as sodium substitutes
  High potassium foods: potato chips, dried apricots[17]
Endogenous potassium loads: most commonly, a result of blood cell product lysis
  Hemolysis
  Rhabdomyolysis: disintegration of muscle associated with excretion of myoglobin in the urine
  Succinylcholine therapy[18]
  Acute tumor lysis syndrome: can occur after chemotherapy in patients with large chemosensitive tumors, such as lymphoma and leukemia[19]

**Causes of
Redistribution
Hyperkalemia**

Hyperkalemia can occur without excess total body potassium when potassium moves from intracellular to extracellular compartments, most commonly seen during acidosis.

Metabolic acidosis[20]
Respiratory acidosis
Hyperkalemic periodic paralysis: adynamia episodica, paralysis periodica paramyotonica[21]
Exercise-induced hyperkalemia: beta-blockers can exacerbate exercise-induced hyperkalemia in both normals and diabetics and patients with renal insufficiency.[22]

References

1. Modder B, Meuthen I: Pseudohyperkalemia in the serum in reactive thrombocytosis and thrombocythemia. Dtsch Med Wochenschr 111 (9):329, 1986.
2. Batlle DC, Arruda JAL, Kurtzman NA: Hyperkalemic distal renal tubular acidosis associated with obstructive uropathy. N Engl J Med 304:373, 1981.
3. Brautbar N, Levi J, Rosler A, et al: Familial hyperkalemia, hypertension, and hyporeninemia with normal aldosterone levels. Arch Intern Med 138:607, 1978.

4. Tan SY, Burton M: Hyporeninemic hypoaldosteronism: an overlooked cause of hyperkalemia. Arch Intern Med 141:30, 1981.

5. Nadler JL, Lee FO, Hsueh W, Horton R: Evidence of prostacyclin deficiency in the syndrome of hyporeninemic hypoaldosteronism. N Engl J Med 314:1015, 1986.

6. Manser TJ, Estep H: Pseudo-Addison's disease. Isolated corticotropin deficiency associated with hyporeninemic hypoaldosteronism. Arch Intern Med 146 (5):996, 1986.

7. Kalin MF, Poretsky L, Seres DS, Zumoff B: Hyporeninemic hypoaldosteronism associated with acquired immune deficiency syndrome. Am J Med 82 (5):1035, 1987.

8. Perez GO, Lespier L, Knowles R, et al: Potassium homeostasis in chronic diabetes mellitus. Arch Intern Med 137:1018, 1977.

9. Rimmer JM, Horn JF, Gennari FJ: Hyperkalemia as a complication of drug therapy. Arch Intern Med 147:867, 1987.

10. Zipser RD, Henrich WL: Implications of nonsteroidal anti-inflammatory drug therapy. Am J Med 80:78, 1986.

11. Findling JW, Beckstrom D, Rawsthorne L, et al: Indomethacin-induced hyperkalemia in three patients with gouty arthritis. JAMA 244:1127, 1980.

12. Narins RG, Chusid P: Diuretic use in critical care. Am J Cardiol 57 (2):26A, 1986.

13. Schwartz SM, Carroll HM, Scharschmidt LA: Sublimed (inorganic) sulfur ingestion. A cause of life-threatening metabolic acidosis with a high anion gap. Arch Intern Med 146:1437, 1986.

14. Swenson ER: Severe hyperkalemia as a complication of timolol, a topically applied beta-adrenergic antagonist. Arch Intern Med 146:1220, 1986.

15. Nicolis GL, Kahn T, Sanchez A, Gabrilove JL: Glucose-induced hyperkalemia in diabetic subjects. Arch Intern Med 141:49, 1981.

16. McIvor ME: Delayed fatal hyperkalemia in a patient with acute fluoride intoxication. Ann Emerg Med 16 (10):1165, 1987.

17. Potassium in foods adapted from Pennington JAT, Church HN, Food Values of Portions Commonly Used. Harper & Row, New York, 1980, as referenced in Med Lett.

18. Frankville DD, Drummond JC: Hyperkalemia after succinylcholine administration in a patient with closed head injury without paresis. Anesthesiology 67 (2):264, 1987.

19. Stark ME, Dyer MC, Coonley CJ: Fatal acute tumor lysis syndrome with metastatic breast carcinoma. Cancer 60 (4):762, 1987.

20. Adrogue JH, Lederer ED, Suki WN, Eknoyan G: Determinants of plasma potassium levels in diabetic ketoacidosis. Medicine 65 (3):163, 1986.

21. Ricker K, Rohkamm R, Bohlen R: Adynamia episodica and paralysis periodica paramyotonica. Neurology 36 (5):682, 1986.

22. Castellino P, Simonson DC, DeFronzo RA: Adrenergic modulation of potassium metabolism during exercise in

normal and diabetic humans. Am J Physiol 252:E68, 1987.

Selected Readings

Cannon-Babb ML, Schwartz AB: Drug-induced hyperkalemia. Hosp Pract 21 (9A):99, 1986.
Treatment with multiple therapeutic agents for multiple underlying medical conditions leads to greater vulnerability to hyperkalemia.

Lee TH, Salomon DR, Rayment CM, Antman EM: Hypotension and sinus arrest with exercise-induced hyperkalemia and combined verapamil/propranolol therapy. Am J Med 80 (6):1203, 1986.
A case of life-threatening hypotension due to sinus arrest is described in a patient in whom exercise-induced hyperkalemia developed during a stable regimen that included verapamil, propranolol, and ibuprofen. Clinicians should be aware of this potential metabolic-drug interaction.

Raymond KH, Lifschitz MD: Effect of prostaglandins on renal salt and water excretion. Am J Med 80 (1A):22, 1986.
Well-referenced review of renal prostaglandin physiology.

Thier SO: Potassium physiology. Am J Med 80 (4A):3, 1986.
Current concepts of potassium physiology.

99

Hyponatremia: Inappropriate Secretion of Antidiuretic Hormone (SIADH) and Other Associations

Hyponatremia can manifest a wide spectrum of clinical symptoms such as anorexia, weakness, lethargy, psychotic reactions, and seizures. Causes of hyponatremia are diverse. Common associations include many medical illnesses; iatrogenic causes, such as administration of certain drugs or excessive free water; and inappropriate secretion of antidiuretic hormone (IADH). Spurious or pseudohyponatremia can be caused by hypertriglyceridemia,[1,2] hyperglycemia, paraproteinemia, or serum taken near an infusion of hypoosmotic fluid.

Conditions Associated with Excess Free Water Intake and Salt-Wasting Mechanisms

Conditions associated with an impairment of water excretion
Shock
Congestive heart failure[3]: poor prognosis observed with severe hyponatremia[4]
Nephrotic syndrome
Hepatic failure: sodium and free water excretion often impaired with cirrhosis[5]
Renal failure: dilutional mechanism
Intensive exercise: marathon runners[6]
Common associations with salt depletion
Gastrointestinal loss: vomiting, diarrhea, nasogastric suction
Excessive perspiration: running
Renal disease: salt-wasting nephropathy is commonly a chronic tubulointerstitial disease.

Drug-induced Hyponatremia

Diuretics,[7] e.g., thiazides[8]: elderly patients may be at higher risk for developing diuretic-induced hyponatremia[9]
Mannitol infusions[10]
Trimethoprim[11]
Captopril[12]
Chlorpropamide: enhances renal ADH sensitivity

Miscellaneous Mechanisms

Myxedema
Adrenal insufficiency
Hypokalemia
Self-induced water intoxication and schizophrenia: usually occurs 5 to 15 years after onset of psychosis[13]
Beer potomania: increased beer consumption in patients with dietary sodium and protein insufficiency[14]
Sick-cell syndrome: osmotic redistribution of water seen in a variety of seriously ill patients[15]

Postoperative hyponatremia: due to hypotonic fluid administration in the presence of nonosmotic secretion of arginine vasopressin,[16] severe postoperative hyponatremia has been reported in previously normal women after elective surgery.[17]
Heatstroke[18]

Inappropriate Secretion of Antidiuretic Hormone: Common and Uncommon Associations

Hyponatremia in seriously ill people should raise the question of inappropriate secretion of antidiuretic hormone (SIADH). The primary abnormality in SIADH is continued secretion of antidiuretic hormone, which inappropriately concentrates sodium in the urine when the serum is hypotonic.[19] Multiple medical disorders, particularly neurologic and pulmonary diseases, and drugs have been associated with SIADH.

Central nervous system disorders
    Infection: bacterial, viral
    Post-head trauma
    Postneurosurgical
    Cerebrovascular disease, e.g., stroke,[20] subarachnoid hemorrhage: hyponatremia may contribute to poor prognosis[21]
    Brain tumors
    Hydrocephalus
    Acute psychosis with or without psychotropic drugs[22]
    Carcinomatous meningitis[23]
    Chronic lymphocytic leukemic meningitis[24]
    Temporal arteritis[25]
Pulmonary disorders
    Infections: tuberculosis, pneumonia, lung abscess, aspergillosis
    Pulmonary carcinoma: bronchogenic carcinoma associated with ectopic ADH, oat cell carcinoma, small cell carcinoma[26,27]
Asthma
Mechanical ventilation-associated complications
Drug associations[8,28]
    Nicotine[29]
    Antineoplastic agents: vincristine, cyclophosphamide, cisplatin,[30] melphalan,[31] vinblastine[32]
    Acetaminophen
    Clofibrate
    Hypoglycemic agents: chlorpropamide, phenformin

Phenothiazines[33]: fluphenazine, thioridazine, chlorpromazine[34]

Carbamazepine: risk of hyponatremia increases with age and carbamazepine serum level.[35]

Antidepressants: desipramine,[36] imipramine[37]

Metabolic-endocrine associations

Myxedema[39]

Hypokalemia[40]

Adrenal insufficiency: mineralocorticoid deficiency

Hypopituitarism

Porphyria

Diabetic amyotrophy[41]

Neoplasms: pancreatic and duodenal carcinoma, lymphoma

Advanced age[42]

Rocky Mountain spotted fever[43]

Chronic schizophrenia: clinical association with polydipsia[44]

Waldenström's macroglobulinemia: report of a patient who developed hyponatremia due to SIADH rather than isotonic hyponatremia from hyperproteinemia[45]

References

1. Ladenson JH, Apple FS, Koch DD: Misleading hyponatremia due to hyperlipemia: a method-dependent error. Ann Intern Med 95:707, 1981.
2. Howard JM, Reed J: Pseudohyponatremia in acute hyperlipemic pancreatitis. A potential pitfall in therapy. Arch Surg 120 (9):1053, 1985
3. Hamilton RW, Buckalew VM Jr: Sodium, water, and congestive heart failure (editorial). Ann Intern Med 100:902, 1984.
4. Packer M, Lee WH, Kessler PD, et al: Role of neurohormonal mechanisms in determining survival in patients with severe chronic heart failure. Circulation 75:IV80, 1987.
5. Arroyo V, Gines P, Rimola A, Gaya J: Renal function abnormalities, prostaglandins, and effects of nonsteroidal anti-inflammatory drugs in cirrhosis with ascites. An overview with emphasis on pathogenesis. Am J Med 81:104, 1986.
6. Frizzell RT, Lang GH, Lowance DC, Lathan SR: Hyponatremia and ultramarathon running. JAMA 255 (6):772, 1986.
7. Abramow M, Cogan E: Clinical aspects and pathophysiology of diuretic-induced hyponatremia. Adv Nephrol 13:1, 1984.
8. Booker JA: Severe symptomatic hyponatremia in elderly outpatients: the role of thiazide therapy and stress. J Am Geriatr Soc 32:108, 1984.
9. Ashouri OS: Severe diuretic-induced hyponatremia in

the elderly. A series of eight patients. Arch Intern Med 146 (7):1355, 1986.

10. Flear CTG, Gill GV: Hyponatremia: mechanisms and management. Lancet 2:26, 1981.

11. Eastell R, Edmonds CJ: Hyponatremia associated with trimethoprim and a diuretic. Br Med J 289:1658, 1984.

12. Al-Mufti HI, Arieff AI: Captopril-induced hyponatremia with irreversible neurologic damage. Am J Med 79 (6):769, 1985.

13. Vieweg WV, David JJ, Rowe WT, et al: Death from self-induced water intoxication among patients with schizophrenic disorders. J Nerv Ment Dis 173 (3):161, 1985.

14. Joyce SM, Potter R: Beer potomania: an unusual cause of symptomatic hyponatremia. Ann Emerg Med 15 (6):745, 1986.

15. Lead article. Sick cells and hyponatraemia. Lancet 1:342, 1974.

16. Chung HM, Kluge R, Schrier RW, Anderson RJ: Post-operative hyponatremia. A prospective study. Arch Intern Med 146 (2):333, 1986.

17. Arieff AI: Hyponatremia, convulsions, respiratory arrest, and permanent brain damage after elective surgery in healthy women. N Engl J Med 314:1529, 1986.

18. Tucker LE, Stanford J, Graves B, et al: Classical heatstroke: clinical and laboratory assessment. South Med J 78 (1):20, 1985

19. Cooke CR, Turin MD, Walker WG: The syndrome of inappropriate antidiuretic hormone secretion (SIADH): pathophysiologic mechanisms in solute and volume regulation. Medicine 58:240, 1979.

20. Joynt RJ, Feibel JH, Sladek CM: Antidiuretic hormone levels in stroke patients. Ann Neurol 9:182, 1981.

21. van Gijn J, Hijdra A, Wijdicks EF, et al: Acute hydrocephalus after aneurysmal subarachnoid hemorrhage. J Neurosurg 63 (3):355, 1985

22. Kramer DS, Drake ME Jr: Acute psychosis, polydipsia, and inappropriate secretion of antidiuretic hormone. Am J Med 75:712, 1983.

23. Oster JR, Perez GO, Larios O, et al: Cerebral salt wasting in a man with carcinomatous meningitis. Arch Intern Med 143:2187, 1983.

24. Stagg MP, Gumbart CH: Chronic lymphocytic leukemic meningitis as a cause of the syndrome of inappropriate secretion of antidiuretic hormone. Cancer 60 (2):191, 1987.

25. Luzar MJ, Whisler RL, Hunder GG: Syndrome of inappropriate antidiuretic hormone secretion in association with temporal arteritis. J Rheumatol 9:957, 1982.

26. Kamoi K, Ebe T, Hasegawa A, et al: Hyponatremia in small cell lung cancer. Mechanisms not involving inappropriate ADH secretion. Cancer 60 (5):1089, 1987.

27. Passamonte RM: Hypouricemia, inappropriate secretion of antidiuretic hormone, and small cell carcinoma of the lung. Arch Intern Med 144:1569, 1984.

28. Moses AM, Miller M: Drug-induced dilutional hyponatremia. N Engl J Med 291:1234, 1974.

29. Blum A: The possible role of tobacco cigarette smoking in hyponatremia of long-term psychiatric patients. JAMA 252:2864, 1984.

30. Littlewood TJ, Smith AP: Syndrome of inappropriate antidiuretic hormone secretion due to treatment of lung cancer with cisplatin. Thorax 39:636, 1984.
31. Greenbaum-Lefkoe B, Rosenstock JG, Belasco JB: Syndrome of inappropriate antidiuretic hormone secretion: a complication of high-dose intravenous melphalan. Cancer 55:44, 1985.
32. Ravikumar TS, Grage TB: The syndrome of inappropriate ADH secretion secondary to vinblastine-bleomycin therapy. J Surg Oncol 24:242, 1983.
33. Kimelman N, Albert SG: Phenothiazine-induced hyponatremia in the elderly. Gerontology 30:132, 1984.
34. Tildesley HD, Toth E, Crockford PM: Syndrome of inappropriate secretion of antidiuretic hormone in association with chlorpromazine ingestion. Can J Psychiatry 28:487, 1983.
35. Lahr MB: Hyponatremia during carbamazepine therapy. Clin Pharmacol Ther 37 (6):693, 1985.
36. Lydiard RB: Desipramine-associated SIADH in an elderly woman: case report. J Clin Psychiatry 44:153, 1983.
37. Liskin B, Walsh BT, Roose SP, et al: Imipramine-induced inappropriate ADH secretion. J Clin Psychopharmacol 4:146, 1984.
38. Finsterer U, Beyer A, Jensen U, et al: The syndrome of inappropriate secretion of the antidiuretic hormone (SIADH)—treatment with lithium. Intensive Care Med 8:223, 1982.
39. Skowsky WR, Kikuchi TA: The role of vasopressin in the impaired water excretion of myxedema. Am J Med 64:613, 1978.
40. Nanji AA: Hypokalemia in the syndrome of inappropriate secretion of antidiuretic hormone (letter). West J Med 134:452, 1981.
41. Osei K, Falko JM: Chronic hyponatremia associated with diabetic amyotrophy. Arch Intern Med 146 (3):534, 1986.
42. Goldstein CS, Braunstein S, Goldfarb S: Idiopathic syndrome of inappropriate antidiuretic hormone secretion possibly related to advanced age. Ann Intern Med 99:185, 1983.
43. Kaplowitz LG, Robertson GL: Hyponatremia in Rocky Mountain spotted fever: role of antidiuretic hormone. Ann Intern Med 98:334, 1983.
44. Kirch DG, Bigelow LB, Weinberger DR, et al: Polydipsia and chronic hyponatremia in schizophrenic inpatients. J Clin Psychiatry 46:179, 1985.
45. Braden GL, Mikolich DJ, White CF, et al: Syndrome of inappropriate antidiuresis in Waldenstrom's macroglobulinemia. Am J Med 80 (6):1241, 1986.

Selected Readings

Anderson RJ, Chung HM, Kluge R, et al: Hyponatremia: a prospective analysis of its epidemiology and the pathogenetic role of vasopressin. Ann Intern Med 102:164, 1985. *Clinical study of etiology, pathogenesis, and prognostic implications of hyponatremia in hospitalized patients.*

Arieff AI: Hyponatremia, convulsions, respiratory arrest,

and permanent brain damage after elective surgery in healthy women. N Engl J Med 314:1529, 1986.
Discussion of severe hyponatremia in previously healthy women undergoing elective surgery. Clinical consequences and autopsy findings are discussed.

Glasgow BJ, Steinsapir KD, Anders K, Layfield LJ: Adrenal pathology in the acquired immune deficiency syndrome. Am J Clin Pathol 84 (5):594, 1985.
Adrenal pathology was examined in 41 autopsied patients with AIDS. Common clinical findings included vomiting, diarrhea, fever, hypotension, and hyponatremia. None of the 32 patients showed characteristic skin hyperpigmentation.

Jamieson MJ: Hyponatremia. Br Med J 290:1723, 1985.
Helpful clinical discussion of evaluation of hyponatremia.

Janz T: Sodium. Emerg Med Clin North Am 4:115, 1986.
A useful discussion of disorders of sodium metabolism in clinical and emergency medicine.

Kovacs L, Nemethova V, Vucalova Y, et al: Simple diagnosis of diabetes insipidus and antidiuretic hormone excess. Exp Clin Endocrinol 85:228, 1985.
Helpful clinical discussion.

Narins RG, Chusid P: Diuretic use in critical care. Am J Cardiol 57 (2):26A, 1986.
The dangers of hyponatremia are reviewed, and the rational use of loop diuretics and hypertonic saline is outlined.

Raymond KH, Lifschitz MD: Effect of prostaglandins on renal salt and water excretion. Am J Med 80 (1A):22, 1986.
The clinical consequences of taking nonsteroidal anti-inflammatory drugs in terms of hyperkalemia, sodium retention with associated edema, and possible hyponatremia are discussed.

Sandifer MG: Hyponatremia due to psychotropic drugs. J Clin Psychiatry 44:301, 1983.
Useful, well-referenced review.

Schrier RW: Pathogenesis of sodium and water retention in high-output and low-output cardiac failure, nephrotic syndrome, cirrhosis, and pregnancy. N Engl J Med 319: 1065;1127, 1988.
Two part, major review article of current concepts.

Whitaker SJ, Meanock CI, Turner GF, et al: Fluid balance and secretion of antidiuretic hormone following transsphenoidal pituitary surgery. A preliminary series. J Neurosurg 63:404, 1985.
Delayed hyponatremia appears to occur most often in patients with hypoadrenalism, as glucocorticoid coverage is decreased.

100
Hyperuricemia: Common and Uncommon Causes

Hyperuricemia, usually defined as a serum urate greater than 7.0 mg/dl in men and 6.0 mg/dl in women, is present in between 2 and 18% of the population. Levels of urate greater than 7.0 mg/dl carry an increased risk of gouty arthritis or nephrolithiasis. The majority of patients with hyperuricemia, however, do not develop these conditions, and one does not usually need to treat asymptomatic hyperuricemia.[1] Hyperuricemia can be caused by increased production of uric acid through inherited enzymatic defects, increased cell turnover, drugs, or dietary factors. More commonly, hyperuricemia results from decreased renal excretion of urate. The etiology of hyperuricemia can be important in the treatment of gouty arthritis. Gout secondary to increased uric acid production is usually treated with a xanthine oxidase inhibitor, and gout due to decreased renal excretion of urate is frequently treated initially with a uricosuric drug.

Increased Production of Urate

Inherited enzymatic defects
Hypoxanthine-guanine phosphoribosyltransferase deficiency[2]: complete deficiency results in the Lesch-Nyhan syndrome, whereas partial enzyme deficiency often results in severe form of gouty arthritis at an early age. The condition is inherited as an X-linked recessive trait. Elevated urate is due to increased purine synthesis.
Phosphoribosylpyrophosphate synthetase overactivity[3]: inherited as an X-linked recessive trait. Elevated urate is due to increased purine synthesis.
Glycogen storage diseases (except with type I disease, elevated urate is due to increased degredation of purine nucleotides): type I (glucose-6-phosphatase deficiency, von Gierke's disease),[4] an autosomal recessive disorder, elevated urate is due to increased purine synthesis; type III

(debrancher deficiency, Cori-Forbes disease)[5]; type V (muscle phosphorylase deficiency, Mc-Ardle's disease)[5]; type VII (muscle phosphofruc-tokinase deficiency)[5]; carnitine palmityltransfer-ase deficiency[6]; muscle phosphoglycerate mutase deficiency[7]; myoadenylate deaminate deficiency[8]

Increased cell turnover
  Myeloproliferative disorders
  Lymphoproliferative disorders: leukemia[9,10]
  Polycythemia vera
  Carcinomatosis
  Hemolytic disorders[11]
  Megaloblastic anemias
  Psoriasis
  Hypoxemia: includes such conditions as seizures, myocardial infarction, and hypotensive epi-sodes.[12] Hyperuricemia can be a marker for severe tissue hypoxia and may be a poor prog-nostic sign in severe acute illness.[13]
  Tissue necrosis
  Infectious mononucleosis[14]

Drugs or dietary factors
  Ethanol[15]: can cause increased degradation of pu-rine nucleotides
  Purine-rich diet
  Pancreatic extract
  Fructose: can cause increased degradation of pu-rine nucleotides
  Cytotoxic drugs[16]: the acute tumor lysis syndrome resulting from rapid cell death in fast-growing tumors treated with cytotoxic drugs can cause massively elevated urate levels and acute renal failure.[17]
  Nicotinic acid
  Ethylamino-1,3,4-thiadiazole
  4-Amino-5-imidazole carboxamide riboside
  Toxins and ingestions causing tissue necrosis and cell death
  Vitamin B_{12}: may occur with acute injections in patients with pernicious anemia
  Theophylline[18]

Mechanism unknown: obesity

Decreased Renal Excretion of Urate

Idiopathic: 80 to 90% of patients with gouty arthritis have hyperuricemia due to decreased renal excre-tion of urate of an unknown etiology
Clinical disorders

Renal: chronic renal failure, lead nephropathy,[19,20] polycystic kidney disease, renal transplantation[21]

Cardiovascular: cyanotic congenital heart disease,[22] hypertension

Endocrine: hyperparathyroidism, hypothyroidism, diabetes insipidus, Bartter's syndrome,[23]

Elevated serum lactate or hydroxybutyrate: muscular exercise, ethanol ingestion, diabetic ketoacidosis, lactic acidosis, starvation, toxemia of pregnancy

Decreased extracellular volume: dehydration, salt restriction, diuretics

Miscellaneous conditions: Down syndrome, chronic beryllium disease, sarcoidosis, obesity

Drugs

Diuretics: acetazolamide, amiloride, chlorthalidone, furosemide, organomercurials, thiazides, and triamterene can all cause hyperuricemia. Diuretics are an important cause of hyperuricemia and may be implicated in three-fourths of women with gouty arthritis.[24] However, diuretics rarely cause gout, and there probably is no reason to lower uric acid pharmacologically in patients on diuretics without gouty arthritis or kidney stones.[25,26]

Ethanol

Salicylates (low dose)

Ethambutol

Laxative abuse (alkalosis)

Levodopa

Methoxyflurane

Pyrazinamide

Cyclosporine[27]

References

1. Campion EW, Glynn RJ, DeLabry LO: Asymptomatic hyperuricemia: risks and consequences in the normative aging study. Am J Med 82:421, 1987.
2. Wilson JM, Kelley WN: Molecular genetics of hypoxanthine-guanine phosphoribosyltransferase deficiency in man. Arch Intern Med 145:1895, 1985.
3. Becker MA, Losman MJ, Rosenberg AL, et al: Phosphoribosyl-pyrophosphate synthetase superactivity: a study of five patients with catalytic defects in the enzyme. Arthritis Rheum 29:880, 1986.
4. Cohen JL, Vinik A, Faller J, Fox IH: Hyperuricemia in glycogen storage disease Type I: Contributions by hypoglycemia and hyperglucagonemia to increased urate production. J Clin Invest 75:251, 1985.
5. Mineo I, Kono N, Hara N, et al: Myogenic hyperuri-

cemia: a common pathophysiologic feature of glycogenosis types III, V, and VII. N Engl J Med 317:75, 1987.

6. Bertorini TE, Shively V, Taylor B, et al: ATP degradation products after ischemic exercise: hereditary lack of phosphorylase or carnitine palmityltransferase. Neurology 35:1355, 1985.

7. DiMauro S, Miranda AF, Khan S, et al: Human muscle phosphoglycerate mutase deficiency: newly discovered metabolic myopathy. Science 212:1277, 1981.

8. DiMauro S, Miranda AF, Hays AP, et al: Myoadenylate deaminase deficiency: muscle biopsy and muscle culture in a patient with gout. J Neurol Sci 47:191, 1980.

9. Maurer HS, Steinherz PG, Gaynon PS, et al: The effect of initial management of hyperleukocytosis on early complications and outcome of children with acute lymphoblastic leukemia. J Clin Oncol 6:1425, 1988.

10. Smith T: Tumor lysis syndrome after steroid therapy for anaphylaxis. South Med J 81:415, 1988.

11. Reynolds MD: Gout and hyperuricemia associated with sickle-cell anemia. Semin Arthritis Rheum 12:404, 1983.

12. Wolliscroft JO, Fox IH: Increased body fluid purine levels during hypotensive events: evidence for ATP degradation. Am J Med 81:472, 1986.

13. Wolliscroft JO, Colfer H, Fox IH: Hyperuricemia in acute illness: a poor prognostic sign. Am J Med 72:58, 1982.

14. Dylewski JS, Gerson M: Hyperuricemia in patients with infectious mononucleosis. Can Med Assoc J 132:1169, 1985.

15. Faller J, Fox IH: Ethanol-induced hyperuricemia: evidence for increased urate production by activation of adenine nucleotide turnover. N Engl J Med 307:1598, 1982.

16. Nanji AA, Mikhael NZ, Stewart DJ: Increase in serum uric acid level associated with cisplatin therapy: correlation with liver but not kidney platinum concentrations. Arch Intern Med 145:2013, 1985.

17. Cohen LF, Balow JE, Magrath IT, et al: Acute tumor lysis syndrome: a review of 37 patients with Burkitt's lymphoma. Am J Med 68:486, 1980.

18. Morita Y, Nishida Y, Kamatani N, Miyamoto T: Theophylline increases serum uric acid levels. J Allergy Clin Immunol 74:707, 1984.

19. Halla JT, Ball GV: Saturnine gout: a review of 42 patients. Semin Arthritis Rheum 11:307, 1982.

20. Reynolds PP, Knapp MJ, Baraf HS, Holmes EW: Moonshine and lead: relationship to the pathogenesis of hyperuricemia in gout. Arthritis Rheum 26:1057, 1983.

21. Najarian JS, Simmons RL: Hyperuricemia after renal transplantation. Am J Surg 156:397, 1988.

22. Ross EA, Perloff JK, Danovitch GM, et al: Renal function and urate metabolism in late survivors with cyanotic congenital heart disease. Circulation 73:396, 1986.

23. Meyer WJ, Gill JR, Bartter FC: Gout as a complication of Bartter's syndrome: a possible role for alkalosis in the decreased clearance of uric acid. Ann Intern Med 83:56, 1975.

24. Lally EV, Ho G, Kaplan SR: The clinical spectrum of gouty arthritis in women. Arch Intern Med 146:2221, 1986.

25. Langford HG, Blaufox MD, Borhani NO, et al: Is thiazide-produced uric acid elevation harmful? Analysis of data from the hypertension detection and follow-up program. Arch Intern Med 147:645, 1987.
26. Takala J, Anttila S, Gref CG, Isomaki H: Diuretics and hyperuricemia in the elderly. Scand J Rheumatol 17:155, 1988.
27. Palestine AG, Nussenblatt RB, Chan CC: Side effects of systemic cyclosporine in patients not undergoing transplantation. Am J Med 77:652, 1984.

Selected Readings

Beck LH: Requiem for gouty nephropathy. Kidney Int 30:280, 1986.
Reviews data supporting and refuting the existence of urate nephropathy and concludes that hyperuricemia does not cause renal insufficiency, thereby eliminating a reason to treat asymptomatic hyperuricemia.

Becker MA: Clinical aspects of monosodium urate monohydrate crystal deposition disease (gout). Rheum Dis Clin North Am 14:377, 1988.
Useful, well-referenced update on the clinical aspects of gout.

Boss GR, Seegmiller JE: Hyperuricemia and gout: classification, complications and management. N Engl J Med 300:1459, 1979.
General subject review.

German DC, Holmes EW: Hyperuricemia and gout. Med Clin North Am 70:419, 1986.
General subject review.

Holmes EW: Clinical gout and the pathogenesis of hyperuricemia. p. 1445. In McCarty DJ (ed): Arthritis and Allied Conditions: A Textbook of Rheumatology. 10th Ed. Lea & Febiger, Philadelphia, 1985.
General subject review.

Kelley WN: Approach to the patient with hyperuricemia. p. 489. In Kelley WN, Harris ED, Ruddy S, Sledge CB (eds): Textbook of Rheumatology, 2nd Ed. WB Saunders, Philadephia, 1985.
Useful chart on workup of hyperuricemia.

Kelley WN, Fox IH: Gout and related disorders of purine metabolism. p. 1359. In Kelley WN, Harris ED, Ruddy S, Sledge CB (eds): Textbook of Rheumatology, 2nd Ed. WB Saunders, Philadelphia, 1985.
Pathophysiology and clinical features of gout, as well as the classification of hyperuricemia.

Wisner DE, Simkin PA: Management of gout and hyperuricemia. Primary care 11:283, 1984.
General subject review.

101
Hypercalcemia: Common and Less Common Causes

The most common presentation of hypercalcemia is an asymptomatic patient with hypercalcemia encountered on a routine biochemical analysis.[1] Malignancy is a common cause in hospital patients[2]; hyperparathyroidism is the most common cause in outpatients.

Malignancy

The number of bony metastases does not necessarily correspond to the level of hypercalcemia in malignancy; humoral and local osteolysis are the two major pathogenic mechanisms in malignancy associated with hypercalcemia.[3-5]

Breast cancer: most common neoplasm associated with hypercalcemia[6]
Lung cancer: in decreasing frequency, squamous carcinoma, adenocarcinoma, and oat cell carcinoma[7]
Multiple myeloma and other hematologic tumors[8]
Urogenital and gynecologic tumors
Pheochromocytoma: usually associated with hyperparathyroidism[9]
Head and neck tumors
Gastrointestinal tract and pancreatic tumors[10]
Hepatic tumors
Lymphoreticular tumors: lymphoma[11]
Squamous cell carcinoma: head and neck,[12] colon[13]
Renal cell carcinoma: hypernephroma[14]

Endocrine Disorders

Primary hyperparathyroidism[15]: parathyroid adenoma is the most common cause followed by parathyroid hyperplasia. Parathyroid carcinoma is a rare cause.[16]
Secondary hyperparathyroidism: renal failure is the most common cause
Multiple endocrine adenomatoses: type I—parathyroid, pituitary, and pancreatic dysfunction; type

II—pheochromocytoma, medullary thyroid carcinoma, and parathyroid hyperplasia
Thyroid dysfunction: hyperthyroidism and hypothyroidism
Adrenal insufficiency
Acromegaly

Drug-Induced Hypercalcemia

Thiazides
Vitamin D: intoxication[17] and hypersensitivity
Calcium supplementation: peptic ulcer patients with milk-alkali syndrome[18]
Vitamin A supplements
Lithium[19]

Less Common Causes of Hypercalcemia

Immobilization hypercalcemia[20]
Paget's disease[21]
Immobilization: usually in young patients
Granulomatous disorders: sarcoidosis,[22] tuberculosis, berylliosis, coccidioidomycosis,[23] eosinophilia[24]
Munchausen syndrome[25]
Acute renal failure: often with rhabdomyolysis
Hypophosphatasia
Familial hypocalciuric hypercalcemia[26]
Dialysis osteomalacia[27]

Causes of Spurious or Artifact-Associated Hypercalcemia

Protein, acid-base, and albumin abnormalities can alter serum calcium levels.
Hemoconcentration: venous stasis with prolonged tourniquet application, dehydration
Calcium contamination of serum sample: cork stoppers, test tube contamination
Protein abnormalities: increased total calcium with normal ionized calcium
Acidosis: decreases the binding of calcium to albumin, raising ionic concentration
Physiologic: during first week of life and in some adult males under 50 years of age[28]

References

1. Juan D: Differential diagnosis of hypercalcemia. Postgrad Med 66 (4):72, 1979.
2. Fisken RA, Heath DA, Somers S: Hypercalcemia in hospital patients. Lancet 1:202, 1981.
3. Insogna KL, Broadus AE: Hypercalcemia of malignancy. Annu Rev Med 38:241, 1987.

4. Martin TJ: Humoral hypercalcemia of malignancy. Bone Miner 4:83, 1988.
5. Burtis WJ, Wu TL, Insogna KL, Stewart AF: Humoral hypercalcemia of malignancy. Ann Intern Med 108:454, 1988.
6. Skrabanek P, McPartlin J, Powell D: Tumor hypercalcemia and "ectopic hyperparathyroidism." Medicine 59:262, 1980.
7. Coggeshall J, Merrill W, Hande K, et al: Implications of hypercalcemia with respect to diagnosis and treatment of lung cancer. Am J Med 80:325, 1986.
8. Mundy GR, Bertolini DR: Bone destruction and hypercalcemia in plasma cell myeloma. Semin Oncol 13:291, 1986.
9. Stewart AF, Hoecker JL, Mallette LE, et al: Hypercalcemia in pheochromocytoma. Ann Intern Med 102:776, 1985.
10. Monno S, Nagata A, Homma T, et al: Exocrine pancreatic cancer with humoral hypercalcemia. Am J Gastroenterol 79:128, 1984.
11. Breslau NA, McGuire JL, Zerwekh JE, et al: Hypercalcemia associated with increased serum calcitriol levels in three patients with lymphoma. Ann Intern Med 100:1, 1984.
12. Dorman EB, Yang H, Vaughan CW, et al: The incidence of hypercalcemia in squamous cell carcinoma of the head and neck. Head Neck Surg 7:95, 1984.
13. Chevinsky AH, Berelowitz M, Hoover HC Jr: Adenosquamous carcinoma of the colon presenting with hypercalcemia. Cancer 60 (5):1111, 1987.
14. Laski ME, Vugrin D: Paraneoplastic syndromes in hypernephroma. Semin Nephrol 7 (2):123, 1987.
15. Scholz DA, Purnell DC: Asymptomatic primary hyperparathyroidism. 10-year prospective study. Mayo Clin Proc 56 (8):473, 1981.
16. Fujimoto Y, Obara T: How to recognize and treat parathyroid carcinoma. Surg Clin North Am 67 (2):343, 1987.
17. Drinka PJ, Nolten WE: Hazards of treating osteoporosis and hypertension concurrently with calcium, vitamin D, and distal diuretics. J Am Geriatr Soc 32:405, 1984.
18. Carroll PR, Clark OH: Milk alkali syndrome. Does it exist and can it be differentiated from primary hyperparathyroidism? Ann Surg 197:427, 1983.
19. Salata R, Klein I: Effects of lithium on the endorine system: a review. J Lab Clin Med 110 (2):130, 1987.
20. Maynard FM: Immobilization hypercalcemia following spinal cord injury. Arch Phys Med Rehab 67:41, 1986.
21. Kanis JA, Gray RE: Long-term follow-up observations on treatment in Paget's disease of bone. Clin Orthop 217:99, 1987.
22. Lufkin EG, DeRemee RA, Rohrbach MS: The predictive value of serum angiotensin-converting enzyme activity in the differential diagnosis of hypercalcemia. Mayo Clin Proc 58 (7):447, 1983.
23. Parker MS, Dokoh S, Woolfenden JM, et al: Hypercalcemia in coccidioidomycosis. Am J Med 76:341, 1984.
24. Jurney TH: Hypercalcemia in a patient with eosinophilic granuloma. Am J Med 76:527, 1984.

25. Frame B, Jackson GM, Kleerekoper M, et al: Acute severe hypercalcemia in a la Munchausen. Am J Med 70:316, 1981.
26. Marx SJ, Fraser D, Rapoport A: Familial hypocalciuric hypercalcemia: mild expression of the gene in heterozygotes and severe expression in homozygotes. Am J Med 78:15, 1985.
27. Drueke T, Cournot-Witmer G: Dialysis osteomalacia: clinical aspects and physiopathological mechanisms. Clin Nephrol 24 (Suppl 1):S26, 1985.
28. Lee DBN, Zawada ET, Kleeman CR: The pathophysiology and clinical aspects of hypercalcemic disorders. West J Med 129:278, 1978.

Selected Readings

Davis PJ, Davis FB: Diagnosis of hyperparathyroidism. Otolaryngol Head Neck Surg 93 (1):62, 1985.
Availability of immunoassays for specific regions of the parathyroid hormone (PTH) molecule allows discrimination between primary hyperparathyroidism and tumoral hypercalcemia states associated with circulating PTH-like substances.

Forster J, Querusio L, Burchard KW, et al: Hypercalcemia in critically ill surgical patients. Ann Surg 202:512, 1985.
A review of 100 patients hospitalized in a surgical intensive care unit found that approximately 15% of critically ill surgical patients developed hypercalcemia. Possible mechanisms are discussed.

Fournier A, Sebert JL, Makdassi R: Stages of the etiological diagnosis of hypercalcemia. Ann Med Interne (Paris) 136 (1):49, 1985.
Helpful clinical overview of state-of-the-art serum assays and radiographic methods useful in the evaluation of hypercalcemia.

Jamieson MJ: Hypercalcemia. Br J Med 290:378, 1985.
Useful and concise clinical discussion of the evaluation and differential diagnosis of hypercalcemia.

Kochersberger G: Primary hyperparathyroidism in the elderly. Compr Ther 14:24, 1988.
Clinical features of primary hyperparathyroidism in elderly women may be confused with normal aging. Author suggests that there are large groups of elderly patients with hyperparathyroidism who are asymptomatic or mildly symptomatic. Secondary renal dysfunction and skeletal disease, particularly osteoporosis, cause significant morbidity. Author suggests that surgical management may be indicated when symptoms are present or repeated serum calcium levels exceed 11.0 mg/dl.

Mundy GR: Hypercalcemia of malignancy revisited. J Clin Invest 82:1, 1988.
Useful review of current concepts.

Mundy GR, Ibbotson KJ, D'Souza SM, et al: The hypercalcemia of cancer: clinical implications and pathogenic mechanisms. N Engl J Med 310:1718, 1984.
Well-referenced review of current concepts of hypercalcemia of cancer.

Mundy GR, Ibbotson KJ, D'Souza SM: Tumor products and the hypercalcemia of malignancy. J Clin Invest 76:391, 1985.
An update of current concepts of hypercalcemia in malignancy.

102
Hypomagnesemia: Common Causes and Associations

Although magnesium deficiency rarely shows specific signs or symptoms,[1] it can cause ventricular ectopy and sudden death in certain high-risk patient populations.[2] Current evidence suggests that magnesium deficiency is implicated in the pathogenesis of atherosclerosis, cardiac arrhythmias, and coronary spasm[3]; yet hypomagnesemia is one of the most underdiagnosed electrolyte deficiencies in current medical practice.[4] Since serum magnesium does not always accurately reflect intracellular magnesium stores,[5] a high index of suspicion for hypomagnesemia must exist in those patients in whom magnesium deficiency cannot be risked and in those patients with electrolyte abnormalities known to be commonly associated with hypomagnesia, such as hypokalemia, hypocalcemia, hyponatremia, and hypophosphatemia.[6] Malabsorption syndromes and excessive urinary losses are common mechanisms of magnesium wasting. Alcoholism and iatrogenic, particularly diuretic use, are common causes; whereas diet related and congenital disorders are less common.[7]

Disorders Associated with Increased Gastrointestinal Magnesium Excretion

Diarrhea, particularly chronic diarrhea[8,9]

Malabsorption syndromes: jejunoileal bypass surgery,[10,11] short bowel syndrome, bowel and biliary fistulae

Alcoholic cirrhosis: combined result of malnutrition, hepatic dysfunction, and hyperaldosteronism; hypomagnesemia can also be a spurious finding because hypoproteinemia can falsely lower serum magnesium levels[12]

Colonic neoplasms

Acute pancreatitis[13,14]

Vitamin deficiency

709

Primary hypomagnesemia: an inherited selective magnesium malabsorption
Cholestatic liver disease

Endocrine and Electrolyte Abnormalities Associated with Increased Renal Magnesium Excretion	Hyperparathyroidism Hyperaldosteronism Diabetes mellitus: particularly during diabetic ketoacidosis Hypercalcemia Hyperthyroidism Pregnancy: particularly the last trimester of pregnancy and in insulin-dependent pregnant women[15] Excessive lactation Phosphate depletion Organic aciduria Vitamin D deficiency[16]
Renal Disorders: Intrinsic, Tubular Injury and Inherited Causes	Chronic renal disease[17,18]: glomerulonephritis, pyelonephritis Recovery phase from acute tubular necrosis and postobstructive nephropathy, such as hydronephrosis[19] Drug-induced renal tubular injuries: aminoglycosides, amphotericin B,[20] cisplatin[21,22] Hereditary renal magnesium wasting[23,24] Renal tubular acidosis[25]
Drugs and Other Iatrogenic Causes	Diuretic therapy[26]: patients with cardiovascular disease who are treated with diuretics and digitalis with both potassium and magnesium deficiency are at high risk for ventricular ectopy. Laxative abuse Antibiotics: ticarcillin, gentamicin,[27] carbenicillin Cyclosporine[28] Blood transfusion[29] Drugs causing cellular shifts: glucose, amino acids, insulin Intravenous therapy with inadequate magnesium replacement Gastric suction Dialysis: magnesium deficient dialysate[30] Acute ethanol use[31]

Diet-Related Conditions and Miscellaneous Associations

Magnesium deficient diets: liquid protein diets[32]
Protein-calorie malnutrition: kwashiorkor
Soft water[33]
Alcoholism: poor magnesium dietary intake is compounded by alcohol's direct inhibitory action on renal tubular reabsorption of magnesium[34,35]
Cystic fibrosis[36]

References

1. Kingston ME, Al-Siba'i MB, Skooge WC: Clinical manifestations of hypomagnesemia. Crit Care Med 14 (11):950, 1986.
2. Berkelhammer C, Bear RA: A clinical approach to common electrolyte problems: 4. Hypomagnesemia. Can Med Assoc J 132:360, 1985.
3. Ryzen E, Elkayam U, Rude RK: Low blood mononuclear cell magnesium in intensive cardiac care unit patients. Am Heart J 111(3):475, 1986.
4. Whang R: Magnesium deficiency: pathogenesis, prevalence, and clinical implications. Am J Med 82(Suppl 3A):24, 1987.
5. Hollifield JW: Magnesium depletion, diuretics, and arrhythmias. Am J Med 82(Suppl 3A):30, 1987.
6. Whang R, Oei TO, Aikawa JK, et al: Predictors of clinical hypomagnesemia. Hypokalemia, hypophosphatemia, hyponatremia, and hypocalcemia. Arch Intern Med 144:1794, 1984.
7. Laban E, Charbon GA: Magnesium and cardiac arrhythmias: nutrient or drug? J Am Coll Nutr 5(6):521, 1986.
8. Lim P, Jacob E: Tissue magnesium level in chronic diarrhea. J Lab Clin Med 80(3):313, 1972.
9. Saunders DR, Wiggins HS: Fecal excretion of soluble magnesium by humans. West J Med 139:655, 1983.
10. Hocking MP, Duerson MC, O'Leary JP, Woodward ER: Jejunoileal bypass for morbid obesity. Late follow-up in 100 cases. N Engl J Med 308:995, 1983.
11. Van Gaal L, Delvigne C, Vandewoude M, et al: Evaluation of magnesium before and after jejuno-ileal versus gastric bypass surgery for morbid obesity. J Am Coll Nutr 6(5):397, 1987.
12. Lim P, Jacob E: Magnesium deficiency in liver cirrhosis. Q J Med 41:291, 1972.
13. Hersh T, Siddiqui DA: Magnesium and the pancreas. Am J Clin Nutr 26(3):362, 1973.
14. Davies M, Klimiuk PS, Adams PH, et al: Familial hypocalciuric hypercalcemia and acute pancreatitis. Br Med J (Clin Res) 282:1023, 1981.
15. Mimouni F, Miodovnik M, Tsang RC, et al: Decreased maternal serum magnesium concentration and adverse fetal outcome in insulin-dependent diabetic women. Obstet Gynecol 70(1):85, 1987.
16. Rude RK, Adams JS, Ryzen E, et al: Low serum concentrations of 1,25-dihydroxyvitamin D in human magnesium deficiency. J Clin Endocrinol Metab 61(5):933, 1985.

17. Randall RE Jr: Magnesium metabolism in chronic renal disease. Ann NY Acad Sci 162(2):831, 1969.
18. Mennes P, Rosenbaum R, Martin K, Slatopolsky E: Hypomagnesemia and impaired parathyroid hormone secretion in chronic renal disease. Ann Intern Med 88:206, 1978.
19. Davis BB, Preuss HG, Murdaugh HV Jr: Hypomagnesemia following the diuresis of post-renal obstruction and renal transplant. Nephron 14:275, 1975.
20. Burgess JL, Birchall R: Nephrotoxicity of amphotericin B, with emphasis on changes in tubular function. Am J Med 53(1):77, 1972.
21. Schilsky RL, Anderson T: Hypomagnesemia and renal magnesium wasting in patients receiving cisplatin. Ann Intern Med 90:929, 1979.
22. Bosl GJ, Leitner SP, Atlas SA, et al: Increased plasma renin and aldosterone in patients treated with cisplatin-based chemotherapy for metastatic germ-cell tumors. J Clin Oncol 4(11):1684, 1986.
23. Evans RA, Carter JN, George CR, et al: The congenital "magnesium-losing kidney." Report of two patients. Q J Med 59(197):39, 1981.
24. Zelikovic I, Dabbagh S, Friedman AL, et al: Severe renal osteodystrophy without elevated serum immunoreactive parathyroid hormone concentrations in hypomagnesemia due to renal magnesium wasting. Pediatrics 79(3):403, 1987.
25. Passer J: Incomplete distal renal tubular acidosis in hypomagnesemia-dependent hypocalcemia. Arch Intern Med 136:462, 1976.
26. Ryan MP: Diuretics and potassium/magnesium depletion. Directions for treatment. Am J Med 82 (Suppl 3A):38, 1987.
27. Bar RS, Wilson HE, Mazzaferri EL: Hypomagnesemic hypocalcemia secondary to renal magnesium wasting. A possible consequence of high-dose gentamicin therapy. Ann Intern Med 82:646, 1975.
28. June CH, Thompson CB, Kennedy MS, et al: Profound hypomagnesemia and renal magnesium wasting associated with the use of cyclosporine for marrow transplantation. Transplantation 39(6):620, 1985.
29. McLellan BA, Reid SR, Lane PL: Massive blood transfusion causing hypomagnesemia. Crit Care Med 12(2):146, 1984.
30. Kenny MA, Casillas E, Ahmad S: Magnesium, calcium and PTH relationships in dialysis patients after magnesium repletion. Nephron 46(2):199, 1987.
31. Mendelson HJ, Ogata M, Mello NK: Effects of alcohol ingestion and withdrawal on magnesium states of alcoholics: clinical and experimental findings. Ann NY Acad Sci 162(2):918, 1969.
32. Licata AA, Lantigua R, Amatruda J, Lockwood D: Adverse effects of liquid protein fast on the handling of magnesium, calcium and phosphorus. Am J Med 71(5):767, 1981.
33. Haring BS, Van Delft W: Changes in the mineral composition of food as a result of cooking in "hard" and "soft" waters. Arch Environ Health 36(1):33, 1981.
34. Flink EB: Nutritional aspects of magnesium metabolism. West J Med 133:304, 1980.

35. Lim P, Jacob E: Magnesium status of alcoholic patients. Metabolism 21(11):1045, 1972.
36. Orenstein SR, Orenstein DM: Magnesium deficiency in cystic fibrosis. South Med J 76(12):1586, 1983.

Selected Readings

Brautbar N, Altura BM: Hypophosphatemia and hypomagnesemia result in cardiovascular dysfunction: theoretical basis for alcohol-induced cellular injury. Alcoholism (NY) 11(2):118, 1987.

Interesting study implicating hypomagnesemia and hypophosphatemia in the pathogenesis of alcoholic cardiovascular disease.

Elin RJ: Magnesium metabolism in health and disease. DM 34:161, 1988.

Current concepts of magnesium in human physiology. Important review of limitations of current clinical laboratory evaluations of magnesium status, which is primarily an intracellular cation that limits our ability to evaluate fully intracellular total body magnesium. Magnesium deficiency can cause weakness, tremors, seizures, arrhythmias, hypokalemia, and hypocalcemia. Risk factors and medical conditions associated with magnesium are reviewed. Comprehensively referenced.

Elkayam U, Rude RK: Low blood mononuclear cell magnesium in intensive cardiac care unit patients. Am Heart J 111(3):475, 1986.

A study measuring blood mononuclear cell magnesium content and serum magnesium concentrations in 104 unselected patients admitted to an intensive cardiac care unit concluded that the incidence of intracellular magnesium deficiency in patients with cardiovascular disease is much higher than the serum magnesium would lead one to suspect, and may contribute to clinical cardiovascular morbidity.

Ferment O, Garnier PE, Touitou Y: Comparison of the feedback effect of magnesium and calcium on parathyroid hormone secretion in man. J Endocrinol 113(1):117, 1987.

This study suggests that magnesium is less potent than calcium in regulating parathyroid hormone secretion in vivo.

Lalor BC, France MW, Powell D, et al: Bone and mineral metabolism and chronic alcohol abuse. Q J Med 59:497, 1986.

In four patients, the development of hyperparathyroidism was probably related to an underlying magnesium deficiency.

Maxwell MH, Waks AU: Cations and hypertension: sodium, potassium, calcium, and magnesium. Med Clin North Am 71(5):859, 1987.

The association between sodium intake and hypertension has been studied for almost a century. More recently, it has been suggested that abnormalities in dietary intake of potassium, calcium, and magnesium may play a major role in the pathogenesis of hypertension.

Packer M, Gottlieb SS, Kessler PD: Hormone-electrolyte interactions in the pathogenesis of lethal cardiac arrhythmias in patients with congestive heart failure. Basis of a new physiologic approach to control of arrhythmias. Am J Med 80(4A):23, 1986.

A useful approach to the prevention of sudden death in patients with congestive heart failure addresses the reversible causes of lethal ventricular arrhythmias in these individuals. Both experimental and clinical evidence indicates that circulating neurohormones and electrolyte deficits (particularly of potassium and magnesium) interact to provoke malignant ventricular ectopic rhythms.

Ryzen E, Wagers PW, Singer FR, Rude RK: Magnesium deficiency in a medical ICU population. Crit Care Med 13(1):19, 1985.

The serum magnesium level was measured in 94 consecutive patients admitted to a medical ICU over a 2-month period. Sixty-five percent of patients with serum creatinine concentrations of 1.1 mg/dl or less were hypomagnesemic.

Sjogren A, Floren CH, Nilsson A: Magnesium deficiency in IDDM related to level of glycosylated hemoglobin. Diabetes 35(4):459, 1986.

Magnesium and potassium were analyzed in plasma, erythrocytes, and urine collected during 24 hours and in muscle biopsies from 25 subjects with insulin-dependent, type I diabetes mellitus (IDDM). Results indicate that some patients with IDDM have lowered contents of magnesium in striated muscle and/or plasma, and that those parameters depend on the degree of diabetic control.

Touitou Y, Godard JP, Ferment O, et al: Prevalence of magnesium and potassium deficiencies in the elderly. Clin Chem 33(4):518, 1987.

This study underlines the large prevalence of magnesium and potassium deficiencies in the elderly, an observation that could not be attributed to pathology or treatment. Routine electrolyte studies, therefore, appear to be justified in the elderly.

Zelikovic I, Dabbagh S, Friedman AL, et al: Severe renal osteodystrophy without elevated serum immunoreactive parathyroid hormone concentrations in hypomagnesemia due to renal magnesium wasting. Pediatrics 79(3):403, 1987.

Calcium deficiency rickets due to primary or secondary renal magnesium wasting in conjunction with moderate renal failure represents a largely unrecognized metabolic bone disease.

103
Hypophosphatemia: Common and Uncommon Associations

Hypophosphatemia is associated with a wide spectrum of acute and chronic clinical disorders. Severe hypophosphatemia occurs most commonly in hospitalized patients and can precipitate respiratory failure, neuromuscular weakness, cardiac arrhythmias, and hemolysis.[1] Though these severe complications usually occur in patients with preexisting wasting illnesses, such as chronic alcoholism and cancer,[2] significant hypophosphatemia can occur even in previously normophosphatemic hospitalized patients, particularly in patients receiving dextrose solutions, phosphate-binding antacids, and in those being treated for alcoholic withdrawal or malnutrition.[3]

Since phosphorus is primarily an intracellular ion, serum phosphorus levels do not always accurately reflect total body phosphorus stores. Multiple chronic, potentially disabling disorders have been linked to hypophosphatemia, such as erythrocyte, leukocyte, and platelet abnormalities and osteomalacia, cardiomyopathies, and skeletal myopathies.[4] Major pathophysiologic mechanisms that cause hypophosphatemia include decreased phosphate intake, increased renal and gastrointestinal phosphate wasting, and transcellular shifts.[5]

Acute and Chronic Medical Disorders Commonly Associated with Hypophosphatemia

Acute medical disorders
  Alcoholic withdrawal: phosphate less than 1.1 mg/dl may precede hemolysis or rhabdomyolysis.[6]
  Diabetic ketoacidosis: insulin and fluid administration can precipitate hypophosphatemia.[7]
  Sepsis
  Acute gout
  Hypothermia[8]
  Burns[9]

Heatstroke[10]
Respiratory infections: muscle enzyme elevations are the most common associated laboratory findings.[11]
Reye's syndrome[12]
Chronic medical disorders
Chronic alcoholism: muscle phosphorus is commonly low, even without low serum phosphorus[13]
Malabsorption syndromes
Vitamin D deficiency[14,15]
Renal tubular disorders
Malnutrition[16]
Malignancy: lymphoma in leukemic phase[17,18]
Osteomalacia
Depression: decreased phosphorus intake[19]
Panic disorders: low inorganic phosphate levels have been associated with panic symptoms during lactate infusions[20]
Cystic fibrosis[21]

Drugs and Treatment

Hyperalimentation[22]
Refeeding after starvation
Phosphate-binding antacids
Carbohydrate loading: parenteral glucose, fructose, and dextrose administration
Volume expansion: including infusions of saline, glycerol, and lactate
Diuretics
Chronic steroid administration
Drugs associated with intracellular shifts: insulin, epinephrine, glucagon, gastrin, bicarbonate
Estrogen therapy[23]
Drug poisonings: salicylates, aminophylline,[24,25] paint sniffing[26]
Hyperthermia treatment[27]

Electrolyte and Endocrine Associations

Hypokalemia
Hypomagnesemia
Adlosteronism
Pregnancy[28]
Hyperparathyroidism[29,30]
Hypothyroidism

Congenital Disorders

Adult hypophosphatasia[31,32]
McCune-Albright syndrome[33]

Idiopathic hypercalciuria and hereditary hypophosphatemic rickets[34]

References

1. Janson C, Birnbaum G, Baker FJ II: Hypophosphatemia. Ann Emerg Med 12(2):107, 1983.
2. Knochel JP: The clinical status of hypophosphatemia. An update. N Engl J Med 313:447, 1985.
3. King AL, Sica DA, Miller G, Pierpaoli S: Severe hypophosphatemia in a general hospital population. South Med J 80(7):831, 1987.
4. Medical Staff Conference, University of California, San Francisco: Hypophosphatemia. West J Med 122:482, 1975.
5. Berkelhammer C, Bear RA: A clinical approach to common electrolyte problems: 3. Hypophosphatemia. Can Med Assoc J 130:17, 1984.
6. Ryback RS, Eckardt MJ, Pautler CP: Clinical relationships between serum phosphorous and other blood chemistry values in alcoholics. Arch Intern Med 140:673, 1980.
7. Hasselstrom L, Wimberley PD, Nielsen VG: Hypophosphatemia and acute respiratory failure in a diabetic patient. Intensive Care Med 12(6):429, 1986.
8. Levy LA: Severe hypophosphatemia as a complication of the treatment of hypothermia. Arch Intern Med 140:128, 1980.
9. Loven L, Larsson L, Nordstrom H, Lennquist S: Serum phosphate and 2,3-diphosphoglycerate in severely burned patients after phosphate supplementation. J Trauma 26(4):348, 1986.
10. Tucker LE, Stanford J, Graves B, et al: Classical heatstroke: clinical and laboratory assessment. South Med J 78(1):20, 1985.
11. Fisher J, Magid N, Kallman C, et al: Respiratory illness and hypophosphatemia. Chest 83(3):504, 1983.
12. Carroll JL, Kanter RK: Hypophosphatemia and Reye's syndrome. Crit Care Med 13(6):480, 1985.
13. Knochel JP: Hypophosphatemia in the alcoholic. Arch Intern Med 140:613, 1980.
14. Hochberg Z, Benderli A, Levy J, et al: 1,25-Dihydroxyvitamin D resistance, rickets, and alopecia. Am J Med 77(5):805, 1984.
15. Gundberg CM, Cole DE, Lian JB, et al: Serum osteocalcin in the treatment of inherited rickets with 1,25-dihydroxyvitamin D_3. J Clin Endocrinol Metab 56(5):1063, 1983.
16. Varsano S, Shapiro M, Taragan R, Bruderman I: Hypophosphatemia as a reversible cause of refractory ventilatory failure. Crit Care Med 11(11):908, 1983.
17. Matzner Y, Prococimer M, Polliack A, et al: Hypophosphatemia in a patient with lymphoma in leukemic phase. Arch Intern Med 141:805, 1981.
18. Wollner A, Shalit M, Brezis M: Tumor genesis syndrome. Hypophosphatemia accompanying Burkitt's lymphoma cell leukemia. Miner Electrolyte Metab 12(3):173, 1986.
19. Maddock RJ, Moses JA Jr, Roth WT, et al: Serum

phosphate and anxiety in major depression. Psychiatry Res 22(1):29, 1987.

20. Gorman JM, Cohen BS, Liebowitz MR, et al: Blood gas changes and hypophosphatemia in lactate-induced panic. Arch Gen Psychiatry 43(11):1067, 1986.

21. Friedman HZ, Langman CB, Favus MJ: Vitamin D metabolism and osteomalacia in cystic fibrosis. Gastroenterology 88(3):808, 1985.

22. Yagnik P, Singh N, Burns R: Peripheral neuropathy with hypophosphatemia in a patient receiving intravenous hyperalimentation. South Med J 78(11):1381, 1985.

23. Citrin DL, Elson P, Kies MS, Lind R: Decreased serum phosphate levels after high-dose estrogens in metastatic prostate cancer. Possible implications. Am J Med 76(5):787, 1984.

24. Hall KW, Dobson KE, Dalton JG: Metabolic abnormalities associated with intentional theophylline overdose. Ann Intern Med 101(4):457, 1984.

25. Robertson NJ: Fatal overdose from a sustained-release theophylline preparation. Ann Emerg Med 14(2):154, 1985.

26. Voigts A, Kaufman CE Jr: Acidosis and other metabolic abnormalities associated with paint sniffing. South Med J 76(4):443, 1983.

27. Gerad H, van Echo DA, Whitacre M, et al: Doxorubicin, cyclophosphamide, and whole body hyperthermia for treatment of advanced soft tissue sarcoma. Cancer 53(12):2585, 1984.

28. Madsen H, Ditzel J: Red cell 2,3-diphosphoglycerate and hemoglobin—oxygen affinity during normal pregnancy. Acta Obstet Gynecol Scand 63(5):399, 1984.

29. Patron P, Gardin JP, Paillard M: Renal mass and reserve of vitamin D: determinants in primary hyperparathyroidism. Kidney Int 31(5):1174, 1987.

30. Kirschbaum BB, Sica DA, Hom BM, Newsome HH: Hypocalciuric hyperparathyroidism with chronic renal failure. South Med J 76(8):1075, 1983.

31. Whyte MP, Teitelbaum SL, Murphy WA, et al: Adult hypophosphatasia. Medicine 58:329, 1979.

32. Fallon MD, Teitelbaum SL, Weinstein RS, et al: Hypophosphatasia: clinicopathologic comparison of the infantile, childhood, and adult forms. Medicine 63:12, 1984.

33. Lee PA, Van Dop C, Migeon CJ: McCune-Albright syndrome. Long-term follow-up. JAMA 256:2980, 1986.

34. Tieder M, Modai D, Shaked U, et al: "Idiopathic" hypercalciuria and hereditary hypophosphatemic rickets. Two phenotypical expressions of a common genetic defect. N Engl J Med 316:125, 1987.

Selected Readings

Aubier M, Murciano D, Lecocguic Y, et al: Effect of hypophosphatemia on diaphragmatic contractility in patients with acute respiratory failure. N Engl J Med 313:420, 1985.
A study of the effects of hypophosphatemia on diaphragmatic func-

tion in eight patients with acute respiratory failure who were artificially ventilated. Authors conclude that hypophosphatemia impairs the contractile properties of the diaphragm during acute respiratory failure, and they emphasize the importance of maintaining normal serum inorganic phosphate levels in such patients.

Berkelhammer C, Bear RA: A clinical approach to common electrolyte problems: 3. Hypophosphatemia. Can Med Assoc J 130(1):17, 1984.

This paper discusses common clinical disorders associated with hypophosphatemia and presents an approach to diagnosis and treatment.

Brautbar N, Altura BM: Hypophosphatemia and hypomagnesemia result in cardiovascular dysfunction: theoretical basis for alcohol-induced cellular injury. Alcoholism (NY) 11(2):118, 1987.

Authors propose several schemes for possible alcoholic-induced myocardial and vascular injury.

Gorman JM, Cohen BS, Liebowitz MR, et al: Blood gas changes and hypophosphatemia in lactate-induced panic. Arch Gen Psychiatry 43(11):1067, 1986.

Low inorganic phosphate levels at baseline appear associated with patients who will panic during subsequent lactate infusion. This finding may reflect hyperventilation or an abnormality in intracellular glycolysis.

Venditti FJ, Marotta C, Panezai FR, et al: Hypophosphatemia and cardiac arrhythmias. Miner Electrolyte Metab 13(1):19, 1987.

In the absence of known causes of cardiac arrhythmias, hypophosphatemia can be associated with significant ventricular ectopic activity.

HEMATOLOGY

104
Normochromic Normocytic Anemia: Common Causes and Associations

Causes of normochromic normocytic anemia include a wide spectrum of disorders. Abnormally-shaped erythrocytes and the degree of reticulocytosis can provide early clues to the etiology of normocytic anemia. The most common cause of normochromic normocytic anemia with increased reticulocytosis is acute blood loss.[1]

Increased reticulocytosis, particularly if spherocytes are evident on peripheral smear, also can reflect an underlying congenital or acquired hemolytic anemia. Chronic normocytic anemia with decreased reticulocytosis often leads to a diagnosis of disorders associated with suppressed bone marrow function. This may be secondary to an apparent primary pathology in hematopoietic progenitors in the bone marrow or secondary pathology with suboptimal production of hematopoietic growth factors, i.e., lack of erythropoietin production in patients who are anephric, or idiosyncratic autoimmunity to the precursors. Although the peripheral smear can sometimes hasten the diagnosis, for example, when schistocyte and burr cells are associated with renal failure, the etiology of inadequate bone marrow function is often difficult and may require multiple studies, including a bone marrow biopsy to rule out possible underlying infectious, inflammatory, and neoplastic disorders.

Posthemorrhagic blood loss: anemia may not be evident for up to 24 to 48 hours because of redistribution of body fluids.[1]
Anemia of chronic disease,[2] chronic infections and inflammation, malignancy,[3] rheumatic diseases[4]
Refractory anemia of the elderly: common causes of

723

anemia in the elderly include marrow aplasia, ineffective iron use, and preleukemic states.[5]

Hypothyroidism: may be associated with a macrocytosis[6]

Other endocrinopathies: hypoadrenalism, hypopituitarism, hypogonadism

Bone marrow suppression: aplastic anemia,[7] toxic suppression, drug-induced suppression, carcinoma

Chronic renal insufficiency: burr cells are often seen with uremia[8]; depressed erythropoietin production in anephric patients

Myeloproliferative disorders: leukemia, myelofibrosis

Sickle cell disorders[9]

Hypersplenism: a combination of splenic sequestration and dilution secondary to expanded plasma volume

References

1. Beissner RS, Trowbridge AA: Clinical assessment of anemia. Postgrad Med 80(6):83, 1986.
2. Roodman GD: Mechanisms of erythroid suppression in the anemia of chronic disease. Blood Cells 13:171, 1987.
3. Dutcher JP: Hematologic abnormalities in patients with nonhematologic malignancies. Hematol Oncol Clin North Am 1:281, 1987.
4. Richert-Boe KE: Hematologic complications of rheumatic disease. Hematol Oncol Clin North Am 1:301, 1987.
5. Gardner FH: Refractory anemia in the elderly. Adv Intern Med 32:155, 1987.
6. Mazzaferri EL: Adult hypothyroidism. 1. Manifestations and clinical presentation. Postgrad Med 79(7):64, 1986.
7. Ammus SS, Yunis AA: Acquired pure red cell aplasia. Am J Hematol 24:311, 1987.
8. Pavlovic-Kentera V, Clemons GK, Djukanovic L, Biljanovic-Paunovic L: Erythropoietin and anemia in chronic renal failure. Exp Hematol 15:785, 1987.
9. Embury SH: The clinical pathophysiology of sickle cell disease. Annu Rev Med 37:361, 1986.

Selected Readings

Brandeau ML, Eddy DM: the workup of the asymptomatic patient with a positive fecal occult blood test. Med Decis Making 7:32, 1987.
Workup protocols for an asymptomatic patient who has a positive fecal occult blood test are evaluated. Two protocols were particularly effective. In the first, a barium enema study is followed by colonoscopy; if colonoscopy is negative, the barium enema study is repeated. In the second, a colonoscopy is performed, and if negative, is followed with a barium enema study.

Cazzola M, Bergamaschi G, Huebers HA, Finch CA: Pathophysiological classification of acquired bone marrow failure based on quantitative assessment of erythroid function. Eur J Haematol 38:426, 1987.

Bone marrow failure encompasses a broad spectrum of disorders including aplastic, dysmyelopoietic, and myelophthistic anemias. This study characterizes these anemias according to the degree of erythroid proliferation and efficiency of erythropoiesis.

Erslev AJ, Wilson J, Caro J: Erythropoietin titers in anemic, nonuremic patients. J Lab Clin Med 109:429, 1987.

Study concludes that erythropoietin titers in these anemias appear to be determined primarily by the degree of anemia and not by any specific effect of these illnesses on the production of erythropoietin.

Fossat C, David M, Harle JR, et al: New parameters in erythrocyte counting. Value of histograms. Arch Pathol Lab Med 111:1150, 1987.

This study rates a new, third-generation automated hematology system that can furnish a full range of values, including erythrocyte parameters and a leukocyte differential count. The value of these parameters in classifying anemias is assessed in a patient population that included those with iron deficiency anemias, thalassemias, and other forms of anemia.

Gaillard HM, Hamilton GC: Hemoglobin/hematocrit and other erythrocyte parameters. Emerg Med Clin North Am 4:15, 1986.

This article discusses the clinical benefits of these two hematologic tests by reviewing what is being measured and how those values can be interpreted, with emphasis on emergency department evaluation.

Murgo AJ: Thrombotic microangiopathy in the cancer patient including those induced by chemotherapeutic agents. Semin Hematol 24:161, 1987.

Current concepts and review of mechanisms causing anemia and thrombocytopenia in cancer patients. Well-referenced clinical review article.

Quaglini S, Stefanelli M, Barosi G, Berzuini A: ANEMIA: an expert consultation system. Comput Biomed Res 19:13, 1986.

ANEMIA is a knowledge-based consultation program for anemic states. It has been built using an artificial intelligence programming scheme, called EXPERT, which was developed at Rutgers University. At present, ANEMIA is able to provide assistance in the diagnosis and management of disease entities, including iron deficiency anemias, anemias due to chronic disorders, thalassemias, hemolytic anemias, and a few other miscellaneous conditions.

105
Hypochromic Microcytic Anemia: Common Causes and Associations

Hypochromic microcytic (mean corpuscular volume [MCV] less than 80 μm^3) anemia reflects inadequate hemoglobin synthesis and is most commonly secondary to iron deficiency or chronic disease. Iron deficiency anemia should be suspected when low serum iron is associated with an elevated iron binding capacity. Absence of stainable iron in the bone marrow and low serum ferritin are diagnostic for iron deficiency anemia. Although rarer, hereditary hemoglobinopathies are an important diagnostic distinction because long-term iron replacement therapy inadvertently given to patients with thalassemia could result in hemochromatosis.[1] When thalassemia is suspected, hemoglobin electrophoresis, hemoglobin A2 levels, fetal hemoglobin levels, and family studies may lead to the diagnosis of beta-thalassemia or one of the variants.[2]

Iron deficiency: laboratory findings (decreased MCV, low serum iron, and increased iron binding capacity) can be delayed up to 4 weeks after onset of blood loss.[3]

Anemia of chronic disease: may be microcytic or normocytic. Common chronic disorders include infections, inflammations, malignancy, and rheumatic diseases.[4-6]

Occult gastrointestinal blood loss: polyps of the colon,[7] Barrett's esophagus,[8] drug-induced gastric bleeding,[9,10] colorectal carcinoma, metastatic disease[11]

Thalassemia: family history and peripheral smear findings, such as target cells, poikilocytosis, and basophilic stippling on peripheral smear, may provide important diagnostic clues.[12,13]
Beta—homozygous
Beta—heterozygous
Alpha trait

Hemoglobin E: consider the diagnosis of hemoglobin E in southeast Asians with microcytosis, whether anemic or not.[14]

Sideroblastic anemia: iron stain of bone marrow discloses ring sideroblasts.[15]

Congenital sideroblastic anemia

Pyridoxine responsive

Preleukemic

Drug-induced: chemotherapy, chloramphenicol, antituberculosis therapy

Lead poisoning: suspect lead poisoning when given a history of lead exposure; basophilic stippling occurs in less than 10% of red blood cells. Elevated serum and urine lead levels may be helpful.[16]

References

1. Beissner RS, Trowbridge AA: Clinical assessment of anemia. Postgrad Med 80(6):83, 1986.
2. Kellermeyer RW: General principles of the evaluation and therapy of anemias. Med Clin North Am 68:533, 1984.
3. Wallerstein RO: Role of the laboratory in the diagnosis of anemia. JAMA 236:490, 1976.
4. Roodman GD: Mechanisms of erythroid suppression in the anemia of chronic disease. Blood Cells 13:171, 1987.
5. Dutcher JP: Hematologic abnormalities in patients with nonhematologic malignancies. Hematol Oncol Clin North Am 1:281, 1987.
6. Richert-Boe KE: Hematologic complications of rheumatic disease. Hematol Oncol Clin North Am 1:301, 1987.
7. Kelly JK, Langevin JM, Price LM, et al: Giant and symptomatic inflammatory polyps of the colon in idiopathic inflammatory bowel disease. Am J Surg Pathol 10:420, 1986.
8. Cooper BT, Barbezat GO: Barrett's esophagus: a clinical study of 52 patients. Q J Med 62:97, 1987.
9. Ivey KJ: Gastrointestinal intolerance and bleeding with non-narcotic analgesics. Drugs 32(Suppl 4):71, 1986.
10. Jaffin BW, Bliss CM, LaMont JT: Significance of occult gastrointestinal bleeding during anticoagulation therapy. Am J Med 83:269, 1987.
11. Yang PM, Sheu JC, Yang TH, et al: Metastasis of hepatocellular carcinoma to the proximal jejunum manifested by occult gastrointestinal bleeding. Am J Gastroenterol 82:165, 1987.
12. Steinberg MH, Embury SH: Alpha-thalassemia in blacks: genetic and clinical aspects and interactions with the sickle hemoglobin gene. Blood 68:985, 1986.
13. Orkin SH: Molecular genetics and potential gene therapy. Clin Immunol Immunopathol 40:151, 1986.
14. Lachant NA: Hemoglobin E: an emerging hemoglobinopathy in the United States. Am J Hematol 25:449, 1987.

15. Pasanen A, Tenhunen R: Heme synthesis in sidero-blastic anemias. Scand J Haematol 45(Suppl):60, 1986.
16. Cullen MR, Robins JM, Eskenazi B: Adult inorganic lead intoxication: presentation of 31 new cases and a review of recent advances in the literature. Medicine 62:221, 1983.

Selected Readings

Cao A, Rosatelli C, Pirastu M: Prenatal diagnosis of inherited hemoglobinopathies. J Genet Hum 34:413, 1986.

This paper reviews the different methods presently available for prenatal diagnosis of hemoglobin disorders and the impact of this technology in the control of beta-thalassemia in several Mediterranean populations.

Robertson JD, Maughan RJ, Davidson RJ: Fecal blood loss in response to exercise. Br Med J (Clin Res) 295:303, 1987.

Interesting report of recent qualitative tests indicating that gastrointestinal bleeding during exercise may be an important contributory factor in sports anemia. Study concludes that use of drugs, particularly analgesics, by marathon runners should be discouraged.

106
Macrocytic Anemia: Megaloblastic Anemias and Other Causes

A routine laboratory finding of macrocytosis (mean corpuscular volume [MCV] greater than or equal to 105 μm^3) can be the first manifestation of vitamin deficiency, preleukemia, or alcoholism.[1] Macrocytic anemia reflects an underlying disordered or increased erythropoiesis associated with conditions often first suspected from abnormal erythrocytes found on peripheral smear. Such helpful findings might include hypersegmented neutrophils associated with B_{12} deficiency; oval and tear drop-shaped erythrocytes seen with myelofibrosis; and predominantly round macrocytes seen with increased reticulocytosis, chronic liver disease, and in aplastic anemias.[2] Macrocytosis can lead to the diagnosis of megaloblastic anemia, which is most commonly caused by deficiency of B_{12} or folate, or by drugs that inhibit the absorption and/or use/metabolism of these vitamins. Although serum B_{12} and red cell folate levels are helpful, only a minority of patients with macrocytosis are found to have a megaloblastic anemia.[3] Alcoholism and disorders that increase reticulocytosis, such as hemolysis and chronic blood loss, are important diagnostic considerations.

Vitamin B_{12} deficiency: pernicious anemia, gastrointestinal disorders,[4] cancer, malnutrition, malabsorption, infestation of *Diphyllobothrium latum* or fish tapeworm associated with eating sushi and tasting raw gefilte fish[5]

Folate deficiency[6]: diet, pregnancy,[7] drugs, malabsorption, alcohol, cancer, malnutrition

Alcoholism: folate deficiency and direct toxic effects are proposed mechanism; however, macrocytosis is also seen in alcoholism without evidence of folate deficiency or liver disease[3]

Myeloproliferative disorders: preleukemia, lymphoma, myelofibrosis with extramedullary myeloid metaplasia, leukemia, multiple myeloma (usually only in the setting of patients receiving cytotoxic drugs, in which case, macrocytosis may be secondary to treatment), other causes of bone marrow failure

Chronic liver disease: round erythrocytes and target cells commonly found in alcoholics

Cytotoxic drugs: chlorambucil, melphalan, methotrexate, azathioprine, cyclophosphamide, procarbazine, busulfan

Gastric bypass surgery[8]

Hypothyroidism

Reticulocytosis: hemolysis or acute blood loss

Normal pregnancy

Healthy neonates: macrocytosis in newborns becomes microcytosis at 3 months.[9]

References

1. Breedveld FC, Bieger R, van Wermeskerken RK: The clinical significance of macrocytosis. Acta Med Scand 209:319, 1981.
2. Rapaport SI (ed): Diagnosis of anemia. p. 10. In Intro-

duction to Hematology. 2nd ed. JB Lippincott, Philadelphia, 1987.

3. Wheby MS: Anemia: classification, mechanisms, diagnosis, and physiologic effects. p. 170. In Thorup OA Jr (ed): Fundamentals of Clinical Hematology. 5th ed. WB Saunders, Philadelphia, 1987.

4. Phillips DL, Keeffe EB: Hematologic manifestations of gastrointestinal disease. Hematol Oncol Clin North Am 1:207, 1987.

5. Goldmann DR: Hold the sushi. JAMA 253:2495, 1985.

6. Davis RE: Clinical chemistry of folic acid. Adv Clin Chem 25:233, 1986.

7. Qvist I, Abdulla M, Jagerstad M, Svensson S: Iron, zinc, and folate status during pregnancy and two months after delivery. Acta Obstet Gynecol Scand 65:15, 1986.

8. Schilling RF, Gohdes PN, Hardie GH: Vitamin B_{12} deficiency after gastric bypass surgery for obesity. Ann Intern Med 101:501, 1984.

9. Beissner RS, Trowbridge AA: Clinical assessment of anemia. Postgrad Med 80 (6):83, 1986.

Selected Readings

Thompson WG, Babitz L, Cassino C, et al: Evaluation of current criteria used to measure vitamin B_{12} levels. Am J Med 82:291, 1987.

Recent improvements in serum vitamin B_{12} assays, indicate a reevaluation of previous serum B_{12} assays.

107
Hemolytic Anemia: Common Causes and Associations

Acute hemolytic anemia can precipitate a medical crisis. Clinical signs of fulminant hemolysis are obvious, such as acute hypotension, hemoglobinuria, and hemoglobinemia, particularly in the clinical setting of transfusion therapy, sepsis, a known lymphoproliferative disorder, or drugs associated with increased risk for immune reactions.[1] Chronic, recurrent hemolytic anemia may not be obvious because symptoms can be intermittent and transient, such as episodic generalized weakness, icterus, dark urine, or dark stools.

Initial laboratory findings can be misleading, for example, significant reticulocytosis can mimic a macrocytic anemia. Other laboratory findings, such as the following however, can be very helpful: spherocytosis, found in both congenital and acquired hemolytic anemias; hypochromic and sickled cells seen in hemoglobinopathies; fragmented cells suggesting vascular damage such as occurs with infections and neoplasms; basophilic stippling seen in lead poisoning and thalassemia; and target cells with liver disease and hemoglobinopathies.[2]

Hereditary
  Membrane defects: hereditary spherocytosis, elliptocytosis, stomatocytosis, Rh null syndrome
  Enzyme defects: pentose phosphate shunt (G-6-PD deficiency), glutathione glycolytic enzyme, and nucleotide enzyme disorders
  Hemoglobinopathies: sickle cell anemia, hemoglobin C disease, thalassemia, and others[3-5]
  Erythropoietic porphyrias[6]
Paroxysmal nocturnal hemoglobinuria: can present with acute anemia, thrombocytopenia and nephropathy, which may simulate hemolytic uremic syndrome[7,8]
Lead poisoning: serum and urine lead levels may be helpful.[9]
Mechanical: prosthetic heart valve associated[10]
Drug-induced: increased incidence of immune hemolytic anemia associated with nonsteroidal anti-inflammatory drugs. Drugs implicated include mefenamic acid, ibuprofen, sulindac, naproxen, tolmetin, and aspirin.[11]
Arsenic hydride: from inhalation of arsine gas (arsenic hydride, AsH_3) formed in the course of many industrial processes
Copper: from ingestion of copper sulfate in suicide attempts and from accumulation of toxic amounts from hemodialysis fluid contaminated by copper pipes
Insect venoms: bee and wasp stings have been associated with severe hemolysis; also reported are spider and scorpion bites.
Heat: severe burns; the acute hemolytic anemia seen

in the first 24 hours after severe second- and third-degree burns is thought secondary to direct effects of heat on circulating erythrocytes.

Transfusion reactions: immediate and delayed (after 10 to 18 days). Two basic mechanisms: (1) direct effect, (2) induction of autoimmune-type reactions Autoantibodies[12]

Hypophosphatemia: important consideration in hospitalized alcoholics and in diabetic ketoacidosis[13]

Infection: with or without signs of disseminated intravascular coagulation (DIC); classic example is malaria. Other infections with pathogenesis involving red blood cell hemolysis include bartonellosis, babesiosis, and *Clostridium welchii*. Also, *Mycoplasma pneumoniae* infections with induction of cold agglutinins.

Liver disease: peripheral smear may contain target cells[14]

Pregnancy

Cancer

Lymphoproliferative disease

Autoimmune hemolytic disease of newborn

References

1. Gregory SA, McKenna R, Sassetti RJ, Knospe WH: Hematologic emergencies. Med Clin North Am 70:1129, 1986.
2. Rapaport SI (ed): Diagnosis of anemia. p. 10. In Introduction to Hematology. 2nd Ed. JB Lippincott, Philadelphia, 1987.
3. Fucharoen S, Winichagoon P: Hemoglobinopathies in Southeast Asia. Hemoglobin 11:65, 1987.
4. Lambotte C: Hemoglobinopathies and related syndromes. General introduction. Personal experience in Africa and Europe. J Genet Hum 34:375, 1986.
5. Wheby MS: Anemia: classification, mechanisms, diagnosis, and physiologic effects. p. 165. In Thorup OA Jr (ed): Fundamentals of Clinical Hematology. WB Saunders, Philadelphia, 1987.
6. Poh-Fitzpatrick MB: The erythropoietic porphyrias. Dermatol Clin 4:291, 1986.
7. Dockter ME, Morrison M: Paroxysmal nocturnal hemoglobinuria erythrocytes are of two distinct types: positive or negative for acetylcholinesterase. Blood 67:540, 1986.
8. Kletzel M, Arnold WC, Berry DH: Paroxysmal nocturnal hemoglobinuria presenting as recurrent hemolytic uremic syndrome. Clin Pediatr 26:319, 1987.
9. Cullen MR, Robins JM, Eskenazi B: Adult inorganic lead intoxication: presentation of 31 new cases and a review of recent advances in the literature. Medicine 62:221, 1983.
10. Carrier M, Martineau JP, Bonan R, Pelletier LC: Clinical

and hemodynamic assessment of the Omniscience prosthetic heart valve. J Thorac Cardiovasc Surg 93:300, 1987.
11. Sanford-Driscoll M, Knodel LC: Induction of hemolytic anemia by nonsteroidal antiinflammatory drugs. Drug Intell Clin Pharm 20:925, 1986.
12. Sokol RJ, Hewitt S: Autoimmune hemolysis: a critical review. CRC Crit Rev Oncol Hematol 4:125, 1985.
13. Shilo S, Werner D, Hershko C: Acute hemolytic anemia caused by severe hypophosphatemia in diabetic ketoacidosis. Acta Haematol (Basel) 73:55, 1985.
14. Ostrowski J: Erythrocyte porphobilinogen deaminase activity in liver disease. Gastroenterology 92:845, 1987.

Selected Readings

Brimijoin S, Hammond PI, Petitt RM: Paroxysmal nocturnal hemoglobinuria: erythrocyte acetylcholinesterase deficit analyzed by immunoassay and fluorescence-activated sorting. Mayo Clin Proc 61:522, 1986.

An immunodisplacement assay based on a specific, solid-phase monoclonal antibody was designed to measure acetylcholinesterase in tissue extracts. Inasmuch as enzyme-deficient cells represent the complement-sensitive population, cell sorting may help in assessing clinical status and, perhaps, in developing new therapeutic modalities for paroxysmal nocturnal hemoglobinuria.

Gregory SA, McKenna R, Sassetti RJ, Knospe WH: Hematologic emergencies. Med Clin North Am 70:1129, 1986.

This article reviews emergencies associated with red cell, white cell, and hemostatic disorders as well as transfusion reactions. Useful clinical data.

Patten E: Immunohematologic diseases. JAMA 258:2945, 1987.

Useful review of current concepts of pathophysiology of autoimmune hematologic disorders highlighting transfusion reactions, cold agglutinin disease, drug-induced immune hemolysis, thrombocytopenia purpura, and autoimmune disorders of neutrophils.

108

Polycythemia: Causes of Primary, Secondary, and Relative Polycythemia

Polycythemia is a laboratory finding of increased erythrocytes. Elevated hematocrits (52% in men, 47% in women) or elevated hemoglobins (17.7 g/dl in men, 15.7 g/dl in women), are often the first clues.[1] Symptoms of mild, chronic polycythemia are usually nonspecific, such as dizziness, headaches, and pruritus. Symptoms of severe polycythemia (hematocrits greater than 60%), however, can be devastating, even manifesting as stroke[2] or myocardial infarction.[3] When confronted with an elevated hematocrit, it is important to distinguish between a relative and absolute polycythemia. Relative and absolute polycythemia are differentiated by measuring the red cell mass and plasma volume.[4] A relative polycythemia reflects a relative volume loss or state of hemoconcentration, whereas an absolute polycythemia reflects an actual increase in red cell volume, which can be a primary or secondary process. Secondary polycythemia can be further categorized as physiologically appropriate or physiologically inappropriate.[1]

Relative Polycythemia

The red cell mass is normal, but the plasma volume is contracted. Dehydration and stress polycythemia are the most common causes of relative polycythemia.

Excessive body fluid losses: vomiting, diarrhea, water deprivation, sweating, burns
Stress erythrocytosis or Gaisböck's syndrome: commonly seen in middle-aged men with cardiovascular risk factors, such as hypertension and coronary artery disease[1]

Absolute-Primary Polycythemia

The red cell mass is increased and the plasma volume is either increased or normal.

Polycythemia vera: a hematopoietic stem-cell disease

of clonal origin associated with hepatosplenomegaly and panhyperplastic marrow, which produces granulocytosis, eosinophilia, and basophilia.[5]

Secondary Physiologically Appropriate Polycythemia

When polycythemia occurs in physiologic response to tissue hypoxia, underlying cardiopulmonary insufficiency is a common cause. Hemoglobinopathies with disordered oxygen-carrying function provide a less common but important diagnostic consideration.[6]

Pulmonary insufficiency: chronic obstructive pulmonary disease,[7] pulmonary arteriovenous fistulae, poorly perfused aerated lung

Hypoventilation: pickwickian syndrome, nocturnal hypoxia,[8] chronic lung disease, congestive heart failure

Cardiovascular disease: right-to-left shunts, congenital heart disease[9]

High altitude[10,11]

Hemoglobins with disordered oxygen binding: acquired or congenital methemoglobinemia, acquired sulfhemoglobinemia, acquired carboxyhemoglobinemia, i.e., smokers' polycythemia, which occurs when excessive smoking causes undue exposure to high levels of carbon monoxide that has a high affinity for hemoglobin and can be measured as carboxyhemoglobin[12,13]

Hemoglobins with increased affinity for oxygen: alpha chain variants include Chesapeake, Capetown; beta chain variants include Rainier, Yakima, Kempsey, Ypsilanti, Hiroshima. More than 30 variants have been described.

Congenitally decreased levels of 2,3-DPG or hemoglobin variants that have altered binding to 2,3-DPG

Autosomal dominant polycythemia[14]

Kidney diseases

Renovascular disease: renal artery stenosis causing local renal hypoxia and resultant increased erythropoietin production

Hypernephroma: check for hematuria

Hydronephrosis

Cystic kidney

Transplant rejection

Exogenous androgen administration

Adrenal hypercorticism

Virilizing tumors

Environmental toxin exposure: nitrites, sulfonamides, coal tar derivatives, others producing met-
hemoglobin and sulfhemoglobin
Cobalt, various alcohols

**Secondary
Physiologically
Inappropriate
Polycythemia**

When polycythemia occurs in response to inappropriately elevated erythropoietin, consider possible
hepatic[15] or renal[16] neoplasms. Such polycythemia
can be the first clue to certain uncommon neoplasms.

Nonmalignant renal disorders: cysts, tumors, hydro-
nephrosis, renal transplantation (during rejection)
Malignant renal disorders: hypernephroma, carci-
noma, adenoma
Pheochromocytoma[17]
Adrenal adenoma
Hepatoma
Cerebellar hemangioblastoma
Uterine leiomyoma
Ovarian carcinoma
Von Hippel-Lindau disease: an inherited disorder
with a wide spectrum of manifestations, including
tumors such as cerebellar hemangioblastoma, renal
cell carcinoma, and pheochromocytoma[18]
Idiopathic or exertional erythrocytosis[19]

References

1. Golde DW, Hocking WG, Koeffler HP, Adamson JW:
   Polycythemia: mechanisms and management. Ann Intern Med 95:71, 1981.
2. Pearce JM, Chandrasekera CP, Ladusans EJ: Lacunar
   infarcts in polycythemia with raised packed cell volumes.
   Br Med J (Clin Res) 287:935, 1983.
3. Yeager SB, Freed MD: Myocardial infarction as a
   manifestation of polycythemia in cyanotic heart disease.
   Am J Cardiol 53:952, 1984.
4. Silverstein MN: Relative and absolute polycythemia.
   How to tell them apart. Postgrad Med 81(5):285, 1987.
5. Adamson JW, Fialkow PJ, Murphy S, et al: Polycythemia
   vera: stem-cell and probable clonal origin of the disease.
   N Engl J Med 295:913, 1976.
6. Imai K: Functional abnormalities in hemoglobin variants: abnormalities in oxygen-transport function. Nippon Ketsueki Gakkai Zasshi 48:1993, 1985.
7. Guidet B, Offenstadt G, Boffa G, et al: Polycythemia
   in chronic obstructive pulmonary disease. A study of
   serum and urine erythropoietin and medullary erythroid progenitors. Chest 92:867, 1987.
8. Moore-Gillon JC, Treacher DF, Gaminara EJ, et al:
   Intermittent hypoxia in patients with unexplained
   polycythaemia. Br Med J (Clin Res) 293:588, 1986.

9. Rosove MH, Perloff JK, Hocking WG, et al: Chronic hypoxemia and decompensated erythrocytosis in cyanotic congenital heart disease. Lancet 2:313, 1986.
10. Fujimaki T, Matsutani M, Asai A, et al: Cerebral venous thrombosis due to high-altitude polycythemia. J Neurosurg 64:148, 1986.
11. Gronbeck C III: Chronic mountain sickness at an elevation of 2,000 meters. Chest 85:577, 1984.
12. Smith JR, Landaw SA: Smokers' polycythemia. N Engl J Med 298:6, 1978.
13. Doll DC, Greenberg BR: Cerebral thrombosis in smokers' polycythemia. Ann Intern Med 102:786, 1985.
14. Prchal JT, Crist WM, Goldwasser E, et al: Autosomal dominant polycythemia. Blood 66:1208, 1985.
15. Desaint B, Conrad M, Florent C, et al: Polycythemia in liver diseases. Ann Gastroenterol Hepatol 22:399, 1986.
16. Hocking WG: Hematologic abnormalities in patients with renal disease. Hematol Oncol Clin North Am 1:229, 1987.
17. Shulkin BL, Shapiro B, Sisson JC: Pheochromocytoma, polycythemia, and venous thrombosis. Am J Med 83:773, 1987.
18. Burns C, Levine PH, Reichman H, Stock JL: Adrenal hemangioblastoma in Von Hippel-Lindau disease as a cause of secondary erythrocytosis. Am J Med Sci 293:119, 1987.
19. Mankad VN, Moore RB, McRoyan D, Zuckerman K: Erythrocytosis associated with spontaneous erythroid colony formation and idiopathic hypererythyropoietinemia. J Pediatr 111:743, 1987.

Selected Readings

Cotes PM, Dore CJ, Yin JA, et al: Determination of serum immunoreactive erythropoietin in the investigation of erythrocytosis. N Engl J Med 315:283, 1986.
Among patients with erythrocytosis with an unknown cause, this assay is useful in identifying patients with secondary erythrocytosis who have inappropriate erythropoietin secretion.

Datz FL, Taylor A Jr: The clinical use of radionuclide bone marrow imaging. Semin Nucl Med 15:239, 1985.
Bone marrow aspiration and biopsy are excellent techniques for evaluating bone marrow, but this evaluation is limited to a small part of the total blood-forming organ. With the introduction of radionuclide bone marrow imaging, a simple technique became available that overcomes marrow sampling error by giving a total body view of functioning marrow.

Grotta JC, Manner C, Pettigrew LC, Yatsu FM: Red blood cell disorders and stroke. Stroke 17:811, 1986.
Helpful clinical review.

Ihde DC: Paraneoplastic syndromes. Hosp Pract 22 (8):105, 1987.
Hematologic and other paraneoplastic syndromes are organized in an interesting clinical review.

Mundy GR: Ectopic hormonal syndromes in neoplastic disease. Hosp Pract 22(4):179, 1987.
Interesting clinical update.

109
Causes of Thrombocytopenia

The evaluation of thrombocytopenia should include questioning the patient for a history of bleeding, either spontaneous or associated with minor surgery. Examination of the blood smear is essential to rule out artifactual or pseudothrombocytopenia (see p. 741). Should thrombocytopenia be confirmed, then distinction into one of two categories is important for diagnosis and therapeutic reasons. These two categories are (1) thrombocytopenia secondary to inadequate megakaryocytopoiesis, and (2) thrombocytopenia secondary to excessive platelet destruction. Examination of the bone marrow is extremely helpful in this regard. Finding normal or enhanced megakaryocytopoiesis in the setting of thrombocytopenia, for example, argues for a shortened platelet survival.

Acquired Aplastic Anemia	General Megakaryocytic aplasia
Autoimmune	Immune thrombocytopenia purpura (ITP) Rheumatoid arthritis: Felty's syndrome Systemic lupus erythematosus
Cyclic Thrombocytopenia[1]	Periodic thrombocytopenia has an average 30 day cycle, with a range of 20 to 40 days. Megakaryocytes are reduced in number when platelet count is lowest. Etiology is unknown. However, it is speculated that cyclic thrombocytopenia is secondary to abnormal responsiveness of the marrow to either positive- or negative-feedback stimuli.
Disseminated Intravascular Coagulation	Look for microangiopathy on blood smear and for presence of fibrin-split products and coagulopathy.
Drug- and Toxin-Induced	Biologic response modifiers: interferon-alpha Cytotoxic drugs

738

Antimetabolites: 6-mercaptopurine, cytosine arabinoside, antifolates
Antracyclines: doxorubicin, daunomycin
Nitrogen mustards: busulfan, procarbazine, cyclophosphamide
Drug reactions (common)
Antibiotics: ristocetin
Antirheumatic drugs: gold salts[2]
Diuretics: thiazide diuretics
Heparin[3,4]
Protamine sulfate
Idiosyncratic drug reactions
Acetaminophen
Allopurinol
Antiarrhythmics: diltiazem, amiodarone[5,6]
Antibiotics: chloramphenicol,[7] isoniazide (INH), sulfonamides, streptomycin, rifampin,[8] cephalosporins
Anticonvulsants: carbamazepine, ethosuximide, paramethadione, phenacemide, phenytoin,[9] trimethadione, sodium valproate
Antihistamines: tripelennamine, cimetidine,[9] ranitidine
Antihypertensives: hydralazine, captopril
Antirheumatic drugs: colchicine, indomethacin, phenylbutazone, aspirin
Cinchona alkaloids: quinidine,[10] quinine
Diuretics: acetazolamide, furosemide
Estrogens: diethylstilbestrol
Hypoglycemics: carbutamide, chlorpropamide, tolbutamide
Sulfhydryl compounds[11]
Tranquilizers: chlordiazepoxide, chlorpromazine, meprobamate, promazine
Vinblastine[12]
Toxins
Abused toxins: ethanol alcohol[13]
Environmental toxins: benzene, trinitrotoluene, arsenic, vinyl chloride, turpentine
Snake bite venom

Hereditary Thrombocytopenia

May-Hegglin anomaly: rare autosomal dominant trait characterized by giant platelets and basophilic inclusions within granulocytes
Factor IX deficiency
Giant platelet syndrome: similar to May-Hegglin anomaly except that granulocytes lack basophilic inclusions

Thrombocytopenia with absent radius syndrome
Thrombocytopenia with normal platelet morphology: i.e., Alport's syndrome—associated with nerve deafness and nephritis.
Thrombopoietin deficiency
von Willebrand's disease
Wiskott-Aldrich syndrome: X-linked disorder seen in males characterized by eczema, thrombocytopenia with microplatelets, and susceptibility to infections secondary to immunodeficiency. Unlike other inherited thrombocytopenias, reduced platelet levels in this syndrome appear secondary in part to accelerated platelet destruction.

Infectious Disease-Related Thrombocytopenia

Bacterial
Meningococcal septicemia
Mycoplasma pneumoniae
Protozoan
Malaria: often in the setting of disseminated intravascular coagulation
Toxoplasmosis
Leishmaniasis: *Leishmania donovani*
Viral
Cytomegalovirus infections, especially in newborns
Early lymphocytic choriomeningitis infection
Infectious mononucleosis: usually during acute phase of early illness[14]
Herpes simplex: with disseminated and severe disease
Human immunodeficiency virus (HIV)
Mumps
Parvovirus infections
Rubella: usually within 1 week of onset of rash and most prominent in newborns
Varicella
Viral hepatitis

Marrow Infiltration

Myelofibrosis
Gaucher's disease
Osteopetrosis

Nutritional

Anorexia
Folic acid deficiency: examine for megaloblastic anemia
Vitamin B_{12} deficiency: in pernicious anemia

Iron deficiency: associated thrombocytopenia is usually seen in children and young adults with severe deficiency

Malignancies

Carcinoma widely metastatic to the bone marrow
Leukemia
Mastocytosis
Myeloma

Paroxysmal Nocturnal Hemoglobinuria

Thrombocytopenia is reflective of stem cell disorder in paroxysmal nocturnal hemoglubinuria (PNH), a predysplastic syndrome. The diagnosis of PNH should be considered in patients with unexplained chronic thrombocytopenia.[15,16]

Physical Factors Possibly Affecting Platelet Survival

Aortic valvular disease
Burns
Extracorporeal perfusion
Fat embolism
Glomerulonephritis
Hemangioma
Primary pulmonary hypertension
Swan-Ganz catheter
Pulmonary embolus[17]
Ionizing radiation

Pregnancy Related

Preeclampsia
Thrombocytopenia of prematurity

Pseudothrombo-cytopenia

It is important to rule out the presence of platelet autoagglutinins causing agglutination in the presence of EDTA.[18] Less commonly, platelet autoagglutinins may act independently to clump platelets after phlebotomy independent of the anticoagulant used. Platelet clumping results in the platelet count being artifactually low by automated particle counters. This condition should be ruled out by carefully examining a well-prepared blood film.

Thrombotic Thrombocytopenic Purpura

A patient with thrombotic thrombocytopenic purpura[19] will have a triad of hemolytic anemia associated with microangiopathic changes in erythrocytes, thrombocytopenia, and fluctuating, often severe, neurologic abnormalities. It is usually associated with fever and renal dysfunction.

References

1. von Schulthess GK, Gessner U: Oscillating platelet counts in healthy individuals: experimental investigation and quantitative evaluation of thrombocytopoietic feedback control. Scand J Haematol 36:473, 1986.
2. Adachi JD, Bensen WG, Kassam Y, et al: Gold induced thrombocytopenia: 12 cases and a review of the literature. Semin Arthritis Rheum 16:287, 1987.
3. Kelton JG, Murphy WG: Acute thrombocytopenia and thrombosis. Heparin-induced thrombocytopenia and thrombotic thrombocytopenic purpura. Ann NY Acad Sci 509:205, 1987.
4. Laster J, Cikrit D, Walker N, Silver D: The heparin-induced thrombocytopenia syndrome: an update. Surgery 102:763, 1987.
5. Baggott LA: Diltiazem-associated immune thrombocytopenia. Mt Sinai J Med (NY) 54:500, 1987.
6. Weinberger I, Rotenberg Z, Fuchs J, et al: Amiodarone-induced thrombocytopenia. Arch Intern Med 147:735, 1987.
7. Feder HM Jr: Chloramphenicol: what we have learned in the last decade. South Med J 79:1129, 1986.
8. Pau AK, Fisher MA: Severe thrombocytopenia associated with once-daily rifampin therapy. Drug Intell Clin Pharm 21:882, 1987.
9. Yue CP, Mann KS, Chan KH: Severe thrombocytopenia due to combined cimetidine and phenytoin therapy. Neurosurgery 20:963, 1987.
10. Reid DM, Shulman NR: Drug purpura due to surreptitious quinidine intake. Ann Intern Med 108:206, 1988.
11. Jaffe IA: Adverse effects profile of sulfhydryl compounds in man. Am J Med 80:471, 1986.
12. Abrahamsen AF, Klepp O, Fossa SD, Snstevold A: Transient vinblastine-induced thrombocytopenia during chemotherapy with vinblastine, cis-platinum and bleomycin. Scand J Haematol 37:44, 1986.
13. Jansen EH, Bieger R: Severe thrombocytopenia due to alcohol abuse. Ned Tijdschr Geneeskd 130:1612, 1986.
14. Purtilo DT: Epstein-Barr virus: the spectrum of its manifestations in human beings. South Med J 80:943, 1987.
15. Solal-Celigny P, Tertian G, Fernandez H, et al: Pregnancy and paroxysmal nocturnal hemoglobinuria. Arch Intern Med 148:593, 1988.
16. Baumann MA, Pacheco J, Paul CC, et al: Paroxysmal nocturnal hemoglobinuria associated with the acquired immunodeficiency syndrome. Arch Intern Med 148:212, 1988.
17. Pesola GR, Carlon GC: Pulmonary embolus-induced disseminated intravascular coagulation. Crit Care Med 15:983, 1987.
18. van Vliet HH, Kappers-Klunne MC, Abels J: Pseudo-thrombocytopenia: a cold autoantibody against platelet glycoprotein GP IIb. Br J Haematol 62:501, 1986.
19. Bowdler AJ: Chronic relapsing thrombotic thrombocytopenia purpura. South Med J 80:507, 1987.

Selected Readings

Aster RH: Quantitative platelet disorders. p.1290. In Williams WJ, Beutler E, Ersley AJ, Lichtman MA (eds): Hematology, 3rd Ed. McGraw-Hill, New York, 1983. *Good general reference.*

Atkinson JL, Sundt TM Jr, Kazmier FJ, et al: Heparin-induced thrombocytopenia and thrombosis in ischemic stroke. Mayo Clin Proc 63:353, 1988. *A retrospective study of patients who underwent carotid endarterectomy to determine the frequency of postoperative occlusions and the role of heparin-induced thrombosis suggests that a potential for increased risk of embolic or thrombotic cerebrovascular events in patients treated with heparin exists.*

Brannan DP, Guthrie TH Jr: Idiopathic thrombocytopenic purpura in adults. South Med J 81:75, 1988. *Idiopathic thrombocytopenic purpura—an immune thrombocytopenia usually manifested by acute bleeding, thrombocytopenia, and normal to increased megakaryocytes in the bone marrow—is often associated with an IgG antibody against the platelet membrane. Pathophysiology, clinical features, and current concepts of management are reviewed.*

Carr ME Jr: Disseminated intravascular coagulation: pathogenesis, diagnosis, and therapy. J Emerg Med 5:311, 1987. *Pathogenesis, diagnosis, and management of disseminated intravascular coagulation are reviewed, including recent laboratory tests and experimental therapy.*

Fruchtman S, Aledort LM: Disseminated intravascular coagulation. J Am Coll Cardiol 8 (6 Suppl B):159B, 1986. *Thrombin generation is the central process that marks disseminated intravascular coagulation. Although this may lead to thrombosis, usually of the microcirculation, hemorrhage can also occur. The pathophysiologic, clinical, and laboratory features of disseminated intravascular coagulation are reviewed, with an emphasis on early recognition of this life-threatening state.*

Harker LA, Fuster V: Pharmacology of platelet inhibitors. J Am Coll Cardiol 8(6 Suppl B):21B, 1986. *Useful pharmacologic review to enhance the choice of suitable platelet-inhibiting drugs.*

Nilsson T, Norberg B: Thrombocytopenia and pseudothrombocytopenia: a clinical and laboratory problem. Scand J Haematol 37:341, 1986. *A review of patients with thrombocytopenia evaluated in a hematologic outpatient clinic found that pseudothrombocytopenia and thrombocytopathies can confuse management of patients with alleged thrombocytopenia. It is suggested that an assessment of platelet morphology and hemostatic testing should be added to platelet function testing.*

Pabinger I: Clinical relevance of protein C. Blut 53:63, 1986. *Heterozygous and homozygous protein C deficiency states are reviewed. Heterozygous protein deficiency is an important risk factor for venous thrombosis and pulmonary embolism.*

110
Coagulation Disorders: Most Common Clinical Associations

Coagulation disorders that cause an increased bleeding tendency generally can be assigned to either of two basic categories: (1) ineffective action of procoagulant proteins, or (2) insufficient platelet activity. Clinical history of hemarthroses, hematomas, hematuria and/or prolonged bleeding after minor trauma generally indicate the former category, whereas history of late bleeding after trauma (4 to 6 hours later), epistaxis, gastrointestinal bleeding and/or presence of petechiae usually correlate with ineffective platelet function.

Clinical history is important in determining whether a bleeding disorder is congenital or acquired. Prior history of an uneventful tooth extraction or major surgery, for example, generally rules out a significant congenital bleeding tendency. Laboratory testing, essential for diagnosis, may reveal subclinical bleeding disorders that may become significant after invasive diagnostic procedures or surgery.

The tests commonly used for screening procoagulant activity assay either of the two classic procoagulant cascades that may generate the thrombin necessary for clot formation—the so-called intrinsic and extrinsic clotting pathways. The former pathway is so named as it uses proteins "intrinsic" to the cell-free plasma, whereas the latter requires "extrinsic" factors presented by tissue following injury. Screening of platelet activity is best achieved using the bleeding time test described below. A normal bleeding time generally rules out insufficient platelet activity.

Prothrombin Time: Causes of Prolonged Prothrombin Time

The prothrombin time (PT) measures the coagulant activity of the "extrinsic system," including fibrinogen, prothrombin, and factors V, VII, and X. Tissue extract, such as brain, and calcium chloride are added to fresh plasma to monitor the PT. This test is the best single test for monitoring patients on warfarin therapy.[1-4]

Inadequate Production of Procoagulants

Hepatic failure
  Severe liver damage: poisoning, hepatitis, cirrhosis
Inadequate vitamin K in diet
  Premature infants
  Newborn infants of vitamin K-deficient mothers: hemorrhagic disease of the newborn, maternal primidone therapy
  Debilitated patients on broad spectrum antibiotics
Inadequate vitamin K absorption
  Poor fat absorption: obstructive jaundice, fistulas, sprue, steatorrhea, celiac disease, colitis, chronic diarrhea
Inherited factor deficiency
  Factor I: fibrinogen
  Factor II: prothrombin
  Factor V: labile factor; Owren's disease or parahemophilia
  Factor VII: stable factor; deficiency causes prolonged PT with normal partial thromboplastin time (PTT)
  Factor X: Stuart-Prower factor
  Protein C inhibitor deficiency resulting in reduction of factors V and VIII
Acquired factor deficiency
  Factor VII deficiency of severe congestive heart failure
  Factor X deficiency of amyloidosis
Drugs: coumarin-type drugs for anticoagulant therapy

Rapid Destruction of Procoagulants

Fibrinolytic states
  Disseminated intravascular coagulation (DIC):
    Postsurgery: especially associated with intraoperative hypotension

Post-trauma
Postpartum
Septicemia
Acute nonlymphocytic leukemia: M3 by the French-American-British classification

Partial Thromboplastin Time: Causes of Prolonged Partial Thromboplastin Time

The partial thromboplastin time (PTT) measures coagulant activity generated in the "intrinsic system." A phospholipid emulsion is added to platelet-poor plasma, which is subsequently recalcified with calcium chloride. The test should be performed as soon as possible after collection to minimize glass activation effects. The best single screening test for disorders of coagulation, it is abnormal in 90% of patients with coagulation disorders.[1] Furthermore, it is a highly useful screen for deficiencies of all major plasma coagulation factors except factors VII and XIII. PTT also may be prolonged in some patients with von Willebrand's disease.

Inadequate Production or Procoagulants

Hepatic failure
Severe liver damage: poisoning, hepatitis, cirrhosis
Severe congestive heart failure
Inherited factor deficiency
Factor I: fibrinogen
Factor II: prothrombin
Factor V: labile factor
Factor VIII: hemophilia factor; classic hemophilia
Factor IX: Christmas factor; Christmas disease or hemophilia B
Factor X: Stuart-Prower factor
Factor XI: Rosenthal's syndrome—activated PTT is prolonged, but PT and bleeding time are normal.
Factor XII: Hageman factor; deficiency not associated with hemorrhagic manifestations

Protein C inhibitor deficiency resulting in reduction of factors V and VIII

Acquired factor deficiency: factor X deficiency of amyloidosis

Circulating Anticoagulants

Testing for a circulating anticoagulant is performed by mixing the test plasma with control plasma at a 1:1 ratio. As any clotting factor must be at concentrations much less than 50% of normal to affect prolongation of PT or PTT, a prolonged coagulation time for a 1:1 mixture of test plasma with control plasma indicates the presence of an anticoagulant in the test plasma.

Autoimmune Disease-Related Anticoagulants

Systemic lupus erythematosus
Rheumatoid arthritis
Ulcerative colitis

Acquired Post-Transfusion of Plasma Proteins

Acquired post-transfusion of plasma proteins is usual in patients treated for congenital clotting factor deficiency.[5]

Drug-induced Anticoagulants

Drugs associated with development of antibodies to factors VIII, XI, XII and V: penicillins, sulfonamides, phenytoin, procainamide, chlorpromazine

Pregnancy

Pregnancy-related factor VIII inhibitors

Malignancy-Related Anticoagulants

Lymphoproliferative diseases: Waldenström's macroglobulinemia, multiple myeloma, benign monoclonal gammopathies

Artifactual Anticoagulants

Lupus-type anticoagulant[6]: antiphospholipid antibodies that interfere with PTT assay—compare PTT of relipidated platelet-poor plasma with PTT of platelet-rich plasma. The latter will often be within the normal range.

Heparin-contamination: plasma with prolonged thrombin time and normal reptilase time

Bleeding Time: Causes of Prolonged Bleeding Time

The bleeding time is the interval between standardized puncture of the skin and cessation of bleeding. This test is a useful screening test for disorders of platelet function, both congenital and acquired, and for von Willebrand's disease.[1,7] The bleeding time is independent of the coagulation mechanism, except in the setting of a severe impairment of the clotting system.

Quantitative Platelet Deficiency

Thrombocytopenia: especially for platelet counts below 50,000/µl of blood. Patients with thrombocytopenia secondary to rapid platelet destruction generally have bleeding times shorter than patients with comparable thrombocytopenia secondary to inadequate megakaryocytopoiesis.

Qualitative Platelet Deficiency

Primary thrombocytopathies
Bernard-Soulier syndrome: giant platelets with dense granules
Thrombasthenia: impaired aggregation by adenosine diphosphate (ADP) constitutes the major functional defect, impaired clot retraction
Storage pool deficiency: platelets with decreased numbers of dense bodies resulting in diminished amounts of platelet adenosine triphosphate (ATP) and ADP.
Platelets with decreased numbers of granules resulting in diminished amounts of various substances, such as thromboglobulin, platelet factor 4 and platelet-derived growth factor
Secondary thrombocytopathies: von Willebrand's disease—best noted 2 hours after dose of 10 grains of aspirin; bleeding time is variable without this aspirin tolerance test
Acquired thrombocytopathies
Myeloproliferative disorders[8]: primary thrombocythemia, polycythemia vera, myeloid metapla-

sia, chronic myelogenous leukemia, acute leukemia

Dysproteinemias: multiple myeloma, macroglobulinemia

Liver disease

Acquired storage pool deficiency: usually in the setting of incipient myeloproliferative disease

Other conditions noted to have associated thrombocytopathy: scurvy, pernicious anemia, infectious mononucleosis, status post-transfusion with cryoprecipitate, status postmajor-surgery, Bartter's syndrome

Drug-induced thrombocytopathies[9]

Aspirin: permanent impairment of circulating platelets

Nonsteroidal anti-inflammatory drugs (NSAIDs): transient impairment of circulating platelets reversed rapidly after discontinuing drug

Plasma expanders: dextran—inhibits platelet factor 3 activity, bleeding time more likely to be affected with a dextran of molecular weight greater than 65,000 daltons; hydroxyethyl starch

Drugs with direct anti-platelet activity: dipyridamole, clofibrate, vitamin E, ticlopidine, furosemide, hydralazine, nitroprusside

Drugs that inhibit through their effects on plasma membranes: ethanol, local and general anesthetics, phenothiazines, tricyclic antidepressants, antihistamines

Drugs that may inhibit by undetermined mechanisms: penicillin, carbenecillin

Warfarin Resistance: Causes of Warfarin Resistance[10]

Drug-induced Warfarin Resistance	Barbiturates
	Ethchlorvynol
	Glutethimide
	Griseofulvin
	Heptabarbital
	Vitamin K
	Adrenocortical steroids

Birth control pills
Cholestyramine
Colchicine
Meprobamate
Rifampin

Hereditary Warfarin Resistance

Protein C deficiency[11,12]: a vitamin K-dependent inhibitor of factors Va and VIIIa; deficiency of which causes warfarin-associated necrosis or enhanced thrombosis during early stages of warfarin therapy before reduction in activities of factors II and X.
Protein S deficiency[13]: vitamin K dependent co-factor of protein C required for full activity of protein C
Antithrombin III deficiency
Idiopathic[14]

Acquired Warfarin Resistance

Disseminated intravascular coagulation[15]: via inhibitors to protein C
Paraneoplastic states[16]
Poor warfarin absorption: short bowel syndrome[17]

Heparin Resistance: Causes of Heparin Resistance

Antithrombin-III deficiency
  Quantitative: classic deficiency
  Qualitative: variant forms of antithrombin-III having low heparin co-factor activity[18,19]

References

1. Angelos MG, Hamilton GC: Coagulation studies: prothrombin time, partial thromboplastin time, bleeding time. Emerg Med Clin North Am 4:95, 1986.
2. Hirsh J, Levine MN: The optimal intensity of oral anticoagulant therapy. JAMA 258:2723, 1987.
3. Hirsh J, Deykin D, Poller L: "Therapeutic range" for oral anticoagulant therapy. Chest 89 (2 Suppl):11S, 1986.
4. Peterson CE, Kwaan HC: Current concepts of warfarin therapy. Arch Intern Med 146:581, 1986.

5. Desposito F, Arkel Y: Inhibitors of coagulation in children. CRC Crit Rev Oncol Hematol 7:53, 1987.
6. Espinoza LR, Hartmann RC: Significance of the lupus anticoagulant. Am J Hematol 22:331, 1986.
7. Day HJ, Rao AK: Evaluation of platelet function. Semin Hematol 23:89, 1986.
8. Rasi V, Lintula R: Platelet function in the myelodysplastic syndromes. Scand J Haematol 45(Suppl):71, 1986.
9. Smith JB: Pharmacology of thromboxane synthetase inhibitors. Fed Proc 46:139, 1987.
10. Bentley DP, Backhouse G, Hutchings A, et al: Investigation of patients with abnormal response to warfarin. Br J Clin Pharmacol 22:37, 1986.
11. McGehee WG, Klotz TA, Epstein DJ, et al: Coumarin necrosis associated with hereditary protein C deficiency. Ann Intern Med 101:59, 1984.
12. Griffin JH, Mosher DF, Zimmerman TS, et al: Protein C, an antithrombotic protein, is reduced in hospitalized patients with intravascular coagulation. Blood 60:261, 1982.
13. Walker FJ: Protein S and the regulation of activated protein C. Semin Thromb Hemost 10:131, 1984.
14. Warrier I, Brennan CA, Lusher JM: Familial warfarin resistance in a black child. Am J Pediatr Hematol Oncol 8:346, 1986.
15. Marlar RA, Endres-Brooks J, Miller C: Serial studies of protein C and its plasma inhibitor in patients with disseminated intravascular coagulation. Blood 66:59, 1985.
16. Salem HH, Mitchell CA, Firkin BG: Current views on the pathophysiology and investigations of thrombotic disorders. Am J Hematol 25:463, 1987.
17. Kearns PJ Jr, O'Reilly RA: Bioavailability of warfarin in a patient with severe short bowel syndrome. J Parenter Enteral Nutr 10:100, 1986.
18. Wolf M, Boyer C, Tripodi A, et al: Antithrombin Milano: a new varient with monomeric and dimeric inactive antithrombin III. Blood 65:496, 1985.
19. Bauer KA, Ashenhurst JB, Chediak J, et al: Antithrombin "Chicago": a functionally abnormal molecule with increased heparin affinity causing familial thrombophilia. Blood 62:1242, 1983.

Selected Readings

Angelos MG, Hamilton GC: Coagulation studies: prothrombin time, partial thromboplastin time, bleeding time. Emerg Med Clin North Am 4:95, 1986.
A practical outline for using coagulation studies to evaluate the bleeding patient in the emergency room setting.

Bentley DP, Backhouse G, Hutchings A, et al: Investigation of patients with abnormal response to warfarin. Br J Clin Pharmacol 22:37, 1986.
Algorithms using plasma warfarin concentration and plasma clearance were developed that correctly predicted the cause of abnormal warfarin sensitivity and resistance in patients. These algorithms may prove useful in the clinical setting.

Espinoza LR, Hartmann RC: Significance of the lupus anticoagulant. Am J Hematol 22:331, 1986.
Lupus anticoagulants are heterogeneous immunoglobulins that may interfere with phospholipid-dependent clotting reactions. Clinical associations include repeated thromboses in patients under the age of 40, systemic lupus erythematosus and other autoimmune disorders, repeated fetal wastage, and drug therapy such as procainamide, phenothiazines, and others.

High KA: Antithrombin III, protein C, and protein S. Naturally occurring anticoagulant proteins. Arch Pathol Lab Med 112:28, 1988.
A review of current concepts and diagnosis of deficiencies of proteins associated with thromboembolic disease. Diagnosis of an anticoagulant protein deficiency has serious implications for a patient and his kindred.

Kane WH, Davie EW: Blood coagulation factors V and VIII: structural and functional similarities and their relationship to hemorrhagic and thrombotic disorders. Blood 71:539, 1988.
Comprehensive, well-referenced review of current concepts of blood coagulation factors V and VIII.

Kaplan AP, Silverberg M: The coagulation-kinin pathway of human plasma. Blood 70:1, 1987.
Well-referenced comprehensive review of the human coagulation-kinin pathway.

Li GC, Greenberg CS, Currie MS: Procainamide-induced lupus anticoagulants and thrombosis. South Med J 81:262, 1988.
Procainamide is commonly associated with autoantibodies and occasionally a lupus-like syndrome. Serologic and coagulation profiles that may be useful in monitoring these patients are discussed.

Perry MO: Anticoagulation: a surgical perspective. Am J Surg 155:268, 1988.
Helpful review of heparin pharmacokinetics and drug interactions, with clinical guidelines for effective anticoagulation therapy.

Sontheimer RD: The anticardiolipin syndrome. A new way to slice an old pie, or a new pie to slice? Arch Dermatol 123:590, 1987.
Antiphospholipid antibodies, such as anticardiolipin, may play a role in clinical associations of systemic lupus erythematosus, such as recurrent thrombosis, spontaneous abortion, and the biologic false-positive VDRL reaction. Interesting review of current concepts.

Wessler S, Gitel SN: Pharmacology of heparin and warfarin. J Am Coll Cardiol 8 (6 Suppl B):10B, 1986.
Aspects of the hemostatic mechanisms relevant to the antithrombotic action of heparin and warfarin are discussed. Drug assays and practical guidelines for their use in low, medium, and high dose regimens are outlined.

111
Deep Vein Thrombosis: Common and Uncommon Associations

Although most venous thrombi and pulmonary emboli that occur in hospitalized patients are asymptomatic,[1] acute pulmonary embolism remains a common cause of morbidity and mortality in hospitalized patients. Immobilization is a well-established major risk factor for the development of venous stasis and thrombosis; however, when deep vein thrombosis or pulmonary emboli occur in previously healthy, unhospitalized, active patients, risk factors are neither well established nor usually obvious. Major pathogenic mechanisms for deep vein thrombosis include direct venous trauma, venous stasis associated with damage to venous endothelium, and venous stasis associated with systemic hypercoagulability.[2] When symptomatic venous thrombi are recognized, if underlying predisposing risk factors, such as prolonged bed rest, trauma, or chronic illness, are not obvious, less common causes, as well as mimics of deep vein thrombosis, should be considered.

Common Conditions Associated with Decreased Mobilization and Deep Vein Thrombosis

Immobility is a major risk for deep vein thrombosis. In bedridden patients, most thrombi begin asymptomatically in the calf. If the thrombus extends from a calf vein into the proximal venous segment, the risk of pulmonary embolism increases.[1]

Prolonged bed rest of chronic illness
Postoperative states: particularly after pelvic, thoracic, or abdominal surgery
Orthopaedic surgery: hip surgery,[3] knee replacement[4,5]
Shock syndromes
Postcerebrovascular infarction: thromboembolic disease in a paralyzed extremity can occur unexpectedly[6]
Long periods of travel

Bone fractures: trauma may cause increased viscosity of blood, predisposing patients to deep vein thrombosis[7]
Head trauma and spinal cord injured patients: heterotopic calcification can masquerade as deep venous thrombosis[8]
Neurosurgical patients[9,10]

Hematologic Disorders Associated with Hypercoagulable States and Deep Vein Thrombosis

Thrombosis can result from hematologic disorders involving the vascular bed, platelets, or plasma procoagulants.[11] Hypercoagulable states can be caused by primary hematologic disorders or occur with hematologic dysfunction secondary to chronic disease.

Platelet disorders: thrombocytosis, thrombocythemia, thrombotic thrombocytopenia purpura
Polycythemia: primary or secondary polycythemias
Hyperglobulinemias: macroglobulinemia, cryoglobulinemia
Miscellaneous hyperviscosity syndromes
Sickle-cell disease
Antithrombin III deficiency
Disseminated intravascular coagulation (DIC): multiple causes and associations such as cancer and sepsis
Homocystinuria
Myeloproliferative syndrome: agnogenic myeloid metaplasia and status postsplenectomy
Paroxysmal nocturnal hemoglobinuria.
Hereditary protein C deficiency[12]

Malignancy Associated with Deep Vein Thrombosis and Thromboembolic Disease

A recent study correlated deep vein thrombosis in otherwise healthy patients with subsequent diagnosis of cancer, including breast, ovary, endometrium, prostate, colon, pancreas, lung, and lymphoma.[13,14] Markers of other thromboembolic disorders commonly associated with underlying malignancy may be present, such as can be seen in DIC, nonbacterial-thrombotic endocarditis, and rarely pulmonary hypertension.[15]

Cacinoma: prostate, breast, stomach, pancreas
Hepatocarcinoma[16]
Adenocarcinoma
Renal cell carcinoma
Choriocarcinoma

Miscellaneous Medical Disorders and Laboratory Findings Associated with Deep Vein Thrombosis

Pregnancy: particularly when associated with serum lupus anticoagulant[17]

Oral contraceptive agents[18,19]

Hypothyroidism

Postmyocardial infarction

Increased antibodies to cardiolipin: elevated levels of antibodies to cardiolipin in young patients status postmyocardial infarction may be associated with increased risk for recurrent myocardial infarction and other thrombotic events, such as cerebrovascular infarction and deep vein thrombosis.[20,21]

More than 60 years old[22]

Obesity[23]

Lupus anticoagulant or inhibitor: its presence correlates with an increased frequency of thrombosis in systemic lupus erythematosus, other connective tissue diseases, and sometimes without connective tissue disease; it is also associated with a biologic false-positive for syphilis and thrombocytopenia[24-26]

Inflammatory bowel disease[27]

Drug abusers: nonseptic deep venous thrombosis in the upper extremities occurs in intravenous drug abusers[28]

Chemotherapy: increased frequency of thrombosis in patients with breast cancer[29]

Mimics of Deep Vein Thrombosis

Symptomatic venous thrombosis is usually associated with large occlusive thrombi in proximal veins.[1] The subsequent swelling and tenderness can be mimicked by infection, inflammation, and trauma causing similar signs.

Popliteal cysts: formed by effusions of synovial fluid, usually in patients with knee joint pathology[30]

Cellulitis

Superficial phlebitis

Chronic venous insufficiency

Osteomyelitis

Lymphangiitis

Arthritis

Bursitis

Lymphedema

Tumors: Kaposi's sarcoma

Hyperalgesic pseudothrombophlebitis in acquired immune deficiency syndrome (AIDS) patients: painful erythematous swelling of the lower extremity mimics deep vein thrombosis in AIDS patients.[31]

Scurvy: adult scurvy can mimic deep vein thrombosis and other hematologic dysfunction.[32]
Heterotopic calcification: spinal cord[33] and head injuries[34]
Status postsclerosant treatment of varicose veins and deep vein thrombosis[35]
Acute alcoholic myopathy: acute, painful, focal swelling can occur after alcoholic binges and can mimic deep vein thrombosis.[36]
Compartment syndromes[37,38]
Calcinosis cutis: heterotopic ossification in burn patients[39]

References

1. Hirsh J, Hull RD, Raskob GE: Epidemiology and pathogenesis of venous thrombosis. J Am Coll Cardiol 8 (Suppl):104B, 1986.
2. Wessler S: Venous thrombosis and pulmonary embolism. Hosp Pract 22 (12):159, 1987.
3. Turpie AG, Levine MN, Hirsh J, et al: A randomized controlled trial of a low-molecular-weight heparin (enoxaparin) to prevent deep-vein thrombosis in patients undergoing elective hip surgery. N Engl J Med 315:925, 1986.
4. Stulberg BN, Insall JN, Williams GW, Ghelman B: Deep-vein thrombosis following total knee replacement. An analysis of six hundred and thirty-eight arthroplasties. J Bone Joint Surg 66:194, 1984.
5. Lovelock JE, Griffiths HJ, Silverstein AM, Anson PS: Complications of total knee replacement. AJR 142:985, 1984.
6. Izzo KL, Aquino E: Deep venous thrombosis in high-risk hemiplegic patients: detection by impedance plethysmography. Arch Phys Med Rehabil 67:799, 1986.
7. Ernst E, Schmidt-Pauly E, Muhlig P, Matrai A: Blood viscosity in patients with bone fractures and long term bedrest. Br J Surg 74:301, 1987.
8. Ragone DJ Jr, Kellerman WC, Bonner FJ Jr: Heterotopic ossification masquerading as deep venous thrombosis in head-injured adult: complications of anticoagulation. Arch Phys Med Rehabil 67:339, 1986.
9. Swann KW, Black PM, Baker MF: Management of symptomatic deep venous thrombosis and pulmonary embolism on a neurosurgical service. J Neurosurg 64:563, 1986.
10. Swann KW, Black PM: Deep vein thrombosis and pulmonary emboli in neurosurgical patients: a review. J Neurosurg 61:1055, 1984.
11. Penner JA: Hypercoagulation and thrombosis. Med Clin North Am 64:743, 1980.
12. Brenner B, Shapira A, Bahari C, et al: Hereditary protein C deficiency during pregnancy. Am J Obstet Gynecol 157:1160, 1987.
13. Aderka D, Brown A, Zelikovski A, Pinkhas J: Idiopathic deep vein thrombosis in an apparently healthy patient

as a premonitory sign of occult cancer. Cancer 57:1846, 1986.
14. Clarke-Pearson DL, Synan IS, Colemen RE, et al: The natural history of postoperative venous thromboemboli in gynecologic oncology: a prospective study of 382 patients. Am J Obstet Gynecol 148:1051, 1984.
15. Kane RD, Hawkins HK, Miller JA, Noce PS: Microscopic pulmonary tumor emboli associated with dyspnea. Cancer 36:1473, 1975.
16. Brisbane JU, Howell DA, Bonkowsky HL: Pulmonary hypertension as a presentation of hepatocarcinoma. Report of a case and brief review of the literature. Am J Med 68:466, 1980.
17. Lubbe WF, Butler WS, Palmer SJ, Liggins GC: Lupus anticoagulant in pregnancy. Br J Obstet Gynaecol 91:357, 1984.
18. Goldzieher JW: Hormonal contraception: benefits versus risks. Am J Obstet Gynecol 157:1023, 1987.
19. Rosenberg L, Kaufman DW, Strom B, Shapiro S: Venous thromboembolism in relation to oral contraceptive use. Obstet Gynecol 69:91, 1987.
20. Hamsten A, Norberg R, Bjorkholm M, et al: Antibodies to cardiolipin in young survivors of myocardial infarction: an association with recurrent cardiovascular events. Lancet 1:113, 1986.
21. Asherson RA, Mackay IR, Harris EN: Myocardial infarction in a young man with systemic lupus erythematosus, deep vein thrombosis, and antibodies to phospholipid. Br Heart J 56:190, 1986.
22. Goldhaber SZ, Hennekens CH, Evans DA, et al: Factors associated with correct antemortem diagnosis of major pulmonary embolism. Am J Med 73:822, 1982.
23. Rawal N, Sjostrand U, Christoffersson E, et al: Comparison of intramuscular and epidural morphine for postoperative analgesia in the grossly obese: influence on postoperative ambulation and pulmonary function. Anesth Analg 63:583, 1984.
24. Fisher M, McGehee W: Cerebral infarct, TIA, and lupus inhibitor. Neurology 36:1234, 1986.
25. Boey ML, Colaco CB, Gharavi AE, et al: Thrombosis in systemic lupus erythematosus: striking association with the presence of circulating lupus anticoagulant. Br Med J (Clin Res) 287:1021, 1983.
26. Kaell AT, Shetty M, Lee BC, Lockshin MD: The diversity of neurologic events in systemic lupus erythematosus. Prospective clinical and computed tomographic classification of 82 events in 71 patients. Arch Neurol 43:273, 1986.
27. Talbot RW, Heppell J, Dozois RR, Beart RW Jr: Vascular complications of inflammatory bowel disease. Mayo Clin Proc 61:140, 1986.
28. Kurtin P, Wagner J: Deep vein thrombosis in intravenous drug abusers presenting as a systemic illness. Am J Med Sci 287:44, 1984.
29. Levine MN, Gent M, Hirsh J, et al: The thrombogenic effect of anticancer drug therapy in women with stage II breast cancer. N Engl J Med 318:404, 1988.
30. MacGuire AM, Cassidy JT: Popliteal cysts. Am Fam Physician 32 (6):139, 1985.

31. Abramson SB, Odajnyk CM, Grieco AJ, et al: Hyperalgesic pseudothrombophlebitis. New syndrome in male homosexuals. Am J Med 78:317, 1985.
32. Reuler JB, Broudy VC, Cooney TG: Adult scurvy. JAMA 253:805, 1985.
33. Sugarman B: Medical complications of spinal cord injury. Q J Med 54:3, 1985.
34. Spielman G, Gennarelli TA, Rogers CR: Disodium etidronate: its role in preventing heterotopic ossification in severe head injury. Arch Phys Med Rehabil 64:539, 1983.
35. Williams RA, Wilson SE: Sclerosant treatment of varicose veins and deep vein thrombosis. Arch Surg 119:1283, 1984.
36. Ford CS, Caldwell SH, Kilgo GR: Acute alcoholic myopathy. Am Fam Physician 29 (5):249, 1984.
37. Graham B, Loomer RL: Anterior compartment syndrome in a patient with fracture of the tibial plateau treated by continuous passive motion and anticoagulants. Report of a case. Clin Orthop 195:197, 1985.
38. Qvarfordt P, Eklof B, Ohlin P: Instramuscular pressure in the lower leg in deep vein thrombosis and phlegmasia cerulae dolens. Ann Surg 197:450, 1983.
39. Heim M, Blankstein A, Friedman B, Horoszowski H: Calcinosis cutis—a rare late complication of burns. Burns Incl Therm Inj 12:502, 1986.

Selected Readings

Appelman PT, DeJong TE, Lampmann LE: Deep venous thrombosis of the leg: US findings. Radiology 163:743, 1987.

In a prospective study, 121 consecutive patients with a clinical diagnosis of deep venous thrombosis of the leg were examined with real-time ultrasonography. The accuracy of detection was not improved by including data from thrombus visualization or the response of the common femoral vein to the Valsalva maneuver.

Broaddus C, Matthay MA: Pulmonary embolism. Guide to diagnosis, treatment, and prevention. Postgrad Med 79 (4):333, 1986.

Useful clinical review.

Brown JG, Ward PE, Wilkinson AJ, Mollan RA: Impedance plethysmography. A screening procedure to detect deep-vein thrombosis. J Bone Joint Surg 69:264, 1987.

Impedance plethysmography was found to be a useful noninvasive screening procedure for potentially fatal proximal venous thrombosis.

Colditz GA, Tuden RL, Oster G: Rates of venous thrombosis after general surgery: combined results of randomized clinical trials. Lancet 2:143, 1986.

Despite evidence that prophylaxis against deep-vein thrombosis is effective, a large proportion of general surgical patients receive no prophylaxis. This study reconfirms the value of prophylaxis to reduce the incidence of deep-vein thrombosis and suggests that combined treatments may be most effective.

Cronan JJ, Dorfman GS, Scola FH, et al: Deep venous thrombosis: US assessment using vein compression. Radiology 162:191, 1987.

In this study, ultrasound had a sensitivity of 89% and a specificity of 100%.

Hull RD, Hirsh J, Carter CJ, et al: Diagnostic efficacy of impedance plethysmography for clinically suspected deep-vein thrombosis. A randomized trial. Ann Intern Med 102:21, 1985.
Results of a study using serial impedance plethysmography alone or combined impedance plethysmography and leg scanning suggest that serial impedance plethysmography used alone is an effective strategy to evaluate such symptomatic patients.

Sy WM, Seo IS: Radionuclide venography: imaging monitor in deep-vein thrombosis of the pelvis and lower extremities. Br J Radiol 59:325, 1986.
A study of 74 adults with documented deep-vein thrombosis of the pelvis and/or lower extremities who had baseline and follow-up radionuclide venography.

van Rijn AB, Heller I, Van Zijl J: Segmental air plethysmography in the diagnosis of deep vein thrombosis. Surg Gynecol Obstet 165:488, 1987.
The diagnostic accuracy of segmental air plethysmography using a pulse volume recorder in the detection of deep-vein thrombosis is assessed.

Vogel P, Laing FC, Jeffrey RB Jr, Wing VW: Deep venous thrombosis of the lower extremity: US evaluation. Radiology 163:747, 1987.
The sensitivity of duplex ultrasonography (US) for detecting deep venous thrombosis of the lower extremity was compared with that of venography in a prospective study of 54 patients. This study concludes that ultrasonography should be the screening examination of choice for evaluating patients with suspected lower extremity deep venous thrombosis.

Wheeler HB, Anderson FA Jr: Diagnostic approaches to deep vein thrombosis. Chest 89 (Suppl):407S, 1986.
This article briefly reviews the advantages and limitations of currently available methods for the diagnosis of deep-vein thrombosis.

Zorba J, Schier D, Posmituck G: Clinical value of blood pool radionuclide venography. AJR 146:1051, 1986.
This clinical study concludes that radionuclide will not replace contrast venography, but may well be used to complement contrast venography when it is technically unsatisfactory or unequivocal, in patients with a history of intolerance to contrast media, and in bed-bound patients.

112

Major Causes of Lymphadenopathy in Patients With and Without Acquired Immune Deficiency Syndrome

Lymphadenopathy manifests as disease that ranges in clinical significance from benign and self-limited to malignant and fatal. The establishment of certain risk factors can help guide the evaluation. If a patient falls within a human immunodeficiency virus (HIV)-risk group or is seropositive for HIV infection, certain categories of infection and neoplasm, such as opportunistic infections and lymphoma, become more probable; therefore, it is important to initially establish or rule out possible HIV or acquired immune deficiency syndrome (AIDS) related illness (see Section VII, Infectious Disease; Chapter 74). In patients without HIV risk factors or established HIV infection, increased age is associated with an increased risk for malignancy, and certain clinical characteristics of lymphadenopathy have been traditionally associated with infection and malignancy. Current concepts of HIV high-risk groups and HIV infection should be incorporated into the traditionally accepted major categories of disorders associated with lymphadenopathy: infectious, neoplastic, and collagen–vascular or immunologic disease.

Persistent Generalized Lymphadenopathy in HIV-Risk Groups and AIDS: Major Clinical Factors To Consider

Persistent generalized lymphadenopathy (PGL) (lymph nodes 1 cm or greater in diameter in 2 or more noncontiguous extrainguinal sites, persisting longer than 3 months) is common in patients at risk and those infected with HIV.[1–5] The adenopathy is usually nontender, soft or nonrubbery, mobile, generalized with symmetric enlargement (1 to 4 cm) and most commonly involves the axilla.[1] When such adenopathy is biopsied, nonspecific follicular hyperplasia is the usual finding.[3,6] Despite abundant recent studies, the exact significance of such adenopathy within the natural course of HIV infection has not been established. However, the following clinically useful facts are emerging regarding PGL in relation to HIV-risk groups and AIDS.

PGL incidence has risen with the incidence of AIDS cases in similar epidemiologic groups.[3,7]

PGL occurs in groups at high risk for HIV infection, but who are seronegative.

PGL occurs in HIV-positive patients who do not meet the Centers for Disease Control (CDC) criteria for AIDS.

PGL occurs in patients meeting the CDC criteria for AIDS.

PGL in patients without specific identified disease probably represents a manifestation of HIV infection, i.e., an early expression of HIV infection that commonly occurs with seroconversion.[1]

Patients with PGL have a high rate of HIV positivity—60 to 100%.[1,5,8,9]

Many immunologic abnormalities have been established in patients with PGL, such as low T-helper cell (CD4) counts, low T-helper/T-suppressor ratios.[5,6,10]

Infectious Disease

Although some infections characteristically involve lymph nodes as a prominent feature, almost any infectious process can be associated with lymphadenopathy. In non-HIV risk groups, soft or firm tender nodes are often signs of infection. In patients with HIV infection, most common infections are opportunistic, such as *Pneumocystis carinii*, *Toxoplasma gondii*, mycobacterial, and fungal. Certain viruses, such as Epstein-Barr and cytomegalovirus, also occur with increased frequency with HIV infections.[11,12]

Bacterial
  Bacterial endocarditis: usually generalized lymphadenopathy
  Bacteremia: generalized adenopathy
  Cellulitis: regional adenopathy
  Anthrax: *Bacillus anthracis* infection usually causes a necrotic cutaneous ulcer or pustule; however, pustules can be absent with disseminated infection and mediastinitis.

Bubonic plague: *Pasteurella pestis (Yersinia pestis)* infection, usually transmitted by a rat or flea bite, is associated with lymphadenopathy and often painful regional adenopathy surrounding the site of infection.[13]

Tularemia: *Francisella (Pasteurella) tularensis* infection most commonly produces tender, erythematous, fluctuant regional adenopathy but less commonly produces generalized lymphadenopathy.[14]

Brucellosis: unexplained fever with generalized lymph node involvement in a systemic granulomatous process, in patients who consume unpasteurized dairy products

Mycobacterial infections: *Mycobacterium avium-intracellulare* complex is the most common mycobacterium found in patients with AIDS.[15]

Pulmonary tuberculosis: in patients with AIDS, disseminated or miliary infiltrates are more frequent than the classic findings of hilar adenopathy and apical and cavitary disease.[16,17]

Extrapulmonary tuberculosis: more common in AIDS patients than the non-AIDS population[18,19]

Scrofula: cervical adenopathy in young children often associated with atypical mycobacterium[20]

Miliary tuberculosis: generalized tuberculosis is present in about 15% of patients with miliary TB; more common in AIDS

Mycobacterium leprae: generalized lymphadenopathy

Spirochetal infection—syphilis: HIV infection has been associated with accelerated syphilitic infection and recurrent neurosyphilis in adequately treated patients.[21,22]

Lyme disease: infection with tick-borne *Borrelia burgdorferi*; worldwide distribution, with manifestations involving the skin, joints, heart, and nervous system[23]

Treponema pertenye: yaws

Cat-scratch disease: regional lymphadenitis in 5 to 10%, nodes tend to be suppurative[24]

Viral

Epstein-Barr virus (EBV): primary infection in normal hosts results in acute infectious mononucleosis; in immunodeficient hosts, however, EBV infection may be associated with a malignant lymphoproliferative disorder.[25,26]

Infectious mononucleosis: may have significant generalized lymphadenopathy, often prominent cervical nodes. Mononucleosis-like syndromes in HIV-risk patients may be associated with sero-conversion of HIV.[27-29]

Lymphoproliferative disorders: when associated with EBV, may have prominent lymphadenopathy[30]

Cytomegalovirus: sometimes called "heterophile negative" mononucleosis in non-HIV patients; a wide clinical spectrum of cytomegalovirus exists in AIDS patients, which can manifest as pneumonia or progressive encephalopathy or be asymptomatic.[31,32]

Rubella: postauricular, suboccipital, or posterior cervical lymphadenopathy

Herpes simplex: oral or genital form causes regional lymphadenopathy

Hemophagocytic syndrome: a rare condition, associated with a variety of infectious agents; lymphadenopathy is prominent in the idiopathic form[33]

Fungal

Histoplasmosis: regional lymphadenopathy as part of the primary infection or generalized lymphadenopathy in the disseminated form[34]

Coccidioidomycosis: lymphadenopathy, particularly in the cervical regions

Sporotrichosis: may cause suppurative lymphadenopathy

Parasitic

Trypanosomiasis: African sleeping sickness[35] and Chagas' disease manifest lymphadenopathy of the head and neck during the acute infection, particularly with generalized involvement.

Filariasis: common cause of lymphadenopathy in tropical regions

Toxoplasmosis: localized and generalized lymphadenopathy[36]; toxoplasmic encephalitis is a frequent neurologic presentation of HIV infection.[37,38]

Neoplasms

Lymphadenopathy, regional or generalized, raises the clinical suspicion of neoplasm, particularly in the older patient, with firm, nontender adenopathy appearing subacutely in cervical or supraclavicular regions. It is unusual for malignancy to present as an isolated inguinal adenopathy. Patients with inherited or acquired immunodeficiency disorders are more vulnerable to B-cell lymphomas, Kaposi's sarcomas, and squamous cell carcinomas.[39]

Lymphomas: characteristically associated with lymphadenopathy; AIDS population at high risk[40]
Hodgkin's disease: most commonly presents as lymph node enlargement; cervical regions are most commonly involved; femoral and inguinal regions are rarely involved; history of lymph nodes waxing and waning over months; lymphadenopathy, particularly predominant in nodular sclerosing and lymphocyte predominant types
Non-Hodgkin's lymphoma: may present with peripheral lymphadenopathy[41]
Angioimmunoblastic lymphadenopathy[42]
Malignant histiocytosis[43]
Leukemia—chronic lymphocytic leukemia, acute myelogenous leukemia: lymphadenopathy is prominent in adult T-cell leukemias that appear to have an association with retrovirus infections.[44]
Sarcomas: particularly the immunoblastic type; AIDS patients at high risk for Kaposi's sarcoma[39]
Solid tumors: usually indicate a systemic spread with other evidence of the primary process usually clinically apparent

Collagen-Vascular/ Immunologic Disorders

Systemic lupus erythematosus: about half of patients have enlarged lymph nodes when the lupus is clinically active. Nodes are usually nontender and histologic examination reveals nonspecific follicular hyperplasia or necrotizing lymphadenitis. Lymphadenopathy may be recurrent, may wax and wane, and may herald flare of disease activity.[45]
Felty's syndrome[46]
Mixed connective tissue disease
Ankylosing spondylitis[47]
Whipple's disease: lymphadenopathy an unusual feature of this disease
Urticarial vasculitis
Serum sickness[48]
Sickle-cell anemia: status posthypertransfusions[49]

Miscellaneous

Sarcoidosis: peripheral lymphadenopathy not uncommon; thoracic lymphadenopathy and pulmonary involvement more typical[50]
Intravenous drug abuse: regional and generalized

lymphadenopathy seen; high risk group for many infections, including HIV infection. Drug impurities can cause systemic lymphadenopathy.[51] Drug-related lymphadenopathy: phenytoin,[52] carbamazepine, quinidine

References

1. Kaslow RA, Phair JP, Friedman HB, et al: Infection with the human immunodeficiency virus: clinical manifestations and their relationship to immune deficiency. A report from the multicenter AIDS cohort study. Ann Intern Med 107:474, 1987.
2. Metroka CE, Cunningham-Rundles S, Pollack MS, et al: Generalized lymphadenopathy in homosexual men. Ann Intern Med 99:585, 1983.
3. Miller B, Stansfield SK, Zack MM, et al: The syndrome of unexplained generalized lymphadenopathy in young men in New York City. Is it related to the acquired immune deficiency syndrome? JAMA 251:242, 1984.
4. Fishbein DB, Kaplan JE, Spira TJ, et al: Unexplained lymphadenopathy in homosexual men: a longitudinal study. JAMA 254:930, 1985.
5. Schechter MT, Boyko WJ, Douglas B, et al: The Vancouver Lymphadenopathy—AIDS Study: 6. HIV seroconversion in a cohort of homosexual men. Can Med Assoc J 135:1355, 1986.
6. Gold JW, Weikel CS, Godbold J, et al: Unexplained persistent lymphadenopathy in homosexual men and the acquired immune deficiency syndrome. Medicine 64:203, 1985.
7. Mathur-Waugh V, Enlow RW, Spigland I, et al: Longitudinal study of persistent generalized lymphadenopathy in homosexual men: relation to acquired immune deficiency syndrome. Lancet 1:1033, 1984.
8. Bayer H, Bienzle U, Schneider J, et al: HTLV III antibody frequency and severity of lymphadenopathy {C}. Lancet 2:1347, 1984.
9. Laurence J, Brun-Vezinet F, Schutzer SE, et al: Lymphadenopathy-associated viral antibody in AIDS. Immune correlations and definition of a carrier state. N Engl J Med 311:1269, 1984.
10. DeShazo RD, Penico JP, Pankey GA, et al: Studies in homosexual patients with and without lymphadenopathy. Relationships to the acquired immune deficiency syndrome. Arch Intern Med 144:1153, 1984.
11. Goebel FD: Clinical manifestations of acquired immunologic deficiency syndrome (AIDS). Acta Med Austriaca 14:1, 1987.
12. Pitchenick AE, Burr J, Suarez M, et al: Human T-cell lymphotropic virus-III (HTLV-III) seropositivity and related disease among 71 consecutive patients in whom tuberculosis was diagnosed. A prospective study. Am Rev Respir Dis 135:875, 1987.
13. Centers for Disease Control: Human plague-US 1983. MMWR 32:329, 1983.
14. Guerrant RL, Humphries MK Jr, Butler JE, et al: Tickborne oculoglandular tularemia: case report and review

of seasonal and vectorial associations in 106 cases. Arch Intern Med 136:811, 1976.

15. Centers for Disease Control, U.S. Department of Health and Human Services: Diagnosis and management of mycobacterial infection and disease in persons with human immunodeficiency virus infection. Ann Intern Med 106:254, 1987.
16. Suster B, Akerman M, Orenstein M, Wax MR: Pulmonary manifestations of AIDS: review of 106 episodes. Radiology 161:87, 1986.
17. Chaisson RE, Schecter GF, Theuer CP, et al: Tuberculosis in patients with the acquired immunodeficiency syndrome. Clinical features, response to therapy, and survival. Am Rev Respir Dis 136:570, 1987.
18. Alvarez S, McCabe WR: Expulmonary tuberculosis revised: a review of experience at Boston City and other hospitals. Medicine 63:25, 1984.
19. Joint Position Paper of the American Thoracic Society and the Centers for Disease Control: Mycobacterioses and the acquired immunodeficiency syndrome. Am Rev Respir Dis 136:492, 1987.
20. Lai KK, Stottmeier KD, Sherman IH: Mycobacterial cervical lymphadenopathy: relation of etiologic agents to age. JAMA 251:1286, 1984.
21. Chapel TA: The signs and symptoms of secondary syphilis. Sex Transm Dis 7:161, 1980.
22. Johns DR, Tierney M, Felsenstein D: Alteration in the natural history of neurosyphilis by concurrent infection with the human immunodeficiency virus. N Engl J Med 316:1569, 1987.
23. Goldings EA, Jericho J: Lyme disease. Clin Rheum Dis 12:343, 1986.
24. Wear DJ, Margileth AM, Hadfield TL, et al: Cat-scratch disease: a bacterial infection. Science 221:1403, 1983.
25. List AF, Greco FA, Vogler LB: Lymphoproliferative diseases in immunocompromised hosts: the role of Epstein-Barr virus. J Clin Oncol 5:1673, 1987.
26. Purtilo DT: Lymphotropic viruses, Epstein-Barr virus (EBV), and human T-cell lymphotropic virus-I (HTLV-I)/adult T-cell leukemia virus (ATLV), and HTLV-III/ human immune deficiency virus (HIV) as etiological agents of malignant lymphoma and immune deficiency. AIDS Res 2(Suppl 1):S1, 1986.
27. Buchanan JG, Goldwater PN, Somerfield SD, Tobias MI: Mononucleosis-like-syndrome associated with acute AIDS retrovirus infection. NZ Med J 99:405, 1986.
28. Sumaya CV, Boswell RN, Ench Y, et al: Enhanced serological and virological findings of Epstein-Barr virus in patients with AIDS and AIDS-related complex. J Infect Dis 154:864, 1986.
29. Valle SL: Febrile pharyngitis as the primary sign of HIV infection in a cluster of cases linked by sexual contact. Scand J Infect Dis 19:13, 1987.
30. Sullivan JL, Byron KS, Brewster FE, et al: X-linked lymphoproliferative syndrome: natural history of the immunodeficiency. J Clin Invest 71:1765, 1983.
31. Hilborne LH, Nieberg RK, Cheng L, Lewin KJ: Direct in situ hybridization for rapid detection of cytomegalovirus in bronchoalveolar lavage. Am J Clin Pathol 87:766, 1987.

32. Post MJ, Hensley GT, Moskowitz LB, Fischl M: Cytomegalic inclusion virus encephalitis in patients with AIDS: CT, clinical, and pathologic correlation. AJR 146:1229, 1986.
33. Risdall RJ, McKenna RW, Nesbit ME, et al: Virus-associated hemophagocytic syndrome: a benign histiocytic proliferation distinct from malignant histiocytosis. Cancer 44:993, 1979.
34. Goodwin RA Jr, Des Prez RM: State of the art: histoplasmosis. Am Rev Respir Dis 117:929, 1978.
35. Foulkes JR: Human trypanosomiasis in Africa. Br Med J 283:1172, 1981.
36. Krick JA, Remington JS: Current concepts in parsitology: toxoplasmosis in the adult—an overview. N Engl J Med 298:550, 1978.
37. Levy RM, Rosenbloom S, Perrett LV: Neuroradiologic findings in AIDS: A review of 200 cases. AJR 147:977, 1986.
38. Berger JR, Moskowitz L, Fischl M, Kelley RE: Neurologic disease as the presenting manifestation of acquired immunodeficiency syndrome. South Med J 80:683, 1987.
39. Purtilo DT: Opportunistic cancers in patients with immunodeficiency syndromes. Arch Pathol Lab Med 111:1123, 1987.
40. Ioachim HL, Cooper MC, Hellman GC: Lymphomas in men at high risk for acquired immune deficiency syndrome (AIDS). A study of 21 cases. Cancer 56:2831, 1985.
41. Devita VT Jr, Jaffe ES, Hellman S: Hodgkin's disease and non-Hodgkin's lymphomas. p. 1644. In Devita VT Jr, Hellman S, Rosenberg SA (eds): Cancer Principles and Practice of Oncology. JB Lippincott, Philadelphia, 1985.
42. Reynaud R, Emberger JM, Ciurana AJ, et al: Angioimmunoblastic lymphadenopathy. Schweiz Med Wochenschr 108:325, 1978.
43. Warnke RA, Kim H, Dorfman RF: Malignant histiocytosis (histiocytic medullary reticulosis). I. Clinicopathologic study of 29 cases. Cancer 35:215, 1975.
44. Frizzera G, Moran EM, Rappaport H: Angio-immuno lymphadenopathy: diagnosis and clinical course. Am J Med 59:803, 1975.
45. Rothfield N: Clinical features of SLE. p. 1083. In Kelly WN, Harris ES Jr, Ruddy S, et al (eds): Textbook of Rheumatology. WB Saunders, Philadelphia, 1985.
46. Goldberg J, Pinals RS: Felty syndrome. Semin Arthritis Rheum 10:52, 1980.
47. Marantz PR, Linzer M: Diffuse lymphadenopathy as a manifestation of ankylosing spondylitis. Am J Med 80:951, 1986.
48. Lawley TJ, Bielory L, Gascon P, et al: A prospective clinical and immunological analysis of patients with serum sickness. N Engl J Med 311:1407, 1984.
49. Morgan J, Waring NP, Daul CB, et al: Persistent lymphadenopathy associated with hypertransfusion in sickle-cell disease. J Allergy Clin Immunol 76:869, 1985.
50. Thomas PD, Hunninghake GW: Current concepts of the pathogenesis of sarcoidosis. Am Rev Respir Dis 135:747, 1987.

51. Carbone A, Manconi R, Poletti A, Volpe R: A histopathologic study of persistent generalized lymphadenoapathy in intravenous drug abusers. Pathol Res Pract 181:195, 1986.
52. Marg E, Kopke E, Schillat I: Lymphadenopathy in phenytoin treatment. Psychiatr Neurol Med Psychol (Leipz) 30:430, 1978.

Selected Readings

Ahmed T, Wormser GP, Stahl RE, et al: Malignant lymphomas in a population at risk for acquired immune deficiency syndrome Cancer 60:719, 1987.
Authors evaluate the occurrence of malignant lymphomas in populations at high risk for AIDS, including prisoners from New York state and nonprisoner intravenous drug abusers. Non-Hodgkin's lymphoma was the most common malignancy seen in intravenous drug abusers with AIDS.

Centers for Disease Control, U.S. Department of Health and Human Services: Diagnosis and management of mycobacterial infection and disease in persons with human immunodeficiency virus infection. Ann Intern Med 106:254, 1987.
Mycobacterial disease occurs commonly in patients with AIDS and HIV infections. M. avium complex was the most frequently identified infection among all patients with AIDS; however, M. tuberculosis was more common in certain groups, such as Haitians and intravenous drug users.

Farthing CF, Henry K, Shanson DC, et al: Clinical investigations of lymphadenopathy, including lymph node biopsies, in 24 homosexual men with antibodies to the human T-cell lymphotropic virus type III (HTLV-III). Br J Surg 73:180, 1986.
Data from 27 lymph node biopsies performed on 24 homosexual patients with lymphadenopathy are presented and correlated with viral studies. Authors suggest that homosexuals with lymphadenopathy, who are human T-cell lymphotropic virus type III (HTLV-III) antibody positive, do not need a routine node biopsy unless an alternative diagnosis is strongly suspected.

Fournier AM, Dickinson GM, Erdfrocht IR, et al: Tuberculosis and nontuberculous mycobacteriosis in patients with AIDS. Chest 93:772, 1988.
Interesting data culled from 36 AIDS patients with culture-proven nontuberculous mycobacteriosis compared to 20 AIDS patients with tuberculosis. Lymphadenopathy was seen primarily with tuberculosis. In a minority of patients with nontuberculous mycobacteriosis, a clinical syndrome with dyspnea, chills, hemoptysis, and chest pain was identified.

Freidig EE, McClure SP, Wilson WR, et al: Clinical-histologic-microbiologic analysis of 419 lymph node biopsy specimens. Rev Infect Dis 8:322, 1986.
Results of culture and histopathologic data of 419 lymph node biopsy specimens obtained from 414 patients with lymphadenopathy of unknown etiology were correlated with clinical histories. Clinical diagnoses in decreasing frequency were lymphadenopathy of unknown etiology, sarcoidosis, malignant lymphoma, metastatic carcinoma, histoplasmosis, tuberculosis, and other miscellaneous

conditions. With one exception, lymph node cultures in immuno-competent patients were positive only when biopsy findings included a granuloma and/or an acute inflammatory lesion.

Jacobson MA, Mills J: Serious cytomegalovirus disease in the acquired immunodeficiency syndrome (AIDS). Clinical findings, diagnosis, and treatment. Ann Intern Med 108:585, 1988.

A review of clinical features and current diagnoses and management of serious cytomegaloviral infection in AIDS patients.

Kaplan MH, Susin M, Pahwa SG, et al: Neoplastic complications of HTLV-III infection. Lymphomas and solid tumors. Am J Med 82:389, 1987.

Neoplastic disease in 29 of 200 patients infected with human T-lymphotropic virus type III (HTLV-III) evaluated at a suburban hospital focuses on the high incidence rate of neoplastic transformation in this population.

Kim JH, Durack DT: Manifestations of human T-lymphotropic virus type I infection. Am J Med 84:919, 1988.

Review update of clinical syndromes associated with human T-lymphotropic virus type I (HTLV-I) infection, which ranges from asymptomatic carrier states to acute T-lymphocytic leukemia (ATLL) with lymphadenopathy, hepatosplenomegaly, hypercalcemia, cutaneous lesions, and systemic immunosuppression.

Muhlemann MF, Anderson MG, Paradinas FJ, et al: Early warning skin signs in AIDS and persistent generalized lymphadenopathy. Br J Dermatol 114:419, 1986.

Skin manifestations, including chronic acneiform folliculitis, extensive cutaneous fungal infections, and neck and beard impetigo, may provide early warning signs of AIDS.

Sunderam G, McDonald RJ, Maniatis T, et al: Tuberculosis as a manifestation of the acquired immunodeficiency syndrome (AIDS). JAMA 256:362, 1986.

Data from 48 cases of mycobacteria disease from a group of 136 AIDS patients is presented. Twenty-nine patients had severe and extrapulmonary manifestations of tuberculosis. Authors suggest that unusual and severe presentations of overwhelming tuberculosis in certain clinical settings may be predictive of the presence of AIDS.

113
Leukopenia: Common Causes and Associations

Leukopenia is defined as white blood cell concentration in the peripheral blood that is below 4,500 leukocytes/μl.[1] Important in the evaluation of leukopenia is examination of the blood smear, which often can rule out artifactual leukopenia secondary to clumping or rupturing of leukocytes in automated counters. Also, by providing a differential white blood cell count, examination of the peripheral smear will help to categorize the leukopenia as a neutropenia (fewer than 1,500 neutrophils/μl blood), lymphopenia (fewer than 1,000 lymphocytes/μl of blood) or combined cytopenia, as seen in pancytopenia. Because of the much shorter half-life of neutrophils compared to that of lymphocytes, neutropenia generally will precede lymphopenia after onset of conditions causing pancytopenia. This in part may explain why neutropenia is much more commonly seen than lymphopenia.

Clinical history is of prime importance in the evaluation. Clinically significant neutropenias often are associated with frequent pyrogenic infections, whereas clinically significant lymphopenia often is associated with depressed immunity to viruses. Also, it is important to establish whether the leukopenia is newly acquired or chronic by examining the patient's former laboratory data. Establishing that the leukopenia is newly acquired indicates an evolving disorder causing either decreased effective leukocyte production, increased leukocyte destruction, or increased leukocyte sequestration. Of course, this also rules out congenital causes of leukopenia, such as benign familial leukopenia. Should a newly acquired neutropenia be documented or suspected, careful review of history for recent infections, administration of drugs, or exposure to toxins is indicated. Although any drug conceivably can cause idiosyncratic leukopenia, drugs listed below have caused leukopenia in more than a few individuals. As a safe rule of thumb, it is best to discontinue all nonessential medication for any patient found to have newly acquired leukopenia.

Anaphylaxis
Autoimmune disease
  Systemic lupus erythematosus
  Various neutropenias
  Thymoma
  Adult Still's disease: after treatment with azathioprine and sulfasalazine[2]
  Rheumatoid arthritis: Felty's syndrome, often associated with splenomegaly
Cachexia

Drugs and Chemicals Biologic response modifiers
  Colony stimulating factor: transient early effect after administration
  Interferons
  Cyclosporin A: may cause dose-related lymphopenia
Cytotoxic drugs
  Antimetabolites: 6-mercaptopurine, cytosine arabinoside, antifolates, azathioprine
  Antracyclines: doxorubicin, daunomycin
  Nitrogen mustards: busulfan, procarbazine, cyclophosphamide
Idiosyncratic drug reactions[3]
  Analgesics: acetaminophen
  Antiarrhythmics: quinidine
  Antibiotics: chloramphenicol, isoniazide (INH), sulfonamides (including topical silver sulfadiazine[4]), piperacillin,[5] vancomycin
  Anticonvulsants: diphenylhydantoin, carbamazepine, ethosuximide, paramethadione, phenacemide, phenytoin, trimethadione
  Antihistamines: brompheniramine, cimetidine, tripelennamine.
  Antihypertensives: captopril, enalapril, hydralazine, methyldopa
  Anti-inflammatory drugs: aspirin, colchicine, gold salts,[6] ibuprofen, indomethacin, phenylbutazone, sulfasalazine
  Antithyroid drugs: carbimazole, thiouracil
  Diuretics: acetazolamide, chlorothiazide, furosemide, hydrochlorothiazide
  Hypoglycemics: carbutamide, chlorpropamide, tolbutamide

Tranquilizers: chlordiazepoxide, chlorpromazine, meprobamate, promazine

Other: allopurinol, chloroquine,[7] isotretinoin[8]

Infectious Disease-Related Leukopenia

Bacterial: brucellosis, miliary tuberculosis, nosocomial (*Corynebacterium*[9]), paratyphoid, septicemia, tularemia, typhoid

Parasitic: kala-azar, malaria

Rickettsial: sandfly fever, scrub typhus

Viral: hepatitis, infectious mononucleosis, influenza, parvovirus infections, psittacosis, rubella

Ionizing Radiation

External: radiotherapy, nuclear accidents

Internal: I^{131} therapy for nodular goiter[10], P^{32} therapy for essential thrombocythemia

Hematopoietic Disorders

AIDS[11]

Acute nonlymphocytic leukemia

Aleukemic leukemia

Aplastic anemia and related conditions

Benign familial leukopenia (Yemenite [Ethiopian] Jews): no progression in degree of leukopenia and unimpressive clinical history of infections

Chédiak-Higashi syndrome: ineffective granulopoiesis with intramedullary destruction of proliferative granulocytic cells secondary to defective cell granules[12]

Evans's syndrome: associated with thrombocytopenia without splenomegaly

Gaucher's disease: usually associated with hepatosplenomegaly

Hairy-cell leukemia

Hypersplenism

Myeloproliferative disease: subacute or smoldering nonlymphocytic leukemia

Pernicious anemia: inadequate vitamin B_{12} absorption; look for neutrophils with hypersegmented nuclei on blood smear (greater than five lobes) and megaloblastic changes in bone marrow.

T-cell leukemia[13]

Thymoma[14]: often associated with autoimmune disease

Miscellaneous

Down syndrome.

Hemodialysis on cellulosie hemodialyzers[15,16]

Severe renal injury

References

1. Keeling RP: Non-neoplastic disorders of granulocytes and monocytes. p. 428. In Thorup OA Jr (ed): Fundamentals of Clinical Hematology. 5th Ed. WB Saunders, Philadelphia, 1987.
2. Bliddal H, Helin P: Leucopenia in adult Still's disease during treatment with azathioprine and sulfasalazine. Clin Rheumatol 6:244, 1987.
3. Finch SC: Neutropenia. p. 773. In Williams WJ, Beutler E, Erslev AJ, Lichtman MA (eds): Hematology. 3rd Ed. McGraw-Hill, New York, 1983.
4. Choban PS, Marshall WJ: Leukopenia secondary to silver sulfadiazine: frequency, characteristics and clinical consequences. Am Surg 53:515, 1987.
5. Bressler RB, Huston DP: Piperacillin-induced anemia and leukopenia. South Med J 79:255, 1986.
6. Bliddal H, Eiberg B, Helin P: Gold-induced leucopenia may predict a similar adverse reaction to sulphasalazine (letter). Lancet 1:390, 1987.
7. Sturchler D, Schar M, Gyr N: Leukopenia and abnormal liver function in travellers on malaria chemoprophylaxis. J Trop Med Hyg 90:239, 1987.
8. Friedman SJ: Leukopenia and neutropenia associated with isotretinoin therapy. Arch Dermatol 123:293, 1987.
9. Riebel W, Frantz N, Adelstein D, Spagnuolo PJ: Corynebacterium JK: a cause of nosocomial device-related infection. Rev Infect Dis 8:42, 1986.
10. Wasserman J, Blomgren H, Petrini B, et al: Changes of the blood lymphocyte subpopulations and their functions following ^{131}I treatment for nodular goiter and ^{32}P treatment for polycythemia vera. Int J Radiat Biol 53:159, 1988.
11. Frontiera M, Myers AM: Peripheral blood and bone marrow abnormalities in the acquired immunodeficiency syndrome. West J Med 147:157, 1987.
12. Barak Y, Nir E: Chediak-Higashi syndrome. Am J Pediatr Hematol Oncol 9:42, 1987.
13. Sohn CC, Blayney DW, Misset JL, et al: Leukopenic chronic T cell leukemia mimicking hairy cell leukemia: association with human retroviruses. Blood 67:949, 1986.
14. Ackland SP, Bur ME, Adler SS, et al: White blood cell aplasia associated with thymoma. Am J Clin Pathol 89:260, 1988.
15. Hoenich NA, Levett D, Fawcett S, et al: Biocompatibility of hemodialysis membranes. J Biomed Eng 8:3, 1986.
16. Cheung AK, Henderson LW: Effects of complement activation by hemodialysis membranes. Am J Nephrol 6:81, 1986.

Selected Readings

Ackland SP, Bur ME, Adler SS, et al: White blood cell aplasia associated with thymoma. Am J Clin Pathol 89:260, 1988.

Interesting case report of acquired hypoplastic neutropenia associated with a thymoma. An autoimmune mechanism is suggested.

Coleman DL: Regulation of macrophage phagocytosis. Eur J Clin Microbiol 5:1, 1986.

State-of-the-art review of current concepts of macrophage phagocytosis, with an emphasis on new approaches emerging for the regulation of phagocytic activity of macrophages.

Keeling RP: Non-neoplastic disorders of granulocytes and monocytes. p. 428. In Thorup OA Jr (ed): Fundamentals of Clinical Hematology. 5th Ed. WB Saunders, Philadelphia, 1987.

Good general reference.

Werman HA, Brown CG: White blood cell count and differential count. Emerg Med Clin North Am 4:41, 1986.

Review of current laboratory methods used to count white cells and to determine differential counts presented within the context of clinical situations.

Index

Page ranges indicate the first to last pages of each chapter.